Enhancing Quality of Life in Patients with Cerebral Palsy

Ana Presedo
Mohammad Hossein Nabian
Nastaran Maghbouli
Editors

Enhancing Quality of Life in Patients with Cerebral Palsy

A Comprehensive Guide

Springer

Editors
Ana Presedo
Neuro-Orthopedics Unit
Hôpital Robert-Debré
Paris, France

Mohammad Hossein Nabian
Center for Orthopedic Trans-Disciplinary
Applied Research
Tehran University of Medical Sciences
Tehran, Iran

Nastaran Maghbouli
Department of Physical Medicine and
Rehabilitation, School of Medicine, Shariati
Hospital
Tehran University of Medical Sciences
Tehran, Iran

ISBN 978-3-032-20966-5 ISBN 978-3-032-20967-2 (eBook)
https://doi.org/10.1007/978-3-032-20967-2

This Springer imprint is published by the registered company Springer Nature Switzerland AG
The registered company address is: Gewerbestrasse 11, 6330 Cham, Switzerland

Acknowledgments

This book is the result of countless shared moments, insights, and collaborations with individuals and teams who have dedicated their lives to improving the quality of life for those with cerebral palsy. It would not have been possible without the unwavering support and contributions of many.

To the caregivers—parents, siblings, partners, and friends—who show extraordinary resilience, love, and advocacy every single day: your voices shaped this book. Your lived experiences, challenges, and triumphs are the heart of this work, and we are deeply grateful for your openness and trust.

To my colleagues in multidisciplinary teams—physicians, therapists, nurses, psychologists, educators, and social workers—thank you for your commitment to holistic, person-centered care. Your collaboration and shared wisdom have enriched every chapter and continue to inspire better practices in rehabilitation.

Special thanks to the individuals with cerebral palsy who have taught us what it truly means to live with courage, dignity, and determination. Your stories remind us that quality of life is not defined by limitations but by possibilities.

I also extend my gratitude to the institutions and mentors who have supported this endeavor, and to the editorial team whose guidance helped bring this vision to life.

This book is a tribute to all of you—and to the power of working together with empathy, purpose, and hope.

About the Book

Ana Presedo

I've been taking care of patients with cerebral palsy for more than 20 years. When I started, without having much knowledge about this neurological condition, I was focused on the biological aspects of the pathology so I tried to get the best possible training regarding diagnosis and management of orthopedic problems. At that time, advances in computer engineering led to the development of motion analysis techniques that allowed for a better comprehension of mechanisms involved in gait. Diagnostic imaging and genetic tests provided insight into the causes of brain lesions. Research in biomechanics improved knowledge about locomotion with a deeper understanding about how the different components of the musculoskeletal system were interacting to produce movement. All this knowledge has implemented the orthopedic clinical decision-making aiming to optimize functional abilities of children with cerebral palsy.

The approach to orthopedic surgery in this population has radically changed during these last two decades. We moved from staged procedures to single-stage multilevel procedures to correct lower limb problems in a comprehensive way for patients who are able to walk. Surveillance programs have been developed in order to ensure regular screening of patients at risk for specific problems like hip disease and scoliosis. In order to consider all possible needs of our patients, multidisciplinary teams cover all steps of management: early diagnosis, physical therapy, preparation for surgery, postoperative care, and rehabilitation. Surgical advancements like minimally invasive surgery (guided growth techniques and percutaneous procedures) and neurosurgical techniques intended to reduce spasticity have brought new perspectives to the global management of these patients.

After being involved in the care of children with cerebral palsy for so many years, I realized that taking into account only the biological aspects of the pathology was not enough to enhance the quality of life of patients. The International Classification of Functioning, Disability and Health (ICF), proposed by the World Health Organization in 2001, combines the medical and social model of disability into a bio-psycho-social model. This classification is a framework for considering the individuals in their context and points out participation as being the main determinant of quality of life. Thus, we should promote treatments oriented to help our patients to take part in life situations as much as possible. With this in mind, integrating the families and the caregivers as part of the therapeutic project would be a necessary condition to obtain outcomes that meet their expectations.

When this young group of researchers, under the coordination of Dr. Hossein Nabian, presented this editorial project to me, I thought it was a necessary update in the field. This book covers all topics related to the global management of children with cerebral palsy, including bio-psycho-social aspects related to patients and families. I sincerely admire the energy and determination of the authors to put all this chapters together into an extraordinary book that should serve as a guide for treatment and also be a motivation for young surgeons to get involved into the specialty of neuro-orthopedics.

Nastaran Maghbouli

Cerebral palsy is not a diagnosis—it is a lifelong journey. For those living with it, and for the families and professionals who walk beside them, the path is often complex, demanding, and deeply personal. As a rehabilitation specialist privileged to work with individuals affected by cerebral palsy, I have witnessed firsthand the transformative power of compassionate, coordinated care. This book is born from that experience.

The concept of "quality of life" transcends clinical outcomes. It encompasses autonomy, dignity, participation, and joy. For individuals with cerebral palsy, achieving a meaningful quality of life requires more than medical intervention—it demands a multidisciplinary approach rooted in empathy, collaboration, and respect. Physicians, therapists, nurses, educators, and—most critically—caregivers must work in concert, not merely to treat symptoms but to nurture potential.

This book stands apart from previous publications by offering dedicated guidance not only for multidisciplinary teams but also for caregivers—based on our practical experience. These two crucial perspectives are often overlooked in academic literature.

Whether you are a physician, a therapist, or a parent navigating this journey, may this book offer clarity, encouragement, and a renewed commitment to improving lives—not just through treatment but through understanding.

Because in the end, quality of life is not measured by milestones alone, but by moments of connection, empowerment, and hope.

Paris, France — Ana Presedo
Tehran, Iran — Nastaran Maghbouli

Contents

1 Introduction to Cerebral Palsy

Simin Khayatzadeh Kakhki, Elham Pourbakhtyaran, and Kiana Tahan

Case

An 8-month-old female infant was referred to our clinic with the chief complaint of motor delay. She was born via cesarean section at 35 weeks of gestation due to maternal preeclampsia. She is the first child of non-consanguineous parents. Birth weight was 2200 g, with Apgar scores of 6 and 9 at 1 and 5 min, respectively. The neonatal course was remarkable for mild respiratory distress syndrome, managed with nasal CPAP for 3 days; she was discharged on day 12 of life in good condition.

At the age of 8 months (corrected age ~ 6.5 months), the parents found that the child was unable to roll over independently and had head lag. On physical examination, the infant showed right-hand preference, while the left upper limb demonstrated decreased spontaneous movements.

Increased tone and hyperreflexia in the left upper and lower limbs were observed, along with the presence of clonus at the left ankle, persistent fisting of the left hand, and cranial nerve deficits. Primitive reflexes were exaggerated on the left side.

MRI of the brain revealed right periventricular leukomalacia with volume loss in the posterior limb of the internal capsule, consistent with perinatal hypoxic-ischemic injury.

S. K. Kakhki (✉)
Division of Pediatric Neurology, Bahrami Children Hospital, School of Medicine, Tehran University of Medical Sciences, Tehran, Iran
e-mail: skhayatzadeh@sina.tums.ac.ir

E. Pourbakhtyaran
Department of pediatrics, Division of Pediatric Neurology, Growth and Development Research Center, Children's Medical Center, Pediatrics Center of Excellence, Tehran University of Medical Sciences, Tehran, Iran

K. Tahan
Medical School, Shahid Beheshti University of Medical Sciences, Tehran, Iran

A. Presedo et al. (eds.), *Enhancing Quality of Life in Patients with Cerebral Palsy*, https://doi.org/10.1007/978-3-032-20967-2_1

1.1 General Concept

Cerebral palsy (CP) is a condition defined as a heterogeneous group of permanent, non-progressive neurodevelopmental disorders of movement and posture that result in motor disability. It arises from disturbances in the developing brain during the fetal or infancy period. Although the primary brain injury is static, functional impairments and musculoskeletal manifestations may evolve throughout life [1]. In addition to motor disability, CP is frequently accompanied by comorbidities such as sensory deficits, cognitive and communication impairments, epilepsy, and musculoskeletal complications.

Historical descriptions of CP were lacking before the nineteenth century. William Little was the first to provide a medical report of CP, and later, William Osler authored the first book dedicated to the condition and named it *zerebrale Kinderlähmung* ("cerebral child paralysis") [2].

Cerebral palsy is the most common type of movement disorder. The estimated prevalence of CP is 2–3 per 1000 live births [3], though prevalence varies by region and healthcare system. Risk factors include prenatal, natal, and postnatal insults. Prenatal etiologies such as prematurity, low birth weight, antenatal complications, intracranial hemorrhage, periventricular leukomalacia, and post-neonatal insults such as meningitis, head trauma, or hypoxic events may result in CP.

A recent 2024 study reported that inherited genetic etiologies play a role in 25% of cases [4], whereas it was believed previously that only 2% of cases were genetically determined.

1.2 Classification

1.2.1 By Motor Involvement

- Spastic CP (about 80%, most common): Characterized by increased tone and hyperreflexia, with stiffness and limitations in movements.
    1. *Spastic hemiplegia*: Affects one side of the body, usually the arm and legs. It is accompanied by delayed walking, circumductive gait, toe-walking, hand preference before 24 months, and asymmetric growth of extremities.
    2. *Spastic monoplegia*: Only one limb is affected. Motor disability challenges appear based on the specific limb involved.
    3. *Spastic diplegia*: Bilateral lower extremities involvement, strongly associated with prematurity and damaged immature brain. The first symptom is often seen during crawling (commando crawl), with symmetric spasticity in the legs.
    4. *Spastic quadriplegia*: The most severe form with significant complications.
- Dyskinetic CP (choreoathetoid and dystonic): Involves involuntary, variable, and uncontrolled movements; Choreoathetoid CP is the result of hyperbilirubinemia and hypoxic-ischemic encephalopathy insulting the basal ganglia (mostly the globus pallidus). In dystonic CP, trunk muscles are more involved than limbs.

- Ataxic CP: The rarest form, presenting with impaired balance, coordination, and hypotonia. Wide-based and irregular gait is often observed in these patients.
- Mixed CP: Combination of features, most commonly spastic–dyskinetic [5].

1.2.2 By Topographic Distribution

- Hemiplegia: One side of the body is involved, typically the arm more than the leg.
- Diplegia: Legs are predominantly involved, often seen in preterm infants.
- Quadriplegia: Bilateral upper and lower extremities are affected and is usually associated with severe disability and multiple comorbidities.
- Monoplegia: One limb affected, rare.
- Triplegia: Rare, affecting three limbs [6].

1.2.3 Functional Classification

Functional classification in CP provides insight into a person's abilities and limitations in movement, manual skills, communication, and feeding.

Functional classification systems include:

- Gross Motor Function Classification System (GMFCS) for movement assessment (Table 1.1): Five-level scale (I–V) describing mobility and independence [7].
- Manual Ability Classification System (MACS) for manual dexterity evaluation (Table 1.2): Five-level scale (I–V) assessing hand use in daily activities (ages 4–18); Mini-MACS is used in younger children [8].
- Communication function classification system (CFCS) (Table 1.3): Focuses on activity and participation levels [9].
- Eating and drinking Ability Classification System (EDACS) for eating (Table 1.4): Identifies aspiration risk in patients with cerebral palsy [10].

Table 1.1 GMFCS is used for infants under 2 years of age up to their eighteenth birthday

Level I	Walks and climbs stairs independently; can run, jump, but speed, balance, and coordination are limited
Level II	Walks but not for long distances, climbs stairs with a railing, and is minimally able to run or jump
Level III	Walks using a device, climbs stairs dependent on supervision, and uses a wheelchair for long distances
Level IV	Requires physical assistance
Level V	Uses a wheelchair and assistance devices in all settings, with limited ability to hold neck and trunk against gravity

Table 1.2 MACS assesses hand skills for tasks like eating, writing, and dressing

Level I	Handles objects easily and perfectly
Level II	Handles most objects with minimal limitations in speed
Level III	Handles objects with difficulty and requires assistance
Level IV	Handles a limited selection of easily managed objects and requires frequent assistance
Level V	Unable to handle objects or to complete even simple actions with hands

Table 1.3 CFCS evaluates the effectiveness of communication in an individual with cerebral palsy in different situations

Level I	A person independently and effectively alternates between being a sender and receiver of information with most people in most environments
Level II	A person independently alternates between being a sender and receiver with most people in most environments, but the conversation may be slower.
Level III	A person usually communicates effectively with familiar communication partners, but not unfamiliar partners, in most environments.
Level IV	The person is not always consistent in communicating with familiar communication partners.
Level V	A person is rarely able to communicate effectively, even with familiar people.

Table 1.4 EDACS scale eating and drinking ability of a patient suffering from cerebral palsy

Level I	Eats and drinks safely and efficiently
Level II	Eats and drinks safely, with some limitations in efficiency
Level III	Eats and drinks with limitations in safety and efficiency
Level IV	Eats and drinks with significant limitations
Level V	Unable to eat and drink, requiring a nasogastric tube or other feeding device

1.3 Physical Examination

1.3.1 History

Prominent findings include delayed motor development (late head control, sitting, and walking), abnormal hand preference before 12 months, or progression from neonatal hypotonia to spasticity.

Perinatal history should document gestational age, birth weight, Apgar scores, complications, family history, and consanguinity [11].

1.3.2 Examination

Evaluation points include: head circumference and growth parameters assessment; posture, tone (spasticity, hypotonia, dystonia), and muscle strength; persistence of primitive reflexes and abnormalities in postural reactions; deep tendon reflexes, contractures, coordination, and gait; presence of involuntary movements, scoliosis, or orthopedic deformities [11].

1.3.3 Standardized Assessments in the Monitoring of Cerebral Palsy

Early and accurate identification of motor disability in infancy is essential for timely intervention. Several tools aid in diagnosis and monitoring:

- *General Movements Assessment* (GMA) is a noninvasive observational tool for identifying neurological issues from birth to about 5 months. It evaluates the presence or absence of fidgety movements and can predict CP [12].
- *Hammersmith Infant Neurological Examination* (HINE) assesses cranial nerve function, neonatal reflexes, and postural and movement at ages 2–24 months. Sensitivity is around 90% [13, 14].
- *Gross Motor Function Measure* (*GMFM*) is used to evaluate functional motor skills of infants, such as rolling, sitting, standing, and walking. It is useful for rehabilitation planning of motor disability [15].

1.4 Diagnosis

The diagnosis of cerebral palsy (CP) is primarily clinical, based on the patient's history and physical examination, in combination with neuroimaging techniques for differential diagnosis. MRI of the brain is the gold standard imaging technique (with a sensitivity of approximately 86%–89%) to assess the severity of lesions and rule out treatable conditions that may mimic CP. In early infancy, cranial ultrasound helps identify intraventricular hemorrhage or periventricular leukomalacia. Other evaluations include an EEG for suspected seizures, and genetic and metabolic tests for unusual cases or a family history of CP. Comorbid conditions, including hearing, vision, speech/language, cognitive abilities, feeding challenges, and musculoskeletal health, should be further evaluated. Achieving an early diagnosis before the age of 2 is ideal for prompt interventions, family guidance, and improved functional outcomes, especially when MRI findings are paired with standardized neurological assessments.

1.5 Medical Comorbidities Associated with Cerebral Palsy

The permanence yet non-progressive nature of Cerebral palsy accounts for a lifelong sequela of diverse comorbidities. The phenotypic motor type of CP (spastic, dyskinetic, ataxic, or mixed), the resulting sensorimotor deficits, and intellectual-behavioral challenges are the core manifestations that evolve and predispose affected individuals to secondary complications. These features, occurring secondarily to motor dysfunctions, affect neurodevelopment, gastrointestinal, musculoskeletal, respiratory, genitourinary, endocrine, and reproductive functions, as well as impairments in communication, vision, and hearing. Furthermore, we delve deeper into the medical significance of these outcomes and underscore the necessity of persistent care and monitoring.

1.5.1 Complications Associated with Neurodevelopment

- *Epilepsy.* Acknowledged for its recurrent and spontaneous seizures, epilepsy is a widespread neurological condition impacting about 0.5% [16]. However, the occurrence of this disorder is augmented as a comorbidity in individuals with CP, as incidence rates are reported to be between 15% and 90% [17]. Shared etiological factors, such as congenital brain malformations and peri- or prenatal asphyxia and infections, explain the heightened co-occurrence between these two disorders [18]. The prevalence of epilepsy in CP varies across its subtypes, being most frequent in hemiplegia (approximately 66%) and quadriplegia/tetraplegia (42%–50%), while less notable in diplegia (15%–27%) and rarely observed in dyskinetic or ataxic CP. These patterns correlate with the extent of cortical involvement and the regions affected [19, 20]. Epilepsy in children with CP most commonly manifests as the generalized form, followed by partial seizures, infantile spasms, and myoclonic jerks [21]. The presentation of epilepsy is also dependent on subtype: quadriplegic/diplegic CP is often accompanied by earlier seizures, predominantly generalized tonic–clonic or West syndrome seizures within the first year, whereas hemiplegic CP typically presents with partial seizures with later onset [21, 22]. Factors such as neonatal seizures, familial epilepsy, abnormalities observed in EEG and cranial imaging, and severe intellectual impairment are linked to the subsequent emergence of epilepsy and poor outcome in CP [17, 23]. Ultimately, epilepsy is a recognized hallmark of severe CP as it adversely impacts the motor and cognitive abilities and, consequently, the overall quality of life. Even among children with severe symptoms, around 30% of cases remit over time, suggesting a positive outlook on effective interventions and therapeutic approaches with AEDs (antiepileptic drugs) [22].
- *Intellectual disability and cognitive/executive problems.* Early insults to the developing brain can disrupt the trajectory of normal development, causing cognitive deficits that impede the social outcome of the child throughout adolescence [24]. The extent of intellectual impairments relies heavily on lesion site, CP subtype, and developmental course. Children with CP display a wide range of intellectual disabilities (ID), from profound cognitive impairment to average or above-average functioning. Notably, severe motor impairments often impede accurate assessment, which may result in overestimating intellectual disability in clinical practice [25]. In a study performed to investigate the risk of ID in children with spastic CP, severe intellectual disability was more prevalent in children with bilateral spastic CP (BSCP) compared with children with unilateral spastic

CP. Compared with very preterm infants with BSCP, the risk of ID was higher in moderately preterm and at-term children with BSCP [26].

Studies have estimated that intellectual impairments, defined as IQ scores below 70, manifest in about 50%–70% of children with CP, though their occurrence varies by subtype and severity [27]. Such impairments present more frequently in dyskinetic and quadriplegic forms, evidently correlating with motor defects and early-onset epilepsy [28]. The prevalence of sleep disturbances, intellectual impairment, and academic challenges complicates the lives of children with CP. Similarly, intellectual disability is frequently seen in those with CP [28]. Notably, cognitive deficits in CP are dynamic, as brain plasticity, environmental factors, and rising demands in society alter their progression over time. A broad range of disabilities is seen across individuals, including speech and language difficulties, visuospatial and perceptual deficits, attention and executive dysfunction, and reduced working memory. These difficulties persist into adulthood, where language, visuospatial, executive functioning, and academic participation remain impaired [29].

- *Behavioral and psychiatric comorbidity.* Children and adolescents with CP have increased odds of mental disorders compared to their able-bodied peers, underscoring the importance of routine psychiatric screening and proper interventions. Factors hindering mental health include age, living status, medication use, mobility, and manual impairments, as well as maladaptive parental dynamics. Difficulties in social engagement, severe motor impairments (GMFCS IV–V), and moderate manual impairments (MACS II–III) predispose individuals to psychiatric complications [30].

Many children with cerebral palsy confront serious challenges in daily life. Some will be highly dependent on their caregivers. While motor deficits are most commonly reported, children with cerebral palsy also experience higher rates of behavioral problems, attention difficulties, social communication issues, and, to a lesser extent, mood disorders in comparison to the general population. Individual risk factors for psychological problems include normal intellect, communication issues, and less functional disability. In a longitudinal study, a strong association between social functioning and Communication Function Classification System (CFCS) levels was documented. At 8–12 years, 35 out of 45 children in CFCS level I had social functioning age expectations. 25 out of 29 in CFCS levels II to V had social functioning below the expected for their age. CFCS and age were stronger determinants of social functioning development than GMFCS or MACS and age [31].

In children, motor and communication impairments can reduce participation in play, sometimes leading to social isolation [32]. Children with speech difficulties face greater challenges in peer communication [33]. Experiences of acceptance versus stigma strongly affect social confidence [34]. In childhood, children often undergo stress, anxiety, depression, and compulsive behavior, along with other comorbid disorders such as autism and ADHD [35, 36]. In adulthood, higher prevalence of almost all mental disorders is observed, especially in depression and anxiety, psychotic, and bipolar disorders. However, substance use disorders are relatively less common. Insufficient sleep, chronic pain and inactivity, social isolation, and conflicts in interpersonal interactions contribute to these struggles [37]. Regular psychiatric screening and management of children with CP can improve psychosocial outcomes and the overall quality of life.

- *Sleep disorders.* Sleep disorders encompass a broad spectrum of disruptions that impair sleep patterns. These disorders are remarkably common in children with CP, with prevalence rates ranging from 13% to 85%, being most frequent in severe phenotypes such as quadriplegia, GMFCS IV–V, or comorbid epilepsy [38]. This range surpasses the 25% observed in normally developing children, even though the types of sleep disorders are similar in both groups and consist of difficulty initiating and maintaining sleep, parasomnias, nocturnal hyperhidrosis, nightmares, bruxism, sleepwalking, and sleep talking [39, 40].

  Although there is no complete consensus on this matter, several factors hypothetically contribute to sleep deprivation. These include physiological factors such as spasticity, postural restrictions, pain, nocturnal seizures, delayed melatonin secretion, airway obstruction and apnea, gastroesophageal reflux, and visual impairment, as well as environmental factors like noise, lighting, temperature, unfamiliar beds, utilization of orthoses, and familial dynamics [38, 41]. Pain resulting from motor spasticity and contractures limits an individual's ability to reposition in bed and leads to constant awakenings, irritability, aggression, hyperactivity, and compulsive behaviors [38, 40]. The importance of proper management should not be neglected, as sleep disorders not only hinder the physical, emotional, and cognitive growth of children but also deprive caregivers of adequate rest. Interventions range from therapeutic and surgical approaches (adenotonsillectomy, respiratory support) to non-pharmacological strategies (optimization of room lightness and temperature, noise reduction) [42, 43].

1.5.2 Feeding, Nutrition, and Gastrointestinal Health

- *Oropharyngeal dysfunction, gastroesophageal reflux disease, constipation.* As a result of the numerous comorbidities, children burdened with CP suffer from complex feeding and gastrointestinal complications, endangering growth, nutrition, and overall health. *Oropharyngeal dysfunction (OPD)* consists of difficulties in the oral, pharyngeal, and esophageal phases of swallowing and affects up to 90% of cases. It typically presents with dysphagia and oral motor incoordination and mostly accompanies younger children and those with greater motor dysfunctions (GMFCS levels III–V). Excessive saliva drooling, coughing, wheezing, choking, and congestion are among the complications concurrent with OPD [44, 45].

  Gastroesophageal reflux disease (GERD) presents in 15%–77% of the population with CP, and contributes to esophagitis, regurgitation, chest infections, and impaired weight gain. These coexisting complications are often exacerbated by conditions such as anticonvulsant medications, spasticity, scoliosis, and prolonged supine positioning [46].

Constipation, occurring in 26%–74% of individuals with CP, proceeds from alterations in intestinal motility. Uncoordinated mechanisms between the central nervous system (CNS), autonomic nervous system, and enteric nervous system, spasticity and reduced abdominal and lower trunk mobility, inadequate fiber and fluid intake, and side effects of anticholinergics and opioids, all contribute to even more discomfort in both patients and caregivers. Alleviation of constipation may involve both therapeutic and non-therapeutic approaches, like consumption of oral and rectal stimulants, increase of dietary fluids and fiber, daily abdominal massage, and stretching or strengthening exercises to facilitate spasticity and mobility [47, 48].

- *Nutrient and micronutrient intake.* These disorders collectively act in concert to cause malnutrition, often from protein-calorie deficiency, which is documented in 46%–90% of cases [49] and threatens growth and development by reducing muscle mass and fat stores, impairing bone mineralization, immune function, circulation, and cardiac function, and attenuating respiratory muscle strength [50–52].

  Nutritional management is achieved through assessment of intake, body composition, and growth trajectories [44]. This aids in early interventions in case of insufficient nutrient intake. Enteral nutrition can be a lifesaving intervention for those with severe oral disabilities: nasogastric feeding and gastrostomy are, respectively, employed for short-term and long-term nutritional support, and in cases of profound dysphagia, post-pyloric feeding is most suitable [52, 53]. Adjusting the diet to tailor to the severity and type of oral dysfunction, such as modifying food textures and fluid thickness, enhancing protein and micronutrient intake, and increasing caloric density with fats while offering a smaller, more manageable portion of food, can help maximize feeding efficiency and minimize aspiration risk [52]. Overall, personalized nutritional care enhances neurodevelopment, bone health, survival, and quality of life in children with CP, while helping families with daily feeding challenges [53].

1.5.3 Musculoskeletal Complications

- *Dystonia.* Dystonia is the condition of unintentional, persistent, or intermittent muscle contractions that lead to repetitive, twisting movements, and atypical postures [54]. Dystonia is responsible for the disability caused by CP and is particularly associated with dyskinetic CP (the second-most common type of CP), where dystonia and choreoathetosis are often co-observed, with dystonia exerting a stronger impact on motility exacerbation [55]. These atypical movements may involve one limb (focal form), specific regions (segmental form), or the entire body (generalized form) and are marked by a rotational element in posture, like equinovarus of the foot. The severity of dystonia increases with arousal, stress, cognitive effort, hunger, or tiredness, but subsides during sleep [55]. Dyskinetic CP stems from perinatal insults that injure thalamocortical pathways, basal ganglia, cerebellum, and their tightly connected network, thereby interfering with the plasticity and integration of normal sensorimotor [56]. Impaired relaxation of muscles and inefficient voluntary control are among the complications of dystonia. The excruciating pain that comes along with dyskinetic CP should be carefully considered, as it is the second-most common cause of moderate-to-severe pain in pediatric CP [54]. Personalized approach of oral, enteral, or transdermal medications, botulinum neurotoxin A (advised for focal or segmental dystonia), and intrathecal baclofen and deep brain stimulation (advised for severe types of dystonia unresponsive to previous medications), are among the methods used to manage this comorbid in CP [57].

The differentiation between dystonia and typical spasticity in CP needs to be carefully addressed to optimize personalized treatment and elicit the desired response. This distinction is of great importance, as interventions such as selective dorsal rhizotomy reduce spasticity but do not alleviate dystonia, which may persist and further continue to limit function [58].

- *Hip displacement.* Hip displacement is one of the most common musculoskeletal complications in children with cerebral palsy (CP), occurring in about 35% of cases, with progression to gross dislocation in 15%–20% of cases if left untreated [59, 60]. The progression of this complication is often associated with pain, increased contractures, deformities, such as windswept deformity and scoliosis, and difficulty with basic daily movements [60]. The likelihood of hip displacement is tightly correlated with gross motor severity, being virtually absent in GMFCS I, but rising to nearly 90% in non-ambulatory children at GMFCS V [61]. Displacement reportedly initiates around 2 and 3 years of age [62], and its pathophysiology is explained by the interplay between spastic hip adductors and flexors, weak abductors and extensors, and delayed or absent weight-bearing, which in turn drives acetabular dysplasia and progressive femoral deformities, such as coxa valga, excessive femoral anteversion, and horizontal physis [61].

  Annual radiographic monitoring is fundamental in early detection and prevention of this burden and is analyzed using Reimer's migration percentage (MP), the gold standard for measuring femoral head lateralization on an anteroposterior pelvis radiograph: an MP greater than 30% designates "hips at risk," a migration value above 40% predicts progressive worsening and the need for surgical intervention [61–63]. National hip surveillance programs, most notably Sweden's CPUP, demonstrate that systematic follow-up with standardized radiographs, GMFCS-based risk stratification, and timely interventions, such as soft-tissue releases, postural care, injection of botulinum A toxin, or reconstructive osteotomies, can prevent further hip dislocations [61, 64].
- *Scoliosis.* Scoliosis is commonly encountered in clinical examination of cerebral palsy, with a prevalence exceeding that of the general population (1%–2% idiopathic scoliosis vs. 15%–80% in CP-related scoliosis) [65]. This comorbid condition is distinct from the idiopathic scoliosis and progresses beyond skeletal maturity, at a rate of about 3°–4° per year in adults [66]. Its course is dependent on functional severity, with nearly half of non-ambulatory children at GMFCS levels IV–V developing severe curves. Moreover, hip displacement

and early onset with a Cobb angle greater than 30° escalate the progression [66, 67]. Not only does severe scoliosis aggravate mobility reserves of an individual but it also compromises the upright posture, a vital position that supports feeding and pulmonary function by reducing reflux and aspiration [65]. Although conservative methods, such as bracing or seating adaptations may slow progression, modern spinal fusion facilitates the regression of spinal deformations and pelvic asymmetry [66]. It is worth mentioning that these operations, however effective, remain hazardous and demand cautious pre- and post-operative care.

- *Low bone mineral density and fragility fractures*. Fractures are complications that are frequently observed among individuals with CP and are reported to have a prevalence of 12%–26% in childhood and up to 60% across the lifespan. It primarily affects the lower extremities, with the femur being the most frequently impacted. Compared to their healthy peers, children with CP present with reduced cortical thickness and fail to achieve the optimal bone mineral accrual, thereby making osteopenia and fragility fractures difficult to avert; this is seen in nearly 80% of GMFCS IV–V cases, in which fractures occur without trauma. Low bone mineral density (BMD) arises from cumulative risk factors, including malnutrition, immobility, impaired growth, use of anticonvulsants or glucocorticoids, and endocrine dysfunction. Dual radiograph absorptiometry (DXA) is the gold standard for the assessment of BMD. Fracture patterns vary by age and mobility: ambulatory children are prone to upper limb fragility, non-ambulatory children are susceptible to distal femur fractures, adults with CP face tibia/fibula injuries in early adulthood, and vertebral or hip fractures later in life. With regard to the need for surveillance and targeted management, interventions like calcium and vitamin D supplementation, bisphosphonate therapy, and weight-bearing exercises could be of use [68–70].

1.5.4 Respiratory Morbidity

Emergency admissions in individuals with CP are often subsequent to respiratory comorbidities, which represent the leading cause of morbidity and mortality in this population. This aligns with epidemiological studies demonstrating an approximately 14-fold increased risk of respiratory morbidity in adults with CP. About one-quarter of emergency admissions for respiratory causes occur in patients with CP [71]. This comorbid condition may range from acute lower respiratory tract infections requiring hospitalization to chronic symptoms such as cough, wheeze, abnormal breath sounds, and voice changes during or following meals [72].

Multiple factors can explain the increased likelihood of this burden: advanced GMFCS level (IV–V), oropharyngeal dysfunctions (dysphagia, gastroesophageal reflux, and consequent aspiration), and salivary aspiration caused by uncontrolled seizures predispose an individual to respiratory infections. Structural deformities like scoliosis and kyphoscoliosis restrict lung volumes, and malnutrition diminishes respiratory muscle strength. Chronic bacterial colonization, together with upper airway obstruction, may afflict an individual with pneumonia. Interventions require a multidisciplinary approach, including scheduled screening, aspiration control, respiratory tract clearance, nutrition, dental hygiene, and prophylactic vaccination and antibiotics [71–73].

1.5.5 Communication, Vision, and Hearing

- *Impaired communication.* Across the CP population, multisensory and communicative impairments have been widely reported. In terms of impaired communication, these challenges manifest as impaired verbal articulation like dysarthria (motor speech disorder), dyspraxia (difficulty coordinating and planning speech), and restricted non-verbal communication. Roughly half of children with CP undergo speech problems, and 25% are diagnosed as non-speaking [74]. Speech and language therapy (SLT) with the goal of optimizing communication skills is deemed an effective intervention [29].
- *Visual disabilities.* Children with CP frequently grapple with visual disabilities, which may be further exacerbated in the presence of seizures, epilepsy, and hydrocephalus. Insults in chiasmatic and cortical regions associated with vision and perception drive the progression of cerebral visual impairment (CVI) and the resultant diminished acuity and visual fields, oculomotor dysfunction, and perceptual deficits. The burden is predominantly attributable to refractive errors, strabismus or "squint," and nystagmus (involuntary, repetitive eye movement). For school-aged children, additional concern arises due to impaired manual coordination and impaired writing ability. Ultimately, ocular abnormalities are documented predominantly in spastic CP [75–77].
- *Hearing.* Complementing sensory deficits, auditory impairments are associated with a notable proportion of children with CP (10%–40%), especially in hyperkinetic subtypes [78]. Sensorineural, conductive, or mixed auditory loss, commonly occurring in this population, further undermines speech and communication, cognition, and psychosocial outcomes [79]. This burden is mostly ascribed to non-genetic factors such as perinatal infections (e.g., cytomegalovirus, meningitis); hypoxic–ischemic injuries; metabolic dysfunctions (e.g., hyperbilirubinemia), prematurity complications (e.g., very low birthweight), and intensive neonatal interventions (e.g., extracorporeal membrane oxygenation) [79].

  Early assessment, as well as prompt interventions including auditory correction, electro-acoustic rehabilitative techniques, and hearing aid support, may substantially influence the child's communicative development [78].

1.5.6 Genitourinary and Endocrine

Over half of those affected with CP face lower urinary tract complications, most often manifesting as urinary incontinence caused by neurogenic detrusor overactivity. Indeed, voiding difficulties such as hesitancy or pelvic floor overactivity are less common, but they pose serious risks for renal complications in individuals with greater motor impairment (GMFCS III or higher) cognitive deficits, or spastic quadriplegia. Communication barriers in expressing the need to void, along with limited mobility, predispose children to retention and possible urinary tract infections. Incontinence continues into adulthood, where leakage and urgency are the most common complaints among women and men, respectively. Obesity is an additional risk factor for the occurrence of incontinence and nocturia [80–82].

Beyond genitourinary complications, endocrine dysfunction is frequently reported, most obviously presenting as growth failure due to low growth hormone and IGF-I/IGFBP-3 secretion. Nutritional support and possible GH therapy, coupled with routine urodynamic testing and endocrine evaluation, hold promise for enhancing overall quality of life in CP [83].

1.5.7 Reproductive System

The reproductive health of individuals with CP has historically been neglected in societies. Women with CP endure multiple gynecological problems. Menstrual management is a common concern, and they may experience earlier menopause. While 20% may become pregnant, elevated rates of complications, including Cesarean delivery, preterm birth, low birth weight, loss of mobility during pregnancy, and postpartum depression, underscore the importance of specialized obstetric care. Men with CP are not spared from these difficulties, as their sexual health is also adversely affected by physical challenges, often resulting in sexual and societal isolation. Proactive counseling and adaptive strategies offering support would be highly beneficial [84, 85].

1.6 Prognosis and Goals of Management

The prognosis of CP depends largely on the type, severity, associated comorbidities, and access to early intervention/rehabilitation. As previously discussed, CP commonly co-exists with epilepsy, especially drug-resistant epilepsy, mental retardation, visual and hearing impairment, as well as feeding and behavioral disorders [86]. Severe CP with profound motor impairment, feeding difficulties, respiratory issues, or cognitive impairment carries a reduced lifespan [87].

Walking ability is influenced by cerebral palsy types (spastic unilateral, spastic bilateral, dyskinetic, and ataxic cerebral palsy), as well as IQ level, active epilepsy, and severe visual and hearing impairment. Severe CP, defined as both the inability to walk and an IQ of <50, was present in 20% of the subjects. The presence of a severe intellectual impairment increased the risk of being unable to walk by 56-fold if the child had unilateral spastic cerebral palsy type and by nine-fold if the child had bilateral spastic cerebral palsy type [88].

As the clinical presentation and predisposing factors for CP are diverse, treatment is also a complex issue. Treatment of spasticity includes botulinum toxin therapies and surgical techniques [89]. Some randomized clinical trials reported that stem cell therapy can offer the potential to treat CP [90–93]. Addressing Associated Problems, including epilepsy, feeding difficulties, speech and language problems, vision/hearing problems, skeletal and respiratory complications, is equally important.

Predicting outcomes in children with CP, establishing realistic goals, and determining the best interventions are pivotal steps in guaranteeing each child a bright future with the utmost potential.

1.7 Conclusion

Cerebral palsy is defined as a permanent, non-progressive disorder affecting movement and posture, often with multiple comorbidities. Early diagnosis, timely intervention, and multidisciplinary care are important. Family education and involvement, along with a multidisciplinary approach, can enhance functional capacity, independence, and psychosocial health and quality of life.

1.8 Recommendation for Parents and Caregivers

1.8.1 Recommendations for Family Education on Monitoring Infant Development and Regular Check-Ups

- *Routine Pediatric Visits:* Parents should know that regular well-baby check-ups are essential. Pediatricians will monitor growth, neurodevelopment, and early signs of delay.
- *Awareness of Developmental Milestones:* Families should be educated about typical milestones in motor, language, social, and cognitive development (e.g., head control by 4 months, rolling over by 4–6 months, sitting by 6–8 months). Any suspicious delay should prompt medical evaluation.
- *Identification of red flags:* Parents should seek medical attention if they notice:
  1. Persistent stiffness or marked hypotonia.
  2. Poor eye fixation and tracking or absence of social smile by 3 months.
  3. Inability to roll or sit by the expected age.
  4. Asymmetrical use of hands or legs.
- *Importance of Screening and Neuroimaging:* In high-risk infants, additional neurodevelopmental follow-up and imaging may be required.

- *Parental Engagement in Stimulation:* Families should be guided in providing age-appropriate stimulation; for instance, tummy time, talking to the baby, interactive play, and encouraging symmetrical use of both hands and legs.
- *Significance of Early Intervention:* Parents should understand that early intervention, such as physiotherapy, occupational therapy, and speech therapy, significantly improves long-term outcomes.
- *Ongoing follow-up beyond the first year:* vision, hearing, speech, cognition, and behavior must be monitored regularly through early childhood.

1.9 Key Takeaways for Parents

Regular pediatric evaluation and careful observation of your baby's development are important. If you notice delays or asymmetry in your child's movements or communication, seek medical advice early, as timely intervention greatly improves outcomes.

1.10 Guide for Multidisciplinary Teams

It is essential for all members of the multidisciplinary team, while caring for a patient with the diagnosis of cerebral palsy, to be aware of conditions that mimic cerebral palsy. Not all motor delays and abnormal movements are due to cerebral palsy. A wide range of metabolic, genetic, neuromuscular, and neurodegenerative disorders may present similar clinical features. "*So, Patients with cerebral palsy should be referred to a pediatric neurologist to rule out other differential diagnoses that may mimic cerebral palsy.*"

References

1. Dan B, Rosenbaum P, Carr L, Gough M, Coughlan J, Nweke N. Proposed updated description of cerebral palsy. Dev Med Child Neurol. 2025;67(6):700–9.
2. Panteliadis C, Panteliadis P, Vassilyadi F. Hallmarks in the history of cerebral palsy: from antiquity to mid-20th century. Brain Dev. 2013;35(4):285–92.
3. Oskoui M, Coutinho F, Dykeman J, Jetté N, Pringsheim T. An update on the prevalence of cerebral palsy: a systematic review and meta-analysis. Dev Med Child Neurol. 2013;55(6):509–19.
4. Wang Y, Xu Y, Zhou C, Cheng Y, Qiao N, Shang Q, et al. Exome sequencing reveals genetic heterogeneity and clinically actionable findings in children with cerebral palsy. Nat Med. 2024;30(5):1395–405.
5. Abate BB, Tegegne KM, Zemariam AB, Wondmagegn Alamaw A, Kassa MA, Kitaw TA, et al. Magnitude and clinical characteristics of cerebral palsy among children in Africa: a systematic review and meta-analysis. PLOS Glob Public Health. 2024;4(6):e0003003.
6. Reid SM, Carlin JB, Reddihough DS. Classification of topographical pattern of spasticity in cerebral palsy: a registry perspective. Res Dev Disabil. 2011;32(6):2909–15.
7. Huroy M, Behlim T, Andersen J, Buckley D, Fehlings D, Kirton A, et al. Stability of the gross motor function classification system over time in children with cerebral palsy. Dev Med Child Neurol. 2022;64(12):1487–93.

8. Eliasson AC, Krumlinde-Sundholm L, Rösblad B, Beckung E, Arner M, Ohrvall AM, et al. The manual ability classification system (MACS) for children with cerebral palsy: scale development and evidence of validity and reliability. Dev Med Child Neurol. 2006;48(7):549–54.
9. Hidecker MJ, Cunningham BJ, Thomas-Stonell N, Oddson B, Rosenbaum P. Validity of the communication function classification system for use with preschool children with communication disorders. Dev Med Child Neurol. 2017;59(5):526–30.
10. Bykova KM, Frank U, Girolami GL. Eating and drinking ability classification system to detect aspiration risk in children with cerebral palsy: a validation study. Eur J Pediatr. 2023;182(7):3365–73.
11. Sarathy K, Doshi C, Aroojis A. Clinical examination of children with cerebral palsy. Indian J Orthop. 2019;53(1):35–44.
12. Novak I, Morgan C, Adde L, Blackman J, Boyd RN, Brunstrom-Hernandez J, et al. Early, accurate diagnosis and early intervention in cerebral palsy: advances in diagnosis and treatment. JAMA Pediatr. 2017;171(9):897–907.
13. Kapil N, Majmudar-Sheth B, Johnson T. Hammersmith infant neurological examination subscores are predictive of cerebral palsy. Pediatr Neurol. 2024;151:84–9.
14. Maitre NL, Chorna O, Romeo DM, Guzzetta A. Implementation of the hammersmith infant neurological examination in a high-risk infant follow-up program. Pediatr Neurol. 2016;65:31–8.
15. Alotaibi M, Long T, Kennedy E, Bavishi S. The efficacy of GMFM-88 and GMFM-66 to detect changes in gross motor function in children with cerebral palsy (CP): a literature review. Disabil Rehabil. 2014;36(8):617–27.
16. Cowan LD, Bodensteiner JB, Leviton A, Doherty L. Prevalence of the epilepsies in children and adolescents. Epilepsia. 1989;30(1):94–106.
17. Gong C, Liu A, Lian B, Wu X, Zeng P, Hao C, et al. Prevalence and related factors of epilepsy in children and adolescents with cerebral palsy: a systematic review and meta-analysis. Front Pediatr. 2023;11:1189648.
18. Szpindel A, Myers KA, Ng P, Dorais M, Koclas L, Pigeon N, et al. Epilepsy in children with cerebral palsy: a data linkage study. Dev Med Child Neurol. 2022;64(2):259–65.
19. Hadjipanayis A, Hadjichristodoulou C, Youroukos S. Epilepsy in patients with cerebral palsy. Dev Med Child Neurol. 1997;39(10):659–63.
20. Bruck I, Antoniuk SA, Spessatto A, Bem RS, Hausberger R, Pacheco CG. Epilepsy in children with cerebral palsy. Arq Neuropsiquiatr. 2001;59(1):35–9.
21. Singhi P, Jagirdar S, Khandelwal N, Malhi P. Epilepsy in children with cerebral palsy. J Child Neurol. 2003;18(3):174–9.
22. Wallace SJ. Epilepsy in cerebral palsy. Dev Med Child Neurol. 2001;43(10):713–7.
23. Mert GG, Incecik F, Altunbasak S, Herguner O, Mert MK, Kiris N, et al. Factors affecting epilepsy development and epilepsy prognosis in cerebral palsy. Pediatr Neurol. 2011;45(2):89–94.
24. Sand K, Starrfelt R, Robotham RJ. Cognitive functioning and assessment in adults with cerebral palsy: a scoping review. Dev Neurorehabil. 2024;27(1–2):57–67.
25. Stadskleiv K. Cognitive functioning in children with cerebral palsy. Dev Med Child Neurol. 2020;62(3):283–9.
26. Cummins D, Kerr C, McConnell K, Perra O. Risk factors for intellectual disability in children with spastic cerebral palsy. Arch Dis Child. 2021;106(10):975–80.
27. Fennell EB, Dikel TN. Cognitive and neuropsychological functioning in children with cerebral palsy. J Child Neurol. 2001;16(1):58–63.
28. Fluss J, Lidzba K. Cognitive and academic profiles in children with cerebral palsy: a narrative review. Ann Phys Rehabil Med. 2020;63(5):447–56.
29. Pennington L, Goldbart J, Marshall J. Speech and language therapy to improve the communication skills of children with cerebral palsy. Cochrane Database Syst Rev. 2004;2004(2):Cd003466.
30. Pizzighello S, Uliana M, Michielotto M, Pellegri A, Vascello MGF, Piccoli S, et al. Psychiatric symptoms in adult patients with cerebral palsy: a cohort study. Front Neurol. 2022;13:998922.

31. Burgess A, Sakzewski L, Whittingham K, Wotherspoon J, Chatfield MD, Ware RS, et al. Development of social functioning in children with cerebral palsy: a longitudinal study. Dev Med Child Neurol. 2023;65(5):674–82.
32. Michelsen SI, Flachs EM, Damsgaard MT, Parkes J, Parkinson K, Rapp M, et al. European study of frequency of participation of adolescents with and without cerebral palsy. Eur J Paediatr Neurol. 2014;18(3):282–94.
33. Hidecker MJ, Paneth N, Rosenbaum PL, Kent RD, Lillie J, Eulenberg JB, et al. Developing and validating the communication function classification system for individuals with cerebral palsy. Dev Med Child Neurol. 2011;53(8):704–10.
34. King G, Law M, King S, Rosenbaum P, Kertoy MK, Young NL. A conceptual model of the factors affecting the recreation and leisure participation of children with disabilities. Phys Occup Ther Pediatr. 2003;23(1):63–90.
35. Downs J, Blackmore AM, Epstein A, Skoss R, Langdon K, Jacoby P, et al. The prevalence of mental health disorders and symptoms in children and adolescents with cerebral palsy: a systematic review and meta-analysis. Dev Med Child Neurol. 2018;60(1):30–8.
36. Bjorgaas HM, Hysing M, Elgen I. Psychiatric disorders among children with cerebral palsy at school starting age. Res Dev Disabil. 2012;33(4):1287–93.
37. McMorris CA, Lake J, Dobranowski K, McGarry C, Lin E, Wilton D, et al. Psychiatric disorders in adults with cerebral palsy. Res Dev Disabil. 2021;111:103859.
38. Simard-Tremblay E, Constantin E, Gruber R, Brouillette RT, Shevell M. Sleep in children with cerebral palsy: a review. J Child Neurol. 2011;26(10):1303–10.
39. Horwood L, Li P, Mok E, Shevell M, Constantin E. A systematic review and meta-analysis of the prevalence of sleep problems in children with cerebral palsy: how do children with cerebral palsy differ from each other and from typically developing children? Sleep Health. 2019;5(6):555–71.
40. Almeida MF, Mello S, Zonta MB, Crippa AC. Cerebral palsy and sleep: nonpharmacological treatment and impact on the life of caregivers—an integrative review. Arq Neuropsiquiatr. 2024;82(3):1–9.
41. Lélis AL, Cardoso MV, Hall WA. Sleep disorders in children with cerebral palsy: an integrative review. Sleep Med Rev. 2016;30:63–71.
42. Dhandayuthapani R, McDougall CM, Gahleitner F, Cunningham S, Urquhart DS. Sleep problems and sleep disordered breathing in children with cerebral palsy. Paediatr Respir Rev. 2025. https://doi.org/10.1016/j.prrv.2025.04.007.
43. Dutt R, Roduta-Roberts M, Brown CA. Sleep and children with cerebral palsy: a review of current evidence and environmental non-pharmacological interventions. Children. 2015;2(1):78–88.
44. Trivić I, Hojsak I. Evaluation and treatment of malnutrition and associated gastrointestinal complications in children with cerebral palsy. Pediatr Gastroenterol Hepatol Nutr. 2019;22(2):122–31.
45. Rogers B, Arvedson J, Buck G, Smart P, Msall M. Characteristics of dysphagia in children with cerebral palsy. Dysphagia. 1994;9(1):69–73.
46. Fernando T, Goldman RD. Management of gastroesophageal reflux disease in pediatric patients with cerebral palsy. Can Fam Physician. 2019;65(11):796–8.
47. Awan WA, Masood T. Role of stretching exercises in the management of constipation in spastic cerebral palsy. J Ayub Med Coll Abbottabad. 2016;28(4):798–801.
48. Faleiros-Castro FS, de Paula ED. Constipation in patients with quadriplegic cerebral palsy: intestinal reeducation using massage and a laxative diet. Rev Esc Enferm USP. 2013;47(4):836–42.
49. Caramico-Favero DCO, Guedes ZCF, Morais MB. Food intake, nutritional status and gastrointestinal symptoms in children with cerebral palsy. Arq Gastroenterol. 2018;55(4):352–7.
50. Kuperminc MN, Stevenson RD. Growth and nutrition disorders in children with cerebral palsy. Dev Disabil Res Rev. 2008;14(2):137–46.
51. Stallings VA, Charney EB, Davies JC, Cronk CE. Nutrition-related growth failure of children with quadriplegic cerebral palsy. Dev Med Child Neurol. 1993;35(2):126–38.

52. Bell KL, Samson-Fang L. Nutritional management of children with cerebral palsy. Eur J Clin Nutr. 2013;67(Suppl 2):S13–6.
53. Rempel G. The importance of good nutrition in children with cerebral palsy. Phys Med Rehabil Clin N Am. 2015;26(1):39–56.
54. Fehlings D, Brown L, Harvey A, Himmelmann K, Lin JP, Macintosh A, et al. Pharmacological and neurosurgical interventions for managing dystonia in cerebral palsy: a systematic review. Dev Med Child Neurol. 2018;60(4):356–66.
55. Monbaliu E, de Cock P, Ortibus E, Heyrman L, Klingels K, Feys H. Clinical patterns of dystonia and choreoathetosis in participants with dyskinetic cerebral palsy. Dev Med Child Neurol. 2016;58(2):138–44.
56. McClelland VM, Lin JP. Sensorimotor integration in childhood dystonia and dystonic cerebral palsy-a developmental perspective. Front Neurol. 2021;12:668081.
57. Fehlings D, Agnew B, Gimeno H, Harvey A, Himmelmann K, Lin J-P, et al. Pharmacological and neurosurgical management of cerebral palsy and dystonia: clinical practice guideline update. Dev Med Child Neurol. 2024;66(9):1133–47.
58. Rice J, Skuza P, Baker F, Russo R, Fehlings D. Identification and measurement of dystonia in cerebral palsy. Dev Med Child Neurol. 2017;59(12):1249–55.
59. Soo B, Howard JJ, Boyd RN, Reid SM, Lanigan A, Wolfe R, et al. Hip displacement in cerebral palsy. J Bone Joint Surg Am. 2006;88(1):121–9.
60. Hägglund G, Lauge-Pedersen H, Wagner P. Characteristics of children with hip displacement in cerebral palsy. BMC Musculoskelet Disord. 2007;8:101.
61. Aroojis A, Mantri N, Johari AN. Hip displacement in cerebral palsy: the role of surveillance. Indian J Orthop. 2021;55(1):5–19.
62. Larnert P, Risto O, Hägglund G, Wagner P. Hip displacement in relation to age and gross motor function in children with cerebral palsy. J Child Orthop. 2014;8(2):129–34.
63. Hermanson M, Hägglund G, Riad J, Rodby-Bousquet E, Wagner P. Prediction of hip displacement in children with cerebral palsy: development of the CPUP hip score. Bone Joint J. 2015;97-b(10):1441–4.
64. Pountney T, Green EM. Hip dislocation in cerebral palsy. BMJ. 2006;332(7544):772–5.
65. Koop SE. Scoliosis in cerebral palsy. Dev Med Child Neurol. 2009;51(s4):92–8.
66. Cloake T, Gardner A. The management of scoliosis in children with cerebral palsy: a review. J Spine Surg. 2016;2(4):299–309.
67. Yoshida K, Kajiura I, Suzuki T, Kawabata H. Natural history of scoliosis in cerebral palsy and risk factors for progression of scoliosis. J Orthop Sci. 2018;23(4):649–52.
68. Houlihan CM. Bone health in cerebral palsy: who's at risk and what to do about it? J Pediatr Rehabil Med. 2014;7(2):143–53.
69. Houlihan CM, Stevenson RD. Bone density in cerebral palsy. Phys Med Rehabil Clin N Am. 2009;20(3):493–508.
70. Presedo A, Dabney KW, Miller F. Fractures in patients with cerebral palsy. J Pediatr Orthop. 2007;27(2):147–53.
71. Gibson N, Blackmore AM, Chang AB, Cooper MS, Jaffe A, Kong WR, et al. Prevention and management of respiratory disease in young people with cerebral palsy: consensus statement. Dev Med Child Neurol. 2021;63(2):172–82.
72. Marpole R, Blackmore AM, Gibson N, Cooper MS, Langdon K, Wilson AC. Evaluation and management of respiratory illness in children with cerebral palsy. Front Pediatr. 2020;8:333.
73. Boel L, Pernet K, Toussaint M, Ides K, Leemans G, Haan J, et al. Respiratory morbidity in children with cerebral palsy: an overview. Dev Med Child Neurol. 2019;61(6):646–53.
74. Kristoffersson E, Dahlgren Sandberg A, Holck P. Communication ability and communication methods in children with cerebral palsy. Dev Med Child Neurol. 2020;62(8):933–8.
75. Black P. Visual disorders associated with cerebral palsy. Br J Ophthalmol. 1982;66(1):46–52.
76. Heydarian S, Abbasabadi MM, Khabazkhoob M, Hoseini-Yazdi H, Gharib M, editors. Vision abnormalities in children and young adults with cerebral palsy; a systematic review. Semin Ophthalmol. 2022;37(4):471–9.

77. Kozeis N, Anogeianaki A, Mitova DT, Anogianakis G, Mitov T, Klisarova A. Visual function and visual perception in cerebral palsied children. Ophthalmic Physiol Opt. 2007;27(1):44–53.
78. Khaydarova GS, Madrimova A, Shaykhova KES. Assessment of hearing in children with cerebral palsy. Int Tinnitus J. 2021;25(1):23–8.
79. Reid SM, Modak MB, Berkowitz RG, Reddihough DS. A population-based study and systematic review of hearing loss in children with cerebral palsy. Dev Med Child Neurol. 2011;53(11):1038–45.
80. Anígìlájé EA, Bitto TT. Prevalence and predictors of urinary tract infections among children with cerebral palsy in Makurdi, Nigeria. Int J Nephrol. 2013;2013:937268.
81. Marciniak C, O'Shea SA, Lee J, Jesselson M, Dudas-Sheehan D, Beltran E, et al. Urinary incontinence in adults with cerebral palsy: prevalence, type, and effects on participation. PM R. 2014;6(2):110–20. quiz 20.
82. Samijn B, Van Laecke E, Renson C, Hoebeke P, Plasschaert F, Vande Walle J, et al. Lower urinary tract symptoms and urodynamic findings in children and adults with cerebral palsy: a systematic review. Neurourol Urodyn. 2017;36(3):541–9.
83. Coniglio SJ, Stevenson RD, Rogol AD. Apparent growth hormone deficiency in children with cerebral palsy. Dev Med Child Neurol. 1996;38(9):797–804.
84. Hayward K, Chen AY, Forbes E, Byrne R, Greenberg MB, Fowler EG. Reproductive healthcare experiences of women with cerebral palsy. Disabil Health J. 2017;10(3):413–8.
85. Wiegerink D, Roebroeck M, Bender J, Stam H, Cohen-Kettenis P, Netherlands TRGSW. Sexuality of young adults with cerebral palsy: experienced limitations and needs. Sex Disabil. 2011;29(2):119–28.
86. Beckung E, Hagberg G, Uldall P, Cans C. Probability of walking in children with cerebral palsy in Europe. Pediatrics. 2008;121(1):e187–92.
87. Strauss D, Brooks J, Rosenbloom L, Shavelle R. Life expectancy in cerebral palsy: an update. Dev Med Child Neurol. 2008;50(7):487–93.
88. Sadowska M, Sarecka-Hujar B, Kopyta I. Cerebral palsy: current opinions on definition, epidemiology, risk factors, classification and treatment options. Neuropsychiatr Dis Treat. 2020;16:1505–18.
89. Liptak GS, Accardo PJ. Health and social outcomes of children with cerebral palsy. J Pediatr. 2004;145(2 Suppl):S36–41.
90. Gu J, Huang L, Zhang C, Wang Y, Zhang R, Tu Z, et al. Therapeutic evidence of umbilical cord-derived mesenchymal stem cell transplantation for cerebral palsy: a randomized, controlled trial. Stem Cell Res Ther. 2020;11(1):43.
91. Chen G, Wang Y, Xu Z, Fang F, Xu R, Wang Y, et al. Neural stem cell-like cells derived from autologous bone mesenchymal stem cells for the treatment of patients with cerebral palsy. J Transl Med. 2013;11:21.
92. Huang L, Zhang C, Gu J, Wu W, Shen Z, Zhou X, et al. A randomized, placebo-controlled trial of human umbilical cord blood mesenchymal stem cell infusion for children with cerebral palsy. Cell Transplant. 2018;27(2):325–34.
93. Zarrabi M, Akbari MG, Amanat M, Majmaa A, Moaiedi AR, Montazerlotfelahi H, et al. The safety and efficacy of umbilical cord blood mononuclear cells in individuals with spastic cerebral palsy: a randomized double-blind sham-controlled clinical trial. BMC Neurol. 2022;22(1):123.

2 Cerebral Palsy: Causes, Prevention, and Perinatal Safety Strategies

Nafiseh Saedi, Sara Ashtri, Amirhossein Ehsani, Amir Ebrahimzadeh Pasha, and Mohammad Mahdi Mehrabi

Case Vignette

A male infant was born via cesarean section at 30 weeks' gestation to a mother with severe pre-eclampsia and required only short-term respiratory intensive care in the neonatal period. The infant exhibited feeding difficulties in the neonatal period and intermittent tone problems, then subsequently exhibited significant global motor delay at 6 months corrected age, along with increased tone in the axial and lower extremities and deficits in postural control. Serial neuroimaging showed progressive changes to the periventricular white matter, and the infant evolved to a phenotype characterized by mostly spastic diplegia, as well as increasing functional and orthopedic concerns. This case is consistent with a multifactorial etiology for the eventual diagnosis of cerebral palsy, primarily placental insufficiency related to the mother's hypertensive disease coupled with extreme prematurity leading to vulnerable white matter injury. Early neonatal instability, particularly related to respiration and feeding, potentially contributed to further aggravation of injuries secondary to hypoxic-ischemic and inflammatory processes. There were also no systematic assessments of process measures outlined in the clinical notes—such as in the serial placental Doppler/growth charts, timing and/or completion of antenatal

N. Saedi (✉)
Obstetrics and Gynecology Department, School of Medicine, Tehran University of Medical Sciences, Tehran, Iran

S. Ashtri
Tehran University of Medical Sciences, Faculty of Medicine, Tehran, Iran

A. Ehsani
Iran University of Medical Sciences, Faculty of Medicine, Tehran, Iran

A. E. Pasha
Kerman University of Medical Sciences, Faculty of Medicine, Kerman, Iran

M. M. Mehrabi
Medical Research Committee, Shahed University, Tehran, Iran

A. Presedo et al. (eds.), *Enhancing Quality of Life in Patients with Cerebral Palsy*, https://doi.org/10.1007/978-3-032-20967-2_2

corticosteroids or magnesium sulphate, details of thorough fetal monitoring measures, and clear records of oxygenation or metabolism measures.

No specific genetic or metabolic tests were actually conducted, limiting the establishment of any precise causation. From a prevention and systems point of view, this case demonstrates biological vulnerabilities (e.g., placental dysfunction and white matter vulnerability associated with prematurity) and care process prompts. The possibilities for addressing the above concerns include: timely antepartum corticosteroid treatment and neuroprotective prevention of preterm birth; thorough antepartum fetal monitoring regarding placental health; careful and thorough intrapartum monitoring regarding maternal-fetal status—consistent monitoring, documentation, or both; strict adherence to resuscitation protocols, the recommendations for neuroprotective care, and anything else that would follow the current best practice; and early developmental surveillance and documentation well before the pediatric or other the pediatricians visit, potentially changing that to developmental screening, prioritized follow up, and existing practice around referral and testing for targeted genetic/metabolic testing.

2.1 Introduction

Cerebral palsy (CP) is a general description of a collection of disorders and conditions that involve posture and movement defects that arise directly following damage to a developing brain, characteristically before birth, during delivery and labor, or shortly after delivery. CP is a neurologic illness that leads to permanent defects of function with an involvement of control of movement (e.g., spasticity, dyskinesia, ataxia). CP is the top child physical impairment with an anticipated incidence of roughly 2–3 per 1000 live births worldwide [7]. Latest figures report that roughly 17 million individuals, or a substantial public health issue, have CP [2]. The extent of CP significantly varies among persons with CP, with some experiencing very minimal impairment of movement and other persons experiencing very serious impairments including potential damage to cognition, speech and language impairment, and seizures.

Pathogenesis of CP is extremely multifactorial and includes perinatal, environmental, and genetic etiologies. Often the etiology of CP is not known. However, with advances in genetics, neonatal intensive care units, and obstetrics, risk factors have been found that coexist with the eventual development of CP. Previously, concern was limited to being within regions of birth asphyxia (inadequate lack of oxygen some during or during labor) and already considered to be a direct cause of CP. The decades have seen a shift to recognize that CP occurred during a multifactorial process, characteristic of prematurity, low birth weight, maternal infection, and genetic mutations, among others, being common pathway factors of pathogenesis [11].

The general purpose of the chapter is to review the etiology of CP with specific attention to genetic and environmental risk factors to disordered development. The chapter further reviews evidence-based preventive interventions to avert exposure to CP. The etiologic progression to CP is a significant consideration with respect to the goal of early identification and intervention but also with respect to guiding public health initiative to prevent CP and reduce severity.

We will specify in this chapter:

- The etiological relevance of genetic elements for CP, such as de novo mutations and single-nucleotide polymorphisms.
- The etiologic significance of factors (prenatal, perinatal, and postnatal) of CP, such as infection of the mother, prematurity and delivery-associated problems.
- Comprehensive prevention programs that span the continuum of care, including primary prevention (prenatal care and maternal health) to secondary and tertiary prevention (neonatal care, early treatment and diagnosis, and therapy).

2.2 Genetic Etiology

The genetic etiologies were the subject of rising studies during the past years as a possible cause of cerebral palsy (CP), with a possible contribution of 14% by genetics [9]. CP was initially considered to be caused by environmental and perinatal risk factors, but with the new literature suggesting that mutations of genes—like de novo mutations and polymorphisms—may play an important role during the formation of the process of developing the brain, and therefore trigger CP without any known damage. This is particularly the case with regard to idiopathic CP where not any known prenatal or perinatal factor exists [9].

2.2.1 Genomic Mutations and CP

With technologies like whole-exome sequencing, various genes that contribute to brain structure and neuronal connection have been found to cause CP when mutated. TUBA1A, CTNNB1, FBXO31, and RHOB are among the examples of the genes that all contribute to early neuronal growth and neuritogenesis too. Since the new mutations interfere with the normal development of the brain, they create malformations that make an individual susceptible to CP. For instance, TUBA1A produces a protein that is an important component of microtubules that make up the structural skeleton of a neuron. Thus, mutations of TUBA1A cause defects of neuronal migration that cause covering structural abnormalities of the brain that would otherwise be common with CP in children [9].

Beyond neurogenesis-induced genes, CP is further linked to other neurogenesis-induced genes that play a part in cell signaling, division, and differentiation such as CTNNB1 and FBXO31. Any type of mutation of these genes can impair the proper growth and development of the synaptic connections between neurons that can make individuals affected by this disease suffer their motor impairments. [9].

2.2.2 Single-Nucleotide Polymorphisms (SNPs)

Except for rare mutations, many common variations of genes or single-nucleotide polymorphisms (SNPs) contribute to CP. SNPs represent small variations in individual DNA building blocks that can influence the function of genes increase the risk of CP by itself and combined with other environmental risk factors like infection or prematurity. Multiple studies indicated that inflammatory and coagulation-related gene SNPs increase the risk of developing CP, particularly among preterm babies infected during pregnancy or delivery [12]. For example, eNOS polymorphisms contribute to low cerebral blood flow during development and thus increase the risk of CP by exposing preterm infants to hemorrhage and damage to the white matter [12].

Polymorphisms of coagulation factor VII (F7), LTA (lymphotoxin-alpha), and PAI-1 (plasminogen activator inhibitor-1) were each associated with coagulation and inflammation that play significant roles during construction of, and repair of, the injured brain during chronically perinatal injury [12].

2.2.3 Genetic Contributions in Familial Cases

Besides new mutations, inherited factor significantly contributes to the genetic etiology of cerebral palsy (CP).

The results show that people with a history of CP among their families have bigger odds of getting the condition themselves, especially if both their parents carry genetic traits that predispose them to illness. For instance, O'Callaghan et al. [13] found that people who have a brother or sister with CP have about a 1.61 times increased chance of contracting the illness, which signifies the risk that their familial history represents. This concentration of CP among families has been considered to be a result of genetic predisposition with the possible addition of the influence of common environmental pressures.

The CP of the majority of cases is not of simple Mendelian transmission patterns, but if one child of the family develops CP, then a limited chance exists to increase the occurrence of such outcomes with future offspring. Thus, families with one child that develops CP can be helped with genetic counseling to learn about possible risk and prepare for future gestations and planning of the family (Table 2.1).

2.2.4 Genetic Testing and Clinical Implications

Detecting genetic mutations involved in CP has important implications for diagnosis and management. Genetic testing has now become an important diagnostic tool for clinicians, especially when a definitive cause of CP is unknown or a child with atypical symptoms does not have obvious causative environmental risk factors. Kindred of researchers and clinicians has helped identify genetic mutations that are causing CP, more accurate diagnosis, and ruling out other genetic or metabolic

Table 2.1 Key genetic risk factors for cerebral palsy

Gene/polymorphism	Associated risk	Study
TUBA1A, CTNNB1, FBXO31, RHOB	14% of CP cases linked to de novo mutations	Jin et al. [9]
eNOS, F7, LTA, PAI-1	Odds ratios 2.1–3.2 (preterm infants)	Nelson et al. [12]
Family history	Odds ratio 1.61	O'Callaghan et al. [13]

disorders that may present with similar symptoms as CP [9]. If a case is discussed that is idiopathic in nature, genetic testing may reveal mutations responsible for disrupting normal brain development. In many cases, these findings can help families, decision making on future pregnancies (e.g., gene mutations that have the potential to recur). For example, if a child is identified with CTNNB1 mutations and diagnosed with CP, the findings could then inform the genetic counseling for the parents after presenting the likelihood of recurrence in future pregnancies related to CTNNB1 mutations [9].

Furthermore, genetic testing may pave the way for new targeted therapies in the future, particularly as personalized medicine evolves. Studies investigating gene and other types of interventions may give us new ways to address or treat underlying changes due to genetic mutations which may contribute to CP, leading to hope for better outcomes for individuals affected by CP.**3.**

2.3 Environmental and Perinatal Risk Factors

Perinatal and environmental factors are important in determining cerebral palsy (CP) characteristics. Most of these factors happen before or during the time of labor and shortly after a child's birth, and they can cause brain injury or corresponding risk factors. Environmental factors such as prenatal infections, maternal health factors, prematurity, and intrapartum complications are the important culprits for CP. To devise approaches and preventive efforts or reduce the impact of CP on a population, a better understanding of these perinatal and environmental factors, particularly among high-risk populations, is important (Table 2.2).

2.3.1 Prenatal Factors

The period of gestation is a crucial time of brain growth, and any disturbances to the pregnant woman and fetus will influence brain development in the fetus. Numerous aspects of the prenatal period are significantly associated with an increased risk for CP.

Preterm Birth

Preterm birth is one of the most consistently identified risk factors for CP, and the earlier an infant is born, the higher the risk for CP. Infants born at less than

Table 2.2 Comprehensive risk factors for cerebral palsy with odds ratios

Risk factor	Risk estimate	Study
Preterm birth (<32 weeks)	Odds ratio 59.2	O'Callaghan et al. [13]
Low birth weight (<2500 g)	Higher risk as birth weight decreases	MacLennan et al. [11]
Multiple gestation (twins, triplets)	Increased risk, often due to prematurity or low birth weight	Bonellie et al. (2005)
Maternal infection (chorioamnionitis)	OR 4.1 (term infants), OR 1.9 (preterm infants)	Wu and Colford [16]
Maternal viral infections (e.g., rubella, CMV, toxoplasmosis)	Increased risk due to fetal brain development disruption	Chen et al. [5]
Placental insufficiency	Increased risk due to inadequate oxygen and nutrient supply	MacLennan et al. [11]
Intrauterine growth restriction (IUGR)	Fourfold increased risk in term infants	Wu et al. (2003)
Preeclampsia and maternal hypertension	OR 1.93 (95% CI 1.48–2.52) for gestational hypertension	MacLennan et al. [11]
Birth asphyxia (HIE)	Risk increases with severe or prolonged asphyxia	Nelson et al. [12]
Emergency cesarean section	OR 1.99 (95% CI 1.63–2.43) due to fetal distress	O'Callaghan et al. [13]
Neonatal stroke	Increased risk for hemiplegic CP	Nelson et al. [12]
Severe neonatal jaundice (kernicterus)	Increased risk of athetoid CP if untreated	MacLennan et al. [11]
Neonatal infections (e.g., meningitis, encephalitis)	Linked to brain injury and CP development	Chen et al. [5]
Head injury (e.g., shaken baby syndrome)	Increased risk from trauma	Nelson et al. [12]
Severe neonatal hypoglycemia	Risk of brain injury and CP if not corrected	Nelson et al. [12]
Anoxic injury (e.g., drowning, choking)	Risk from lack of oxygen leading to CP	Nelson et al. [12]
TUBA1A, CTNNB1, FBXO31, RHOB	14% of CP cases linked to de novo mutations	Jin et al. [9]
eNOS, F7, LTA, PAI-1 SNPs	Odds ratios 2.1–3.2 (preterm infants)	Nelson et al. [12]
Family history of CP	Odds ratio 1.61 for siblings of CP-affected children	O'Callaghan et al. [13]
Sex (male)	Higher risk in males, especially in preterm infants	O'Callaghan et al. [13]
Socioeconomic status (low SES)	Higher risk in low-SES populations	Donald et al. [7]
Assisted reproductive technology (ART)	Slight increase in risk, especially for multiple births	Bearden et al. [2]

32 weeks gestation are at the greatest risk for brain injury that will lead to CP, and CP occurs in 10% of extremely preterm infants [11]. In a meta-analysis, it was shown preterm birth increases the odds of developing CP by approximately 2.9-fold [13]. Preterm infants are at greater risk for intra-ventricular hemorrhaging, white matter injury, and periventricular leukomalacia (PVL), all of which are precursors to CP [13].

Low Birth Weight
A further significant risk factor is low birth weight (LBW) for CP. Infants born who weigh less than 2500 grams are at increased risk for developing CP, with the highest risk associated with infants weighing less than 1500 grams [11]. LBW usually co-occurs with preterm birth, which contributes to brain injury risk. LBW infants are at risk for complications that lead to CP, including an increased rate of intracranial hemorrhage, intraventricular hemorrhage (IVH), and periventricular leukomalacia [11].

Maternal Infections
Maternal infections, especially those that infect the fetal brain, are some of the most critical prenatal contributors to CP. Chorioamnionitis, an infection of the placental membranes, has been linked to an increased risk of CP. A meta-analysis compared the relative risk of CP in term infants [4.7] and preterm infants (1.9), with infection [16]. Pregnant maternal infections such as rubella, cytomegalovirus (CMV), and toxoplasmosis have the potential to infect the fetus, cross the placenta, and cause congenital defects in the fetal brain, which have been linked to CP [5].

Placental Insufficiency
Placental insufficiency is another significant risk factor for CP, which occurs when the placenta cannot provide sufficient oxygen and nutrients to the fetus. Preeclampsia, gestational hypertension, and intrauterine growth restriction problems can also impede the placenta and cause fetal hypoxia, which raises the likelihood of brain injury and CP [11].

2.3.2 Perinatal Factors

Perinatal factors are events that happen surrounding labor that could include complications that cause injuries to the brain.

Birth Asphyxia
Birth asphyxia, or hypoxic-ischemic encephalopathy (HIE), is a major factor for CP onset, particularly in term infants. Perinatal HIE is due to oxygen deprivation during labor and delivery resulting in damage to the developing brain. Birth asphyxia was once thought to be a major cause of CP, although it has been shown to account for only a fraction of cases. In term infants, birth asphyxia alone accounts for less than 10% of CP cases [12]. When combined with other risk factors, such as prematurity or low birth weight, however, the incidence of CP rises substantially [12].

Emergency Cesarean Section
Emergency cesarean sections take place very frequently due to fetal distress or complications that occur during labor. The attribution of the birth as an emergency cesarean usually suggests that the infant was under considerable stress during delivery (e.g., prolonged labor, hypoxic). O'Callaghan et al. [13] studied the rate of CP associated with emergency cesarean births and found increased rates with an odds ratio (OR) of 1.99 (95% CI 1.63–2.43). This suggests that fetal distress, which often leads to an emergency cesarean section, can contribute to brain injury and CP.

Neonatal Stroke
A neonatal stroke takes place when there is a disruption or impediment to blood flow to the infant's brain, either from a clot or by hemorrhaging. Neonatal strokes are a significant cause of hemiplegic CP, especially when the stroke occurs in one hemisphere of the brain. Risk factors for neonatal stroke include maternal coagulation disorders, maternal thrombophilias, and any complications associated with delivery. A stroke during the perinatal period can lead to irreversible brain injury, usually resulting in CP [12].

2.3.3 Postnatal Factors

Postnatal factors are defined as circumstances that impact the newborn's progression after birth during the neonatal period.

Severe Neonatal Jaundice (Kernicterus)
Severe neonatal jaundice leading to kernicterus is a preventable cause of CP. Kernicterus occurs when elevated levels of bilirubin in the blood cause brain damage in the infant. Phototherapy and exchange transfusions are common interventions to help prevent this type of brain injury. Risk factors for kernicterus include blood type incompatibility (e.g., Rh or ABO incompatibility) or decreased levels of G6PD enzyme, which creates a failure to metabolize red blood cells, leading to jaundice [11].

2.3.3.1 Neonatal Infections
An infant may have permanent brain damage that leads to CP from infections such as meningitis or encephalitis in the neonatal period. A neonatal infection may be bacterial (e.g., Group B Streptococcus) or viral (e.g., herpes simplex virus). It is critical to treat these infections promptly with antibiotics or antivirals to prevent brain injury and reduce the risk of CP [12] .

2.4 Interactions Between Genetic and Environmental Factors

Both genetic and environmental factors can each, in isolation, contribute to the development of cerebral palsy (CP), but risk is often exacerbated when genetic vulnerability coincides with environmental factors. These interactions are indicative of the multifactorial nature of CP, where a convergence of both genetic and environmental factors may increase the risk of brain injury consistent with CP.

2.4.1 Genetic Susceptibility and Inflammatory Responses

Recent studies have proven that inflammatory gene polymorphisms play a key role in CP risk in most cases in premature-born or infection-exposed intrauterine babies. For instance, coagulation, inflammation, and vessel control gene polymorphisms may lead to an elevated risk of brain injury if the infant is at risk of maternal infection or perinatal asphyxia [12].

Perhaps the best-documented association is between maternal infection and genetic susceptibility. Certain SNPs in the eNOS gene (which regulates nitric oxide production) have been associated with susceptibility to intraventricular hemorrhage (IVH) and periventricular leukomalacia (PVL) among preterm infants exposed to chorioamnionitis. Inflammatory mechanisms disrupt normal brain development, leading to CP [12].

2.4.2 Family History and Perinatal Complications

The risk of CP is also increased if the child comes from a family with a history of CP. Literature indicates that siblings of children with CP are at higher risk of developing CP, especially if they have multiple perinatal complications in the form of preterm and asphyxia at birth. For example, O'Callaghan et al. [13] indicated that children with CP had siblings with an OR of 1.61, which supports a genetic role in the causality of CP.

In offspring of CP-involvement families, we can then propose that the combination of the child's genetic susceptibilities and insults environmentally (e.g., prenatal issues or perinatal insults that may discover happening at birth) is responsible for the increase risk. Finally, what is reached is the conclusion that we cannot necessarily assign a genetic or an environmental or perinatal risk factor independently, but the risk is mediated by a set of all genetic/environmental factors.

2.4.3 The Contribution of Preterm Birth to Genetic Risk

Preterm birth, itself an environmental risk for CP, is compounded by genetic mutations that put the brain at risk of damage. Variants of genes that indicate risk

Table 2.3 Interaction between genetic and environmental risk factors for cerebral palsy

Genetic risk factor	Environmental risk factor	Combined effect	Study
eNOS polymorphism	Chorioamnionitis (maternal infection)	Increased risk of intraventricular hemorrhage (IVH) and PVL in preterm infants	Nelson et al. [12]
TUBA1A mutation	Preterm birth (<32 weeks)	Increased risk of periventricular leukomalacia (PVL) and CP in preterm infants	Jin et al. [9]
CTNNB1 mutation	Birth asphyxia	Increased risk of spasticity and hemiplegia in term infants	Jin et al. [9]
Family history of CP	Preterm birth	OR 1.61 for siblings of children with CP	O'Callaghan et al. [13]

of CP, for example, TUBA1A or CTNNB1, are thought to influence processes, for example, neuronal migration, which, perinatal processes, for example, prematurity, may disturb. In fact, such gene mutations in preterm infants increase the risk of white matter injury in the form of PVL, which in turn considerably [7, 8] increases the risk for CP [9]. Preterm birth can be an inducer for such infants to the degree that the question is more specific. Such interaction supports the hypothesis that preterm infants with gene variation are at greater risk for CP. In the context of neuroprotection (with treatments such as magnesium sulfate) for preterm infants, it is a move toward eliminating the potential environmental risk factor (premature birth, in this case) and the influence of genetic susceptibility [6] (Table 2.3).

2.5 Prevention Strategies

Though CP prevention in all cases is not possible, there are various strategies that can curb its incidence and intensity. CP prevention is a comprehensive intervention, addressing the aforementioned risk factors on multiple levels, from pregnancy to the neonatal period. Intervention measures belong to the categories of primary prevention, secondary prevention, and tertiary prevention.

2.5.1 Primary Prevention

Primary prevention is preventing CP from occurring, generally through treating reversible risk factors during pregnancy and improving maternal health.

2.5.1.1 Prenatal Education

One of the most important primary prevention interventions is prenatal education. Pregnant women's health education programs are found to decrease unnecessary risk factors for CP, especially in low-resource settings [1]. Educational programs focus on educating women regarding preterm routine prenatal visits, diet, avoiding infection, and harmful drugs such as tobacco and alcohol. Furthermore, prenatal education programs promote the management of existing maternal medical conditions, such as hypertension or diabetes, that result in CP risk.

Magnesium Sulfate

Magnesium sulfate is a very helpful neuroprotective treatment for preterm infants with high-risk preterm labor.

Several studies have proven that magnesium sulfate lowered the incidence of CP in preterm infants by modulating neuronal membranes and inflammation within the immature brain [3]. Research indicates that magnesium sulfate lowers the risk of preterm babies to CP due to IVH and PVL [6]. The intervention has to be administered at 24–32 weeks of gestation and is today an established part of the treatment of preterm birth.

Infection Prevention and Treatment

Maternal infection, including chorioamnionitis and urinary tract infection, is are critical risk factor for CP.

Prevention of maternal infection through appropriate prenatal care, screening, and antibiotic prophylaxis may decrease the risk of infectious brain damage [16]. Rubella, varicella, and influenza immunization preconception and during pregnancy can decrease the risk for congenital infection to causes CP. Reducing exposure to environmental toxins (e.g., safe handling of cat litter to avoid toxoplasmosis infection) will also decrease maternal infections that have the potential to bias normal fetal brain development [16].

Decreasing Multiple Gestations with Assisted Reproductive Technology (ART)

Infertility therapies such as IVF tend to result in multiple gestations, and there is a higher risk of preterm birth and CP. It is also possible to transfer fewer embryos during IVF, or elective single-embryo transfer can lower the risks of multiple gestations and risks of CP significantly [2]. This has become common practice to recommend for women being treated under ART.

2.5.2 Secondary Prevention

Secondary prevention aims at early detection and treatment to prevent worsening of CP following birth. Medical treatment in infancy will decrease brain damage, especially for at-risk infants for CP.

Therapeutic Hypothermia

Cooling treatment or therapeutic hypothermia is now an accepted practice in neonates with hypoxic-ischemic encephalopathy (HIE).

Therapeutic hypothermia needs to be initiated within 6 h of birth. The therapy reduces the body temperature of the infant to prevent secondary brain injury due to oxygen lack [10]. Different research claims that therapeutic hypothermia improves infant survival and outcome considerably when CP risk due to asphyxia during delivery is present, while preventing inflammation and neuronal damage in the brain. Evidence reveals that therapeutic hypothermia reduced CP by 20%–30% in neonates compared to control [10].

Immediate Obstetric Intervention

Immediate Antibiotic Intervention can prevent oxygen deficit to the fetus through interventions like emergency cesarean delivery, especially when fetal distress or complicated labor is present.

Intrapartum monitoring can assist obstetric personnel to show evidence of distress in the mother or baby and can initiate early intervention to avoid inflicting injury on the brain [15]. Elective cesarean delivery in certain situations, such as breech presentation, avoids birth trauma and CP as a result of mechanical injury [15].

2.5.3 Tertiary Prevention

Tertiary prevention refers to rehabilitation and treatment to maximize quality of life and functional outcome in children with CP following early diagnosis, rehabilitation, and supportive therapy.

2.5.3.1 Early Intervention Programs

Other than a CP diagnosis at 6 months, CP infants are free to initiate an early intervention program. Early intervention programs may be a combination of physical therapy, occupational therapy, and speech therapy to aid motor development, communication, and social interaction. It has been established that therapy early is for those children who are capable of showing marvelous functional outcomes and independence [4].

2.5.3.2 Nutritional Support

CP children are predisposed to feeding and swallowing disorders and thus may experience malnutrition and failure to thrive. Dietary care via special foods or feeding tube support can prevent effective caloric intake and growth. Nutrition program also contributes to muscle strength, immunity, and general growth [4].

2.5.3.3 Assistive Devices and Technologies

With an increase in the number of children with CP, assistive devices and equipment like wheelchairs, adaptive utensils, and communication devices may be required to increase independence in activities of daily living. Speech-generating devices and mobility devices increase independence and facilitate participation in school and community settings, and also improve the overall quality of life of children [10].

Rehabilitation and Advanced Therapies

Over the past few years, technical programs and multidisciplinary rehabilitation interventions have been found to be very effective in maximizing outcomes in children with CP. Task-oriented training (TOT) is linked with the greatest gains in gross motor function and in changes of mobility. Virtual reality (VR) therapy enhances balance, postural control, and activities of daily living—especially at a dosage of 101–200 min/week. Robot-aided gait training (RAGT) improved the velocity of walking, standing balance, and the capacity to walk [14]. Stimulation interventions like whole-body vibration (WBV) and functional electrical stimulation (FES) have good-quality evidence to improve gait, step length, and reductions in balance problems. Aerobic exercise, hippotherapy, and muscle strengthening improve mobility, endurance, and spasticity, but moderate evidence is available to recommend these interventions.

2.5.3.4 Pharmacological and Biological Interventions

Pharmacologic intervention remains an important part of symptom management.

BoNT-A injections are commonly used to reduce spasticity and enhance mobility, but safety concerns, such as muscle weakness or respiratory infection, need to be strictly monitored [14]. Biologically, SCT has promise to improve medium-term gross motor outcomes and developmental achievements, but the quality of evidence is low, and larger trials would need to be conducted to confirm safety and long-term efficacy [14].

Indications

Clinical indications for specific or targeted intervention, if they exist, need to be valued as evidence-based choices in the framework of a multidisciplinary decision-making process—not as a prescription.

Intervention is most commonly warranted where there is unequivocal deterioration in a problem that is impairing function, causing pain, or compromising safety despite optimal conservative treatment. Progressive increasing hip displacement with or without pain or loss of function, intractable chronic focal spasticity resistant to vigorous goal-directed physiotherapy, and recurrent aspiration risk or severe bulbar impairment requiring nutritional support with proven failure to thrive are some indications in expert practice. In either situation, there needs to be a registered, clear indication of why there are indications for intervention based on objective measures (imaging, functional test, scales), and the indication needs to be made available during the team meeting with the physician, surgeon, rehabilitation specialist, and the involved members of the family. Where a decision has to be made on a procedural or surgical intervention, the indication should be directly linked with the stated functional goals, attainable expectations of outcome, and the child and family's priority in mind.

For example, a decision to have or not have orthopedic surgery should explicitly balance against each other the potential benefits of greater mobility and/or pain relief against any risks that could come to fruition as a result of the operation (short-term and long-term) and the risk of needing rehabilitation afterward. Similarly, there is consideration of a direct treatment plan involving pharmacologic intervention or procedure intervention (e.g., botulinum toxin for disabling focal spasticity) when outcome measurement is demonstrated to identify substantial improvement in activity or participation and when a reasonable trial of treatment has taken place. There are other intervention drugs that are contraindicated or not effective. It is hoped that any recommendation will be supported by an outcome measurement, follow-up, and staged reassessment, where there is a suitable planning strategy. In the absence of conclusive trials providing evidence to underpin clinical efficacy, clinicians are not able to overestimate clinical indications but use consensus practice, on an individual basis, with the overall goal of doing no harm and maximizing function.

This chapter is meant to explain and support clinical judgment: all clinical subsections must contain some data, a clinical overview of the data given, and, if available, evidence, support provided by high-grade evidence or recommendations provided in a guideline. Unless your chapter is documenting clinical numbers or levels that represent evidence-based practice clinical evidence, either leave it alone if it does not apply, or present it as expert consensus recommendations to prevent findings from being taken out of context (Table 2.4).

Table 2.4 Summary of prevention strategies for cerebral palsy

Level	Strategy	Target group	Effect/outcome
Primary prevention	Prenatal education	Pregnant women	Reduces preventable risks (infections, malnutrition, substance use, unmanaged comorbidities)
	Magnesium sulfate (24–32 weeks)	At-risk preterm labor	Neuroprotection reduces IVH/PVL and CP incidence
	Infection prevention and treatment	Pregnant women	Vaccination + antibiotics reduce intrauterine infections causing CP
	Reducing multiple gestations in ART	Women using IVF/ART	Single-embryo transfer decreases preterm birth and CP risk
Secondary prevention	Therapeutic hypothermia	Neonates with HIE	Cooling within 6 h lowers CP risk by 20%–30%
	Timely obstetric intervention	Fetuses in distress/ complicated labor	C-section or monitoring prevents hypoxia and mechanical injury

(continued)

Table 2.4 (continued)

Level	Strategy	Target group	Effect/outcome
Tertiary prevention	Early intervention programs	Infants ≤6 mo diagnosed with CP	PT, OT, speech → better motor, communication, social outcomes
	Nutritional support	CP children with/ feeding issues	Prevents malnutrition; supports growth & muscle strength
	Assistive devices and technologies	Growing children with CP	Mobility + communication aids improve independence, QoL
	Task-oriented training (TOT)	Children with CP	Large gains in gross motor and mobility (SMD up to 1.06)
	Virtual reality (VR) therapy	Children with CP	High evidence: Improves GMF, balance, ADL (best at 101–200 min/ week)
	Robot-assisted gait training (RAGT)	Children with CP	Improves GMFM-D/E, gait velocity, and balance
	Whole-body vibration (WBV)	Children with CP	High evidence: Large gains in balance, gait velocity, GMFM-D/E
	Functional electrical stimulation (FES/ NMES)	Children with CP	Improves gait velocity, step length, and hand function (high credibility)
	Hippotherapy & aerobic exercise	Children with CP	Moderate effects on GMF, mobility, and participation
	Muscle strength training	Children with CP	Improves balance, gait, and spasticity (low evidence)
	Botulinum toxin A (BoNT-A)	Spastic CP	Improves gait; monitor for adverse events
	Stem cell therapy (SCT)	CP children (trial settings)	GMFM improvements at 6–12 months; evidence is very low

2.6 Practical Guidance for Carers

Early detection of developmental challenges and straightforward access to specialist therapy are pertinent aspects of the functional outcome of the child. Families ought to receive simple, easy-to-use, culturally sensitive signs of urgent referral and developmental screening. Clinicians ought to continue emphasizing considerable emphasis on family-managed education concerning visible developmental accomplishments, feeding capacity, and indicators of loss of previously reached skills or persistence of asymmetry.

Regarding practice, children can be assisted with a developmental check-up schedule, be attended to in an early intervention system and physiotherapy in the community where it is available, and receive their immunization in order to prevent secondary medical complications. Social support, caregiver well-being, and express pathways to clinical service should also be given special care to allow them to respond timely in case of concern.

2.7 Plain and Clear Prevention Advice

Reduction in chronic neonatal brain injury leading to CP in a newborn begins with the antenatal woman receiving routine antenatal care, being treated for fever and infection throughout pregnancy, and not being exposed to teratogenic substances like alcohol, illegal drugs, and cigarette smoking. Avoidance of preterm delivery through individualized obstetrical management and evidence-based antenatal care is a key population-based intervention for the reduction of the incidence.

At birth and early post-partum, stabilization and neonatal resuscitation are immediately and evidence-based, early treatment and recognition of hypoxia or severe metabolic distress, and vigilant monitoring of respiratory and feeding function are essential. Prevention of each instance of CP is not possible, but overall, this type of intervention minimizes risk for perinatal destruction and creates the best opportunity for neurodevelopment.

Critical Clinical Factors in Multidisciplinary Management

Orthopedic clinicians must watch closely and look for progression of musculoskeletal complications, i.e., fixed contractures, hip displacement, and deformities that can limit function and/or pain. Changes in musculoskeletal complications, i.e., acute progression of augmentation of muscle tone, asymmetrical loss of motor milestones or limb growth, should be investigated by imaging and multidisciplinary evaluation in a timely manner. Surgery has to be case by case, depending on rehabilitation goals, and in an overall long-term plan of participation, pain, and mobility. Regular standardized functional assessment has to be performed by neurologists and the entire multidisciplinary team, evidence-based treatments have to be implemented, e.g., selective botulinum toxin injections for focal spasticity, and a goal-directed physiotherapy plan constructed. There should be periodic case conferences along the multidisciplinary team—speech and language therapy, occupational therapy, physiotherapy, orthopedics, nutrition, and social work—to tie short-term problem-solving with engaging longer term involvement goals and with the transition streams.

2.8 Conclusion

Prevention of cerebral palsy (CP) will be a multiple and coordinated effort. Primary prevention is about maternal health, antenatal care, and modifiable risk factors like prematurity and maternal infection. Secondary prevention focuses on early intervention to reduce the severity of CP among at-risk infants, and tertiary prevention focuses on preparing children with CP for the most achievable quality of life possible, e.g., early diagnosis, rehabilitation, and assistive technology. Prevention of every case of CP is not possible, but these levels of prevention are useful methods of reducing the incidence and burden of this chronic disorder.

Disclosure We utilized Grammarly for grammar style and checking for readability of this work.

References

1. Abdullahi A, Zakariyya A, Abba M. An education program for prevention of cerebral palsy for pregnant women attending anti-natal clinics: a descriptive survey. Arch Physiother Glob Res. 2016;20(1):7–18. https://doi.org/10.15442/apgr.20.1.1
2. Bearden D, Monokwane B, Khurana E, Baier J, Baranov E, Westmoreland K, et al. Pediatric cerebral palsy in Botswana: etiology, outcomes, and comorbidities. Pediatr Neurol. 2016;59:23–9. https://doi.org/10.1016/j.pediatrneurol.2016.03.002.
3. Binder C, Schmid P, Abele H, Graf J. Does antenatal $MgSO_4$ administration to the mother in the event of imminent premature birth reduce the occurrence of infantile cerebral palsy in the child?—An umbrella review. Geburtshilfe Frauenheilkd. 2023;83(5):602–11. https://doi.org/10.1055/a-2049-2976.
4. Chanie E, Moges N, Baye F, Mekonnen G, Fekadie M, Bazezew L, et al. Estimate the burden of malnutrition among children with cerebral palsy in Sub-Saharan Africa: a systematic review with meta-analysis. Sci Rep. 2024;14(1):6494. https://doi.org/10.1038/s41598-024-55730-1.
5. Chen D, Huang M, Yin Y, Gui D, Gu Y, Zhuang T, et al. Risk factors of cerebral palsy in children: a systematic review and meta-analysis. Transl Pediatr. 2022;11(4):556. https://doi.org/10.21037/tp-22-78.
6. Crowther CA, Hutton EK, Alfirevic Z, et al. Antenatal magnesium sulphate for neuroprotection in preterm infants—individual patient data meta-analysis. PLoS Med. 2017;14(10):e1002398. https://doi.org/10.1371/journal.pmed.1002398.
7. Donald K, Kakooza A, Wammanda R, Mallewa M, Samia P, Babakir H, et al. Pediatric cerebral palsy in Africa. J Child Neurol. 2014;30(8):963–71. https://doi.org/10.1177/0883073814549245.
8. Gibson CS, MacLennan AH, Goldwater PN, Dekker GA. Antenatal causes of cerebral palsy: associations between inherited thrombophilias, infection, and susceptibility. Obstet Gynecol Surv. 2003;58(8):507–11. https://doi.org/10.1097/01.OGX.0000055205.21611.6E.
9. Jin SC, Lewis SA, Bakhtiari S, Zeng X, Sierant MC, Shetty S, et al. Mutations disrupting neuritogenesis genes confer risk for cerebral palsy. Nat Genet. 2020;52:1046–52. https://doi.org/10.1038/s41588-020-0695-1.
10. Korzeniewski SJ, Slaughter J, Lenski M, Haak P, Paneth N. The complex aetiology of cerebral palsy. Nat Rev Neurol. 2018;14(9):528–43. https://doi.org/10.1038/s41582-018-0043-6.
11. MacLennan AH, Reddihough DS. Cerebral palsy: causes, pathways, and the role of genetic variants. Am J Obstet Gynecol. 2015;213(6):779–88. https://doi.org/10.1016/j.ajog.2015.06.064.

12. Nelson KB, Dambrosia JM, Iovannisci DM, Cheng S, Grether JK, Lammer EJ. Genetic polymorphisms and cerebral palsy in very preterm infants. Pediatr Res. 2005;57(4):494–9. https://doi.org/10.1203/01.PDR.0000156477.00386.E7.
13. O'Callaghan ME, MacLennan AH, Gibson CS, McMichael G, Haan E, Broadbent JL, et al. Epidemiologic associations with cerebral palsy. Obstet Gynecol. 2011;118(3):576–82. https://doi.org/10.1097/AOG.0b013e31822ad2dc.
14. Ren J, et al. Efficacy and safety of interventions for cerebral palsy: an umbrella review of 35 meta-analyses. Glob Meta-Anal J. 2025;1:1. (Attached article; evidence for VR, RAGT, WBV, FES, BoNT-A, SCT.)
15. Shepherd E, Salam RA, Middleton PF, Makrides M, McIntyre S, Badawi N, et al. Antenatal and intrapartum interventions for preventing cerebral palsy: an overview of Cochrane systematic reviews. Cochrane Database Syst Rev. 2017;2017(8):CD012077. https://doi.org/10.1002/14651858.CD012077.pub2.
16. Wu YW, Colford JM. Chorioamnionitis and cerebral palsy in term and near-term infants. JAMA. 2000;284(11):1417–24. https://doi.org/10.1001/jama.284.11.1417.

Diagnosing Cerebral Palsy

3

Aidin Shahilooy and Siamak Abdi

A 2-year-old girl was referred to the pediatric neurology clinic for evaluation of delayed motor milestones and progressive gait worsening. She was born at 35 weeks gestation via spontaneous vaginal delivery with an unremarkable neonatal course. Her parents reported that she achieved motor milestones late, sitting independently at 9 months and walking at 22 months. From the onset of ambulation, her gait was characterized by toe-walking. She experienced frequent falls, particularly later in the day. On physical examination, she was an alert and engaging child with age-appropriate language and cognitive skills. Neurological examination was notable for significant posturing in the lower extremities, more pronounced distally, with a velocity-independent increase in tone. Deep tendon reflexes were normal at the knees and ankles. Upper extremity tone and reflexes were normal. Given the history of mild prematurity and the clinical findings, a provisional diagnosis of spastic diplegic cerebral palsy was made. A brain MRI, ordered to confirm the etiology, was reported as unremarkable, a finding considered atypical for classic spastic diplegia but not sufficient to overturn the strong clinical diagnosis. The patient was started on a regimen of intensive physical and occupational therapy.

3.1 Introduction

Cerebral palsy (CP) is a heterogenous group of disorders originating from a non-progressive pathology in fetal or infantile neuro development and affect movement, posture, and muscle tone [1]. Additional symptoms including intellectual disability,

A. Shahilooy
Department of Genetics, MOM-Gene Personalized Medicine Center, Tehran, Iran

S. Abdi (✉)
Center for Orthopedic Trans-disciplinary Applied Research (COTAR), Tehran University of Medical Sciences (TUMS), Tehran, Iran

A. Presedo et al. (eds.), *Enhancing Quality of Life in Patients with Cerebral Palsy*, https://doi.org/10.1007/978-3-032-20967-2_3

seizures and behavioral disorders can accompany the main symptoms and complicate the diagnosis, which is more based on a combination of clinical signs rather than the etiology of the disorder [2]. CP is the most common pediatric motor disorder, occurring approximately 1 in every 500 births in high-income countries [3]. Prevalence in low-income countries is less certain, with worse disability and quality of life because of greater prevalence of infectious diseases and pre/peri-natal care differences [4]. Considering etiology, CP is an umbrella term involving many etiologies [5]. Because of the changing nature of symptoms of CP as the patients grow up despite the disorder being non-progressive, it is crucial to differentiate CP from progressive diseases [6]. It is a process that has shifted from a practice of prolonged observation and delayed confirmation to an early identification [7]. This evolution is not merely a change in timeline but a fundamental paradigm shift driven by advances in neuroimaging and a deeper understanding of developmental neurobiology [8]. The modern diagnostic journey is a multimodal process that requires the clinician to act as a synthesizer of evidence, integrating information from clinical history, standardized assessments, and neuroimaging to arrive at a conclusion that is both accurate and timely [9].

3.1.1 Defining Cerebral Palsy

For decades, CP was often misattributed almost exclusively to perinatal asphyxia. It is now understood that the etiology is highly varied and multifactorial, with the majority of cases (up to 80%) originating from prenatal factors such as infection, stroke, or brain malformation [10].

The conceptual framework for CP was formally updated by an international consensus, culminating in a definition that now serves as the global standard. This definition states:

> Cerebral palsy (CP) describes a group of permanent disorders of the development of movement and posture, causing activity limitation, that are attributed to non-progressive disturbances that occurred in the developing fetal or infant brain [11].

3.1.2 The Importance of Accurate and Early Diagnosis

The shift from a passive "wait-and-see" approach to a proactive strategy of early diagnosis is arguably the most significant clinical advance in the field of cerebral palsy in the twenty-first century [12]. Historically, the diagnosis was often delayed until a child was 12–24 months of age, a time when motor deficits became undeniable [13]. Today, international guidelines and a wealth of supporting evidence establish that an accurate diagnosis of CP, or a designation of "high risk of CP," can and should be made before 6 months corrected age, and often as early as 3 months [14]. Early diagnosis allows for the immediate implementation of interventions designed to counteract this process [15]. Early, intensive, and task-specific therapies, such as Goals-Activity-Motor Enrichment (GAME) and Constraint-Induced Movement Therapy (CIMT), are a means to actively drive and guide the brain's neuroplastic potential [14]. Early diagnosis is also critical for preventing the cascade of secondary musculoskeletal complications and allows for the immediate initiation of surveillance programs, such as regular hip monitoring via physical examination and radiography [2]. This monitoring can detect the earliest signs of subluxation, allowing for timely and often less invasive interventions that can prevent the development of severe deformities [16].

3.1.3 Overview of the Diagnosis

The three pillars of diagnosis:

- *Clinical history*: The diagnosis process begins with a review of potential risk factors across the developmental timeline [5]. This includes prenatal factors (e.g., intrauterine infections, maternal conditions, multiple gestation), perinatal events (e.g., prematurity, low birth weight, hypoxic-ischemic encephalopathy, perinatal stroke), and postnatal insults (e.g., meningitis, traumatic brain injury) [10].
- *Standardized neurological and motor assessment*: The standard requires the use of validated, quantitative assessment tools that evaluate an infant's neurological status and motor function against age-specific normal ranges [17].
- *Neuroimaging*: Visualizing the brain allows the clinician to identify the structural basis of the motor disorder, which can confirm the diagnosis and offer prognostic information [18]. Magnetic resonance imaging (MRI) is the neuroimaging modality of choice [19]. It has a sensitivity of 86–89% for identifying a relevant brain lesion in children with a confirmed diagnosis of CP [20].

International guidelines have also identified a set of high-yield tools that, when used in combination, provide high diagnostic accuracy [14]:

- *General movements assessment* (*GMA*): This non-invasive, observational tool is a cornerstone of diagnosis in early infancy (from birth to 20 weeks corrected age). It assesses the quality of an infant's spontaneous, endogenously generated movements [21, 22].
- *Hammersmith infant neurological examination* (*HINE*): The HINE is a standardized, scorable neurological examination for infants aged 2–24 months. It systematically assesses posture, tone, reflexes, and motor function [23, 24].

While each tool is strong in isolation, their combined predictive power is exceptional [25]. An infant with an abnormal brain MRI, absent fidgety general movements in GMA, and an abnormal HINE score has a greater than 98% probability of having CP [14].

The diagnostic process is not static but follows an age-dependent algorithm that uses the right tools at the right time [26]:

For infants younger than 5 months corrected age: The diagnostic pathway prioritizes the GMA, particularly during the "fidgety" period, in combination with the HINE and an MRI performed at term-equivalent age or as soon as feasible [27].

For infants older than 5 months corrected age: After the fidgety period, the GMA is no longer applicable. The diagnostic focus shifts to serial HINE assessments to track neurological status over time, supplemented by standardized motor assessments (such as the parent-reported Developmental Assessment of Young Children (DAYC)) to quantify motor delay, alongside MRI findings {Table 3.1} [26].

This pathway should be initiated whenever clinical red flags are present [28]. In older infants, these include persistent head lag after 4 months, fisting of the hands after 4 months, inability to sit independently by 9 months, or the development of a clear hand preference before 12 months of age [2].

3.1.4 Early Diagnosis

Although many etiologies have been suggested to cause CP, the exact mechanism in many patients remain unknown in clinical setting [29]. There is a wide-spread belief in medical communities that birth asphyxia is the primary pathology behind CP [30]. But large-scale studies have reported that asphyxia is the cause in less than

Table 3.1 The multimodal toolkit for early diagnosis of cerebral palsy

Assessment modality	Specific tool/ component	Optimal timing (Corrected age)	Key contribution to diagnosis & predictive value
Neuroimaging	Magnetic resonance imaging (MRI)	Term-equivalent or as early as feasible	Identifies anatomical substrate of motor disorder. Sensitivity: 86%–89%
Standardized motor assessment	General movements assessment (GMA)	Birth to 20 weeks (fidgety period: 9–20 weeks)	Assesses quality of spontaneous movement. Absent fidgety GMs sensitivity: 98%
Standardized neurological exam	Hammersmith infant neurological examination (HINE)	2–24 months	Quantifies neurological dysfunction via scorable exam. Sensitivity: 90%
Standardized developmental assessment	Developmental assessment of young children (DAYC)	>5 months	Quantifies motor delay via parent-report checklist. Predictive accuracy: 80%–89%

Morgan et al. [14], Bosanquet et al. [17], Springer et al. [20], Einspieler and Prechtl [21], Romeo et al. [23], Mendoza-Sengco et al. [26]

10% of patients [5]. In about 80% of cases, the specific cause remains unclear and only risk factors are identified through history taking [10]. Studies in past years had reported 14% of CP cases to have a genetic component [31]. More recent studies have raised the genetic component in CP etiology to about 30% [32]. It seems that a growing body of evidence is suggesting a strong genetic component in CP pathology [33].

Four types of motor dysfunction exist which may change as the newborn grows [11]:

- Spasticity which is seen in 85%–91% of cases
- Dyskinesia, including Dystonia and athetosis in 4%–7% of cases
- Ataxia in 4%–6% of patients
- Hypotonia in 2% of cases [34, 35]

Typically, diagnosis occurred between 12 and 24 months and the time period before that was considered the silent period [13]. Now the age of diagnosis or high suspicion is before 6 months of age. There are three tools which now are used to detect CP before the age of 5 months are MRI (86%–89% sensitivity), the Prechtl qualitative assessment of general movements (GMs) (98% sensitivity) and the Hammersmith infant neurological examination (HINE) (90% sensitivity) [14]. Tools most frequently used for risk assessment after 5 months of age are MRI (86%–89% sensitivity) (where safe and feasible), the HINE (90% sensitivity), and the developmental assessment of young children (DAYC) (83% C index) [26]. Utilizing a combination of results generated by these tools and the clinical data can result in a significantly more accurate diagnosis than isolated clinical assessments [36].

3.2 The Clinical Diagnostic Process

3.2.1 Recognizing Early Indicators: Signs and Symptoms

The diagnostic process is typically initiated by the recognition of clinical signs that deviate from the expected trajectory of infant development [28]. A primary indicator that often raises concern is a delay in reaching motor milestones. Key warning signs include:

- Head lag beyond 4 months of age.
- Inability to roll over by 6 months.
- Inability to sit independently by 9 months.
- Asymmetric crawling (e.g., lopsided crawl, scooting on buttocks) or failure to crawl on all fours by 10–12 months [2].

Clinicians should be alert for:

- Abnormalities of muscle tone: Truncal hypotonia with appendicular hypertonia is a common pattern.
- Persistent fisting beyond 4 months of age.
- Early hand preference: The development of a consistent hand preference before 12 months of age is abnormal and strongly suggests a unilateral motor deficit.
- Abnormal postures: Opisthotonus (arching of the back and neck) when held, or scissoring of the legs when picked up.

The persistence of primitive reflexes beyond their expected age of disappearance is also a key clinical characteristic of CP. Clinicians should assess for the persistence of reflexes such as the Moro reflex beyond 6 months, the asymmetric tonic neck reflex (ATNR), and the palmar grasp reflex [2].

3.2.2 Systematic History Taking

A good history is the first pillar of diagnosis [19]. The history should cover prenatal, perinatal, and postnatal periods. Prenatal history inquires about maternal health (e.g., thyroid disease, infections like CMV or toxoplasmosis), multiple gestations, use of assisted reproductive technology, and any known congenital brain malformations [10]. Perinatal history documents gestational age, birth weight, labor and delivery complications (e.g., uterine rupture, cord problems), and evidence of hypoxic-ischemic encephalopathy (HIE) or perinatal stroke. Postnatal history elicits any history of significant postnatal events such as meningitis, encephalitis, traumatic brain injury, or severe jaundice (kernicterus) [5]. The physician should carefully document the age of reaching key motor milestones, noting any delays or asymmetries [28]. A detailed family history may reveal clues to a potential genetic etiology [37].

3.2.3 Validated Standardized Assessments for Early Detection

General movements assessment (*GMA*): The Prechtl qualitative assessment of general movements (GMA) is a non-invasive tool that has become a cornerstone of early CP detection from birth to 20 weeks corrected age. The assessment involves video recording an infant's spontaneous movements for 3–5 min while they are awake, calm, and lying supine. The absence of normal, small, elegant "fidgety movements" between 9 and 20 weeks of corrected age is highly predictive of a later diagnosis of CP, with a sensitivity of 98% [14, 21].

Hammersmith infant neurological examination (*HINE*): The HINE is a standardized neurological examination designed for infants between 2 and 24 months of age with a predictive accuracy of 90%. The HINE consists of 26 items that assess cranial nerve function, posture, movements, tone, and reflexes and gives a total score out of 78. An asymmetry score can also be calculated, which is particularly useful for detecting hemiplegic CP [23]. Serial HINE assessments are valuable for tracking an infant's neurological trajectory over time [24].

Other predictive tools and their clinical utility: While the GMA and HINE are primary diagnostic tools, other assessments can provide supplementary information to strengthen the diagnosis [17]. The TIMP (Test of Infant Motor Performance) assesses the functional motor behavior of infants from 34 weeks postconceptional age to 4 months post-term. It can predict CP with 61%–90% accuracy and is useful for identifying infants who may benefit from early intervention [25]. The DAYC (Developmental assessment of young children) is a parent-reported checklist that quantifies motor delay and can be used for children older than 5 months. It has a predictive accuracy of 80%–89%. A decline in scores between 6 and 12 months is a particularly predictive pattern [26]. The AIMS (Alberta infant motor scale) is an observational tool that assesses gross motor maturation in infants up to 18 months [38]. It has a more than 85% predictive value for an abnormal motor outcome and can be a useful adjunct in monitoring motor development [39, 40].

3.3 The Role of Neuroimaging in Cerebral Palsy Diagnosis

While CP remains a clinical diagnosis, neuroimaging provides crucial information about the underlying neuropathology, helps to confirm the timing and nature of the brain insult, and can offer valuable prognostic information [18]. Magnetic resonance imaging (MRI) is the preferred neuroimaging modality, and an abnormal MRI is found in approximately 85%–90% of children with CP. For term-born infants with suspected injury, an MRI in the first week of life is recommended. If an acute insult like HIE is suspected, waiting 3–5 days before imaging can maximize the visibility of abnormal findings. For preterm infants, a term-equivalent age (TEA) MRI is recommended [19]. Common findings include:

Predominant White Matter Injury: This is the most common finding, particularly in children born preterm. Periventricular leukomalacia (PVL) is a classic finding strongly associated with spastic diplegia [41].

Predominant Grey Matter Injury: Insults occurring closer to term, when metabolic activity is highest in deep grey matter structures, often result in injury to the basal ganglia and thalamus. This pattern is typically associated with dyskinetic CP. Cortical and subcortical lesions, often from a perinatal arterial stroke, are also common and are the typical substrate for spastic hemiplegia.

Brain Malformations: MRI can reveal underlying congenital anomalies of brain development, such as lissencephaly or polymicrogyria, which point to an early prenatal etiology (Table 3.2) [41].

Table 3.2 Correlation of MRI findings with clinical CP phenotypes

MRI finding	Typical timing of insult	Associated clinical phenotype
Periventricular leukomalacia (PVL)	20–34 weeks gestation (preterm)	Spastic diplegia
Basal ganglia/thalamic injury	Late gestation/term	Dyskinetic (dystonic/ Choreoathetoid) CP
Focal arterial infarct (e.g., MCA territory)	Perinatal/term	Spastic hemiplegia
Multi cystic encephalomalacia/ widespread injury	Term	Spastic quadriplegia
Cerebellar injury/malformation	Variable	Ataxic CP

Himmelmann et al. [41]

To standardize the reporting of neuroimaging findings, classification systems have been developed. The MRI classification system (MRICS) proposed by the surveillance of cerebral palsy in Europe (SCPE) is a reliable and widely used tool. It categorizes findings into five main groups based on the presumed timing and nature of the insult:

- Group A: Maldevelopments (insult in early gestation)
- Group B: Predominant white matter injury (lesions in the late second/early third trimester)
- Group C: Predominant grey matter injury (lesions late in gestation/term)
- Group D: Miscellaneous findings
- Group E: Normal findings on conventional MRI

There is a correlation between the location of the brain lesion on MRI and the resulting clinical subtype of CP.

3.3.1 Utility of Cranial Ultrasound (CUS) in Specific Contexts

Cranial ultrasound is a valuable tool in the neonatal intensive care unit (NICU) for high-risk preterm infants. Sequential CUS can effectively detect major abnormalities like grade III/IV intraventricular hemorrhage (IVH) and cystic PVL, which have high specificity for predicting CP. CUS is less sensitive than MRI for detecting more subtle white matter injury, cerebellar lesions, or cortical malformations, and its utility diminishes as the anterior fontanelle closes [42].

3.3.2 Emerging Neuroimaging Techniques

Diffusion tensor imaging (*DTI*): DTI allows for the visualization and quantitative assessment of white matter tracts, such as the corticospinal tracts. It can provide more precise information about the integrity of these pathways than conventional MRI [18].

Magnetic resonance spectroscopy (*MRS*): MRS provides information about the biochemical composition of brain tissue, allowing for the mapping of metabolites that may be altered in the context of brain injury.

Functional MRI (*fMRI*): fMRI can be used to map motor and language areas of the brain and to study functional connectivity between different brain regions, offering insights into neural reorganization after injury [18].

3.4 The Expanding Role of Genetic Testing

The understanding of cerebral palsy etiology is undergoing a significant paradigm shift. Historically viewed as a condition resulting primarily from perinatal environmental insults like birth asphyxia, it is now clear that genetic factors play a substantial role [29]. This recognition has profound implications for the diagnostic process, family counseling, and future therapeutic strategies [37].

3.4.1 The Shift Toward Recognizing Genetic Contributions to Cerebral Palsy

Recent meta-analyses and cohort studies have consistently shown that a pathogenic or likely pathogenic genetic variant can be identified in a substantial portion of individuals with CP [12]. Estimates suggest that an identifiable genetic cause may be present in up to 30%–35% of CP cases [32, 43]; The diagnostic yield is even higher in individuals with "cryptogenic" CP—that is, those without traditional risk factors (e.g., prematurity, HIE) or with normal brain imaging [44]. Importantly, genetic variants are also found in up to 16% of individuals who have a known risk factor, suggesting that a genetic predisposition may increase an infant's vulnerability to an environmental or perinatal insult [33].

The genetic architecture of CP is heterogeneous, involving a wide range of genes and variant types involved in diverse biological processes crucial for brain development, including neuronal migration, ion channel function, and nervous system connectivity [45]. Both single nucleotide variants (SNVs) and larger copy number variants (CNVs), such as deletions or duplications, have been reported, many of which are de novo mutations [46, 47]. There is significant genetic overlap with other neurodevelopmental disorders with clinical pictures of intellectual disability, epilepsy, and autism [48]. Many single-gene disorders, such as certain hereditary spastic paraplegias, Rett syndrome, and Angelman syndrome, can present with a clinical picture that meets the criteria for CP [49]. The mutations listed below represent a list of the CP clinical picture associated types of variants found and are drawn from published literature and their documentation in the OMIM database (Table 3.3).

Table 3.3 Frequent genetic variants reported in CP patients

Gene	OMIM Phenotype	Locus	Common clinical presentation(s)	Example allelic variants (Mutations)
AP4M1	Spastic paraplegia	7q22.1	Congenital spastic tetraplegia, intellectual disability, thin corpus callosum, cerebellar atrophy. Described as a genetic model for congenital cerebral palsy	Homozygous or compound heterozygous loss-of-function mutations
AP4B1	Spastic paraplegia	1p13.2	Early-onset developmental delay, hypotonia followed by spasticity (diplegia or tetraplegia), intellectual disability, thin corpus callosum	Homozygous or compound heterozygous mutations
AP4E1	Spastic paraplegia	15q21.2	Neonatal hypotonia progressing to spasticity, severe intellectual disability, underdeveloped or absent speech, microcephaly	Homozygous or compound heterozygous loss-of-function mutations. Novel mutations have been identified
AP4S1	Spastic paraplegia	14q24.1	Early-onset developmental delay, intellectual disability, hypotonia followed by spastic diplegia or tetraplegia	Homozygous or compound heterozygous mutations
KANK1	Cerebral palsy, spastic quadriplegic	9p24.3	Spastic quadriplegia, intellectual disability, nystagmus, cerebral atrophy. Inheritance is autosomal dominant with maternal imprinting (paternally inherited deletions cause the phenotype)	Paternally inherited microdeletions on chromosome 9p24.3 involving the KANK1 gene
TUBA1A	Lissencephaly/ Tubulinopathy	12q13.12	Severe brain malformations (lissencephaly, pachygyria) leading to severe-to-profound intellectual disability, spastic tetraplegia, and epilepsy. The severe motor impairment falls under the cerebral palsy spectrum	Wide range of de novo missense mutations that disrupt microtubule structure and function
COL4A1	Porencephaly	13q34	Highly variable, from asymptomatic to severe prenatal brain destruction (porencephaly, hydranencephaly) due to hemorrhage, leading to hemiplegic or quadriplegic cerebral palsy, seizures, and intellectual disability	De novo or inherited heterozygous mutations, often missense mutations affecting glycine residues or splice site mutations

Wilson et al. [45], Bi et al. [50], Vanzo et al. [51], Moreno-De-Luca et al. [52], Winkler et al. [53], Jameel et al. [54], Wang et al. [55]

3.4.2 Clinical Scenarios Warranting Genetic Evaluation

While there is a growing argument that all individuals with CP may merit genomic testing, certain clinical scenarios have a particularly high yield and should prompt strong consideration for a genetic workup [56]. These include:

- CP of unknown cause, with no clear history of perinatal risk factors.
- A normal or non-specific brain MRI that does not explain the clinical picture.
- A family history of CP or other neurodevelopmental disorders.
- The presence of dysmorphic features or congenital anomalies outside the central nervous system.
- The presence of significant co-occurring conditions, such as severe intellectual disability or autism, that seem disproportionate to the motor impairment.

3.4.3 Methodologies in Genetic Testing for Cerebral Palsy

Genetic testing has moved beyond single-gene analysis to more comprehensive genomic approaches [9]. Chromosomal Microarray (CMA) is effective at detecting CNVs (deletions and duplications) but has a relatively low diagnostic yield in CP, around 5%–10% [13].

Whole exome sequencing (WES) or whole genome sequencing (WGS) are now considered first-line tests in many cases [43]. These powerful techniques analyze all protein-coding genes (exome) or the entire genetic code (genome) and have a much higher diagnostic yield, identifying a cause in 23%–35% of cases [12]. Testing the child along with both biological parents (trio-based sequencing) is the preferred approach as it greatly facilitates the identification of de novo variants [32].

3.5 Classifying Cerebral Palsy

3.5.1 Classification by Predominant Motor Abnormality (Physiological)

Spastic CP (80%–90%): This is the most common type, caused by damage to the brain's motor cortex and pyramidal tracts [34]. It is characterized by hypertonia (increased muscle tone) that is velocity-dependent, hyperreflexia, and other upper motor neuron signs [11].

Dyskinetic CP (7%): This type mainly results from injury to the basal ganglia [41]. It is characterized by involuntary, uncontrolled, and recurring movements. Muscle tone is often variable, fluctuating from hypertonia to hypotonia [11]. Dyskinetic CP can be further subdivided:

- Dystonic: Dominated by sustained or intermittent muscle contractions causing twisting and repetitive movements or abnormal postures.

- Choreoathetoid: A combination of chorea (unpredictable, irregular movements) and athetosis (slow, writhing movements).

Ataxic CP (4%): This is one of the least common types, resulting from damage to the cerebellum [34]. It is characterized by a primary disorder of balance and coordination. Movements are clumsy, and individuals often have a wide-based, unsteady gait and intention tremor.

Mixed CP: It is common for individuals to present with features of more than one motor type (e.g., spasticity with dystonia). In these cases, the diagnosis should specify the component motor disorders [11].

3.5.2 Topographical Classification of Motor Impairment (Anatomical)

Monoplegia: One limb is affected (rare).

Hemiplegia: One side of the body (one arm and one leg) is affected.

Diplegia: All four limbs are affected, but the legs are more significantly impaired than the arms.

Quadriplegia/Tetraplegia: All four limbs, and often the trunk and face, are involved [11].

3.5.3 Functional Classification Systems: Describing Abilities and Limitations

Recognizing the limitations of classifications based solely on impairment, a suite of functional classification systems has been developed. These systems focus on what a child *can do* in their daily life, providing a much more meaningful description of their abilities and needs [57]. Each system uses a five-level ordinal scale, where Level I represents the highest level of function and Level V represents the most significant limitation (Table 3.4).

- *Gross motor function classification system* (*GMFCS*): Describes self-initiated movement, with a focus on sitting, transferring, and mobility.
- *Manual ability classification system* (*MACS*): Describes how children use their hands to handle objects in daily activities.
- *Communication function classification system* (*CFCS*): Describes everyday communication performance, including all methods of communication (speech, gesture, assistive technology).
- *Eating and drinking ability classification system* (*EDACS*): Describes the safety and efficiency of eating and drinking.

Table 3.4 Overview of the five-level functional classification systems for CP

Level	GMFCS (Mobility)	MACS (Hand use)	CFCS (Communication)	EDACS (Eating/Drinking)
I	Walks without limitations	Handles objects easily and successfully	Effective sender and receiver with unfamiliar partners	Eats and drinks safely and efficiently
II	Walks with limitations	Handles most objects but with reduced quality and/or speed	Effective, but with a slower pace, with unfamiliar partners	Eats and drinks safely, but with some limitations to efficiency
III	Walks using a hand-held mobility device	Handles objects with difficulty; needs help to prepare/modify activities	Effective sender and receiver with familiar partners	Eats and drinks with some limitations to safety
IV	Self-mobility with limitations; may use powered mobility	Handles a limited selection of easily managed objects in adapted situations	Inconsistent sender and/or receiver with familiar partners	Eats and drinks with significant limitations to safety
V	Transported in a manual wheelchair	Does not handle objects; has severely limited ability to perform even simple actions	Seldom effective sender and receiver even with familiar partners	Unable to eat or drink safely; tube feeding is required

From Paulson and Vargus-Adams [11], licensed under CC-BY 4.0

Historically, CP has been described using severity labels of "mild," "moderate," or "severe." While simple, these terms are subjective, poorly defined, and not used reliably across clinicians. The functional classification systems, particularly the GMFCS, provide a much more objective and standardized method for describing the level of functional limitation and have largely replaced these older, less precise terms [11].

3.6 The Differential Diagnosis

The diagnosis of cerebral palsy, while clinical, is not one of exclusion in the traditional sense [36]. Rather, it is a diagnosis of inclusion based on a specific constellation of symptoms [28]. because many other neurological conditions can present with motor dysfunction in infancy, a thoughtful and systematic approach to differential diagnosis is a cornerstone of diagnostic accuracy [49].

The most critical distinction in the differential diagnosis is between the static encephalopathy of CP and a progressive neurological disorder [6]. The defining feature of CP is that the underlying brain lesion is non-progressive. While the clinical manifestations of CP can change over time—for example, spasticity may increase during growth spurts, or musculoskeletal deformities like contractures and scoliosis can worsen—these changes are secondary consequences of the initial, static injury on a growing body [2].

In contrast, a progressive disorder is characterized by the ongoing loss of previously acquired skills (developmental regression) or a functional decline that cannot be explained by growth and secondary impairments alone. A child who was able to sit independently and then loses this ability, or whose gait deteriorates beyond what is expected for their GMFCS level, should be urgently evaluated for an alternative, progressive diagnosis. This distinction is paramount, as many neurodegenerative and neurometabolic disorders have specific treatments that can halt or slow disease progression, making a delayed diagnosis a critical missed opportunity [49].

3.6.1 Important Conditions Mimicking Cerebral Palsy

A growing number of genetic and metabolic conditions can present with early motor impairment and be misdiagnosed as CP. These "CP mimics" often meet the initial clinical criteria but have a distinct underlying pathophysiology that may have implications for prognosis, genetic counseling, and, in some cases, specific treatment [49]. Key categories of mimics include:

Hereditary spastic paraplegias (*HSPs*): This is a large, genetically heterogeneous group of disorders characterized by progressive lower limb spasticity and weakness due to corticospinal tract degeneration. While some forms are "pure" with only spasticity, many "complex" forms include ataxia, cognitive impairment, or epilepsy, creating significant phenotypic overlap with spastic CP.

Inborn errors of metabolism: Many metabolic disorders can present with motor signs that mimic CP. Examples include:

- Glutaric Aciduria Type 1: Can cause an acute dystonic crisis following a catabolic illness, leading to permanent basal ganglia injury and a dyskinetic movement disorder.
- Arginase Deficiency: A urea cycle disorder that can present with progressive spastic diplegia, often without the neonatal hyperammonemia seen in other urea cycle defects.
- Lesch–Nyhan Syndrome: An X-linked disorder of purine metabolism causing dystonia, choreoathetosis, and characteristic self-injurious behaviors.
- Mitochondrial Disorders: These can present with a wide array of neurological signs, including ataxia, dystonia, and spasticity, often with a fluctuating course.

Leukodystrophies: These are genetic disorders affecting the white matter of the brain. While many are rapidly progressive, some, like Pelizaeus–Merzbacher disease, can have a slow course initially, presenting with nystagmus, hypotonia, and later spasticity and ataxia, mimicking CP.

Dopa-responsive dystonia (*Segawa disease*): This is a critical diagnosis not to miss, as it is highly treatable with levodopa. It typically presents with foot dystonia and gait difficulty, often with marked diurnal fluctuation (worse in the afternoon/evening).

Neurogenetic syndromes: Numerous single-gene disorders can have motor impairment as a prominent feature. Examples include Angelman syndrome (ataxia, jerky movements), Rett syndrome (loss of hand skills, stereotypies), and various pontocerebellar hypoplasias [49].

3.6.2 Clinical and Investigational Clues to Alternative Diagnoses

A systematic approach to identifying red flags can guide the clinician toward an alternative diagnosis [28]. The presence of one or more of the following features listed in (Table 3.5) should prompt a more extensive diagnostic evaluation beyond the standard CP workup.

Table 3.5 Clinical and investigational red flags for conditions mimicking cerebral palsy

Category	Red flag/Clue	Potential alternative diagnoses	Key investigations
History	Developmental regression: Loss of previously acquired motor or cognitive skills	Neurodegenerative disorders, Leukodystrophies, mitochondrial disease	Serial developmental assessments, neuroimaging, metabolic/genetic testing
	Strong family history: Consanguinity or multiple family members with similar disorders	Hereditary spastic paraplegias, genetic syndromes, mitochondrial disease	Detailed pedigree, genetic testing (trio-exome)
	Fluctuating course/diurnal variation: Symptoms worsen with illness or throughout the day	Dopa-responsive dystonia, mitochondrial disease, GLUT-1 deficiency	Trial of levodopa, CSF glucose/lactate, genetic testing
	Absence of risk factors: Term birth with no clear perinatal insult, especially in spastic diplegia	Hereditary spastic paraplegias, genetic mimics	Neuroimaging, genetic testing
Physical examination	Dysmorphic features: Unusual facial features or congenital anomalies outside the CNS	Genetic syndromes (e.g., Angelman), metabolic storage diseases	Genetic consultation, chromosomal microarray, exome sequencing
	Pure motor signs: Isolated dystonia or ataxia without spasticity or other mixed features	Primary dystonias, hereditary ataxias	Neuroimaging, genetic testing
	Peripheral nervous system signs: Areflexia, sensory loss	Peripheral neuropathies, spinocerebellar ataxias	Nerve conduction studies/EMG, genetic testing
	Oculomotor abnormalities: Oculomotor apraxia, ophthalmoplegia, nystagmus	Ataxia-telangiectasia, Joubert syndrome, Pelizaeus-Merzbacher disease	Ophthalmologic evaluation, neuroimaging
Investigations	Normal brain MRI: In the context of significant motor impairment	Hereditary spastic paraplegias, Dopa-responsive dystonia, some genetic mimics	Spine MRI, genetic testing, trial of levodopa if indicated
	Specific progressive MRI findings: Iron deposition in basal ganglia, progressive white matter changes, pontocerebellar hypoplasia	Neurodegeneration with brain iron accumulation (NBIA), Leukodystrophies, genetic syndromes	Targeted genetic testing based on MRI pattern

From Friedman et al. [28] and Lewis et al. [49], licensed under CC-BY 4.0

3.7 Recognizing Associated Conditions

Core motor disorder in cerebral palsy is *often accompanied* by a range of other disturbances. These are not incidental findings; they are direct or indirect consequences of the same early brain insult and are integral to the child's clinical picture. The presence and severity of these comorbidities can have a greater impact on a child's daily function, quality of life, and participation than the motor impairment itself [16].

Key associated conditions that must be screened for include:

- *Pain*: Affects up to 75% of individuals with CP. Pain can arise from multiple sources, including spasticity, dystonia, orthopedic issues like hip subluxation, gastrointestinal problems, and procedures.
- *Intellectual disability*: Occurs in approximately 50% of children with CP. The range is broad, from mild learning disabilities to profound intellectual impairment.
- *Epilepsy*: Seizures are present in 25%–50% of the CP population. The risk is highest in those with spastic quadriplegia and hemiplegia. Early identification and management are critical to prevent seizure-related complications and cognitive effects.
- *Communication disorders*: As many as 75% of individuals with CP may have a communication disorder, including dysarthria (due to impaired motor control of speech muscles), apraxia, or language processing difficulties. About 25% may be nonverbal.
- *Visual impairment*: Affects approximately 40% of children. This includes refractive errors, strabismus (in up to 50%), visual field defects (especially in hemiplegia), and cortical visual impairment (CVI).
- *Hearing impairment*: While less common than visual problems, hearing deficits occur in up to 20% of children with CP and can significantly impact language development.
- *Dysphagia*: Impaired oral-motor function is common and can lead to poor nutrition, failure to thrive, prolonged feeding times, and a significant risk of aspiration pneumonia.
- *Gastrointestinal issues*: Gastroesophageal reflux, constipation, and delayed gastric emptying are frequent and can be significant sources of pain and discomfort.
- *Behavioral and emotional problems*: Approximately one in four children with CP will experience behavioral or emotional challenges, such as ADHD, anxiety, or depression. These can be a primary manifestation of the brain injury or a secondary reaction to the challenges of living with a disability.
- *Sleep disorders*: Affecting up to 40% of children, sleep problems can be caused by pain, spasticity, seizures, respiratory issues, or behavioral factors and can have a significant impact on the child and family [2].
- *Secondary musculoskeletal problems*: These are near-universal consequences of abnormal tone and movement on a growing skeleton. Proactive surveillance for hip displacement (affecting up to 33%), scoliosis, and joint contractures is a mandatory part of management from the time of diagnosis [16].

The American academy of neurology and other professional bodies recommend that screening for these conditions should be an integral part of the initial assessment of any child with suspected CP [19].

3.8 Synthesizing Information: The Diagnostic Statement and Communication

A simple label of "cerebral palsy" is insufficient. The diagnostic statement should be a rich, multi-axial summary that provides a clear and functional picture of the child's condition [11, 16]. A complete diagnostic statement should include:

1. *The core diagnosis*: "Cerebral palsy."
2. *Motor type*: The predominant motor abnormality (e.g., Spastic, Dyskinetic-dystonic, Ataxic).
3. *Topographical distribution*: The body parts affected (e.g., Hemiplegia, Diplegia, Quadriplegia), specifying unilateral or bilateral involvement.
4. *Functional classification*: The child's current functional level on standardized scales, most importantly the GMFCS, but also the MACS, CFCS, and EDACS where applicable. For example: "GMFCS Level IV."
5. *Etiology*: The known or presumed cause, if identified (e.g., "secondary to perinatal arterial ischemic stroke," or "associated with a pathogenic variant in the *AP4E1*gene").
6. *Associated conditions*: A comprehensive list of all diagnosed comorbidities (e.g., "with epilepsy, cortical visual impairment, and dysphagia").

An example of a comprehensive diagnostic formulation would be: "Cerebral Palsy, Spastic Hemiplegia (Right), GMFCS Level II, MACS Level II, secondary to a left middle cerebral artery territory infarction, with associated focal epilepsy and a right homonymous hemianopia."

Looking back at the patient described at the beginning of this chapter, over the subsequent 2 years, despite adherence to therapy, the patient's gait continued to deteriorate. She developed increasing postural instability and new, intermittent, jerky tremors in her hands, particularly with action. Upon careful re-evaluation of her history, her parents described a marked diurnal fluctuation of her symptoms; she was able to walk with relative ease upon waking in the morning, but her stiffness, scissoring, and instability would become progressively more severe throughout the day, often requiring her to be carried by evening. This pathognomonic feature, inconsistent with the static encephalopathy of cerebral palsy, prompted consideration of a Dopa-responsive dystonia (DRD) [49]. A therapeutic trial of low-dose carbidopa-levodopa (initiated at 4 mg/kg/day of the levodopa component) was started. Within 1 week, the response was dramatic and sustained: her gait normalized to a heel-toe pattern, the hypertonia resolved, and the tremors disappeared. Molecular genetic testing identified a heterozygous pathogenic mutation in the *GCH1* gene, confirming the diagnosis of autosomal-dominant Dopa-responsive dystonia, also known as Segawa syndrome. It is crucial to recognize clinical red flags, such as symptom progression and diurnal fluctuation, that differentiate neurometabolic mimics from cerebral palsy, as the diagnostic distinction leads to a profoundly effective and life-altering treatment [49].

3.9 Conclusion: Current Paradigms and Future Horizons in Diagnosing Cerebral Palsy

The diagnosis of cerebral palsy has evolved from a delayed, observational conclusion to a proactive, evidence-based process centered on early and accurate identification. This paradigm shift is driven by a deeper understanding of neurodevelopment, the critical importance of early intervention, and a commitment to family-centered care [58]. Ongoing research and technological advancements continue to refine our ability to diagnose earlier, understand underlying pathology more deeply, and predict outcomes more accurately. Future horizons in diagnosis include:

- *Advanced neuroimaging*: Techniques such as diffusion tensor imaging (DTI), magnetic resonance spectroscopy (MRS), and functional MRI (fMRI) are moving from research into clinical practice. These tools provide quantitative data on white matter tract integrity, brain biochemistry, and functional connectivity, offering a more granular understanding of the brain injury and its consequences than conventional MRI alone [18].
- *Genomic medicine*: The role of genetics in CP is now firmly established, with pathogenic variants identified in up to a third of cases [32]. The increasing accessibility of whole-exome and whole-genome sequencing will likely become a standard component of the diagnostic workup, especially in cases without clear perinatal risk factors [56]. This will not only elucidate etiology but will also identify actionable genetic findings that can guide targeted therapies and management [44].
- *Artificial intelligence/Machine-learning algorithms*: The complexity of CP lends itself to analysis by advanced computational methods [59]. Machine-learning algorithms are being developed to integrate multimodal data—including clinical assessments, neuroimaging, and gait analysis—to improve diagnostic accuracy, predict functional outcomes, and personalize intervention strategies [60, 61].

3.10 A Guide for Parents and Caregivers

What does this diagnosis mean? At its core, cerebral palsy is a condition that affects a child's ability to move and maintain posture. CP is caused by an injury or problem with the brain that happened before, during, or shortly after birth. This injury affects the parts of the brain that control muscles and movement. CP is the most common motor disorder in children. The brain lesion itself is static. However, this does not mean that your child's symptoms or challenges will stay the same.

As your child grows, the effects of that initial brain injury on their developing body can change. For example, muscles can become tighter (spasticity), joints can become stiff (contractures), or the alignment of bones can be affected (like hip displacement or a curve in the spine). Understanding this distinction is vital: the underlying condition is not worsening, but the physical manifestations require ongoing management and therapy to optimize function and prevent complications [2, 3, 10, 11, 16].

Why is an early diagnosis so important? The first few months of life is a critical window of opportunity when the brain is most adaptable. An early diagnosis allows for the immediate start of specialized therapies designed to utilize this neuroplasticity. Therapies like Goals-Activity-Motor Enrichment (GAME) and Constraint-Induced Movement Therapy (CIMT) actively encourage the brain to form new connections and pathways to improve motor skills and function. Starting these interventions early can have a significant positive impact on a child's long-term development. An early diagnosis is also essential for preventing future health problems. It allows child's medical team to begin surveillance programs for common secondary issues associated with CP [7, 14, 60].

Could it be something else? Because the definition of CP is based on problems with movement and posture, there are other medical conditions that can look very similar in the early stages. These are often called "CP mimics." Signs like developmental regression can mean that the diagnosis might be different than CP [28, 49].

What other health conditions are associated with CP that you should pay attention to? Cerebral palsy is a disorder of movement, but the early brain disturbance that causes it can also lead to a range of other health challenges, often called "associated conditions" or "comorbidities." These comorbidities can include pain, intellectual disabilities, epilepsy, visual and hearing impairment, sleep disorders, etc. A comprehensive approach to care means being aware of, screening for, and managing these conditions from the very beginning [2, 58].

3.11 Summary

- The diagnostic process has transitioned from a passive, "wait-and-see" model with confirmation at 12–24 months of age, to an active, evidence-based approach emphasizing identification before 6 months corrected age.
- There are three Core Diagnostic Pillars: Clinical history and developmental trajectory– encompassing prenatal (maternal health, infections, multiple gestation), perinatal (prematurity, HIE, perinatal stroke), and postnatal (meningitis, trauma, kernicterus) events, Standardized neurological and motor assessments, notably the General Movements Assessment (GMA) and the Hammersmith Infant Neurological Examination (HINE), and neuroimaging.
- While the MRICS classification system is currently a standardized framework, emerging modalities (DTI, MRS, fMRI) hold promise for more precise lesion characterization and prognostication.

- Up to one-third of CP cases are attributable to pathogenic genetic variants, which are increasingly viewed as integral to the diagnostic formulation.
- Genomic testing—particularly trio-based whole-exome and whole-genome sequencing—has supplanted targeted single-gene approaches, with yields highest in cryptogenic cases, normal MRI phenotypes, and individuals with disproportionate comorbidities or syndromic features.
- Three complementary dimensions are described in context of classification: Physiological classification (spastic, dyskinetic, ataxic, and mixed forms.), Topographical classification (monoplegia, hemiplegia, diplegia, and quadriplegia/tetraplegia), and Functional classification systems (GMFCS, MACS, CFCS, and EDACS).
- Conditions frequently misclassified as CP include hereditary spastic paraplegias, inborn errors of metabolism (e.g., glutaric aciduria type I, arginase deficiency), leukodystrophies, mitochondrial disorders, and dopamine-responsive dystonia.
- Red flags for CP mimics include developmental regression, diurnal fluctuation, or clinical deterioration not attributable to secondary orthopedic complications.
- Motor impairment in CP rarely occurs in isolation, and systematic screening is warranted for epilepsy, intellectual disability, communication disorders, cortical visual impairment, hearing loss, dysphagia, gastroesophageal reflux, sleep disturbance, behavioral disorders, and secondary musculoskeletal deformities.
- Clinicians are encouraged to provide a comprehensive, multi-axial diagnostic statement incorporating Core diagnosis, Motor type and topographical distribution, Functional classification, Etiology and Associated comorbidities. Such formulations ensure clarity for multidisciplinary teams, facilitate prognostication, and enhance family-centered counseling.
- Incorporation of advanced neuroimaging, genomic medicine, and artificial intelligence into diagnostic workflows promises to further refine early detection, improve precision in etiology, and enable tailored interventions.

References

1. Dan B, et al. Proposed updated description of cerebral palsy. Dev Med Child Neurol. 2025;67(6):700–9.
2. Patel DR, et al. Cerebral palsy in children: a clinical overview. Transl Pediatr. 2020;9(Suppl 1):S125.
3. McIntyre S, et al. Global prevalence of cerebral palsy: a systematic analysis. Dev Med Child Neurol. 2022;64(12):1494–506.
4. Khandaker G, et al. Bangladesh cerebral palsy register (BCPR): a pilot study to develop a national cerebral palsy (CP) register with surveillance of children for CP. BMC Neurol. 2015;15(1):173.
5. Nelson KB. Causative factors in cerebral palsy. Clin Obstet Gynecol. 2008;51(4):749–62.
6. MacLennan AH, et al. Genetic or other causation should not change the clinical diagnosis of cerebral palsy. J Child Neurol. 2019;34(8):472–6.
7. Maitre NL, et al. Network implementation of guideline for early detection decreases age at cerebral palsy diagnosis. Pediatrics. 2020;145(5):e20192126.

8. Cooper MS, Fahey MC, Mackay MT. Making waves: the changing tide of cerebral palsy. J Paediatr Child Health. 2022;58(11):1929–34.
9. Lee RW, et al. A diagnostic approach for cerebral palsy in the genomic era. NeuroMolecular Med. 2014;16(4):821–44.
10. Blair E, Watson L. Epidemiology of cerebral palsy. In: Seminars in fetal and neonatal medicine, vol. 11. Elsevier; 2006.
11. Paulson A, Vargus-Adams J. Overview of four functional classification systems commonly used in cerebral palsy. Children. 2017;4(4):30.
12. Gonzalez-Mantilla PJ, et al. Diagnostic yield of exome sequencing in cerebral palsy and implications for genetic testing guidelines: a systematic review and meta-analysis. JAMA Pediatr. 2023;177(5):472–8.
13. Srivastava S, et al. Molecular diagnostic yield of exome sequencing and chromosomal microarray in cerebral palsy: a systematic review and meta-analysis. JAMA Neurol. 2022;79(12):1287–95.
14. Morgan C, et al. Early intervention for children aged 0 to 2 years with or at high risk of cerebral palsy: international clinical practice guideline based on systematic reviews. JAMA Pediatr. 2021;175(8):846–58.
15. Pham R, et al. Definition and diagnosis of cerebral palsy in genetic studies: a systematic review. Dev Med Child Neurol. 2020;62(9):1024–30.
16. Cantero MJP, et al. Comprehensive approach to children with cerebral palsy. An Pediatr Engl Ed. 2021;95(4):276.e1–276.e11.
17. Bosanquet M, et al. A systematic review of tests to predict cerebral palsy in young children. Dev Med Child Neurol. 2013;55(5):418–26.
18. Gosling AS. Recent advances in the neuroimaging and neuropsychology of cerebral palsy. Appl Neuropsychol Child. 2017;6(1):55–63.
19. Ashwal S, et al. Practice parameter: diagnostic assessment of the child with cerebral palsy: report of the Quality Standards Subcommittee of the American Academy of Neurology and the Practice Committee of the Child Neurology Society. Neurology. 2004;62(6):851–63.
20. Springer A, et al. Profile of children with cerebral palsy spectrum disorder and a normal MRI study. Neurology. 2019;93(1):e88–96.
21. Einspieler C, Prechtl HF. Prechtl's assessment of general movements: a diagnostic tool for the functional assessment of the young nervous system. Ment Retard Dev Disabil Res Rev. 2005;11(1):61–7.
22. Chirigos AJ, et al. Prechtl's general movements assessment at writhing age guides MRI use in clinical implementation network. Pediatr Res. 2024;95(5):1188–90.
23. Romeo DM, et al. Use of the Hammersmith infant neurological examination in infants with cerebral palsy: a critical review of the literature. Dev Med Child Neurol. 2016;58(3):240–5.
24. Burton VJ, et al. Longitudinal Hammersmith infant neurological examination (HINE) trajectories in children with cerebral palsy identified in high-risk follow-up. J Clin Med. 2025;14(5):1572.
25. Caesar R, et al. Clinical tools used in young infants born very preterm to predict motor and cognitive delay (not cerebral palsy): a systematic review. Dev Med Child Neurol. 2021;63(4):387–95.
26. Mendoza-Sengco P, Chicoine CL, Vargus-Adams J. Early cerebral palsy detection and intervention. Pediatr Clin. 2023;70(3):385–98.
27. Philippi H, et al. Computer-based analysis of general movements reveals stereotypies predicting cerebral palsy. Dev Med Child Neurol. 2014;56(10):960–7.
28. Friedman JM, van Essen P, van Karnebeek CD. Cerebral palsy and related neuromotor disorders: overview of genetic and genomic studies. Mol Genet Metab. 2022;137(4):399–419.
29. MacLennan AH, Thompson SC, Gecz J. Cerebral palsy: causes, pathways, and the role of genetic variants. Am J Obstet Gynecol. 2015;213(6):779–88.
30. Ellenberg JH, Nelson KB. The association of cerebral palsy with birth asphyxia: a definitional quagmire. Dev Med Child Neurol. 2013;55(3):210–6.

31. Schaefer GB. Genetics considerations in cerebral palsy. In: Seminars in pediatric neurology, vol. 15. Elsevier; 2008.
32. McMichael G, et al. Whole-exome sequencing points to considerable genetic heterogeneity of cerebral palsy. Mol Psychiatry. 2015;20(2):176–82.
33. Lewis SA, et al. Insights from genetic studies of cerebral palsy. Front Neurol. 2021;11:625428.
34. Smithers-Sheedy H, et al. A special supplement: findings from the Australian Cerebral Palsy Register, birth years 1993 to 2006. Dev Med Child Neurol. 2016;58:5–10.
35. Galea C, et al. Cerebral palsy trends in Australia (1995–2009): a population-based observational study. Dev Med Child Neurol. 2019;61(2):186–93.
36. Aravamuthan BR, et al. Variability in cerebral palsy diagnosis. Pediatrics. 2021;147(2):e2020010066.
37. Elliott AM, Guimond C. Genetic counseling considerations in cerebral palsy. Mol Genet Metab. 2022;137(4):428–35.
38. Piper MC, et al. Construction and validation of the Alberta Infant Motor Scale (AIMS). Can J Public Health. 1992;83:S46–50.
39. Albuquerque PLD, et al. Accuracy of the Alberta Infant Motor Scale (AIMS) to detect developmental delay of gross motor skills in preterm infants: a systematic review. Dev Neurorehabil. 2015;18(1):15–21.
40. Ko J, Lim HK. Reliability study of the items of the Alberta Infant Motor Scale (AIMS) using kappa analysis. Int J Environ Res Public Health. 2022;19(3):1767.
41. Himmelmann K, et al. MRI classification system (MRICS) for children with cerebral palsy: development, reliability, and recommendations. Dev Med Child Neurol. 2017;59(1):57–64.
42. Delin S, et al. Prognostic value of cranial ultrasonography in comparison with magnetic resonance imaging in children with cerebral palsy: a population-based study. Acta Clin Croat. 2020;59(2):260.
43. van Eyk CL, et al. Yield of clinically reportable genetic variants in unselected cerebral palsy by whole genome sequencing. NPJ Genom Med. 2021;6(1):74.
44. Matthews AM, et al. Atypical cerebral palsy: genomics analysis enables precision medicine. Genet Med. 2019;21(7):1621–8.
45. Wilson YA, et al. Clinically relevant genes identified in cerebral palsy cohorts following evaluation of the clinical description and phenotype: a systematic review. J Child Neurol. 2024;39(13–14):500–9.
46. Oskoui M, et al. Clinically relevant copy number variations detected in cerebral palsy. Nat Commun. 2015;6(1):7949.
47. Van Eyk C, et al. Targeted resequencing identifies genes with recurrent variation in cerebral palsy. npj Genom Med. 2019;4(1):27.
48. Fahey MC, et al. The genetic basis of cerebral palsy. Dev Med Child Neurol. 2017;59(5):462–9.
49. Lewis SA, Shetty S, Wilson BA, Huang AJ, Jin SC, Smithers-Sheedy H, Fahey MC, Kruer MC. Insights from genetic studies of cerebral palsy. Front Neurol. 2021;11:625428.
50. Bi D, et al. Association of COL4A1 gene polymorphisms with cerebral palsy in a Chinese Han population. Clin Genet. 2016;90(2):149–55.
51. Vanzo RJ, et al. Clinical significance of copy number variants involving KANK1 in patients with neurodevelopmental disorders. Eur J Med Genet. 2019;62(1):15–20.
52. Moreno-De-Luca A, et al. Adaptor protein complex-4 (AP-4) deficiency causes a novel autosomal recessive cerebral palsy syndrome with microcephaly and intellectual disability. J Med Genet. 2011;48(2):141–4.
53. Winkler I, et al. A new family with spastic paraplegia type 51 and novel mutations in AP4E1. BMC Med Genet. 2021;14(1):131.
54. Jameel M, et al. A novel AP4M1 mutation in autosomal recessive cerebral palsy syndrome and clinical expansion of AP-4 deficiency. BMC Med Genet. 2014;15(1):133.
55. Wang H, et al. Genetic association study of adaptor protein complex 4 with cerebral palsy in a Han Chinese population. Mol Biol Rep. 2013;40(11):6459–67.

56. May HJ, et al. Genetic testing in individuals with cerebral palsy. Dev Med Child Neurol. 2021;63(12):1448–55.
57. Chan, E., C. Frisina, and D. Gaebler-Spira, A resource guide to understanding cerebral palsy: commentary on collaboration to support health literacy and shared decision making. 2021, Sage: London. p. 173–182.
58. Schuengel C, et al. Parents' reactions to the diagnosis of cerebral palsy: associations between resolution, age and severity of disability. Child Care Health Dev. 2009;35(5):673–80.
59. Bahado-Singh RO, et al. Deep learning/artificial intelligence and blood-based DNA epigenomic prediction of cerebral palsy. Int J Mol Sci. 2019;20(9):2075.
60. Bertoncelli CM, et al. Using artificial intelligence to identify factors associated with autism spectrum disorder in adolescents with cerebral palsy. Neuropediatrics. 2019;50(03):178–87.
61. Duran I, et al. Artificial intelligence to improve efficiency of administration of gross motor function assessment in children with cerebral palsy. Dev Med Child Neurol. 2022;64(2):228–34.

Personalized Treatments

4

Aidin Shahilooy and Elahe Motevaseli

The patient is an 8-year-old boy with a diagnosis of spastic diplegic cerebral palsy, classified at a Gross Motor Function Classification System (GMFCS) level III. His medical history is significant for premature birth at 28 weeks gestation, with neonatal MRI revealing periventricular leukomalacia. Clinically, he presents with marked spasticity and hyperreflexia, predominantly in the lower extremities, leading to a scissoring gait pattern and equinus foot deformity bilaterally. He is ambulatory for short distances within the home and classroom using posterior walker-style crutches but requires a manual wheelchair for community distances due to significant fatigue and postural instability. His cognitive function is normal, and he is highly motivated to improve his mobility. The family's primary goals are to decrease the effort of walking, improve his endurance and balance, and enhance his ability to participate in peer-group recreational activities with greater independence.

4.1 Introduction: The Evolving Paradigm of Cerebral Palsy Management

The management of cerebral palsy (CP) is undergoing an important transformation. For decades, the clinical approach has been mostly reactive, focusing on the management of symptoms and secondary impairments such as spasticity, contractures, and movement disorders as they come up. This approach, while beneficial, often addressed the consequences of the underlying neuropathology rather than its cause

A. Shahilooy
Department of Genetics, MOM-Gene Personalized Medicine Center, Tehran, Iran

E. Motevaseli (✉)
Department of Molecular Medicine, School of Advanced Technologies in Medicine, Tehran University of Medical Sciences, Tehran, Iran
e-mail: e_motevaseli@tums.ac.ir

A. Presedo et al. (eds.), *Enhancing Quality of Life in Patients with Cerebral Palsy*, https://doi.org/10.1007/978-3-032-20967-2_4

or individual variability. Traditional interventions, such as orthopedic surgery and therapies aimed at normalizing movement patterns, are applied based on broad clinical phenotypes. The landscape of neurodevelopmental medicine is shifting from this generalized model to a proactive, etiology-driven, and personalized framework. The modern approach to CP care aims to improve development and function by capitalizing on the principles of neuroplasticity.

The genomic revolution has uncovered a genetic basis for a substantial portion of CP cases, opening the door for molecular diagnosis and targeted interventions [1, 2]. Advances in neuroimaging provide unprecedented windows into brain structure and function, allowing for more precise prognostication and selection of therapies [3, 4]. The rise of data science— including artificial intelligence and machine learning—is enabling the synthesis of complex, multi-modal patient data to predict outcomes and guide clinical decisions [5–7]. This is complemented by an explosion in technology-enhanced rehabilitation, including robotics, virtual reality, and wearable sensors [8–10].

This chapter will explore these advancements in detail and the scientific basis and clinical application of personalized treatments for children with CP.

4.2 Redefining the Etiologies: The Genomic Revolution in CP

For over a century, the medical consensus considered CP to result almost exclusively to environmental factors around the time of birth, with hypoxic-ischemic encephalopathy (HIE) or birth asphyxia considered the primary cause.

While perinatal events such as prematurity, infection, and oxygen deprivation are main risk factors, recent large-scale studies have demonstrated that birth-related asphyxia accounts for fewer cases of CP than considered before. This has prompted a re-evaluation of the disorder's etiology, revealing that for as many as one-third of individuals, the condition may be rooted in their genetic makeup [1, 11].

This paradigm shift is supported by evidence from cohort-based whole-exome sequencing (WES) and whole-genome sequencing (WGS) studies, which have identified pathogenic single nucleotide variants (SNVs) and copy number variants (CNVs) in a significant proportion of individuals with CP [11, 12], which supports a move toward integrating genomic testing into the diagnostic work-up for all children with CP, not only those with an absence of risk factors (cryptogenic CP). Meta-analyses have shown that WES provides a molecular diagnosis in approximately 23%–35% of cases, a rate four times greater than that of chromosomal microarray (CMA), which has a yield of around 5% [13, 14]. Targeted gene panels, while useful in some cases, are often insufficient for a disorder with such vast genetic heterogeneity, as they risk missing pathogenic variants in newly discovered or less common genes.

A critical component of this diagnostic strategy is the use of trio sequencing. This approach is essential for identifying de novo mutations. Studies have shown a significant enrichment of de novo mutations in individuals with CP [11, 12].

4.2.1 Gene–Environment Interactions

Finding a genetic basis for CP does not negate the importance of environmental risk factors; rather, it frames the relationship between them. Emerging evidence suggests a complex interplay where an underlying genetic variant may not directly cause CP but instead confers a heightened vulnerability to a perinatal insult [1, 2]. For example, a genetic variant that impairs neuronal development or the brain's ability to respond to and recover from a hypoxic or inflammatory event. This model of a double hit, combining genetic predisposition with an environmental trigger, explains why genetic testing can be valuable even in children with a clear history of prematurity, infection, or HIE [11].

4.2.2 Genotype-Phenotype Correlations and Clinical Implications

Identifying a specific genetic etiology has profound implications that extend far beyond a simple label. For families, a molecular diagnosis can provide closure, end the diagnostic odyssey and sometimes alleviate parental guilt associated with presumed birth-related causes [15]. It allows for accurate genetic counseling regarding recurrence risk in future pregnancies, which can be very different for a de novo mutation versus a recessively inherited one. For instance, if a patient is found to have the condition due to a homozygous recessive mutation, the parents are definite carriers, and the recurrence risk for any future offspring is 25% (this scenario usually occurs in consanguineous marriages). This contrasts sharply with an autosomal dominant inherited mutation from an affected parent or an autosomal dominant inherited mutation with partial penetration from an unaffected parent, where the risk of transmitting the mutation to each child is 50% and risk of developing symptoms depend on the penetration rate in each generation. This necessitates careful clinical evaluation and potential genetic testing of the transmitting parents, who may be unaffected or have a milder or variable presentation of the same disorder.

The most distinct scenario involves a de novo (almost always dominant) mutation, where the genetic variant has arisen for the first time in the affected child and is absent in the parents' somatic DNA. While this finding often brings relief, as the recurrence risk is not 50%, it is not zero. The risk is typically low, in the range of 1%–2%, that accounts for the possibility of parental germline mosaicism. Accurately distinguishing between these inheritance patterns is crucial for providing precise recurrence risk assessment and discussing reproductive options, such as prenatal diagnosis or preimplantation genetic testing (Table 4.1).

Many genes implicated in CP, such as those involved in neurite extension, cytoskeletal dynamics, and Rho GTPase function, are crucial to brain development and are also linked to other conditions. This recognition reframes CP as part of a broader spectrum of neurodevelopmental disorders, often with multi-system involvement [1].

Table 4.1 Comparison of recurrence risk and genetic counseling approach for monogenic cerebral palsy

	Autosomal recessive	Inherited autosomal dominant	Apparent De Novo autosomal dominant
Parental status	Unaffected heterozygous carriers	One affected heterozygous parent (phenotype may be variable)	Unaffected parents (somatic testing may be required)
Sibling recurrence risk	25%	50%	~1%–2%
Key complicating factor	Consanguinity; Pseudodominance; rare de novo + inherited allele combination	Variable expressivity; incomplete penetrance	Parental germline mosaicism (raises risk up to 50%)
Primary counseling focus	Carrier status of parents and extended family; 1-in-4 risk per pregnancy	Clinical evaluation of the affected parent's full phenotypic spectrum; 1-in-2 risk	Discussion of mosaicism possibility; advanced parental testing to refine risk from 1%–2% to either negligible or high
PGT-M indication	Necessary; clear indication	Necessary; clear indication	Considered if germline mosaicism is suspected/ confirmed

PGT-M Preimplantation Genetic Testing for Monogenic disorders

For example, identifying a pathogenic variant in the *COL4A1* gene, which is associated with porencephaly and perinatal stroke, alerts the clinical team to a systemic risk of hemorrhage and may prompt surveillance of other organ systems [16]. Similarly, a diagnosis of *CTNNB1*-related syndrome, which can initially present as spastic diplegic CP, carries a high likelihood of severe intellectual disability and specific movement disorders, allowing for anticipatory guidance and early implementation of targeted developmental therapies [17]. This genotype-driven approach is essential for moving toward precision medicine, where treatment is tailored to the underlying molecular pathology (Table 4.2).

Historically composed of pediatric neurologists, physiatrists, orthopedic surgeons, and physical and occupational therapists, this management model is no longer sufficient to manage the complexity of the modern CP diagnosis. The integration of clinical geneticists and genetic counselors is now essential.

Furthermore, the discovery of shared molecular pathways between CP and other neurodevelopmental disorders breaks down traditional diagnostic silos and creates novel therapeutic opportunities. If a gene like *SCN2A* is known to cause both a form of epilepsy and a CP phenotype, it suggests a common underlying channelopathy [18]. Consequently, a therapeutic agent developed to target that specific ion channel for epilepsy could be repurposed for a subset of CP patients with the same genetic variant. This opens the door to a new paradigm for clinical trials in CP, where cohorts may be defined not by their motor phenotype (e.g., spastic diplegia) but by their molecular etiology (e.g., a trial for individuals with *KIF1A*-related neurodevelopmental disorders), reshaping the landscape of therapeutic development [19].

Table 4.2 Key genes implicated in cerebral palsy and associated phenotypes

Gene symbol	Function	Inheritance pattern	Primary CP motor type	Key associated features	Clinical pearl/ management implication
CTNNB1	β-Catenin signaling, cell adhesion	De novo (AD)	Spastic diplegia/ quadriplegia	Causes spastic diplegia, developmental delay, severe ID, microcephaly, limited speech, visual impairment, dystonia.; often misdiagnosed as CP	Often presents as "cryptogenic" CP. Early diagnosis allows for targeted communication strategies and management of visual deficits.
KIF1A	Axonal transport of synaptic vesicles	De novo (AD), AR	Spastic paraplegia, ataxic CP	Optic nerve atrophy, epilepsy, cognitive impairment, peripheral neuropathy, motor dysfunction, spasticity, ataxia resembling CP	Phenotype can be progressive. Monitor for visual changes and neuropathy. Gene-specific therapies are in development.
GNAO1 [20]	G protein signaling in neurons	De novo (AD)	Dyskinetic CP (chorea, dystonia)	Early-onset epilepsy, severe ID, movement disorder can be paroxysmal, hyperkinetic movement disorder, dystonia, developmental delay mimicking CP	Consider for severe, early-onset dyskinesia. May respond to deep brain stimulation (DBS)
TUBA1A	Microtubule formation, neuronal migration	De novo (AD)	Spastic quadriplegia, mixed	Lissencephaly, microcephaly, epilepsy, brainstem dysfunction, cortical malformations, motor impairment	Associated with severe cortical malformations visible on MRI. Diagnosis confirms a primary brain malformation etiology.

(continued)

Table 4.2 (continued)

Gene symbol	Function	Inheritance pattern	Primary CP motor type	Key associated features	Clinical pearl/ management implication
COL4A1	Vascular basement membrane integrity	AD	Hemiplegic CP	Porencephaly, intracranial hemorrhage, infantile hemiplegia, spasticity; mimics CP	Associated with fragile blood vessels. Consider systemic surveillance (e.g., renal cysts) and caution with anticoagulants.
RHOB	Cytoskeletal regulation, cell migration	De novo (AD)	Mixed spastic-dystonic CP	ID, microcephaly; causes CP via lipid dysregulation	Recently confirmed CP gene involved in cytoskeletal dynamics.
FBXO31	Neuronal polarity, protein degradation	De novo (AD)	Mixed spastic-dystonic CP	ID, developmental delay, spastic-dystonic CP phenotype	Recently confirmed CP gene involved in cell cycle regulation.

AD Autosomal Dominant, AR Autosomal Recessive, ID Intellectual Disability
Refs. [16, 21]

4.3 Precision Diagnostics and Prognostication for Personalized Intervention

4.3.1 Beyond the Clinical Exam: Advanced Neuroimaging as a Biomarker

Neuroimaging has transitioned from merely detecting brain lesions to comprehensively evaluating their effects on neural networks and forecasting functional outcomes. While conventional Magnetic Resonance Imaging (MRI) is the main modality for identifying structural abnormalities like periventricular leukomalacia (PVL) or cortical malformations, advanced techniques provide deeper functional and structural insights.

In CP, Diffusion Tensor Imaging (DTI) is used to assess the integrity of motor pathways, particularly the corticospinal tracts (CSTs). The degree of asymmetry or damage to the CSTs as measured by DTI metrics like fractional anisotropy (FA) has been shown to correlate strongly with the severity of motor impairment, especially in hemiplegic CP [4]. This information can be used to predict long-term motor outcomes and has been explored as a biomarker to predict response to specific rehabilitation programs.

Task-based fMRI can map the pattern of motor cortex reorganization that occurs in response to an early brain lesion. For example, in a child with unilateral CP, fMRI can determine whether motor control of the affected hand is primarily driven by the damaged contralesional hemisphere or has reorganized to the ipsilateral (unaffected) hemisphere. This pattern of activation is a powerful predictor of response to therapies like Constraint-Induced Movement Therapy (CIMT), with evidence suggesting that individuals with preserved contralesional activation may have a better prognosis for functional gains [3].

4.3.2 Quantitative and Data-Driven Phenotyping

The personalization of treatment requires objective, reliable, and valid measures of function that can precisely quantify a child's movement patterns and track changes. This marks a shift from subjective clinical scales—such as the Modified Ashworth Scale, which suffers from low inter-rater reliability—toward objective, quantifiable metrics [22].

Three-Dimensional Gait Analysis (3DGA) is now one of the most important tools for the assessment of walking abnormalities in ambulatory children with CP [23, 24]. Using high-resolution cameras, force plates, and electromyography, 3DGA provides detailed, quantitative data on joint kinematics (angles), kinetics (forces and moments), and muscle activity throughout the gait cycle. This granular data allow for the classification of pathological gait patterns (e.g., true equinus, crouch gait) and the identification of the specific biomechanical and neuromuscular impairments responsible. This information is crucial for personalizing complex orthopedic procedures and for the precise design and tuning of ankle-foot orthoses (AFOs).

Wearable Sensors, such as inertial measurement units (IMUs) and accelerometers, can be worn on the limbs or trunk to continuously record movement data during daily activities [9, 25]. This provides an ecologically valid picture of a child's real-world mobility, activity levels, and gait quality, which can be more informative than a brief snapshot during a clinic visit. This data can be used to monitor the effects of an intervention, track disease progression, and provide real-time feedback to personalize home therapy programs.

4.3.3 AI and Machine Learning in CP Care

Data sets generated by genomics and advanced imaging are suited for analysis by artificial intelligence/machine-learning (ML) algorithms. These tools aim to integrate multimodal data sets to generate predictive models that inform personalized care, including:

Early Diagnosis: A critical window for intervention exists in early infancy when brain plasticity is at its peak. ML models are being trained to analyze video footage of an infant's spontaneous movements (e.g., the General Movements Assessment) [7]. These algorithms can detect subtle abnormalities indicative of a high risk for CP with relatively high accuracy, offering a scalable and accessible method for early screening and diagnosis.

Predicting Treatment Response: The ultimate purpose of personalized medicine is to predict, for an individual patient, which treatment will be most effective. Researchers are developing ML models that integrate clinical, imaging, and biomechanical data to forecast the likely outcome of interventions such as rehabilitation, botulinum toxin injections, or orthopedic surgery [5, 26, 27]. Such models can help clinicians move beyond a trial-and-error approach and select the optimal therapeutic pathway from the start.

Clinical Decision Support Systems (CDSS): The application of these technologies is the development of AI-driven CDSS. These systems will function as a tool for the multidisciplinary team, synthesizing a patient's entire data set—genomic profile, DTI tractography, 3DGA report, and clinical history—to generate evidence-based, personalized treatment recommendations and predicted outcomes [6].

4.4 Personalized Pharmacotherapy for Spasticity and Dystonia

4.4.1 Pharmacogenomics (PGx) of Baclofen

Oral baclofen, a GABA-B receptor agonist, is one of the most frequently prescribed medications for generalized spasticity. Its clinical use, however, its clinical utility is often limited by variable efficacy and a narrow therapeutic window with common side effects including sedation, hypotonia, and fatigue that can limit functional gains.

Baclofen undergoes minimal hepatic metabolism via the cytochrome P450 system and is primarily eliminated by the kidneys. PGx research has focused on genes encoding drug transporters. A key finding in children with CP comes from a multicenter study that identified a specific single-nucleotide polymorphism (SNP), rs11046232, in the *ABCC9* gene, which encodes an ATP-binding cassette transporter. Individuals heterozygous for this variant were found to have a twofold increase in the oral clearance of baclofen compared to those with the common genotype. This accelerated clearance results in subtherapeutic plasma levels, reducing clinical effectiveness at standard doses. Furthermore, clinical response, as measured by a reduction in spasticity, has been associated with variants in other genes. SNPs in *ABCC12*, *SLC28A1*, and *PPARD* have been linked to the degree of improvement in spasticity, seemingly independent of drug clearance (Table 4.3) [28].

4.4.2 Stratifying Botulinum Neurotoxin (BoNT-A) Therapy

Intramuscular injections of Botulinum Neurotoxin-A (BoNT-A) are a first-line treatment for focal spasticity in CP [29, 30]. They act by blocking acetylcholine

Table 4.3 Pharmacogenomic markers influencing oral baclofen response in CP

Gene	Genetic variant (SNP)	Pharmacokinetic/ pharmacodynamic effect	Clinical recommendation
ABCC9	rs11046232	~Twofold increase in oral clearance, leading to lower plasma concentrations.	Patient may be a "fast metabolizer." Consider starting with a higher dose range or have a lower threshold to transition to intrathecal baclofen (ITB) if clinical response is poor.
ABCC12	rs16945874	Associated with a greater reduction in spasticity (improved clinical response).	May predict a more favorable pharmacodynamic response. Can be used to manage family expectations and set more ambitious therapy goals.
SLC28A1	rs1542283, rs16974641	Associated with varied clinical response (spasticity reduction).	Further research needed, but suggests transporter genetics influence drug effect at the target site, not just systemic clearance.
PPARD	rs7770619, rs6906237	Associated with varied clinical response (spasticity reduction).	Highlights the complexity of the drug response pathway beyond simple pharmacokinetics.

Ref. [28]

release at the neuromuscular junction to produce a temporary, localized chemo denervation. Personalization of BoNT-A therapy is evolving beyond muscle selection and now incorporates physiological and pharmacological considerations.

One approach involves stratifying patients based on the underlying pathophysiology of their hypertonia which is assessed using instrumented stretch reflex analysis: velocity-dependent (VD) and length-dependent (LD). A prospective study demonstrated that BoNT-A injections were significantly more effective at reducing stretch reflex hyperactivity in muscles classified pre-treatment as having a VD pattern [31].

Another aspect of personalizing BoNT-A therapy involves mitigating the risk of treatment failure. While primary resistance is rare, secondary non-response is a known clinical issue. The immunogenicity of BoNT-A is thought to be increased by the presence of accessory complexing proteins found in some commercial formulations. Newer formulations that contain the pure 150-kDa neurotoxin without these complexing proteins have a lower protein load and are associated with a reduced risk of antibody formation. Therefore, a personalized strategy for a child requiring long-term, high-dose BoNT-A therapy might involve selecting a formulation with lower immunogenicity from the outset to help preserve long-term treatment efficacy [32].

4.4.3 A Personalized Algorithm for Dystonia Management

The American Academy for Cerebral Palsy and Developmental Medicine (AACPDM) has developed a Care Pathway that provides a framework for a personalized, tiered approach [33].

The algorithm begins with an assessment to confirm the diagnosis of dystonia, differentiate it from spasticity, and classify its distribution as focal, segmental, or generalized. The management plan is then personalized based on this classification and the functional goals of the individual and family.

For Focal or Segmental Dystonia, Targeted injections of BoNT-A are the suggested first-line intervention.

For Generalized Dystonia, the approach involves a systematic, trial-based evaluation of oral medications. Oral baclofen is suggested as a first-line option. If this is ineffective or poorly tolerated, second-line agents such as trihexyphenidyl or benzodiazepines can be considered. A critical step in this pathway is a diagnostic trial of Levodopa. This is essential to identify individuals with Dopa-responsive dystonia (DRD), a distinct genetic disorder that can mimic the phenotype of CP and is highly treatable with Levodopa supplementation.

In Severe, Refractory Generalized Dystonia**,** for individuals whose generalized dystonia is severe and does not respond adequately to oral medications, more invasive therapies are considered. The choice between Intrathecal Baclofen (ITB), which involves a surgically implanted pump delivering baclofen directly to the cerebrospinal fluid, and Deep Brain Stimulation (DBS), which involves surgical implantation of electrodes into the basal ganglia (typically the globus pallidus internus), is considered:

- Focal/Segmental → BoNT-A
- Generalized → Oral meds + levodopa trial
- Severe/Refractory → ITB or DBS [33]

4.5 Rehabilitative and Surgical Interventions

4.5.1 Personalized, High-Intensity Therapies

Constraint-Induced Movement Therapy (CIMT): This is an intervention designed mainly for children with hemiplegic CP. It involves placing a cast or restraint on the less-affected upper limb for several hours a day over a period of weeks, while engaging the child in intensive, structured therapy with the more-affected limb [34]. This forced use drives use-dependent cortical reorganization in the brain's motor areas, leading to significant and lasting improvements in function.

Hand-Arm Bimanual Intensive Therapy (HABIT): As an alternative to CIMT, HABIT focuses on improving the coordinated use of both hands through intensive, structured play and functional activities [35]. It is a personalized choice for children who tolerate the constraint of CIMT poorly or for whom bimanual functional goals (e.g., dressing, catching a ball) are a priority.

Goal-Activity-Motor Enrichment (GAME): This is a home-based program where therapists work with parents to identify specific, meaningful functional goals for their child (e.g., "I want to be able to feed myself with a spoon"). The therapist then trains the parents to be the primary agents of therapy, embedding enriched motor-learning opportunities into the family's daily routines [36–38]. This approach is highly personalized to the child's environment and motivations and has demonstrated improvements in both motor and cognitive domains.

4.5.2 Technology-Enhanced Rehabilitation

Robotics and Biofeedback: Robot-assisted therapy utilizes robotic devices to guide a child's limbs through repetitive movements, allowing for a much higher number of practice repetitions than is possible in conventional therapy. These systems can provide assistance when needed and resistance as the child's strength improves, and they objectively quantify performance. When combined with electromyographic biofeedback, the child can see a visual representation of their own muscle activation on a screen and learn to voluntarily increase activation in a target muscle or decrease co-contraction of an antagonist, providing real-time, patient-driven motor learning [10].

Virtual Reality (VR): VR technology allows for the creation of immersive, interactive, and highly motivating virtual environments for therapy [8, 39]. A key advantage of VR is its near-infinite customizability. A therapy session can be designed as an engaging game that is personalized to the child's interests, cognitive level, and specific motor goals [40]. For a child working on balance, the VR environment could simulate walking across a narrow bridge; for upper limb function, it could be a game of virtual fruit-slicing. Gamifying therapy enhances engagement and adherence. The difficulty of the tasks can be precisely graded to ensure an optimal challenge point for motor learning. The emergence of affordable, home-based VR systems also offers a new avenue for telerehabilitation and increasing the total dose of therapy a child receives.

Wearable Sensors: wearable sensors provide objective data on real-world movement. In a therapeutic context, these data are used to monitor home exercise programs. A therapist can remotely review a child's activity data. This allows the therapist to intervene in a timely manner, providing feedback and adjusting the home program via telehealth to get the child back on track [9].

4.5.3 Data-Driven Surgical Decision-Making

Pre-operative 3DGA is now regarded as a standard of care for planning complex orthopedic procedures, most notably Single Event Multi-Level Surgery (SEMLS) [23, 24, 41]. Quantitative data from 3DGA allow the surgical team to identify the primary drivers of the gait deviation, which may be different from what is apparent on clinical examination. This leads to a highly personalized surgical plan, where each procedure is chosen to address a specific, objectively identified biomechanical problem.

This data-driven approach not only helps in deciding what surgery to perform but also in personalizing the decision *not* to operate. For instance, data from a large cohort of patients who underwent SEMLS showed that individuals with lower pre-surgical functional levels (e.g., slower gait speed) and who required a greater number of individual procedures were at a significantly higher risk of losing their ability to run post-operatively [23].

4.6 The Future Horizon: Neuroprotective and Regenerative Medicine

One of the main goals of personalized medicine in the context of CP management is to target the underlying neurobiology of the brain injury itself. The future horizon of CP treatment involves a move toward neuroprotective, neuroregenerative, and neuromodulatory therapies that aim to prevent, repair, or bypass the damage in the developing brain [42].

The first step in this direction is neuroprotection. One established example of this is therapeutic hypothermia for newborns with moderate to severe hypoxic-ischemic encephalopathy (HIE), which reduces the brain's metabolic rate, suppresses excitotoxicity and inflammation, decreasing the risk of death or major disability, including CP.

Emerging pharmaceutical strategies aim to build on this principle by targeting specific molecular pathways involved in secondary brain injury. These include anti-inflammatory agents, antioxidants, and neurotrophic factors.

The most ambitious future therapies are those that aim to regenerate or repair damaged brain tissue:

Stem Cell Therapy: This approach involves the administration of various types of stem cells with the goal of replacing damaged cells, providing trophic support to surviving neurons, and modulating the neuro-inflammatory environment to promote endogenous repair. While the theoretical potential is enormous and early-phase clinical trials have shown some promise, stem cell therapy for CP remains experimental [43]. Further research is required to determine the optimal cell type, dose, timing, and delivery route, and also to ensure long-term safety and efficacy [44].

Gene Therapy: For the growing number of children with a known monogenic cause of CP, gene therapy represents a form of personalized medicine. The therapeutic goal is to use viral vectors to deliver a functional copy of the defective gene to the relevant cells in the central nervous system. This approach is still in the preclinical phase for CP but holds transformative potential for future interventions [45].

Finally, neuromodulation techniques offer a way to enhance the brain's own capacity for adaptive plasticity. Non-invasive methods like transcranial Direct Current Stimulation (tDCS) and repetitive Transcranial Magnetic Stimulation (rTMS) deliver electrical or magnetic stimulation to the scalp to modulate the excitability of the underlying motor cortex. When paired with intensive rehabilitation, these techniques augment the effects of therapy [46–48]. The application of neuromodulation can be highly personalized, using fMRI to map an individual's specific pattern of motor cortex activation to guide the precise placement of the stimulation coil or electrodes.

4.7 Conclusion

Revisiting the case of the 8-year-old boy with GMFCS level III spastic diplegia, a personalized, multi-modal treatment plan is essential to address his specific impairments and achieve his functional goals. Identifying a specific genetic variant through genomic sequencing can have profound clinical implications, potentially altering the entire treatment paradigm [1, 15].

For our patient, with his focal spasticity in the gastrocnemius and hamstring muscles, targeted injections of botulinum toxin A is a prime consideration [29, 31]. Personalization also involves using dynamic ultrasound guidance to ensure precise injection into the most active muscle regions, with dosages meticulously calculated based not only on muscle mass but also on objective spasticity measurements and the patient's specific functional goals. Genetic variations in drug metabolism pathways can significantly influence a patient's response and susceptibility to side effects [28]. Identifying these variants beforehand would allow for the a priori adjustment of baclofen dosing to maximize therapeutic benefit while minimizing adverse effects like sedation.

Furthermore, personalized treatment requires personalized monitoring. While instrumented gait analysis provides an objective baseline and post-intervention assessment, emerging technologies like wearable inertial sensors are revolutionizing long-term monitoring [9, 23]. By equipping the patient with discreet sensors, we can capture continuous, real-world data on his movement quality, energy expenditure, and participation in daily activities outside the clinic. This objective data stream allows for the fine-tuning of his high-intensity physical therapy regimen and AFO design in near real-time. Ultimately, the therapeutic pathway is not a static prescription, but a dynamic, iterative process [49]. It is determined by a multidisciplinary team that integrates genomic data, precision-guided interventions, and continuous objective monitoring, all in close collaboration with the patient and his family to weigh the benefits and risks against their specific, participation-focused goals.

4.8 For Parents and Caregivers

In the context of CP management instead of a "one-size-fits-all" approach, the focus is now on personalized medicine; This means creating a treatment plan that is uniquely tailored to your child. To do this, doctors and therapists are using new tools to understand the exact cause and specific challenges of CP. This includes Looking at genes, Advanced brain imaging, and High-tech movement analysis. By putting all this information together, the goal is to choose the most effective therapies, medications, and surgeries to help your child gain independence, reduce the effort of moving, and participate more easily in activities with friends and family.

Key Points to Remember

- Your child's CP is unique. The old way of treating CP often meant waiting for problems to appear and then managing them. The new approach tries to understand the root cause from the beginning to be more proactive.
- Answers may be in the genes. Finding a genetic cause doesn't change who your child is, but it can end a long search for answers. It helps your family understand the chances of CP happening in a future pregnancy and may even point toward specific treatments in the future.
- Technology makes treatment smarter. Using tools like virtual reality (VR) can make therapy feel like a game, which helps kids stay motivated. Robotics can help a child practice a movement hundreds of times perfectly. Wearable sensors can track progress at home, giving therapists a real-world view of how your child is doing.
- You are the expert on your child. A personalized plan is always created with the family's goals considered.

4.9 Summary

- Genomic analyses now identify a genetic basis in as many as one-third of individuals with CP [1, 11, 13].
- The "double hit" hypothesis is an emerging model, suggesting that an underlying genetic variant confers heightened vulnerability to a perinatal environmental trigger like hypoxia or infection [1, 2].
- The discovery of shared molecular pathways (e.g., channelopathies involving *SCN2A*) between CP phenotypes and other neurodevelopmental disorders is reframing CP as part of a broader spectrum, breaking down traditional diagnostic silos [1, 18].
- Identifying the underlying gene (e.g., *COL4A1*, *CTNNB1*) provides critical anticipatory guidance for managing multi-system involvement (e.g., systemic hemorrhage risk) and associated neurodevelopmental outcomes (e.g., severe intellectual disability) [16, 17].

- Diffusion Tensor Imaging (DTI) is used to assess corticospinal tract integrity, with metrics like fractional anisotropy (FA) correlating with motor impairment severity. Task-based fMRI maps motor cortex reorganization (contralesional vs. ipsilateral control) and is a powerful predictor of response to therapies like Constraint-Induced Movement Therapy (CIMT) [3, 4].
- Three-Dimensional Gait Analysis (3DGA) provides objective kinematic and kinetic data and is considered standard of care for pre-operative planning of complex orthopedic procedures like Single Event Multi-Level Surgery (SEMLS) [23, 24, 41].
- Relying on subjective clinical scales like the Modified Ashworth Scale for spasticity is limited by low inter-rater reliability; objective, quantitative measures are superior for tracking changes and guiding treatment [22].
- While holding theoretical promise, stem cell therapy for CP remains experimental. Further research is required to establish the optimal cell type, dose, timing, and delivery route and to confirm long-term safety and efficacy [41, 42].
- For monogenic forms of CP, gene therapy is a transformative future direction but remains in the preclinical phase of development [45].

References

1. van Eyk CL, Fahey MC, Gecz J. Redefining cerebral palsies as a diverse group of neurodevelopmental disorders with genetic aetiology. Nat Rev Neurol. 2023;19(9):542–55.
2. Lewis SA, et al. Insights from genetic studies of cerebral palsy. Front Neurol. 2021;11:625428.
3. Schertz M, et al. Imaging predictors of improvement from a motor learning–based intervention for children with unilateral cerebral palsy. Neurorehabil Neural Repair. 2016;30(7):647–60.
4. Jiang Y, et al. White matter lesions and DTI metrics related to various types of dysfunction in cerebral palsy: a meta-analysis and systematic review. PLoS One. 2025;20(1):e0312378.
5. Ahmadi MN, et al. Machine learning to quantify physical activity in children with cerebral palsy: comparison of group, group-personalized, and fully-personalized activity classification models. Sensors. 2020;20(14):3976.
6. Chia K, et al. A decision support system to facilitate identification of musculoskeletal impairments and propose recommendations using gait analysis in children with cerebral palsy. Front Bioeng Biotechnol. 2020;8:529415.
7. Gao Q, et al. Automating general movements assessment with quantitative deep learning to facilitate early screening of cerebral palsy. Nat Commun. 2023;14(1):8294.
8. Ökmen BM, et al. Effect of virtual reality therapy on functional development in children with cerebral palsy: a single-blind, prospective, randomized-controlled study. Turk J Phys Med Rehab. 2019;65(4):371.
9. Khaksar S, et al. Application of inertial measurement units and machine learning classification in cerebral palsy: randomized controlled trial. JMIR Rehabil Assist Technol. 2021;8(4):e29769.
10. Conner BC, Lerner ZF. Improving ankle muscle recruitment via plantar pressure biofeedback during robot resisted gait training in cerebral palsy. In: 2022 International Conference on Rehabilitation Robotics (ICORR). IEEE; 2022.
11. Fehlings DL, et al. Comprehensive whole-genome sequence analyses provide insights into the genomic architecture of cerebral palsy. Nat Genet. 2024;56(4):585–94.

12. Jin SC, et al. Mutations disrupting neuritogenesis genes confer risk for cerebral palsy. Nat Genet. 2020;52(10):1046–56.
13. Srivastava S, et al. Molecular diagnostic yield of exome sequencing and chromosomal microarray in cerebral palsy: a systematic review and meta-analysis. JAMA Neurol. 2022;79(12):1287–95.
14. Yechieli M, et al. Diagnostic yield of chromosomal microarray and trio whole exome sequencing in cryptogenic cerebral palsy. J Med Genet. 2022;59(8):759–67.
15. Lewis SA, et al. Clinical actionability of genetic findings in cerebral palsy: a systematic review and meta-analysis. JAMA Pediatr. 2025;179(2):137–44.
16. Güvener O, et al. Are COL4A1 and COL4A2 gene polymorphisms associated with cerebral palsy? Turk J Phys Med Rehab. 2021;67(2):242.
17. Kayumi S, et al. Genomic and phenotypic characterization of 404 individuals with neurodevelopmental disorders caused by CTNNB1 variants. Genet Med. 2022;24(11):2351–66.
18. Wilson YA, et al. Clinically relevant genes identified in cerebral palsy cohorts following evaluation of the clinical description and phenotype: a systematic review. J Child Neurol. 2024;39(13–14):500–9.
19. Nicita F, et al. Heterozygous KIF1A variants underlie a wide spectrum of neurodevelopmental and neurodegenerative disorders. J Med Genet. 2021;58(7):475–83.
20. Figueiredo TMAC, et al. GNAO1: description of three distinct cases with the same genotype and literature review. Arq Neuropsiquiatr. 2024;82(S 02):A0718.
21. Dzinovic I, et al. Variant recurrence confirms the existence of a FBXO31-related spastic-dystonic cerebral palsy syndrome. Ann Clin Transl Neurol. 2021;8(4):951–5.
22. Yoo M, et al. Reliability of the modified Ashworth and modified Tardieu scales with standardized movement speeds in children with spastic cerebral palsy. Children. 2022;9(6):827.
23. McGrath M, et al. The impact of three-dimensional gait analysis in adults with pathological gait on management recommendations. Gait Posture. 2023;105:75–80.
24. Ma N, et al. Three-dimensional gait analysis in children undergoing gastrocsoleus lengthening for equinus secondary to cerebral palsy. Medicina. 2021;57(2):98.
25. Vanmechelen I, et al. Reliability and discriminative validity of wearable sensors for the quantification of upper limb movement disorders in individuals with dyskinetic cerebral palsy. Sensors. 2023;23(3):1574.
26. Choisne J, et al. An unsupervised data-driven model to classify gait patterns in children with cerebral palsy. J Clin Med. 2020;9(5):1432.
27. Yang J, et al. Harnessing multimodal data and deep learning for comprehensive gait analysis in pediatric cerebral palsy. IEEE Trans Consum Electron. 2024;70:5401.
28. McLaughlin MJ, et al. Pharmacogenomic variability of oral baclofen clearance and clinical response in children with cerebral palsy. PM R. 2018;10(3):235–43.
29. Li M, et al. Baclofen and botulinum toxin a use in tone management for children with cerebral palsy: a review of current literature and research gaps in pre-and peri-operative care. Pediatr Neurol. 2025;172:28–34.
30. Yang H, et al. Safety and efficacy of botulinum toxin type a in children with spastic cerebral palsy aged <2 years: a systematic review. J Child Neurol. 2023;38(6–7):454–65.
31. Bar-On L, et al. Treatment response to botulinum neurotoxin-a in children with cerebral palsy categorized by the type of stretch reflex muscle activation. Front Neurol. 2020;11:378.
32. Carr WW, Jain N, Sublett JW. Immunogenicity of botulinum toxin formulations: potential therapeutic implications. Adv Ther. 2021;38(10):5046–64.
33. Fehlings D, et al. Pharmacological and neurosurgical management of cerebral palsy and dystonia: clinical practice guideline update. Dev Med Child Neurol. 2024;66(9):1133–47.
34. Ramey SL, et al. Constraint-induced movement therapy for cerebral palsy: a randomized trial. Pediatrics. 2021;148(5):e2020033878.
35. Gardas SS, et al. Bimanual movement characteristics and real-world performance following hand–arm bimanual intensive therapy in children with unilateral cerebral palsy. Behav Sci. 2023;13(8):681.

36. Novak I, et al. Early, accurate diagnosis and early intervention in cerebral palsy: advances in diagnosis and treatment. JAMA Pediatr. 2017;171(9):897–907.
37. Morgan C, et al. Early intervention for children aged 0 to 2 years with or at high risk of cerebral palsy: international clinical practice guideline based on systematic reviews. JAMA Pediatr. 2021;175(8):846–58.
38. Gündoğmuş E, Bumin G, Yalçın SS. Effect of early intervention on developmental domains and parent–child interaction among children with developmental delay: a randomized controlled study. Am J Occup Ther. 2024;78(6):7806205110.
39. Fandim JV, et al. Effectiveness of virtual reality in children and young adults with cerebral palsy: a systematic review of randomized controlled trial. Braz J Phys Ther. 2021;25(4):369–86.
40. Demers M, et al. Integration of motor learning principles into virtual reality interventions for individuals with cerebral palsy: systematic review. JMIR Serious Games. 2021;9(2):e23822.
41. Ma N, et al. Single-event multi-level surgery in cerebral palsy: a bibliometric analysis. Medicina. 2023;59(11):1922.
42. Salomon I. Neurobiological insights into cerebral palsy: a review of the mechanisms and therapeutic strategies. Brain Behav. 2024;14(10):e70065.
43. Lv Z-Y, Li Y, Liu J. Progress in clinical trials of stem cell therapy for cerebral palsy. Neural Regen Res. 2021;16(7):1377–82.
44. Qu J, et al. Efficacy and safety of stem cell therapy in cerebral palsy: a systematic review and meta-analysis. Front Bioeng Biotechnol. 2022;10:1006845.
45. Jensen TL, Gøtzsche CR, Woldbye DP. Current and future prospects for gene therapy for rare genetic diseases affecting the brain and spinal cord. Front Mol Neurosci. 2021;14:695937.
46. Ko EJ, et al. Effect of anodal transcranial direct current stimulation combined with cognitive training for improving cognition and language among children with cerebral palsy with cognitive impairment: a pilot, randomized, controlled, double-blind, and clinical trial. Front Pediatr. 2021;9:713792.
47. He W, et al. Safety and effects of transcranial direct current stimulation on hand function in preschool children with hemiplegic cerebral palsy: a pilot study. Front Behav Neurosci. 2022;16:925122.
48. Sun Y-Y, et al. Effects of repetitive transcranial magnetic stimulation on motor function and language ability in cerebral palsy: a systematic review and meta-analysis. Front Pediatr. 2023;11:835472.
49. Kolaski K, et al. Quality appraisal of systematic reviews of interventions for children with cerebral palsy reveals critically low confidence. Dev Med Child Neurol. 2021;63(11):1316–26.

5 An Orthopedic Approach to Cerebral Palsy

Kamran Shirbache, Nazanin Anaraki, Ana Precedo, Nastaran Maghbouli, Ahmadreza Nezameslami, and Mohammad Hossein Nabian

5.1 Definition and Classification

Cerebral palsy (CP) is a group of movement disorders that affect a person's posture, balance, and gait. This clinical manifestation is caused by permanent and non-progressive damage to the brain. But the clinical symptoms of CP can change over time [1]. CP is the most common childhood physical disability with an average of 2.08 per 1000 live births and has a heavy socio-economic burden with implications for society and healthcare systems [2, 3]. So far, many classifications have been proposed for CP. Here, according to the purpose of the chapter, we use the topographical classification in order to guide the clinical examination and FMS, the Gross Motor Function Classification System (GMFCS), and the Manual Ability Classification System (MACS) to determine the functional level of the patient in order to provide the most appropriate treatment [4–6].

K. Shirbache
Robert Debré University Hôpital, Paris, France
e-mail: ana.presedo@aphp.fr

N. Anaraki · N. Maghbouli
Tehran University of Medical Sciences, Tehran, Iran

A. Precedo
Robert Debré University Hospital, Paris, France, USA

A. Nezameslami
Department of Orthopedics, Emory University, Atlanta, GA, USA

M. H. Nabian (✉)
Center for Orthopedic Trans-Disciplinary Applied Research, Tehran University of Medical Sciences, Tehran, Iran
e-mail: mh-nabian@sina.tums.ac.ir

A. Presedo et al. (eds.), *Enhancing Quality of Life in Patients with Cerebral Palsy*, https://doi.org/10.1007/978-3-032-20967-2_5

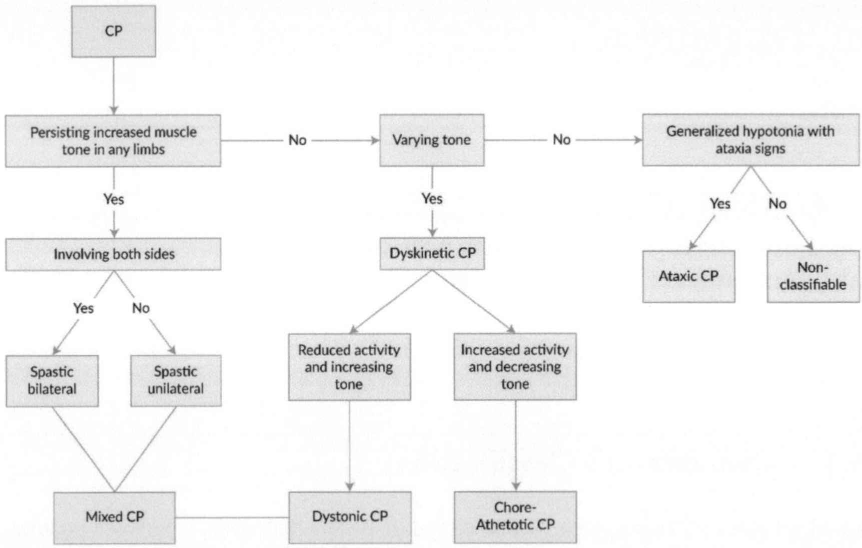

Fig. 5.1 Cerebral Palsy Classification

Cerebral Palsy (CP) is classified into five main types based on motor impairments and neurological characteristics: spastic, dyskinetic, dystonic, ataxic, and mixed. Spastic CP, the most common form, includes two topographic subtypes: unilateral spastic CP (hemiplegic), affecting one side of the body, and bilateral spastic CP (diplegic or quadriplegic), involving both sides, with varying degrees of limb involvement. Dyskinetic CP is characterized by involuntary and fluctuating movements, including choreoathetoid CP, which presents with a combination of rapid, dance-like contractions and slow, writhing movements, often associated with decreased muscle tone. Dystonic CP features sustained, involuntary muscle contractions that cause twisting, repetitive movements and abnormal postures, typically accompanied by increased muscle tone and reduced voluntary control. Ataxic CP is marked by poor coordination, unsteadiness, and hypotonia, resulting in clumsy or shaky movements. Mixed CP refers to cases where patients exhibit a combination of motor types, most commonly spasticity and dystonia; classification is generally based on the dominant motor pattern [2, 5, 7] (Fig. 5.1).

GMFCS and MACS classification are explained in the related section.

5.2 History

As an orthopedic specialist, it is very important to know whether you are visiting a patient with a diagnosis of CP or not. When evaluating a new patient, especially one under 2 years of age, you should consider other possible differential diagnoses and carefully assess for any co-morbidities [1]. Diagnosing CP requires an extensive interview, analysis of the child's development, multiple tests, and CNS imaging. It should be noted that some neurodevelopmental disorders in early life can be improved or even treated and their timely diagnosis is crucial [8]. Several progressive movement disorders, especially in the first period of the disease, may have similar clinical manifestations. Therefore, it may be necessary to refer the patient to a pediatric neurologist for further evaluations. To be aware of this issue, it is helpful to pay attention to some points in the patient's history [9].

Absence of prenatal, perinatal, or postnatal risk factors in CNS damage such as hypoxia, infection, asphyxia, premature birth <32 weeks or <2500 g, instrumented delivery, seizures within 48 h of birth, cerebral infarction, hyperbilirubinemia, meningitis, and head injury underdiagnose CP, so other causes should be considered. If the patient's symptoms are purely spastic or dystonic, usually the disorder is caused by etiologies other than CP, such as spinal cord lesions, hereditary spastic paraparesis, and metabolic disorders [10]. Patients with CP often show a dominant motor type disorder but with a combination of other types and there is usually a subtle involvement of the arm, even in leg dominant patterns [11]. Deteriorating signs or fluctuation of the disorders are rare in CP. Diurnal variation is another point we should be cautious about. If there is a family history of a similar disease, genetic causes should be suspected [12]. Also, dysmorphic features are typical of other resembling syndromes like Angelman, molybdenum, Lesch–Nyhan, lysosomal, etc. If the functional level of the patient does not match with his/her classification, one should think about the causes of cognitive impairment rather than physical injury [8]. The inconsistency of the patient's neuroimaging with his/her symptoms is very decisive in doubting the diagnosis of CP and may lead to other diagnoses [13]. For further information look at Table 5.1.

Otherwise, if the patient is a known case of CP, we can focus on musculoskeletal problems and their related complications. The history of the child's developmental milestones is very helpful in making subsequent decisions. Having a good knowledge of the child's developmental process and his current level of functional activity, it is possible to predict the natural history of the patient and set goals for follow-up and treatment [14]. It is about the time matter, the sooner the child reaches the standing balance, the better the result will be from the correction of pelvic abnormalities and other complications [15, 16].

Knowledge of the previous history of the related medical diseases, the history of physiotherapy, botulinum toxin (BT) injection, and previous surgeries of the patient enables us to evaluate the existing abnormalities and the opportunities for compensation as accurately as possible [17]. Asking about the other medical problems co-existing with Motor Disability in CP Patients is a must. The history of epilepsy is important to consider the possible risk of falling for the patient according to his/her musculoskeletal condition. The related drug history should be checked in order not to interfere with our prescriptions [18]. Intellectual disability is another common impairment in CP that has the potential to affect daily activities, burden of care, quality of life, effectiveness of our interventions, and educations [19]. The majority of children with CP suffer from feeding difficulties and gastrointestinal problems such as oropharyngeal dysfunction,

Table 5.1 Red flags and differential diagnosis of CP

Red flags	DDx	Plan
History	*True muscle weakness*	Neurologist referral Genetic assessment Enzymatic assessment Metabolic assessment
Similar disease in the family Parental relatedness No risk factors No sentinel events Stoppage or regression in neurodevelopment Fluctuation in motor functions Episodic deterioration	Myopathies, Duchenne muscular dystrophy, hereditary motor sensory neuropathy Mitochondrial cytopathies Cerebral white matter diseases: hypo-myelinating, Leukodystrophies Infantile neuroaxonal dystrophy—INAD	
	Spastic diplegia or quadriplegia	
	Adrenoleukodystrophy (ALD) Metachromatic leukodystrophy Hereditary progressive spastic paraplegia Arginase deficiency Holocarboxylase synthetase deficiency Pre-natal iodine deficiency (neurological cretinism) TORCH infections	
Clinical exam	*Significant dystonia or involuntary movements*	
Dysmorphic facies Neurocutaneous lesions Systemic signs Retinopathy or optic atrophy Isolated muscular hypotonia Paraparesis Peripheral nervous system impairments (pes cavus)	DOPA responsive dystonia Mitochondrial disorders Pantothenate kinase-associated neurodegeneration (PKAN) Pyruvate dehydrogenase deficiency Leigh syndrome Glutaric organic acidurias Juvenile neuronal ceroid lipofuscinoses Rett syndrome Pelizaeus-Merzbacher disease Lesch-Nyhan syndrome	
Para clinic	*Ataxia*	
Normal brain MRI Isolated abnormal globus pallidus signals Incompatible imaging findings with cp symptoms Cerebellar atrophy Demyelination	Ataxia-telangiectasia Angelman syndrome Niemann-Pick disease type C Pontocerebellar hypoplasia or atrophy Chronic/adult GM2 gangliosidosis Mitochondrial cytopathy (NARP mutation) Posterior fossa tumors Joubert's syndrome	
	Other CN dysfunctions	
	Polymicrogyria Zellweger syndrome	

Table 5.2 Functional mobility scoring

	Grade	Walking distance	Score		Description
1	Home	5 m	Score for each grade	1	Mostly use wheelchair/ able to stand for transfer/some stepping by caretaker or walker support
				2	Using a walker or frame for walking
2	School	50 m		3	Walking independently by a crutch support
				4	Walking independently by stick help (one or two)
				5	Walking independently but on level surfaces
3	Community	500 m		6	Walking independently on all surfaces
				C	Crawling for mobility
				N	Not applicable for 500 m distances

The same context is defined more specifically for lower and upper limbs as GMFCS and Manual Ability Classification System (MACS), respectively, both of which are explained in the clinical exam section [23]

gastroesophageal disease, and constipation. Since malnutrition causes growth failure and the subsequent orthopedic complications, such as osteomalacia and joint deformity, definitely it should be improved [16, 20].

5.2.1 Functional Mobility Scale (FMS)

A person's performance at home, school, and in the community, as well as skills, such as walking, running, and climbing stairs, should also be carefully questioned. Functional Mobility assessment evaluates the motor efficiency of CP children based on the disabilities and compensatory reactions, which includes different classifications. This index is related to the use of assistive devices and in three environments: home, school, and community. It is very important to evaluate its course in annual examinations and also for targeting treatment. FMS changes provide a relatively accurate prognosis of the child's future status and social educational opportunities. The classification of FMS is mentioned in Table 5.2 [21, 22].

5.3 Clinical Exam

CP patient's examination consists of two dimensions, static and dynamic aspects. Since the information collected from the physical examination is considered a static finding, one should not miss the analysis of functional activities, such as walking, to have a more comprehensive insight. By obtaining this dynamic information, we will have a more accurate picture of the problems of children with CP. Here, we explain both parts practically. First, examine each limb anatomically [24].

5.3.1 Hip

Hip examination in CP is important because late dislocation may occur in this joint following abnormal muscular balance, loss of selective motor control, and muscle tone abnormalities. Therefore, screening children, especially non-walkers and late walkers, is very important [13].

Thomas' hip flexion test: This test is performed in supine position and determines the flexion contracture of the hip. The examiner corrects excessive lumbar lordosis by flexing the contolateral hip. Hip flexion contracture is defined based on the angle between the horizontal axis of the thigh and the floor line [25] (Fig. 5.2e).

Staheli test: This test is performed in the prone position to evaluate hip flexion contracture, especially in bilateral hip pathologies. The patient lies on the edge of the

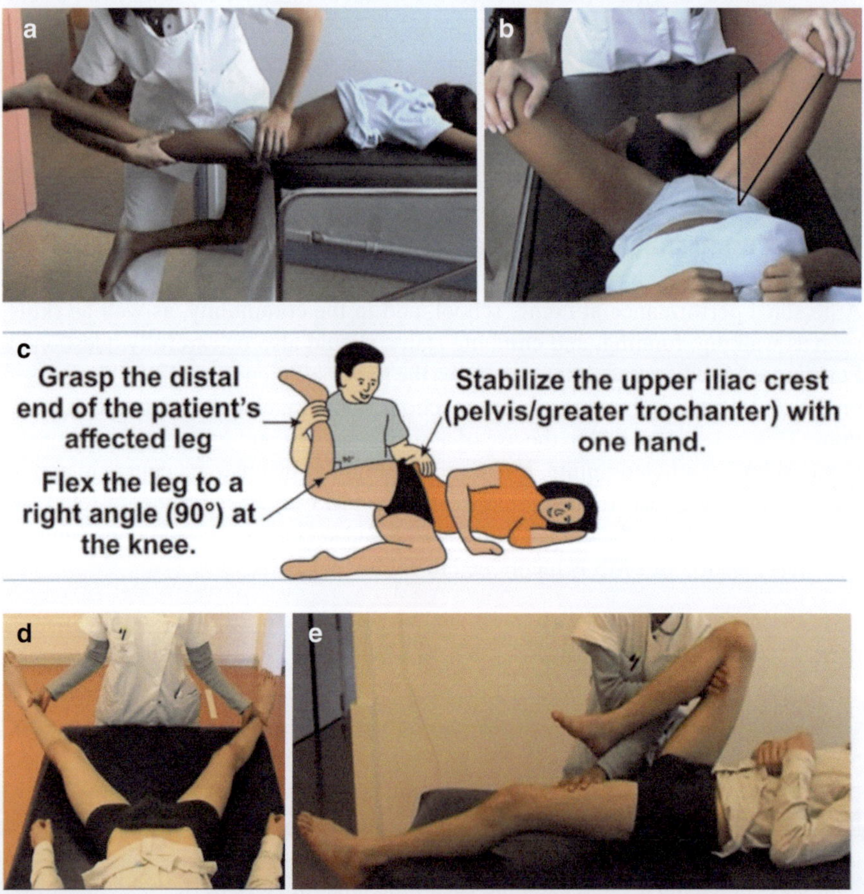

Fig. 5.2 (**a**) Staheli test, (**b**) Phelp's test (flexed knee), (**c**) Ober's Test, (**d**) Phelp's Test (extended Knee), (**e**) Thomas' hip flexion test

couch and the examiner stabilizes the pelvis with one hand, extends the thigh with the other hand, and monitors the lumbar lordosis at the same time, stopping the extension at the point where the patient's pelvis rises. The angle between the long axis of the thigh and the floor line indicates the flexion contraction. This test is more accurate compared to Thomas test in CP patients [25] (Fig. 5.2a).

Phelp's Test: This examination is performed in supine position to evaluate the amount of adductor contracture in such a way that the examiner conducts passive abduction of the thigh with extended knee and flexed knee at 90°. If there is no difference in the two positions, the pathology is in the adductor muscles and if abduction is corrected by knee flexion, the problem is in the internal hamstring and gracilis muscles. The future risk of hip subluxation and chronic hip pain is very likely if a noticeable hip flexion contracture in combination with hip abduction of <30° occurs [25] (Fig. 5.2b, d).

Ober test: This test is performed to check Tensor Fasciae Latae (TFL) and Iliotibial Band (ITB) in CP patients in terms of tightness, contracture, and inflammation. First, ask the patient to lay on his/her side so that the desired side is up. Place the knee and hip of the patient in a flexed position so that the curve of the spine is flattened. Stand behind the patient and hold the pelvis and greater trochanter firmly with one hand. Take the end of the examined leg with the other hand and flex the leg at the right angle of the knee, extend and abduct the hip joint, then lower the limb toward the table until the movement is limited. Note that the hip joint should not be allowed to flex or rotate internally during the examination. If the leg is adducted with the thigh without pain or restriction and falls below the horizon line, the ITB is normal and the test is negative. If the limb remains in abduction and the patient mentions the lateral knee pain, the test is positive and ITB involvement is considered [26] (Fig. 5.2c).

5.3.2 Knee

The first step in dealing with a flexion contracture of the knee is to differentiate the real contracture from spasticity or muscle stiffness [27].

Joint contracture test: The patient is supine; the hip joint is in extension and the ankle is in plantar flexion in the direction of gravity. If there is any residual knee flexion relative to the floor surface, it shows true knee contracture [25].

Popliteal angle test: This testing is performed unilaterally and bilaterally in the supine position. In the one-sided examination, we flex the hip joint 90° with one hand and restrain the opposite limb with the other hand. We extend the knee as much as possible, the amount of residual knee flexion indicates stiffness or muscle contraction. In the bilateral examination, both hips are flexed at 90 ° and the residual knee flexion of each limb is measured while the other limb is folded into the abdomen. Whether the residual knee flexion is due to hip flexion contracture or anterior pelvic tilt can be distinguished from the difference of popliteal angle in unilateral and bilateral examination. Bilateral examination is more accurate

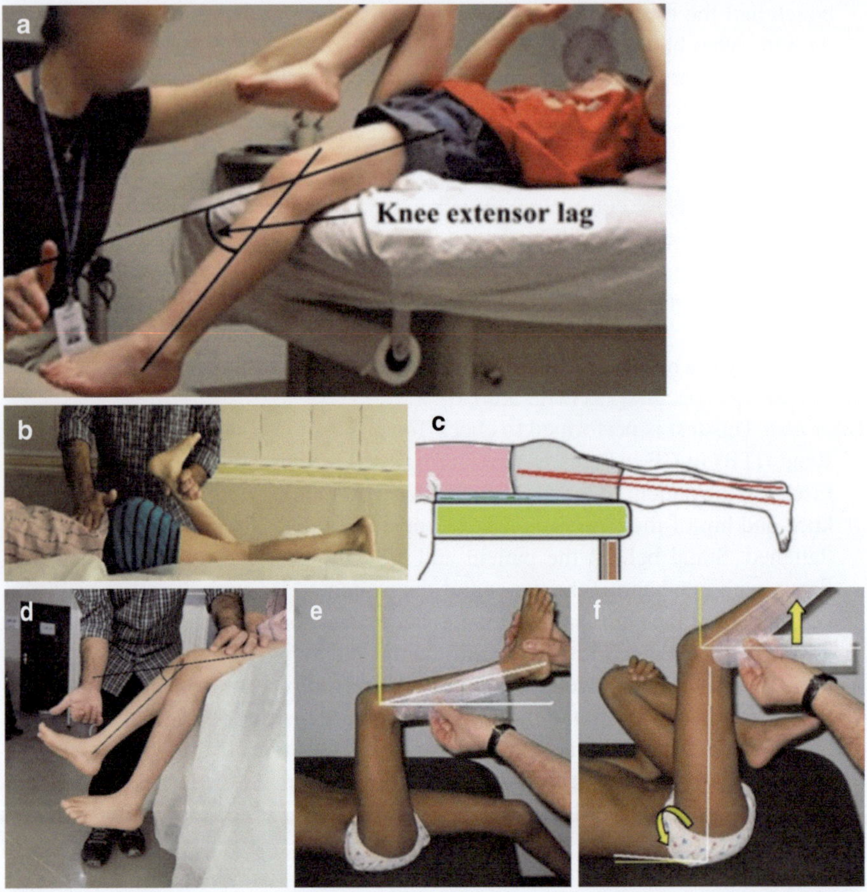

Fig. 5.3 (**a**) Active Knee extension, (**b**) Duncan-Ely's test, (**c**) Prone Passive Lag test, (**d**) Sitting active lag test, (**e**) Popliteal angle test, (**f**) Bilateral popliteal angle

than unilateral, distinguishing hamstring tightness; however, unilateral examination has false positives in anterior pelvic tilt caused by psoas muscle contracture. Also, hamstrings length could be evaluated by popliteal angle measurement [25] (Fig. 5.3e, f).

Duncan-Ely's/Prone Rectus test: This test is performed to examine the rectus femoris in such a way that the child is lying prone and the knee is brought into flexion so that it reaches the pelvis. If the pelvis rises while performing this movement, spasticity of the rectus femoris is considered. Since this disorder requires a different approach to treatment, it is important to pay attention to its association with hamstring contracture [25] (Fig. 5.3b).

Knee Extension Lag is a phenomenon that can indicate hamstring tightness or a diminished efficiency of the knee extensor mechanism in CP patients. Therefore, it is essential to examine this issue in CP [28].

Sitting and Passive Lag test (SAPLT): To check Knee Extension Lag actively, first the person is placed in a sitting position with legs hanging from the edge of the bed, then he/she is asked to extend both knees completely while the ankles are maximally dorsiflexed. For active examination, the person lays prone with the knees passing the edge of the bed and the patient's thighs are fixed on the bed, then the knees extend completely. If each of knees are not fully extended, the degree and the difference between the active and passive examination should be recorded. An active lag could be aroused from muscle strengthening while a passive lag might be a sign of tight restraints in the posterior knee capsule, gastrocnemius, hamstrings, iliopsoas [29] (Fig. 5.3a, c, d).

5.3.3 Ankle and Foot

The most concentration in this part is on checking equino-varus and plano-valgus, which are the most common manifestations in CP [30].

Confusion test: This test is performed to check dorsiflexion in CP patients by asking the child to flex the hip joint against resistance. If the ankle is dorsiflexed during this test due to tibialis anterior contracture, the test is positive. This test is also important for checking selectivity because it shows whether children with strong flexor patterns (hip, knee, ankle) can flex each joint separately or not. Confusion test shows the activity of the swing phase of tibialis anterior muscle and could be an indication for necessity of tendon transfer operation [31] (Fig. 5.4a).

Coleman Block Test: This test is used in children with cavo-varus foot deformity to differentiate between fixed or flexible deformity and to check foot pronation. In this test, we place the affected foot on a block above the surface, place the first metatarsal outside the edge of the block, and ask the child to dorsiflex the first metatarsal. The medial metatarsals are flexed and out of the block, but the other parts of the foot remain on the block, and the first metatarsal cannot cause varus, so if the deformity of the heel while weight bearing during this test is corrected, it is flexible, and if it is not corrected, it is a rigid deformity. In flexible deformity, surgery is aimed at pronation of the hindfoot caused by plantar flexion of the first metatarsal, and in fixed deformity, surgical correction of both the forefoot and hindfoot is necessary [32] (Fig. 5.4d).

Silverskiold test: In this test, the ankle is dorsiflexed passively in both the knee extension and the knee flexed at 90°. If there is a difference of 20–30, it indicates a gastrocnemius contracture and differentiates it from an Achilles tendon contracture [25] (Fig. 5.4e, f).

In the investigation of foot deformities and abnormal movements of the ankle while walking, examination of Extensor Hallucis Longus, Flexor hallucis longus, Posterior tibialis, Anterior tibialis, Peroneus longus, and Peroneus brevis separately are important. Here, we mention the tests related to each [11].

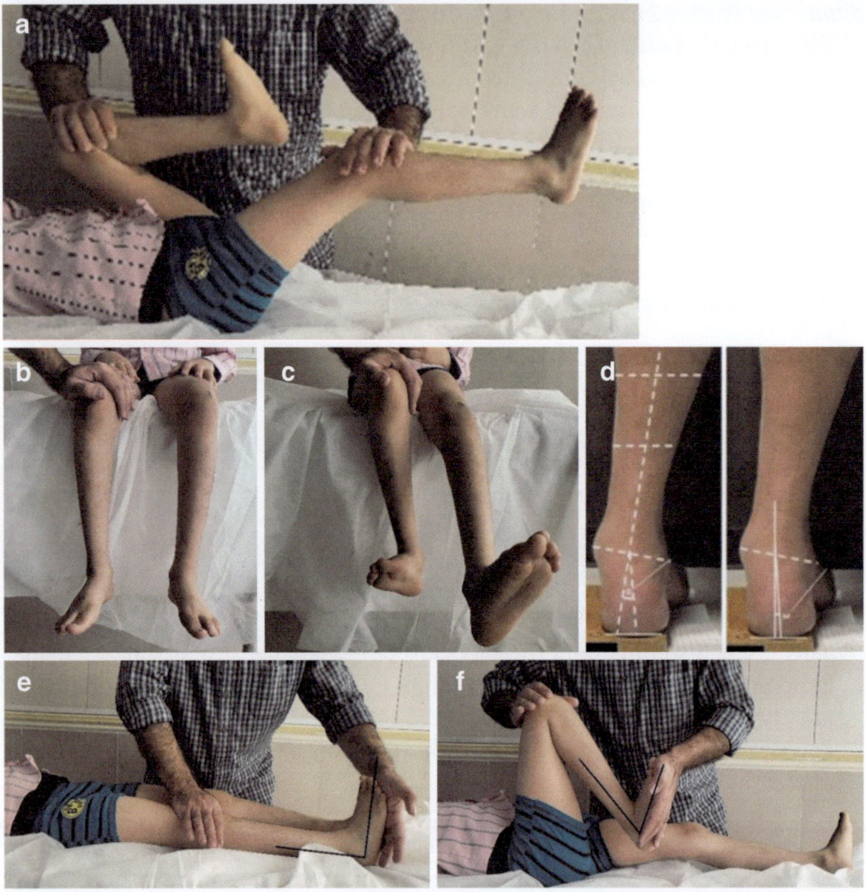

Fig. 5.4 (**a**) Confusion test, (**b**) Flexor hallucis longus test, (**c**) extensor hallucis longus test, (**d**) Coleman Block Test, (**e**) Silverskiold test (Extended knee), (**f**) Silverskiold test (flexed knee)

Extensor Hallucis Longus test: While the child is lying down or sitting, we ask him to extend the metatarsophalangeal and interphalangeal joints of the big toe. In order to check the muscle force, we can put pressure on the back surface of the end phalanges of the big toe in the direction of bending. While the child is lying down or sitting, we ask him to extend the metatarsophalangeal and interphalangeal joints of the big toe. In order to check the muscle force, we can put pressure on the dorsal surface of the distal phalanges of the big toe in the flexion direction [33] (Fig. 5.4c).

Flexor Hallucis Longus test: In addition to bending all joints of the big toe and maintaining stability of the first metatarsal head, this muscle also plays a role in maintaining the medial longitudinal arch during walking. Although it is a deep muscle and its function overlaps with other muscles, applying pressure against the plantar flexion of the big toe helps to examine it [33] (Fig. 5.4b).

Tibialis Anterior test: This is the first dorsiflexor muscle of the ankle, and for its examination, applying pressure on the inner part of the foot against the direction of dorsiflexion and inversion of the foot is helpful [33].

Tibialis Posterior: In addition to plantar flexion and inversion of the ankle, this muscle plays a significant role in keeping the inner arch of the foot, and in the examination, in addition to checking the functional movements of the muscle, it is also important to pay attention to the flatfoot [33].

Peroneal compression test: This test is to check the Peroneus brevis and Peroneus longus muscles. First, we lay the patient in a semi-lateral position on the non-involved side, and the ankle is in the neutral position. To test the peroneus brevis, we hold the end of the leg with one hand, and with the other hand, we turn the side of the leg into eversion. Then we ask the patient to return the foot to the neutral position. It should be noted that the fingers are slightly flexed, the ankle is fixed and the long extensors are relaxed so that only the peroneus brevis muscle is involved during the movement of the talocalcaneonavicular joint. To examine the Peroneus longus muscles, plantarflex the ankle in the same position and while keeping it fixed, elevate the head of the first metatarsal, invert the foot and move the ankle to the dorsiflexion position. Then ask the patient to evert the ankle and make it plantarflexed. Again, in this test, other extensors must be relaxed [34].

5.4 Lever Arm Dysfunction

Lever arm dysfunction should be investigated in all children with CP because it describes a group of the most common disorders that lead to insidious complications such as hip subluxation, torsional deformities of long bones, and/or foot deformities. The locomotion of body is according to muscles and ground reaction forces (GRFs); however, these factors in CPs are not efficient because of bone modelling, reconstruction. or traumatic abnormalities that take the ability to walk from the child (Fig. 5.5a–c). Excessive Femoral Anteroversion (FAV), Tibial Torsion, and Coxavalga are categorized in lever arm dysfunction and result in in-toeing gait and hip instability [35] (Fig. 5.5e, f).

Craig's test (Netter maneuver): This test is for checking FAV, and it is also called the trochanteric protrusion test. With the patient in the prone position and both knees in 90° of flexion, the angle between the vertical line and the long axis of the leg at the greatest prominence of the greater trochanter is palpated laterally, which determines the FAV value. The combination of this test with the x-ray of the internal rotation view of the pelvis gives a more accurate prediction of the angle and axis of the femoral neck (Neck shaft angle) [34] (Fig. 5.5h).

To assess *tibial torsion* inconsistency, there are three methods as below:

1. *Thigh foot angle test*: we make the patient prone and flex the knees 90° to determine the angle between the thigh and the foot. We put the ankle and hind foot in a neutral position and consider the angle between the thigh axis and the foot axis

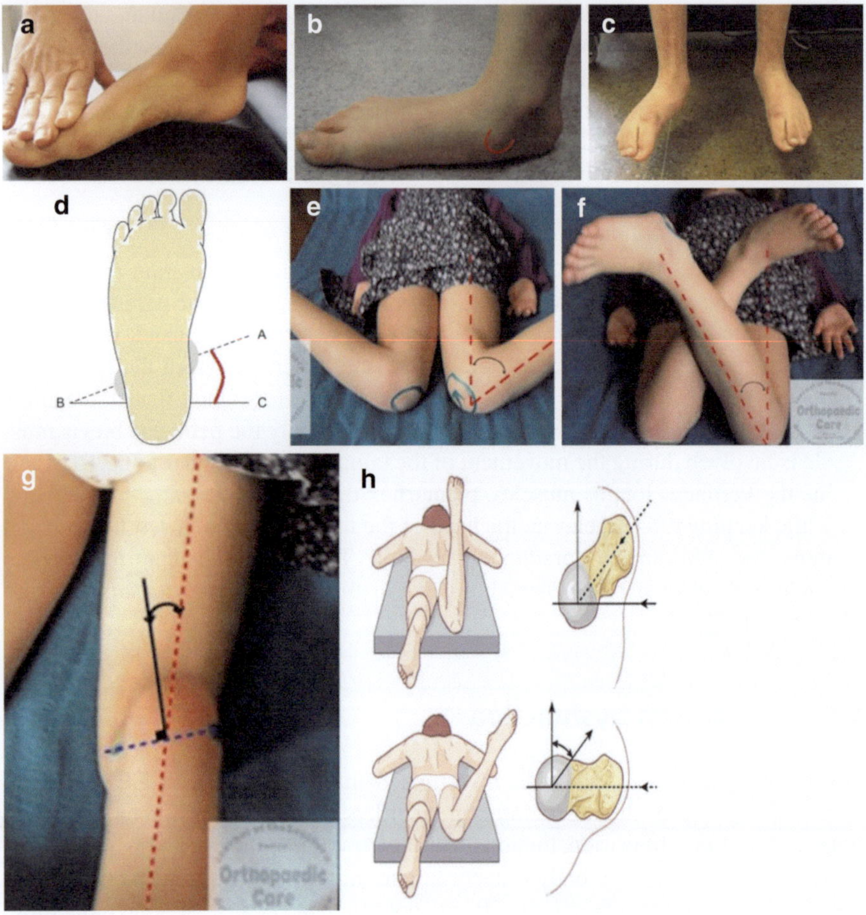

Fig. 5.5 (**a–c**) Foot alignment in sitting and standing position, (**d**) Bi-malleolar axis in tibial torsion, (**e**, **f**) Lower limb alignment, (**g**) Thigh foot angle test, (**h**) Craig's test (Netter maneuver)

as tibial torsion. It should be noted that the axis of the foot is defined by the line between the second and third metatarsals and the midpoint of the heel [25] (Fig. 5.5g).

2. *Bi-malleolar axis test*: With fully extended knees, we rotate the leg to align horizontally with the bi-condylar axis of the femur. The angle between the horizontal axis and the two malleolus indicates tibial torsion [25] (Fig. 5.5d).
3. *Second toe test:* the patient is placed in the prone position and the second toe is placed perpendicular to the floor, then the thigh is restrained and the knee is flexed, the angle between the perpendicular to the floor and the axis of the tibia represents tibial torsion [25].

Anteversion is evaluated during hip examination mentioned before and with the complementary imaging exact cause could be diagnosed [33].

5.4.1 Gait Analysis

Instrumented gait analysis is very useful to evaluate gait deviations and can help to indicate the most appropriate intervention for the patient. There are several techniques used to analyze gait in patients with CP based on new technologies such as videographic gait analysis and instrumented 3D gait analysis [36]; Edinburgh Visual Gait Score (EVGS) is a practical method using two cameras to record CP children's gait specially for postoperative outcomes evaluation. It focuses on 17 observational parameters for lower limbs and is scored on a three-point scale, for further information about the scoring system and interpretation visit www.oandp.org (Edinburgh Visual Gait Score (EVGS): Reference Guide) [37]; however, to offer something useful for all examiners in daily clinics without any equipment, we introduce observational gait analysis based on topographical aspects of CP. In this technique, we ask the child to walk in a private room several times and evaluate him/her in sagittal and coronal planes. The gait cycle and joint ROM at different time frames should be observed carefully [38]. We categorize gait analysis into two types.

Spastic hemiplegia: It stands for spasticity of one side of the body consisting of more impairment at the distal parts, including true equinus which is described in four types [38].

Spastic diplegia: This motor disorder affects both sides consisting of more impairment at the proximal parts, including apparent equinus and crouch gait, which is described in four types, with or without a stiff knee [38].

Some children with CP drag their feet while walking and sometimes even trip, due to reduced toe clearance, which is caused by insufficient flexion of the knee during swing phase. This phenomenon is called "Stiff-knee" gait which could be detected in all types of spastic gait [11].

Recurvatum refers to the increase in knee extension during the standing phase of walking. This pattern can be observed in equinus and jump knee types of gaits. There are two types of recurvatum, early and late, which occur in the first and second halves of stance, respectively. In the first type, the dynamic contraction of the Gastroc-soleus causes rise of heel and hyperextension of knee while the forefoot contacts the floor. The late type occurs after the foot is placed flat on the floor [21, 30].

A more complete explanation of spastic gate types is in Tables 5.3 and 5.4.

Table 5.3 Spastic gait analysis

Type		Name	Sign	Pathology
Spastic hemiplegia				
Type 1		Drop foot	Lack of first rocker at initial contact	Weakness or underactivity of the anterior tibial muscle; overactivity of the gastrocnemius and soleus muscles
Type 2	A	True equinus (without recurvatum)	Drop foot in swing phase and fixed plantarflexion in stance	Static or dynamic contracture of the gastrocnemius and soleus muscles
	B	True equinus with recurvatum knee	Same as 2A, with additional knee hyperextension	Static contracture of gastroc-soleus; weak quadriceps; knee joint instability
Type 3		True equinus/ jump knee	Drop foot, equinus, limited knee flexion in swing, hip hyperflexion, increased lumbar lordosis	Gastroc-soleus spasticity or contracture; hamstring and quadriceps co-contraction (stiff knee gait)
Type 4		Equinus/jump knee/flexed hip	Drop foot, equinus, flexed stiff knee, flexed/adducted hip, anterior pelvic tilt, compensated pelvic lordosis	Proximal involvement; spasticity or contractures in gastroc-soleus, hamstrings, quadriceps, psoas, and adductors
Spastic Diplegia				
Type 1		True equinus	Plantarflexed ankles throughout stance; extended hips and knees	Bilateral contracture of gastrocnemius and soleus
Type 2		Jump knee gait	Equinus at ankle, flexion at knee and hip, anterior pelvic tilt, lumbar lordosis, often with stiff knee gait	Bilateral spasticity or contracture of gastroc-soleus; hamstring and rectus femoris co-contraction
Type 3		Apparent equinus	Normal ankle dorsiflexion but excessive hip/knee flexion; child walks on toes	Spasticity or contracture of hamstrings, quadriceps, psoas/ adductors; normal or minimal gastroc involvement
Type 4		Crouch gait	Excessive dorsiflexion at ankles, and excessive flexion of knees and hips	Lengthened or weak plantarflexors; contractures of hamstrings, quadriceps, and psoas/adductors; may be worsened by isolated heel cord lengthening in younger children

Table 5.4 Different types of spastic gait

Gait	Type I	Type II A	Type II B	Type III	Type IV
Spastic hemiplegia	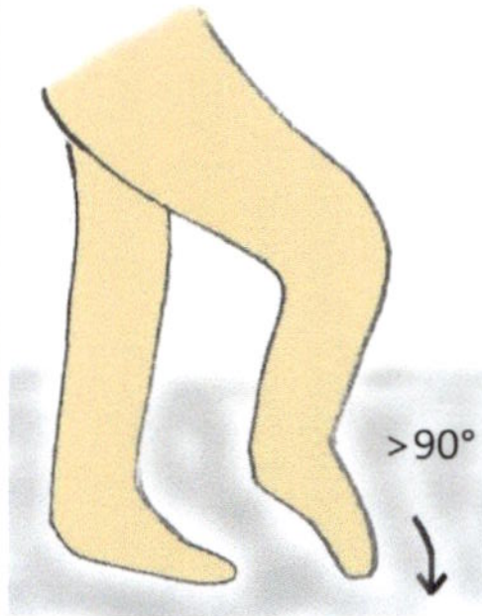 Drop foot	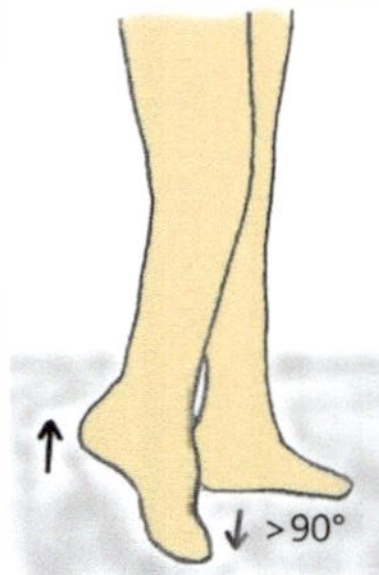 True equinus	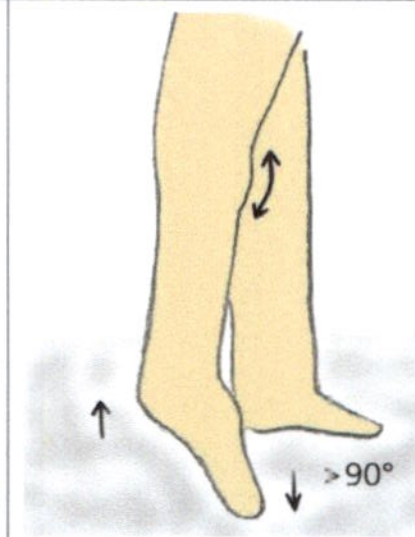 Recurvatum knee	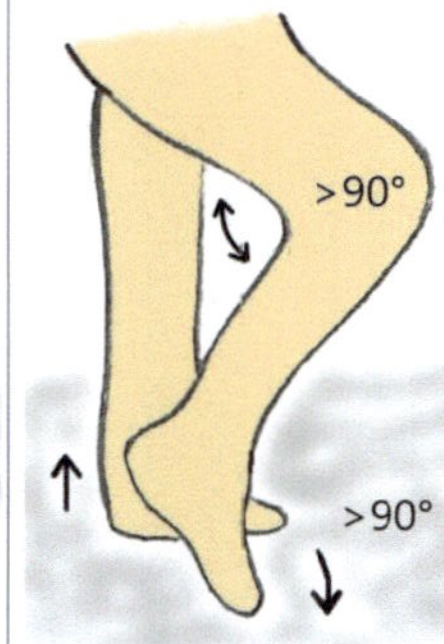 True equinus/jump knee	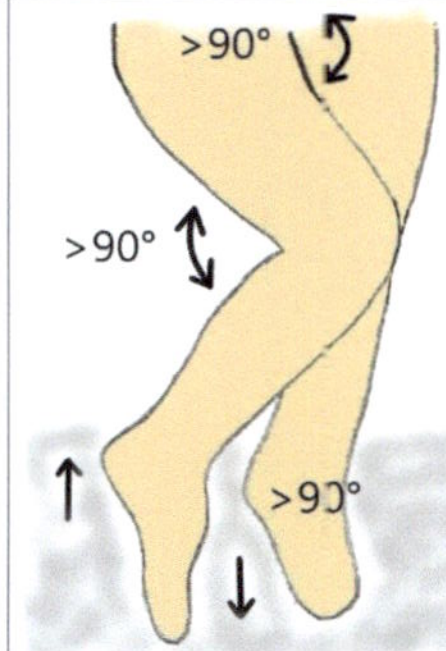 Equinus/jump knee/flexed hip
Spastic diplegia	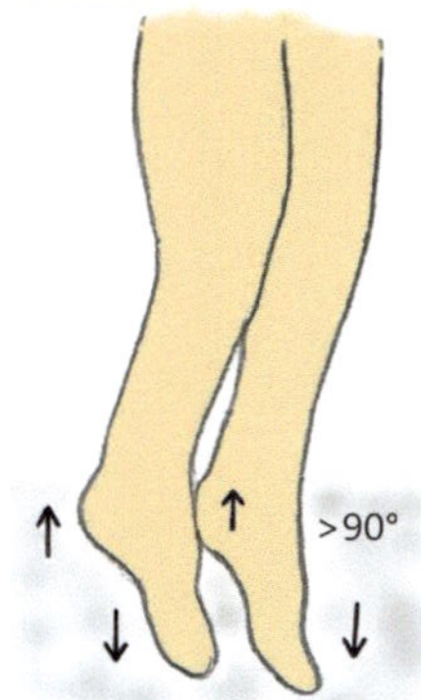 True equinus	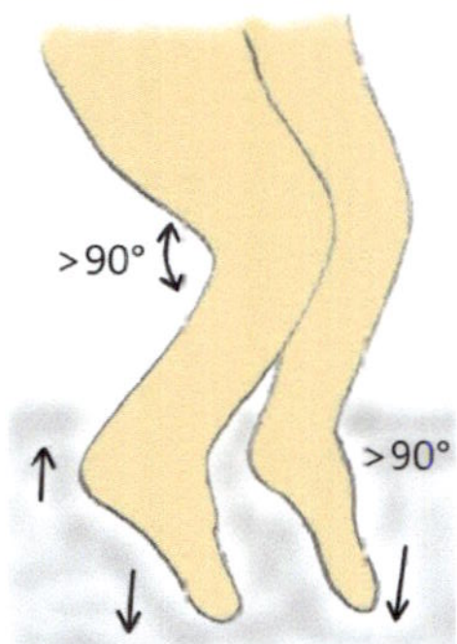 Jump gait		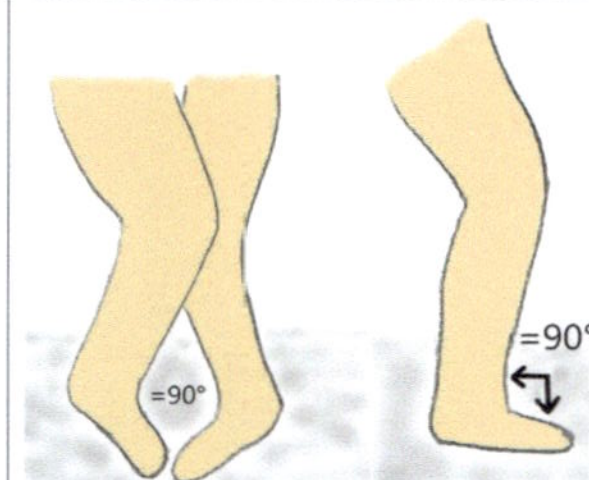 Apparent equinus	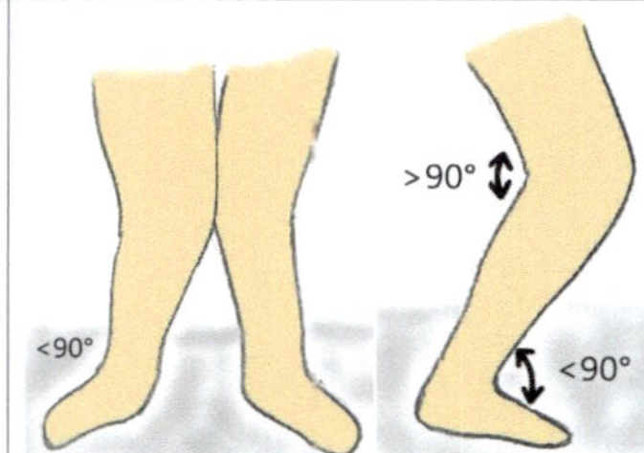 Crouch gait

5.5 Gross Motor Function Classification System (GMFCS)

The GMFCS is a valuable tool for assessing lower body function and selecting the best therapeutic intervention for each child. Children are classified into levels 1–5 based on their assistive device use (e.g., wheelchair, cane, walker) and quality of daily activity performance, with age bands (6–12 and 12–18 years) considered to account for environmental and personal factors affecting capability and performance [22, 39, 40] (Table 5.5).

Table 5.5 Gross Motor Function Classification System (GMFCS)

Level	Age	Description
Level I	6–12	Walking independently in all settings; climbs stairs without assistance. Runs and jumps, but with limited speed, balance, and coordination.
	12–18	
Level II	6–12	Walking in most settings with some difficulty on uneven terrain or long distances. May use railing, assistance, or mobility aids; limited ability to run or jump.
	12–18	Walking in most settings but may use mobility aids for safety or distance. Environmental and personal factors influence mobility; gross motor skills are limited.
Level III	6–12	Walking with a hand-held mobility device indoors; uses wheeled mobility for long distances. Needs assistance for transfers and stairs; may require wheelchair for participation.
	12–18	Walking with a hand-held mobility device; uses wheelchair or powered mobility for distance. Requires assistance for transfers and stairs; mobility varies by setting and ability.
Level V	6–12	Relying on physical assistance or powered mobility and adaptive seating for trunk and pelvic support across settings. They use floor mobility and body support walkers at home, and manual or powered wheelchairs at school and in the community, requiring adaptations for active participation.
	12–18	Using wheeled mobility with adaptive seating and require physical assistance for transfers, sometimes supporting weight during standing. They walk short distances indoors with help, operate powered wheelchairs when possible, and use manual wheelchairs or body support walkers as needed, with adaptations for participation in activities.
Level IV	6–12	Relying on manual wheelchairs and full adult assistance for transfers due to limited head, trunk, and limb control. They may use powered mobility with extensive adaptations and require support to participate in physical activities and sports.
	12–18	Using manual wheelchairs and need physical assistance or mechanical lifts for transfers due to limited head, trunk, and limb control. They may operate powered mobility with extensive adaptations and require support for participation in physical activities and sports.

5.6 Upper Limb

Upper limb involvement includes several patterns that have different appearances depending on the affected muscles, the degree of spasticity or dystonia, and the age of the patient. For this purpose, in the ROM examination of the joints of the upper limb, indicators are considered (Table 5.6) based on which the contracture of that joint is defined. Common patterns include shoulder adduction-internal rotation contraction, elbow flexion contraction and wrist flexion-pronation contraction, thumb internal or external muscle contraction, and palm deformity. In the fingers, the reaction of the long extensors of the finger against the flexion of the wrist or the inherent spasticity of the hand causes the deformation of the swan's neck. Another pattern is the interlocking of the fingers [41, 42].

After evaluation of muscle force and ROM of the shoulder, elbow, forearm, wrist, hand, and finger joints and checking muscle tone based on the scale, we examine the function of the upper limb which we mention the *Manual Ability Classification System (MACS)* for this purpose here. MACS focuses on the ability of children with CP to manipulate objects and define it according to their daily activities [43]. There are five levels in this classification as follows (Table 5.7):

Table 5.6 Upper limb contractures

Contracture type			Description
1	Shoulder	Internal rotation	Unable to perform external rotation of shoulder beyond 0° passively
		Adduction	Unable to perform abduction beyond 45° passively at the glenohumeral joint
2	Elbow flexion		Fixed flexion contracture of elbow more than 30°
3	Wrist flexion		Unable to extend wrist beyond neuter position (0°) passively
4	Wrist pronation		Unable to supinate wrist beyond neuter position (0°) passively while the elbow is by the side at 90°
5	Thumb in palm		Unable to abduct the thumb passing the level of index finger
6	Swan neck		Hyperextension of PIP joints beyond the 0°
7	Interlocking fingers		Unable to abduct fingers beyond 0°

Table 5.7 Manual Ability Classification System scoring system

Level		Description
1	Level I	The child can handle objects easily. Speed and accuracy are the only limitations of their manual task performance in this level.
2	Level II	The child can handle most objects. Low quality and speed of performance in some tasks is acceptable and some complex ones might be avoided or replaced by alternative ways.
3	Level III	The child can handle objects hardly; he/she is in need of help to conduct the task or replace it by alternative ways.
4	Level IV	The child can handle a few numbers of easily managed objects in familiar situations and with continuous support of others.
5	Level V	The child cannot handle objects, severely disabled to perform elementary tasks. Depended to others support completely

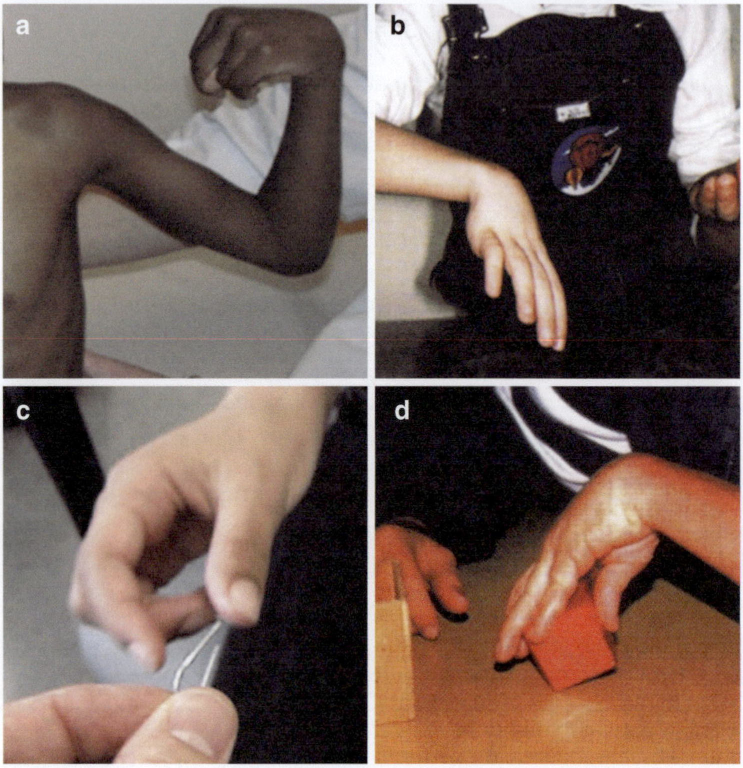

Fig. 5.6 Upper limb function tests; (**a**) Grasp and release, (**b**) Dexterity, (**c**) Pinching test, (**d**) Bimanual tasks

ABILHAND-Kids score is another measurement to check upper limb function that is more complete, includes 21 tasks rating three-point and covers most daily activities (Fig. 5.6). You can get the questionnaire by visiting the relevant site (www.abilhand.org). Parents should fill in the form, then by uploading the results on the website, the child's performance is analyzed via online software and a logit score based on Rasch analysis [44].

5.6.1 Axial Skeleton

Scoliosis, kyphosis, lordosis, pelvic obliquity, or a combination of these can be expected in CP patients. Scoliosis is very common in patients with GMFCS IV–V. Scoliosis starting at a young age (<15 years) has a poorer prognosis. Usually, the onset of puberty, loss of neurologic function, or long-term use of a wheelchair accelerates the development of deformity. It is important to pay attention to the changes and complications caused by spinal deformities in periodical examinations [45].

In this part, we should first determine the severity and flexibility of the spinal deformity, because the flexible curve in childhood can be managed by prescribing wheelchair supports and/or thoracolumbar bracing, provided that the upright sitting position of the child be maintained. After that, it is important to identify any pelvic obliquity, because if this phenomenon is left untreated, it will cause harmful consequences such as pressure points and buttock ulcers, sitting balance disorder, and significant hip joint deformities. Pelvic obliquity is called coronal rotation of the pelvis, which causes asymmetry in the height of the iliac crest. Eventually, determining the presence of muscle contractions in the lower limbs and the adequacy of sitting are also important indicators that must be checked [46].

For examination, we expose the child and place him in a sitting position on the examination table, with one of the parents standing facing him, holding the armpits bilaterally and supporting the child. The assisting parent is asked to apply only mild axial traction to the spine, and we observe the spine from the opposite side, recording the direction and location of the apex of the curve and the presence of any associated pelvic obliquity. In order to determine the severity of the abnormality in appearance, it is necessary to pay attention to the impingement of the lower rib cage on the iliac crest. Then, while applying manual pressure on the top of the deformity and the pelvis on the same side, we ask the parent to apply more axial traction to remove the deformity. If the scoliosis is removed or reduced, it is flexible and otherwise the curve is rigid. Both types of abnormalities can include variable severity [47] (Fig. 5.8a, b).

Scoliosis is divided into two groups based on the number and type of curves. Group I includes double thoracic and lumbar curves, and Group II has single curves in the thoracic or lumbar spine. Group I is mostly in ambulatory patients and has slight pelvic deviation, while Group II has more curves and is more severe in quadriplegic patients with pelvic obliquity [46].

Pelvic obliquity is divided into two categories: supra-pelvic (spine/trunk disorder), pelvic or infra-pelvic (pelvic joint and lower limb) and its differentiation is important for diagnosis and treatment. Large thoracolumbar curves are seen in supra-pelvic obliquity and asymmetric contractions of the lower limbs in infra-pelvic obliquity, therefore, in addition to spinal deformity, hip contractures, leg length discrepancy, or a combination of these factors should also be considered in this section [48] (Fig. 5.7).

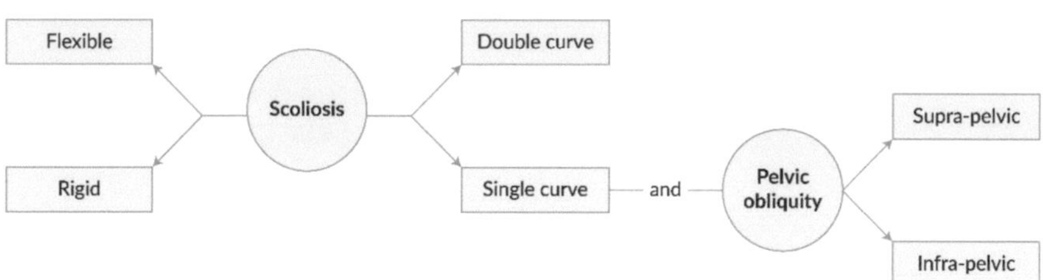

Fig. 5.7 Scoliosis classification

5.6.2 Core Stability

Examining core in CP patients is important because this factor plays a significant role in maintaining the spine, stabilizing the trunk, transferring force from the torso to the lower body and vice versa, and also other functional movements of the upper and lower limbs. By correcting Core stability, a great correction can be achieved in the child's movements. The core includes two groups of superficial and deep muscles, each of which has its own tests, but they overlap [49] (Table 5.8). Here, we mention one test for each group.

Abdominal drawing-in maneuver: This maneuver is used to evaluate the local/deep muscles of the core. In this test, we ask the patient to lie on all fours and contract the Transvers abdominis, internal abdominal oblique, and external abdominal oblique muscles by contracting the abdominal wall. The inability of a person to perform this maneuver indicates the weakness of these muscles. This test, also, is a correction exercise to strengthen the mentioned muscles and improve the stability of the core [50] (Fig. 5.8d).

Pelvic bridging test: In this test, the patient lies prone and flexes the knees completely so that the soles of the feet stick to the ground and are close to the buttock. Ask the patient to raise the hip as high as possible. The inability to perform this maneuver shows the weakness of the surface muscles of the core such as internal oblique, external oblique, erector spinae muscles, and gluteus maximus [49] (Fig. 5.8c).

The list of practical examination tests are presented in Fig. 5.9.

Table 5.8 Core muscles

Core	Inner muscles	Pelvic floor Transversus abdominis Internal Abdominal Obliques Multifidus Diaphragm Deep fibers of the psoas Deep hip rotators
	Outer muscles	Rectus abdominis External obliques Erector spinae Quadratus lumborum Hip muscle groups (Gluteal muscles)

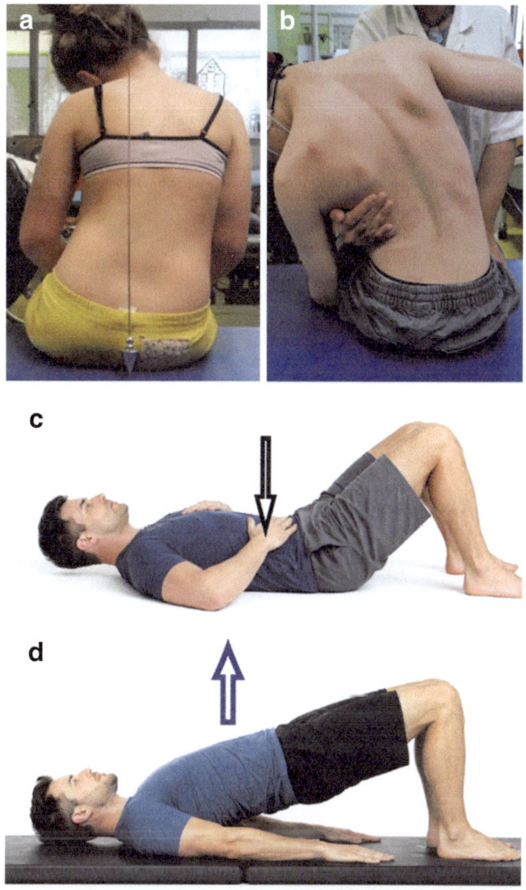

Fig. 5.8 (**a**, **b**) Axial Skeleton Examination, (**c**) Pelvic bridging test, (**d**) Abdominal drawing-in maneuver

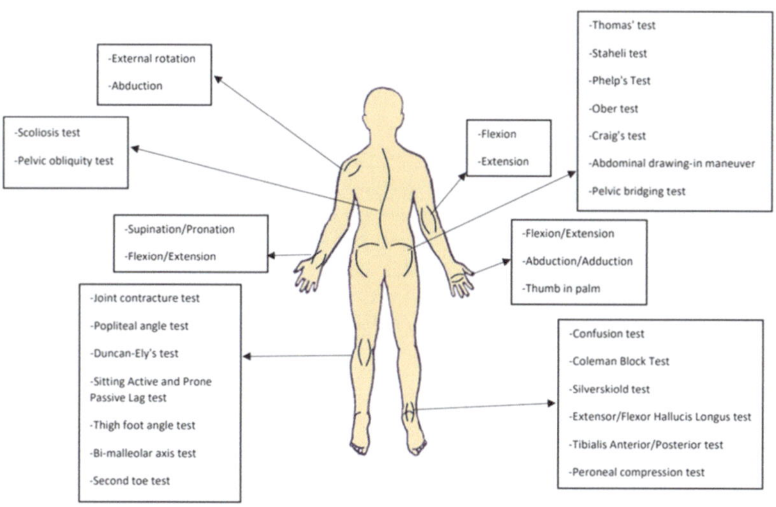

Fig. 5.9 Routine tests in CP

5.7 Analysis of Muscle Strength and Selective Motor Control

First, the general condition of the person, the involved organs, how to walk, and how to adapt to the disability should be considered.

Muscle strength and selective motor control are two indicators not only useful for evaluating the efficiency of surgical interventions but also necessary for providing assistant devices and activity recommendations. For this purpose, the Medical Research Council (MRC) grading system assigns six grades (0–5 scale) in relation to the maximum range of expectation for each muscle [24] (Table 5.9).

In patients with CP, with severe intellectual disability and poor comprehension, Kendall scale should be used manually. It consists of 10 scores as mentioned in Table 5.5. All these scores should be recorded to define the present condition of the patient precisely and compare in post-surgical follow-ups [25] (Table 5.10).

Table 5.9 Medical Research Council (MRC)

Grade	Description
0	Complete paralysis of the muscle
1	Flickering of contraction is detected
2	Able to move in absence of gravity
3	Able to move against gravity but cannot stand resistance
4	Able to move against resistance but not normal power
5	Normal power of the muscle

Table 5.10 Kendall scale

Score	Description
10	The child can hold test position against strong pressure
9	The child can hold test position against moderate-to-strong pressure
8	The child can hold test position against moderate pressure
7	The child can hold test position against slight-to-moderate pressure
6	The child can hold test position against slight pressure
5	The child cannot hold test position against any pressure
4	The child gradually release from test position
3	The child can hold against resistance through full ROM in absence of gravity or he/she can conduct less than 100% ROM against gravity
2	The child can move through full ROM in absence of gravity
1	The child can move through 100% ROM with reduced gravity
T	Just muscle contraction is visible or palpable
0	No muscle contraction is detected

Table 5.11 Muscle group selectivity scoring

Score	Description
0	Not able to move an isolated muscle /only patterned movement could be conducted
1	Able to move an isolated muscle partially
2	Able to move an isolated muscle completely

Selective voluntary motor control (SVMC) means that the child can activate each muscle separately in a selected pattern in response to the demands of a voluntary movement or position. Not having this ability is a sign of a forced joint activation of partner muscles to meet the needs of the patient. SVMC is essential for efficient movement and fine skill acquisition and can be used as a measurement tool for the outcome of subsequent interventions [51].

This scale could be used for each muscle as below (Table 5.11).

This index for the lower limb of spastic patients is measured more specifically under the title of *Selective Control Assessment of the Lower Extremity (SCALE)*. This tool is used to examine the hip, knee, ankle, subtalar and toe joints bilaterally, and according to the grading instructions, each test is recorded in the score sheet. To evaluate the selective voluntary motor control of each joint, a reciprocating movement (flex, extend, flex) different from the dominant movement pattern of that joint is selected. In order to facilitate the examination and comfort of the patient, examinations are evaluated in a sitting position and in the case of the hip joint in a lying position. Moving each joint separately, the ability to perform reciprocal movement, paying attention to involuntary movements in the opposite limb and other joints, and evaluating the speed and power of movement considering the full ROM of the joint are among the things that are considered in scoring [51].

First, the desired movement is passively performed on the patient at a speed of 3 s, and then he is asked to perform the same movement at a similar speed without additional movement in other parts of the body, and the patient is allowed to try it several times. In the hip examination, the examiner helps the child bear the weight of the limb without moving it, and the child flexes, extends, and flexes the hip again while the knee is extended. Flexion and extension of the hip joint with the knee flexed is an alternative test in cases of severe hamstring stiffness. In the continuation, the other four examinations are performed while sitting at a speed of 3 s. Each joint is given a score from 0 to 2 based on performance (Table 5.12). By summing the points obtained from the five mentioned movements, each lower limb gets a maximum SCALE score of 10 [51].

5.7.1 Spasticity vs Dystonia

There are two types of hypertonia in CP patients, and their differentiation is important in terms of diagnosis and treatment. First is spasticity, in which hypertonicity increases in resistance to passive movement with increasing speed. This increase in tone changes with the change of movement direction, and if the movement is

Table 5.12 SCALE scoring

Score	Condition	Description	Examinations	Left	Right
0	Disabled	The requested movement is not performed or significant synergy is observed in other muscles to perform the movement	1.Hip flexion and extension		
1	Impaired	Incomplete performance of the maneuver, i.e. performing only one-way movement, showing less than 50% ROM of passive movement, occurrence of additional movement in another joint and/or slow movement speed for more than 3 s	2.Knee extension and flexion		
			3.Ankle dorsiflexion and plantar flexion		
			4.Subtalar inversion and eversion		
			5.Toe flexion and extension		
2	Normal	Accurate performance of the maneuver without additional movement in other parts	Total SCALE score=	/10	/10

Table 5.13 Spasticity vs Dystonia

		Spasticity	Dystonia
1	Criteria	Increased resistant with increasing velocity of movement	Constant resistant with increasing velocity of movement
		Hyperreflexia, reflex overflow	No hyperreflexia, disappear with sleep
		Clonus, positive Babinski sign	Simultaneous agonist and antagonist contraction
2	Pathology	Pyramidal distribution weakness Extensors of upper extremity Flexors of lower extremity	Disruption of the basal ganglia
3	Treatment	Baclofen Botulinum toxin Selective dorsal rhizotomy Orthopedic surgery Resultant contractures Balancing of muscle/tendo forces	Intrathecal baclofen Botulinum toxin Limited orthopedic surgeries Split tendon transfers for bone surgery for lever arm dysfunctions Note: Selective dorsal rhizotomy is useless Tendon lengthening and transfer are contraindicated

performed at a speed higher than normal or outside the normal range of joint movement, it increases dramatically. Dystonia is the other type which meets persistent or intermittent involuntary contractions of muscles. These contractions cause twisting and repetitive movements and/or abnormal posture [4]. Table 5.13 shows the differences between these two types of hypertonicity for better differentiation. To determine the severity of spasticity, the *Ashworth scale* and the amount of contracture is used, which is mentioned in the relevant part [52]. To assess the severity of dystonia, the criterion *Burke-Fahn-Marsden Rating Scale* is introduced, the indices related to the limbs and trunk are explained in Table 5.14 in this tool [53].

Table 5.14 Modified Burke-Fahn-Marsden scale

<table>
<tr><th>Region</th><th>Provoking factor</th><th></th><th>Severity factor</th><th>weight</th><th>product</th><th colspan="2">Provoking factor:</th></tr>
<tr><td>Neck</td><td>0–4</td><td>×</td><td>0–4</td><td>0.5</td><td>0–8</td><td colspan="2" rowspan="6">0 = no dystonia at rest or with action
1 = dystonia on particular action
2 – dystonia on many actions
3 = dystonia on distant part of body or intermittently at rest
4 = dystonia present at rest</td></tr>
<tr><td>R arm</td><td>0–4</td><td>×</td><td>0–4</td><td>1.0</td><td>0–16</td></tr>
<tr><td>L arm</td><td>0–4</td><td>×</td><td>0–4</td><td>1.0</td><td>0–16</td></tr>
<tr><td>Trunk</td><td>0–4</td><td>×</td><td>0–4</td><td>1.0</td><td>0–16</td></tr>
<tr><td>R leg</td><td>0–4</td><td>×</td><td>0–4</td><td>1.0</td><td>0–16</td></tr>
<tr><td>L leg</td><td>0–4</td><td>×</td><td>0–4</td><td>1.0</td><td>0–16</td></tr>
<tr><td>Severity factor</td><td colspan="2">Neck:
0 = no dystonia present
1 = slight occasional pulling
2 = obvious torticollis but mild
3 = moderate pulling
4 = extreme pulling</td><td colspan="3">Arm:
0 = no dystonia present
1 = slight dystonia, clinically insignificant
2 = mild obvious dystonia but not disabling
3 = moderate, able to grasp, with some manual function
4 = severe, no useful grasp</td><td>Trunk:
0 = no dystonia present
1 = slight bending, clinically insignificant
2 = definite bending, but not interfering with standing or walking
3 = moderate bending, interfering with standing or walking
4 = extreme bending, preventing standing or walking</td><td>Leg:
0 = no dystonia present
1 = slight dystonia, but not causing impairment, clinically insignificant
2 = mild dystonia, walks briskly and unaided
3 = moderate dystonia, severely impairs walking or requires assistant
4 = severe, unable to stand or walk on involved leg</td></tr>
<tr><td colspan="8">Total modified Burke-Fahn-Marsden score= /88</td></tr>
</table>

5.8 Assessment of Muscle Tone

Resistance of muscle in relaxed state or passive stretch of muscle is defined as "Tone." Assessing muscle tone is important to distinguish spasticity and stiffness from dystonia or to diagnose a combination of these conditions. However, it is difficult to determine this condition in children with CP, from the point of view that following stress or excitement, muscle tone is more falsely shown, so it is important to check it in a safe and calm condition. In order to measure the tone, first the muscle contraction is felt in the resting state and then the limb is moved slowly so that the muscle is not involved and its resistance is compared with the previous state. Finally, the muscle tone is felt in passive movement with different speeds and the resistance of the body against the movement. For this purpose, the "Modified Ashworth scale" is provided [25].

Table 5.15 Modified Ashworth Scale

Score	Description
0	There is no increase in muscle tone during passive motion
1	There is slight increase in muscle tone during passive motion, detectable as a catch and release or at the end of the ROM
+1	There is slight increase in muscle tone during passive motion, detectable as a catch after which minimal resistance happens throughout less than half of the ROM.
2	There is more increase in muscle tone during the ROM, although motion is possible in high tone sections easily
3	There is significant increase in muscle tone and passive movement is difficult in high tone sections
4	There is constant rigidity in affected sections during flexion or extension

This test is designed to measure muscle resistance, which is done manually during passive stretching. In modified Ashworth scale, the speed of the test is important because it affects spasticity, so it is suggested that the entire examination be performed in the same way at a speed of 3 s and in the full range of motion [54]. The scoring is as follows (Table 5.15).

5.9 Joint Range of Motion (ROM)

ROM also indirectly indicates muscle length and gives a good estimate of joint contracture, so measuring this parameter with a manual goniometer could be valuable in CP's clinical exam, both statically and dynamically [54].

5.10 Balance

Finally, in order to register a general evaluation about the child's motor control and the compensatory mechanisms of the body, it is necessary to carry out a detailed analysis of the patient's balance at all levels by examining the trunk position, body balance, pelvis, and lower limb position while sitting, standing, and walking [49].

For sitting balance investigation, *Trunk Control Measurement Scale (TCMS)* is used. For this purpose, the child puts aside all accessories, such as orthotics, shoes, or body braces, and sits on the edge of the treatment table without support. The thighs are completely in contact with the table and the hands are placed on the legs. First, the most vertical position of the patient is recorded and considered as the base position. Balance items according to Table 5.16, each one is done three times, and the best performance is recorded. If the child is young, support is done only with one hand to maintain balance [55].

Total TCMS scores in patients with different age groups, topographies, and GMFCS are very different. But the median subscale of this parameter in children aged 8–15 years is defined as an average of 38.5 out of 58 (18 out of 20 for static sitting balance, 16 out of 28 for dynamic sitting balance, and 6 out of 10 for dynamic

Table 5.16 Trunk Control Measurement Scale check list

STATIC SITTING BALANCE
Explain verbally or demonstrate if needed

Item		Score	Bilat/ left	Right
1	**Sit upright and hold this position for 10 s** If score = 0, then total score = 0	Patient falls or can only maintain upright sitting with double arm support	☐0	
		Patient can only maintain upright sitting with single arm support for 10 s	☐1	
		Patient can maintain upright sitting without arm support for 10 s	☐2	
2	**Lift both arms at eye level in 1 s and return**	Patient falls or cannot lift arms	☐0	
		Patient can lift arms but with compensations (backward lean, increase of trunk flexion, lateral flexion, other)	☐1	
		Patient lifts arms without compensations	☐2	
3	**Therapist crosses one leg over the other**	Patient falls, cannot cross legs or can only maintain sitting with double arm support	☐0	☐0
		Patient can maintain sitting with single arm support for 10 s	☐1	☐1
		Patient can maintain sitting without arm support for 10 s	☐2	☐2
4	**Patient crosses one leg over the other (assistance with one hand is allowed)** ***'Minimal'*** *= small trunk movements* *Without signs of imbalance of trunk* *During movement of leg.* ***'Clear'*** *= clear signs of imbalance* i.e. *Lateral flexion or flexion of trunk*	Patient falls, cannot cross legs or can only cross legs with double arm support	☐0	☐0
		Patient can only cross legs with single arm support	☐1	☐1
		Patient crosses legs without arm support but with clear trunk displacement	☐2	☐2
		Patient crosses legs with minimal trunk displacement	☐3	☐3

(continued)

Table 5.16 (continued)

STATIC SITTING BALANCE Explain verbally or demonstrate if needed					
5	**Patient abducts one leg over 10 cm and returns to starting position** *(10 cm width = width of the knee)*		Patient falls, cannot abduct leg or can only abduct leg with double arm support	□0	□0
			Patient can only abduct leg with single arm support	□1	□1
			Patient abducts leg without arm support but with clear trunk displacement	□2	□2
			Patient abducts leg with minimal trunk displacement	□3	□3
Total static sitting balance score=				**/20**	
DYNAMIC SITTING BALANCE (Selective movement control) **1. Explain verbally or demonstrate the item 2. Demonstrated on the patient with manual guidance 3. Asked the patient to perform the item under manual guidance, then start.**					
6	**Lean forward with a fixed trunk for approximately 45° and return** (arms crossed over chest) Normal righting reaction of the head is needed but limited head extension is not scored as a compensation	a	Patient falls or cannot reach target position	□0	
			Patient can lean forward (If score = 0, then item 6b = 0)	□1	
		b	Patient compensates (increased head extension, increased trunk flexion, increased lumbar lordosis, increased knee flexion, other)	□0	
			Patient leans forward without compensations	□1	
7	**Lean backward with a fixed trunk for approximately 45° and return** (arms crossed over chest)	a	Patient falls or cannot reach target position	□0	
			Patient can lean backward (If score = 0, then item 7b = 0)	□1	
		b	Patient compensates (increased head flexion, increased trunk flexion, increased knee extension, other)	□0	
			Patient leans backward without compensations	□1	

(continued)

Table 5.16 (continued)

STATIC SITTING BALANCE Explain verbally or demonstrate if needed					
8	**Touch the table with the elbow at level of the femoral head (by shortening the ipsilateral side and lengthening the contralateral side) and return**	a	Patient falls or does not touch the table with the elbow	□0	□0
			Patient can touch the table with the elbow *(If score = 0, then item 8b and 8c = 0)*	□1	□1
		b	Patient demonstrates (no shortening/lengthening, opposite shortening/lengthening)	□0	□0
			Patient demonstrates expected shortening/lengthening (If score = 0, then item 8c = 0)	□1	□1
		c	Patient compensates (increased trunk flexion, forward or backward lean, pelvic lift, other	□0	□0
			Patient touches the table without compensations	□1	□1
9	**Lift the pelvis at one side and return** No lifting of the thigh is allowed.	a	Patient falls or cannot lift the pelvis	□0	□0
			Patient can lift the pelvis (If score = 0, then item 9b and 9c = 0)	□1	□1
		b	Patient demonstrates no shortening/lengthening	□0	□0
			Patient demonstrates partially expected shortening/lengthening (partial = short and/or small ROM)	□1	□1
			Patient demonstrates expected shortening/lengthening (If score = 0, then item 9c = 0)	□2	□2
		c	Patient compensates (contralateral head flexion, marked lateral trunk displacement, other)	□0	□0
			Patient lifts the pelvis without compensations	□1	□1

(continued)

Table 5.16 (continued)

STATIC SITTING BALANCE Explain verbally or demonstrate if needed					
10	**Rotate the upper trunk three times with head fixated** (arms crossed over chest) **Note:** The movement is initiated from the shoulder Girdle. *Partial = asymmetrical, small ROM, more shoulders than trunk*	a	Patient falls/cannot rotate the upper trunk (patient can not perform the rotation movement, even not with the entire trunk)/ demonstrates no selective rotation of the upper trunk	□0	
			Patient demonstrates partial selective rotation of the upper trunk	□1	
			Patient demonstrates expected selective rotation of the upper trunk (If score = 0, then item 10b = 0)	□2	
		b	Patient rotates the upper trunk with head rotation	□0	
			Patient rotates the upper trunk without head rotation	□1	
11	**Rotate the lower trunk three times with head fixated** (arms crossed over chest) **Note:** The movement is initiated from the pelvic Girdle.	a	Patient falls/ cannot rotate the lower trunk (patient can not perform the rotation movement, even not with the entire trunk)/ demonstrates no selective rotation of the lower trunk	□0	
			Patient demonstrates partial selective rotation of the lower trunk	□1	
			Patient demonstrates expected selective rotation of the lower trunk (If score = 0, then item 11b = 0)	□2	
		b	Patient compensates with pelvic tilt	□0	
			Patient rotates the lower trunk without compensations	□1	

(continued)

Table 5.16 (continued)

STATIC SITTING BALANCE Explain verbally or demonstrate if needed					
12	**Shuffle the pelvis three times in a forward direction and return backwards in three times** (arms crossed over chest) **Shuffle movement** = combination of lateral flexion and rotation with the pelvis, alternated left and right *Partial = with mainly lateral flexion and little rotation; small ROM; takes a lot of effort*	a	Patient falls or cannot shuffle the pelvis in forward and backward direction i.e. no displacement of the body in either direction	□0	
			Patient can partially shuffle the pelvis	□1	
			Patient can shuffle the pelvis by use of both lateral flexion and rotation in one direction and partially in the other direction	□2	
			Patient can shuffle the pelvis by use of both lateral flexion and rotation in both directions	□3	
		b	Patient compensates with excessive trunk displacement	□0	
			Patient shuffles pelvis without compensations	□1	
Total selective movement control=				**/28**	
Dynamic reaching (equilibrium reactions) **Explain verbally then patient perform three times.**					
13	**Reach forward with both arms straight to target at eye level positioned at a distance, corresponding with the forearm length and return** (arms straight forward)		Patient falls or cannot reach target	□0	
			Patient reaches target, but has difficulties in performance. *(difficulties = takes a lot of effort,* i.e., *slow and with difficulty/ uses some support of hand when approaching the starting position)*	□1	
			Patient reaches target and returns to starting position without difficulties	□2	
14	**Reach sideward with one arm straight to target at eye level positioned at a distance, corresponding with the forearm length and return** (one arm straight sideward and other hand on leg)		Patient falls or cannot reach target	□0	□0
			Patient reaches target, but has difficulties in performance.	□1	□1
			Patient reaches target and returns to starting position without difficulties	□2	□2
15	**Reach across the midline with one arm (the opposite side) and return** (one arm straight sideward and other hand on leg) *The target is positioned at eye level at a distance corresponding with half the forearm length of the reaching arm.*		Patient falls or cannot reach target	□0	□0
			Patient reaches target but has difficulty in performance.	□1	□1
			Patient reaches target and returns to starting position without difficulties	□2	□2
Total dynamic reaching=				**/10**	
TOTAL TCMS score =				**/58**	

Table 5.17 Time up and go scoring

Timing	Description
<10 s	The patient is completely independent for the daily activities, with or without walking aid. The balance is in normal range.
<20 s	The patient is independent for main transfers, with or without walking aid. He/she could manage his/her daily activities carefully. The balance is acceptable.
<30 s	The patient is dependent in most activities and requires assistance for his/her daily activities. The balance is poor.

reaching). This index is useful for checking the progress of the child in annual examinations, as well as evaluating the efficiency of the surgery, comparing the score before and after the surgery [55, 56].

Time up and go test (TUG) is used to evaluate CP patients' balance while standing and walking. This test can be used for ages 3–12, provided the child understands the instructions. Time up and go is understandable for most people, and by integrating transitions and walking skills can provide a reliable assessment of children's functional mobility. To start the test, we should determine a 3-meter path free from any obstruction and place a chair with arms at one end of the path for support if needed. First explain the procedure for the child and ask him/her to stand up from chair, walk to the mark on floor, turn around, walk back to chair, and sit down as soon as you said start. Reassure that the patient understood the instruction and use a stopwatch for timing [57, 58].

The results are construed as below (Table 5.17).

5.11 Imaging

Considering the many and sometimes hidden deformities that exist in CP patients, it is very important to take images of the damaged and healthy limbs to compare and evaluate the spine in terms of scoliosis and other deviations. For this purpose, simple X-ray is the best option for initial examination, and more specialized imaging is chosen accordingly. In this section, we mention the imaging and practical views of each part [59].

5.11.1 Hip

Since hip abnormalities are common in children with CP, an AP pelvic X-ray is recommended to evaluate hip displacement and dislocation. To determine the migration percentage, Hilgenreiner's line, Perkins' line, and their parallel lines are drawn following standard guidelines and Reimers Index is calculated [26].

First, Hilgenreiner's line is drawn horizontally through the upper part of the hip cartilage (or the inferior points of the acetabular teardrops in mature children). Perkins' line is then drawn perpendicular to Hilgenreiner's line at the lateral edge of the acetabulum. Two additional parallel lines are drawn along the inner and outer

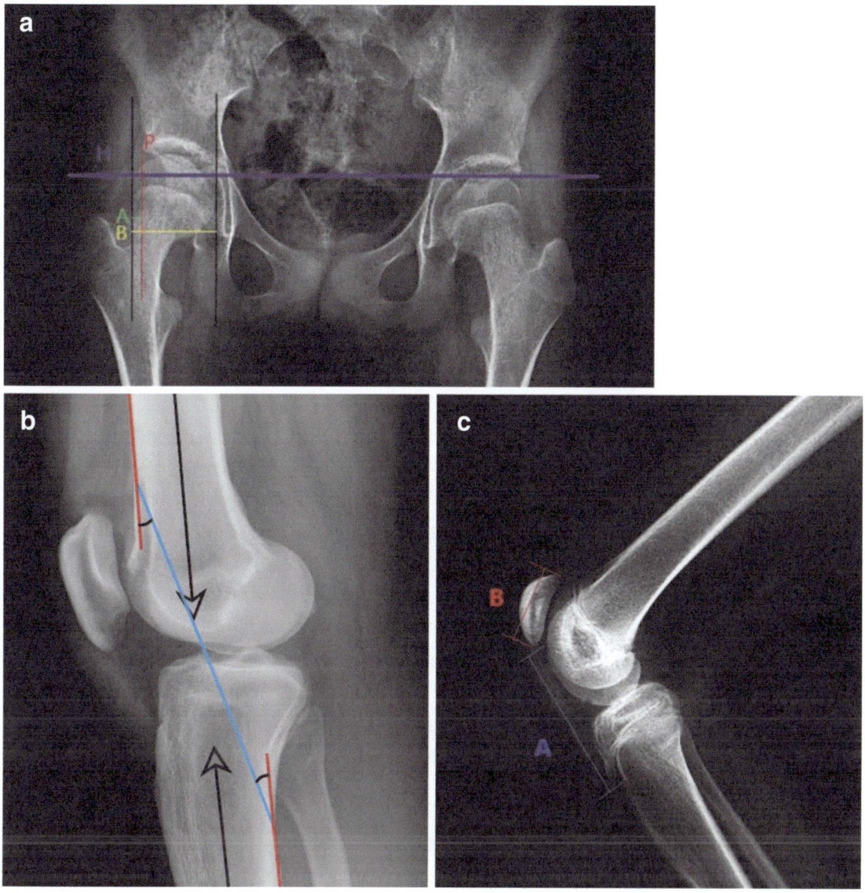

Fig. 5.10 (**a**) Hilgenreiner's line (H), Perkin's line (P), (**b**) Maximum extension lateral knee, (**c**) line Insall-Salvati Index

edges of the femoral head. The width of the femoral head (B) and the distance from Perkins' line to the outer edge of the femoral head (A) are measured, and the migration percentage is calculated as (A/B) × 100%.

A migration percentage of less than 33% is considered normal or mild displacement; 33–50% indicates moderate displacement, and over 50% represents severe displacement, often requiring surgical intervention.

Reimers index offers several advantages over other measurements like the Center-Edge Angle (CEA) or Acetabular Index (AI). It provides a direct measurement of femoral head coverage and better reflects hip stability in children with CP. This method is simpler, more reliable in neurological conditions, and widely validated for monitoring hip displacement, facilitating consistent communication and comparison across studies and clinical settings [59, 60] (Fig. 5.10a).

5.11.2 Knee

To evaluate knee deformities, three views are used as follows:

AP view: standard view for general evaluation of the knee joint [59].
Sunrise view: used in suspected cases of subluxation or dislocation of patella or patellar maltracking [59].
30° lateral view: used in suspected cases of inferior patellar pole fractures or superior displacement of the patella within the trochlear groove of the femur, which is called patella alta [59].

There are several criteria to evaluate the patella alta, here we will mention the Insall-Salvati Index. This index measures the ratio of the length of the patellar tendon to the length of the patella by considering the length of the patellar tendon from the inferior pole of the patella to the tibial tubercle and measuring the length of the patellar from the superior pole to the inferior pole. Then divide the length of the patellar tendon by the length of the patella. The normal range of this index is 0.74–1.5. If ISI is more than 1.5, it is considered patella alta [28, 59] (Fig. 5.10c).

Maximum extension lateral knee view is used to measure the amount of contracture in cases of crouch gait or knee flexion contractures. This imaging view should be done with the patient's cooperation in extending the knee as much as possible or with the help of another person in this movement during imaging. In this view, the angle between the tangent line on the anterior femoral cortex and the tangent line on the posterior tibial cortex is measured, or the angle between the mid-diaphysis of the femur and the mid-diaphysis of the tibia is considered [59] (Fig. 5.10b).

5.11.3 Ankle

In this part, the imaging is to investigate the cause of the pain, confirm the findings of the examination, and evaluate the corrective surgery. AP and lateral views are generally performed and oblique, mortis, and weight-bearing AP views are performed in cases of ankle valgus, distal tibia malalignment, and equinus. For each view, indicators for pediatric foot alignment have been defined, and here we will discuss the practical ones [28, 59].

Weight-bearing AP view: In this view, the talo-first metatarsal angle with a range of 10° ± 7° is considered to evaluate the forefoot alignment (Fig. 5.11f), and the talocalcaneal angle with a range of 10°–56° is used to check the hindfoot alignment (Fig. 5.11d). Although this indicator cannot be measured accurately and reliably. The amount of coverage of the talar head by the navicular is one of the other cases that should be manifested as lateral subluxation in valgus foot deformities and medial subluxation of the navicular on the head of the talus in varus deformities. The normal range of talonavicular coverage angle is 20° ± 9.8° [59] (Fig. 5.11e).

Lateral view: In this view, the lateral talocalcaneal angle is evaluated to check hindfoot deviations, so that its normal range is 49° ± 6.9°, an angle greater than that indicates valgus hindfoot and less than that indicates varus hindfoot. The lateral talus-first metatarsal angle is used to evaluate the midfoot. The normal range of this index is 13° ± 7.5°. To determine the intensity of planus and cavus of the ankle, it is helpful to pay attention to this index, so that the first metatarsal dorsiflex position is considered positive, and the larger the angle, the more midfoot planus, and vice versa, the first metatarsal plantar flexion position is negative and indicates midfoot cavus [59] (Fig. 5.11c).

The next important index in this view is the tibiocalcaneal angle, the normal range of which is 69° ± 8.4°, its higher values are found in equinus and other plantarflexion deformities, and lower values are seen in calcaneus and other dorsiflexion deformities (Fig. 5.11a). The calcaneal pitch index also has a function similar to the tibiocalcaneal angle with a normal range of 39° ± 7° [59] (Fig. 5.11b).

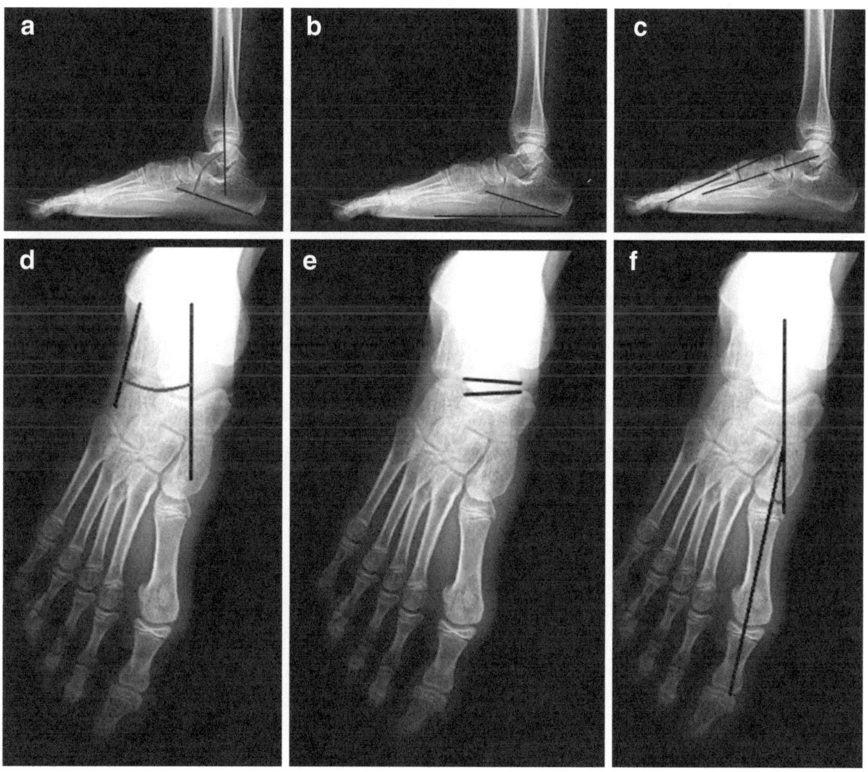

Fig. 5.11 (**a**) Tibiocalcaneal angle, (**b**) Calcaneal pitch, (**c**) Lateral talus-first metatarsal angle, (**d**) Talocalcaneal angle, (**e**) Talonavicular coverage angle, (**f**) Talo-first metatarsal angle

There are some other additional views used for malalignments in CP patients. Teleogram is a view that shows all three joints of the hip, knee, and ankle on both sides in one film, and it is used in cases of leg length inequality [59].

For coronal deformities, orthoroentgenography or scanogram, which adds a ruler next to the graphs of the three pelvic joints, gives the doctor the ability to assess valgus and varus and determine their severity by drawing a line called mechanical axis from the center of the femoral head to the center of the ankle joint. If the mechanical axis passes through the outer third of the knee joint, it is considered valgus alignment and if it passes through the inner third of the knee, it is considered varus alignment [59].

5.12 Spine

Confirmation of any pathological findings in the examination of the spine is with radiography. For this purpose, a simple posteroanterior and lateral view is recommended while standing and if not possible, sitting. It is more accurate to use a standardized sitting frame with side supporting strips for imaging with the least external force [46]. It is helpful to use supine bending and traction films while enforcing manual traction to check the flexibility of the spine. Since the degree of deviation is essential in its pathological definition, it is necessary to use the Cobb method in the interpretation of graphs. In this method, first, we select the upper axis of the deviated spine and draw an intersecting perpendicular line on it, then draw another similar line on the lower axis and measure the angle of the intersection of the two lines (Fig. 5.12a). A curvature of more than 10° in the posteroanterior view is considered as scoliosis, and in the sagittal view, according to the normal lordosis in the cervical and lumbar section and normal kyphosis in the thorax, a curvature of more than 50° is considered abnormal kyphosis or lordosis [45, 59] (Fig. 5.12b).

5.12.1 Computed Tomography (CT)

CT can be a valuable imaging modality in children with cerebral palsy (CP), particularly when detailed visualization of joints and bones is needed. However, due to its high radiation exposure, it is not routinely recommended unless challenging abnormalities cannot be identified through plain radiographs or clinical examination [59]. For preoperative planning, CT offers cross-sectional images of key anatomical landmarks—including the femoral neck, femoral condyles, tibial plateau, and ankle—allowing for precise rotational measurements [61]. Femoral rotation is typically assessed by calculating the angle between a line parallel to the femoral neck and another along the posterior femoral condyles. Similarly, tibial rotation is measured using the angle formed between a line parallel to the tibial plateau and a line connecting the posterior aspects of the medial and lateral malleoli. In the context of spastic hip dysplasia (SHD), a common and disabling complication in CP, CT is essential for measuring femoral anteversion and guiding surgical planning.

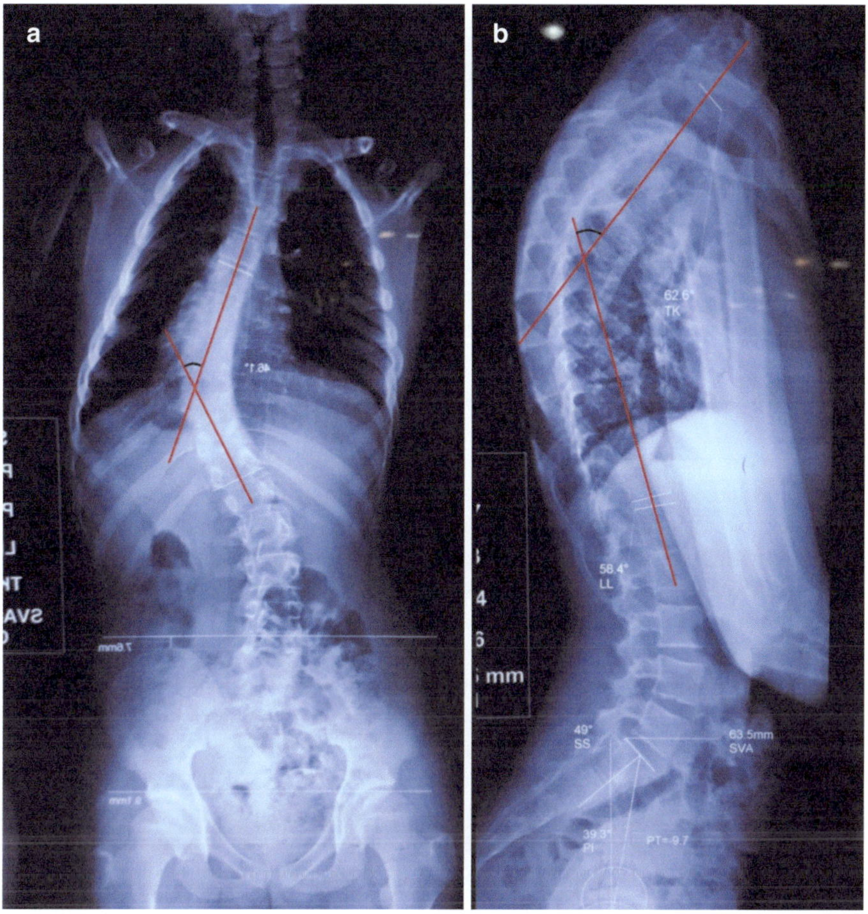

Fig. 5.12 (**a**) AP Spine—Cobb method, (**b**) Lateral spine

Additionally, CT may be indicated when conventional imaging is inconclusive or when prior surgical hardware limits the utility of MRI due to metal artifact [62, 63].

Three-dimensional (3D) CT reconstruction has significantly improved the ability to assess bone geometry in children with CP, addressing many of the limitations associated with traditional two-dimensional imaging. Notably, 3D CT enables direct measurement of femoral anteversion, even in cases with complex flexion, adduction, or rotational contractures—common in advanced stages of CP. This method offers high intraobserver and interobserver reliability and accuracy, regardless of femoral neck-shaft angle or non-anatomic limb positioning, which is often altered by spastic contractures. Such precision is critical in preoperative planning, as misjudgment of rotational deformities can lead to inadequate correction, recurrence, or increased surgical morbidity. Moreover, 3D CT provides valuable cross-sectional detail in evaluating acetabular morphology, including orientation, depth, and femoral head containment—information that is essential when planning corrective osteotomies [62, 64]. It is equally useful in the assessment of complex spinal deformities, allowing for detailed evaluation of fusion status, hardware positioning, and subtle structural anomalies. While CT is used less frequently than MRI for the initial diagnostic workup of CP—due to MRI's superior sensitivity for detecting brain malformations and white matter injury—it maintains a crucial role in specific orthopedic contexts [65]. In particular, CT is a highly effective tool for postoperative evaluation of reconstructive hip surgeries, such as Dega osteotomy, enabling detailed assessment of joint congruity, graft positioning, acetabular containment, and union status in remodeled or previously incongruent joints [62].

5.12.2 Magnetic Resonance Imaging (MRI)

Brain MRI is recommended as the first-line neuroimaging modality for children with suspected or confirmed CP, owing to its superior sensitivity in detecting a wide range of brain abnormalities. Over 80% of children with CP exhibit abnormal MRI findings, which often reveal the underlying neurological insult or malformation responsible for both motor and orthopedic impairments [66]. In the orthopedic context, MRI plays a crucial role in elucidating the etiology of motor dysfunction, characterizing the extent and nature of brain injuries—such as periventricular leukomalacia, white matter damage, or cortical-subcortical lesions—and supporting accurate CP classification. It also assists in identifying candidates for surgical interventions and stratifying the risk of musculoskeletal complications, especially in scoliosis. Additionally, MRI is indicated in cases presenting with atypical features, progressive symptoms, or when metabolic or genetic causes are suspected—particularly when clinical findings do not align with common CP patterns or known perinatal risk factors are absent [67, 68]. Functional MRI has also begun to reveal altered cortical activation and patterns of neuroplasticity in CP, offering promising applications in individualized orthopedic treatment planning and postoperative evaluation [66].

5.12.3 Ultrasonography

ultrasonography can assist orthopedics in CP management in monitoring hip displacement, subluxation, or dysplasia—complications that are more prevalent in children with severe gross motor impairment. Evidence supports that structured hip surveillance programs incorporating regular imaging are associated with improved long-term joint outcomes and reduced risk of progressive deformities [65, 69].

Furthermore, musculoskeletal ultrasound enables real-time evaluation of muscle and tendon structures, facilitating the detection of spasticity-related contractures, muscle atrophy, and altered muscle architecture—although ultrasound has high reliability and validity in evaluating the CP muscle architecture, but this is mainly supported by moderate and limited levels of evidence [70].

Another important application of ultrasound is in neonatal and early pediatric care, where trans-fontanellar ultrasound remains valuable for detecting central nervous system lesions and predicting future orthopedic risks. Abnormal findings—such as parenchymal cysts or echodensities in preterm infants—are closely associated with the later development of specific CP subtypes and related musculoskeletal complications. This supports early risk stratification and proactive orthopedic follow-up. Ultrasound is especially well-suited for repeated use in growing children and for point-of-care assessments in patients with limited mobility or medical fragility [71].

Its non-invasive nature and ease of repeatability make it ideal for ongoing monitoring, as recommended in structured hip surveillance and bone health programs. For instance, early detection of hip migration through ultrasound enables timely non-surgical interventions—such as BT injections or orthotic bracing—or early surgical referral, which can significantly improve functional outcomes and quality of life [72]. In addition, ultrasonography is a valuable tool in both the planning and follow-up of orthopedic procedures. It assists in guiding BT injections, informing decisions on tenotomy or tendon transfers, and monitoring post-procedural muscle morphology and joint alignment. Compared to conventional radiographs, ultrasound offers superior sensitivity in detecting subtle joint effusions and early subluxation, and it can typically be performed without the need for sedation, making it especially advantageous in younger pediatric populations [70].

5.12.4 Data Collection

Systematic data archiving and longitudinal follow-up are foundational to high-quality orthopedic management in children with CP, a condition marked by considerable variability in motor function and orthopedic complications over the lifespan [73]. Long-term data collection enables clinicians and researchers to monitor disease progression, evaluate treatment outcomes, and refine clinical decision-making in a dynamic and individualized manner [10]. Exemplifying this model is the Swedish Cerebral Palsy Follow-up Program (CPUP), widely regarded as a benchmark for comprehensive national surveillance. The CPUP integrates annual multidisciplinary evaluations—including orthopedic, physiotherapy, and occupational therapy assessments—with radiographic hip surveillance and records of interventions, supported by six evidence-based quality indicators [74]. Similar registry frameworks exist in Sweden and Australia, all of which increasingly utilize digital platforms to support data entry, sharing, and analysis [65]. Clinical gait analysis laboratories also contribute valuable biomechanical data, directly influencing surgical planning and serving as a resource for institutional benchmarking and retrospective research [38]. The strategic benefits of meticulous data archiving are numerous: it facilitates benchmarking and quality assurance through comparative outcome analyses, enhances the refinement of clinical algorithms based on longitudinal intervention data, and supports early detection of complications such as hip migration, enabling timely preventive measures [74]. Moreover, archived data contribute to research and innovation, underpinning epidemiological studies, outcome evaluations, predictive modeling, and multicenter clinical trials. Importantly, such data systems also promote patient- and family-centered care by allowing for individualized goal setting, personalized prognostic counseling, and alignment with frameworks such as the "six Fs" (function, family, fitness, fun, friends, future) [75]. Finally, these registries provide critical insights for healthcare policy, enabling informed resource allocation and service planning. In sum, data archiving and longitudinal tracking are essential pillars of modern CP orthopedic care, advancing both clinical excellence and ongoing improvement through evidence-based practice [15].

We provided two checklists for examination and classification of orthopedic information of the CP patients which facilitate case presentation, choosing treatment, comparing outcomes before and after intervention, and data collection for future research (Figs. 5.13 and 5.14).

5.12.5 Promoting Economic Efficiency

The importance of economic considerations in the orthopedic management of CP is increasingly acknowledged, reflecting the disorder's lifelong nature and the complexity of interventions required to optimize function, prevent complications, and enhance quality of life [52]. As the most common cause of severe physical disability in childhood, CP often necessitates long-term orthopedic care, including surgical procedures, orthotic support, spasticity management (such as BT injections), physiotherapy, and participation in structured surveillance programs. These comprehensive care needs result in significant cumulative resource demands over the patient's lifetime, highlighting the critical need for cost-effective and sustainable approaches in both clinical and policy contexts. Emerging research emphasizes that the economic burden of CP extends beyond direct medical costs—such as hospitalizations, interventions, and specialized equipment—to include substantial indirect costs. These may involve lost caregiver productivity, out-of-pocket expenditures, and psychosocial stressors that impact family well-being [76]. For instance, a study in Malaysia estimated the annual cost for a family caring for a child with CP at nearly RM30,000, reflecting a combination of healthcare, developmental, and non-medical expenses. Such findings illustrate the considerable financial strain placed on families and underscore the broader societal and economic impact of CP, reinforcing the imperative for equitable funding models and resource allocation strategies that support long-term, multidisciplinary care [77].

Achieving economic efficiency in the orthopedic management of CP has become a growing priority, with recent literature advocating for systematic cost-effectiveness analyses and value-based decision-making. Health technology assessments are increasingly used to compare the economic and clinical impact of various interventions—such as surgical versus non-surgical approaches, orthotic options, or BT injections—guiding resource allocation toward strategies with the greatest functional benefit per unit cost [76]. Early identification and

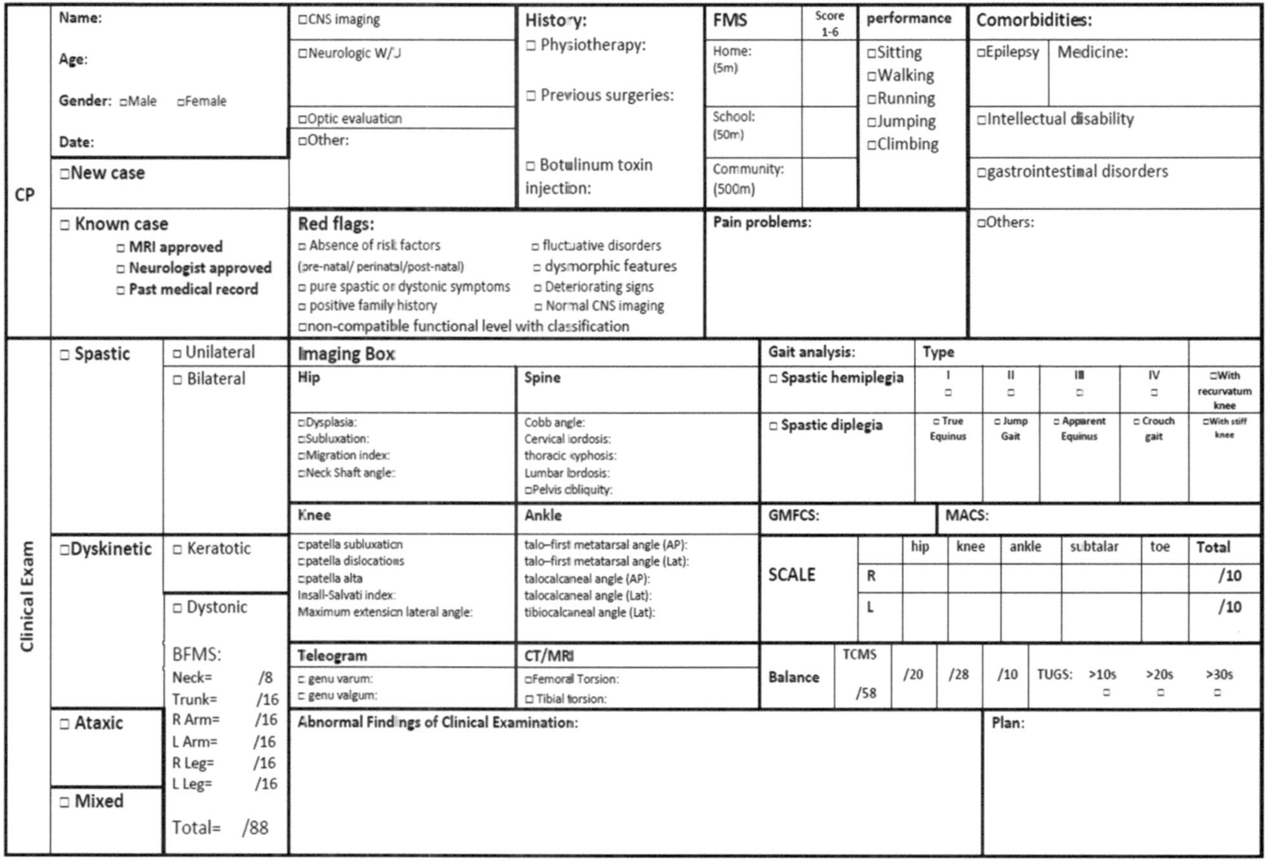

CP

Name:
Age:
Gender: □Male □Female
Date:
□New case
□ Known case
□ MRI approved
□ Neurologist approved
□ Past medical record

□CNS imaging
□Neurologic W/U
□Optic evaluation
□Other:

History:
□ Physiotherapy:
□ Previous surgeries:
□ Botulinum toxin injection:

FMS	Score 1-6
Home: (5m)	
School: (50m)	
Community: (500m)	

performance
□Sitting
□Walking
□Running
□Jumping
□Climbing

Comorbidities:
□Epilepsy
Medicine:
□Intellectual disability
□gastrointestinal disorders
□Others:

Red flags:
□ Absence of risk factors (pre-natal/ perinatal/post-natal)
□ pure spastic or dystonic symptoms
□ positive family history
□ fluctuative disorders
□ dysmorphic features
□ Deteriorating signs
□ Normal CNS imaging
□non-compatible functional level with classification

Pain problems:

Clinical Exam

□ Spastic
□ Unilateral
□ Bilateral
□Dyskinetic
□ Keratotic
□ Dystonic
□ Ataxic
□ Mixed

BFMS:
Neck= /8
Trunk= /16
R Arm= /16
L Arm= /16
R Leg= /16
L Leg= /16
Total= /88

Imaging Box

Hip
□Dysplasia:
□Subluxation:
□Migration index:
□Neck Shaft angle:

Spine
Cobb angle:
Cervical lordosis:
thoracic kyphosis:
Lumbar lordosis:
□Pelvis obliquity:

Knee
□patella subluxation
□patella dislocations
□patella alta
Insall-Salvati index:
Maximum extension lateral angle:

Ankle
talo–first metatarsal angle (AP):
talo–first metatarsal angle (Lat):
talocalcaneal angle (AP):
talocalcaneal angle (Lat):
tibiocalcaneal angle (Lat):

Teleogram
□ genu varum:
□ genu valgum:

CT/MRI
□Femoral Torsion:
□ Tibial torsion:

Gait analysis:	Type				
□ Spastic hemiplegia	I □	II □	III □	IV □	□With recurvatum knee
□ Spastic diplegia	□ True Equinus	□ Jump Gait	□ Apparent Equinus	□ Crouch gait	□With stiff knee

GMFCS:
MACS:

SCALE		hip	knee	ankle	subtalar	toe	Total
	R						/10
	L						/10

Balance	TCMS /58	/20	/28	/10	TUGS:	>10s □	>20s □	>30s □

Abnormal Findings of Clinical Examination:

Plan:

Fig. 5.13 CP information check list

Name: Gender: □male □female Age: **Cerebral Palsy Examination Checklist** Date:

Hip		Right					Left				
		Range of motion		Selectivity	Strength	Tone	Range of motion		Selectivity	Strength	Tone
		Passive	Active		MRC/Kendall	Ashworth	Passive	Active		MRC/Kendall	Ashworth
Flexion											
Extension											
Abduction											
Adduction											
Int Rotation											
Ext Rotation											
Thomas test											
Duncan-Ely's test											
Ober test											
Phlep's test	Knee 0										
	Knee90										
Knee		Right					Left				
Flexion											
Extension											
Popliteal angle											
Patella alta											
Extension lag		Active:		Passive:			Active:		Passive:		
TF angle											
Ankle		Right					Left				
Dorsiflexion	Knee0										
	Knee90										
plantarflexion											
Inversion											
Eversion											
Ext Hallucis Longus											
Flex hallucis longus											
Tibialis Anterior											
Tibialis Posterior											
Confusion test											
Colman test											
Peroneal compression test											
Shoulder		Right					Left				
Flexion											
Extension											
Adduction											
Abduction											
Rotation											
Elbow		Right					Left				
Flexion											
Extension											
Supination											
Pronation											
Wrist		Right					Left				
Flexion											
Extension											
Thumb in palm											
Phalanx		Right					Left				
Flexion											
extension											
Swan neck											
Interlocking fingers											
Axial Skeleton	□Kyphosis □Lordosis □Scoliosis (□flexible □Rigid) □Pelvic obliquity (□Supra-pelvic □Infra-pelvic)										
Core Stability	Abdominal drawing-in maneuver: Pelvic bridging test: Standing Posture:										

Fig. 5.14 CP examination Check list

structured surveillance programs, like the Danish CPUP and other registries, exemplify cost-efficient models that detect orthopedic complications such as hip dysplasia, contractures, and scoliosis at a stage when less invasive and less costly interventions are effective [74]. These prevention-focused strategies not only improve outcomes and delay the need for complex surgeries but also reduce long-term healthcare expenditures [78]. Likewise, the use of advanced technologies such as three-dimensional gait analysis enables individualized treatment planning, optimizing surgical decision-making, avoiding unnecessary procedures, and enhancing the cost-benefit profile of orthopedic care. Integrating standardized outcome classification systems such as GMFCS further supports risk stratification and efficient resource prioritization [79].

In addition, economic value can be realized through the thoughtful optimization of non-surgical interventions. Effective use of orthoses and BT injections has been shown to improve mobility, reduce spasticity, and delay major surgeries when combined with physiotherapy and regular follow-up [78]. Customization of orthotic devices based on clinical need and economic impact enhances treatment outcomes while minimizing waste [76]. Broader policy considerations are equally vital: economic strategies must also account for indirect costs borne by families, including lost productivity and psychosocial burdens. Incorporating family-centered metrics and quality-of-life outcomes into economic evaluations helps ensure that resource allocation not only improves clinical care but also promotes equity, accessibility, and long-term sustainability in CP management [79].

5.13 Goals of Treatment

When evaluating children with CP, the ultimate goal is to reduce disability and enhance independence, enabling greater participation in daily life and society. Early intervention is crucial to address developing complications such as contractures, joint subluxation, bone torsion, and spinal deformities like scoliosis before they become fixed and functionally limiting [80, 81]. Management also targets pain relief, improved hygiene, and ease of caregiving—especially in the context of spasticity or postoperative discomfort. Achieving a satisfactory goal requires a thorough understanding of the different types of motor impairments [82]. Primary impairments are directly related to central nervous system damage and are present from the onset. These include abnormalities in muscle tone and strength, poor balance, and selective motor control deficits. Orthopedic intervention in these cases is generally limited and often managed medically. Secondary impairments, on the other hand, develop over time as a consequence of primary impairments. These include muscle contractures—more frequently in distal biarticular muscles—and bone deformities resulting from abnormal muscle forces caused by spasticity, weakness, and restricted muscle growth. In this context, orthopedic surgery plays a more prominent role, helping to correct evolving musculoskeletal issues and prevent long-term disability. As children grow, they often develop tertiary impairments—adaptive but maladaptive biomechanical strategies such as joint hyperextension—which arise in response to primary spasticity and secondary contractures in an effort to maximize limb function. A proactive, individualized approach that considers motor severity (e.g., GMFCS level), comorbidities, and family goals is essential to optimize outcomes and support long-term participation and independence [52, 83, 84] (Fig. 5.15).

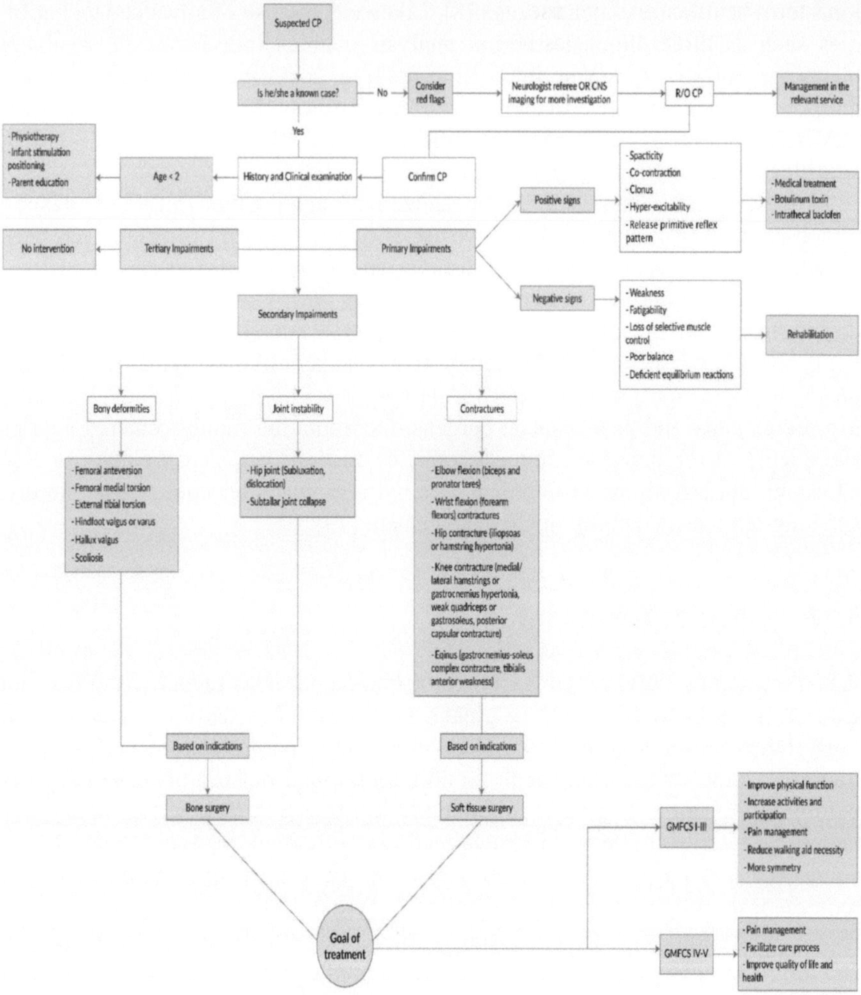

Fig. 5.15 Orthopedic approach to cerebral palsy

5.13.1 Timing Considerations

The timing of orthopedic intervention in children with CP should be considered a cornerstone for maximizing functional outcomes, preventing secondary musculoskeletal complications, and enhancing quality of life [1]. Although the neurological damage in CP is non-progressive, musculoskeletal complications such as spasticity, contractures, deformities, hip displacement, and scoliosis tend to evolve as the child grows. Prompt and well-planned orthopedic strategies—ranging from conservative to surgical treatments—can help address these challenges early and minimize the need for invasive procedures later [82]. Early conservative management, including physiotherapy and orthotic use, is especially important. Initiating physiotherapy soon after diagnosis leverages neuroplasticity to promote motor development and prevent deformities. Likewise, introducing orthoses like ankle-foot orthoses (AFOs) during the early walking stages, improves gait efficiency and delays structural abnormalities. Studies show that early AFO use significantly enhances stride length and dorsiflexion, highlighting the importance of timely intervention before permanent deformities develop [85].

In terms of minimally invasive interventions, Botulinum toxin type A (BTX-A) is most effective when administered before the onset of fixed contractures or skeletal deformities, typically between ages 2 and 8, or when clinical assessment identifies dynamic rather than static tone abnormalities. Early BTX-A use has been shown to enhance gait patterns and improve gross motor function [86]. When integrated into a comprehensive treatment plan alongside physiotherapy and orthotic support, timely BTX-A can extend the interval between interventions and help sustain functional gains. Similarly, selective dorsal rhizotomy (SDR), when performed at a younger age (2–4 years), is linked to a reduced lifetime need for orthopedic surgery, reinforcing the importance of early minimally invasive management [52, 87].

Surgical intervention becomes essential when conservative or minimally invasive treatments can no longer address established musculoskeletal deformities. However, timing is critical—intervening too early increases the risk of recurrence, while late surgeries may result in irreversible structural damage. Studies show that children with more severe motor impairment (higher GMFCS levels) tend to require surgery at younger ages due to faster disease progression [81]. Hip surveillance is particularly vital in nonambulatory children; regular imaging enables early soft tissue or bony procedures before dislocation, ideally when migration exceeds 30–40%, to avoid complex salvage operations. Single-Event Multilevel Surgery (SEMLS) is best performed between ages 8 and 12, once gait patterns stabilize, to ensure long-term functional improvement. Similarly, timely spinal fusion for scoliosis—before the deformity becomes severe—helps preserve sitting balance, lung function, and overall quality of life. Delaying surgery until deformities are fixed increases complication risks, particularly in children with severe CP [78].

Ultimately, the success of orthopedic management in CP hinges on timing: early conservative care can prevent complications, minimally invasive treatments can optimize function, and surgery is most effective when conducted before permanent deformity. Ongoing surveillance ensures these interventions are appropriately timed, supporting improved mobility, independence, and quality of life [88].

5.13.2 Botulinum Toxin Type A (BoNT-A)

BoNT-A is a well-known pharmacological treatment for managing spasticity in children with CP, with extensive orthopedic applications both as a stand-alone intervention and as an adjunct to other therapies [86]. Its primary role in orthopedic management is to reduce muscle spasticity that contributes to joint deformities, contractures, pain, and functional impairment. BoNT-A works by inhibiting acetylcholine release at the neuromuscular junction, resulting in temporary muscle relaxation lasting several months [89, 90]. It is particularly indicated for focal or segmental spasticity that interferes with mobility, daily function, or caregiving. Common orthopedic indications include dynamic equinus deformity of the ankle—most often in ambulatory children (GMFCS I–III)—where gastrocnemius-soleus overactivity impairs dorsiflexion and gait. In non-ambulatory children (GMFCS IV–V), BoNT-A is used to manage hip adductor spasticity by targeting muscles such as the adductor longus and gracilis to reduce the risk of hip subluxation or dislocation [90]. In the upper limbs, injections into muscles like the flexor carpi radialis/ulnaris, biceps brachii, and pronator teres can improve hand function, hygiene, and grasp by relieving wrist and finger flexion [91].

Although earlier concerns existed regarding the use of BoNT-A in children under 2 years of age, recent studies have affirmed its safety, with most adverse events being mild and transient [92, 93]. BoNT-A has demonstrated significant benefits in children with CP, particularly in improving gross and fine motor function. When administered early, it may delay or reduce the need for orthopedic surgery by slowing the progression of contractures and mitigating hip displacement. Additionally, BoNT-A facilitates therapy goals by temporarily reducing spasticity in targeted muscles, thereby enhancing the effectiveness of stretching, orthotic use, and physical therapy [86]. Both caregivers and patients report increased satisfaction due to improved hygiene, decreased pain, and reduced caregiving burden. The treatment is also customizable and reversible, with targeted muscle injections providing individualized therapeutic effects that wear off over several months, allowing for safe and repeatable cycles [88].

Despite its overall safety and efficacy, several considerations remain essential in clinical practice. Excessive localized muscle weakness may occur if muscle selection or dosing is not optimal, potentially impairing function temporarily [91]. Local side effects such as pain, swelling, or bruising at the injection site are common, and sedation or anesthesia is often required for young children. Though rare, systemic adverse events—such as respiratory infections, incontinence, generalized weakness, aspiration, and seizures—are reported more frequently in the CP population. Repeated or high-dose use may lead to the development of neutralizing antibodies and diminished response, and some studies suggest potential long-term effects on muscle health, including atrophy or increased stiffness [87]. Moreover, BoNT-A is less effective in treating fixed contractures or muscles with significant fibrosis, with the best outcomes observed in dynamic deformities. These considerations underscore the importance of individualized assessment and dosing, ensuring that BoNT-A is used judiciously within a multidisciplinary care framework [88].

5.13.3 Pain Management in CP

As far as pain is prevalent in CP patients (74%), and this phenomenon prevents children from participating in social activities and also reduces their quality of life, asking about pain and its management is so important in approaching CP children [19]. The pain caused in CP patients includes hip subluxation, hypertonia, muscle spasm, constipation, gastroesophageal reflux, as well as medical interventions, such as physical therapy, BT intramuscular injection, and serial casting [84].

It is recommended to administer ITB and BoNT injection for hypertonia-associated pain. There is less evidence of the efficiency of massage therapy, intraspinal gabapentin injection, and radiofrequency lesions of the dorsal root ganglion. In cases the pain originated from hip dislocation/subluxation, hip salvage and hip repair surgery are helpful. The type of surgery and osteotomy should be decided based on the patient's condition. To control the pain caused by the procedures, inhale nitrous oxide with topical anesthetic cream, ketamine with midazolam, and clown care therapy is used. For post-operative pain in lower limb surgeries, we could use epidural analgesia with bupivacaine and continuous infusion of magnesium sulfate, as well as preoperative popliteal block. After selective dorsal rhizotomy, use of morphine intrathecally and epidurally has been introduced as the best option. Fewer evidence has been found for the usefulness of other options such as laser therapy, massage therapy, and physiotherapy. Cyclic intravenous pamidronate infusions are effective for osteoporotic fractures in CP patients [94, 95].

5.13.4 Orthopedic Surgery in CP

Orthopedic surgeries play a small role in this group of complications. Therefore, the importance of history, examination, and paraclinic in the approach to the CP patient is to find secondary complications and distinguish them from primary and tertiary disorders, so that the patient's treatment plan can be selected more precisely [23, 84]. The orthopedic surgery plans for CP patients depend on myriads of factors such as age, type of CP, mental status, FMS, and socioeconomic condition of patients, so it is rational to individualize each patient plan, but we introduce some typical interventions for each complication in Table 5.18 [46, 96–98].

Surgical correction of lower limb deformities in children with CP often begins with soft tissue procedures aimed at lengthening tight muscles. Achilles tendon lengthening is frequently performed to correct equinus deformity by elongating the gastrocnemius–soleus complex, thereby improving heel strike and gait [73]. Care is taken to avoid excessive lengthening, which could compromise push-off power and result in a calcaneal gait. For crouch gait marked by persistent knee flexion, medial hamstring lengthening (particularly semitendinosus and gracilis) is commonly employed. However, caution is advised to prevent overcorrection and pelvic imbalance. Tight hip adductors and iliopsoas may also be lengthened to manage hip subluxation and scissoring gait, ultimately improving hip stability and range of motion. Tendon transfers, such as the Split Anterior Tibialis Tendon Transfer (SPLATT), aim to rebalance foot movement by redistributing tendon forces [98, 99]. In selected cases, hamstring transfers may aid hip extension and knee control, although their long-term benefits remain under discussion. Additionally, the Strayer procedure—a gastrocnemius recession preserving soleus integrity—is an effective option for ambulatory children with equinus deformity and adequate muscle strength [26].

When rotational deformities or fixed skeletal abnormalities are present, bony procedures such as osteotomies are often necessary. Femoral derotation osteotomy (FDO) addresses excessive femoral anteversion and internal rotation gait by rotating the femur into a more neutral alignment. Tibial derotation osteotomy (TDO) may accompany FDO when tibial torsion contributes to gait dysfunction. In cases of hip instability, femoral varus osteotomy improves femoral head coverage and is

Table 5.18 Surgery indications for CP

Impairment	Indications for surgery	Procedure
LOWERLIMBS		
Hip flexion contracture: Psoas	Ambulatory child Reduced hip extension in terminal stance Excessive anterior pelvic tilt + lordosis Hip flexion contracture >20° Hip subluxation Kinematic: Excessive anterior pelvic tilt with double-bump pattern in diplegia; single-bump pattern in hemiplegia Kinetics: Delay in transition from hip extensor (internal) moment to hip flexor (internal) moment (beyond the typical 25% of gait cycle)	Selective intramuscular lengthening of the psoas tendon over the brim of the pelvis (spare the iliacus) *Note: Proximal femoral derotational osteotomy done above the lesser trochanter can functionally lengthen the psoas*
	Nonambulatory child As part of the management of hip displacement	Iliopsoas tenotomy or release of the lesser trochanter
	If not:	
Hip adduction contracture: adductors *Note: During normal gait the arc of hip motion in the coronal plane is from 10° of abduction to 10° of adduction. 15° of abduction is sufficient for normal gait*	Ambulatory child Decreased abduction in swing phase (scissoring) Adduction contracture: <15°	Percutaneous or open release of adductor longus alone is usually sufficient
	Nonambulatory child Adduction contracture interfering with care: dressing, toileting, perineal hygiene As part of the management of hip displacement	Open release of adductor longus, adductor brevis, gracilis + iliopsoas tenotomy
	If not:	

(continued)

Table 5.18 (continued)

Impairment	Indications for surgery	Procedure
Hip internal rotation: Anteversion	*Ambulatory child* Excessive internal rotation of the hip due to increased femoral anteversion Increased "scissoring" with knees rubbing Internal foot progression angle—causing tripping	Proximal femoral (intertrochanteric) derotational osteotomy with internal fixation Alternative: Distal femoral derotational osteotomy
	Nonambulatory child As part of the management of hip displacement	Combined proximal femoral derotation + varus osteotomy with stable internal fixation
	If not:	
Proximal femur: Coxa valga and hip subluxation	Increased neck-shaft angle Migration percentage >30% Break in Shenton's arc Increased anteversion	Proximal femoral (intertrochanteric) varus and external derotational osteotomy (VDRO)
	If not:	
Pelvis: Acetabular dysplasia	Acetabular index >30° Subluxated hip Older than 5 years	Periacetabular pelvic osteotomy (e.g., Dega) to restore posterolateral coverage
	If not:	
Knee flexion: Hamstrings	Ambulatory child Decreased knee extension in terminal swing Increased popliteal angle, provided that Bilateral popliteal angle >30° Kinematics: Posterior pelvic tilt Decreased knee extension in terminal swing	Medial hamstring lengthening: Intramuscular tenotomies of the gracilis, semitendinosus; aponeurotic lengthening (striping) of semimembranosus lateral hamstring lengthening: Fascial striping of the biceps femoris aponeurosis. This is avoided unless there is posterior pelvic tilt present to prevent excessive weakness of hip extensors.
	Nonambulatory child Knee flexion contractures due to hamstring contracture interfering with care, dressing, seating, and positioning. Goal is to decrease contracture (and popliteal angle) and not to straighten the knee entirely	Percutaneous or open hamstring lengthening: Medial and lateral
	If not:	

(continued)

Table 5.18 (continued)

Impairment	Indications for surgery	Procedure
Knee flexion contracture	Knee flexion contractures >20° despite hamstring lengthening Hamstring length is sufficient (normal) Older children (closer to skeletal maturity): >12 years Significant crouch pattern in gait (GMFCS II–III) or during standing for transfers (GMFCS IV)	Distal femoral extension osteotomy: This must be accompanied by patella tendon shortening or patellar tendon distal advancement to re-tension the elongated knee extensors following the extension osteotomy
	If not:	
Stiff knee: Rectus femoris	Stiff knee pattern: Limited fl exion at initial swing Foot drag resulting in poor clearance Positive Duncan–Ely sign Kinematic: Peak knee fl exion in initial swing is decreased in amplitude and delayed EMG: RF active throughout gait cycle Avoid in more severe GMFCS III and IV	Rectus femoris tendon is separated from the underlying vasti and the detached tendon is tenodesed to the semitendinosus, gracilis, or sartorius
	If not:	
Tibial torsion: External	External torsion: Bimalleolar axis >30° external Out-toeing: External foot progression angle >30° Foot drag With planovalgus/abducted foot Relatively normal foot progression angle in the presence of increased femoral anteversion that is being corrected by external derotation of the femur	Distal tibial internal derotational osteotomy to correct bimalleolar axis to 10° external (concomitant fibular osteotomy may not be needed for derotations of <30°)
	If not:	
Tibial torsion: Internal	Internal torsion: Bimalleolar axis >10° internal Intoeing: Internal foot progression angle >10° internal Tripping	Distal tibial external derotational osteotomy to correct bimalleolar axis to 10° external (concomitant fibular osteotomy may not be needed for derotations of <30°)
	If not:	

(continued)

Table 5.18 (continued)

Impairment	Indications for surgery	Procedure
Equinus: Gastrocnemius-soleus	Ambulatory child Equinus in stance phase: Poor stability Equinus in swing: Poor clearance Tripping and falling Increased shoe wear	Gastrocnemius contracture alone (Silfverskiold): Isolated lengthening of the gastrocnemius (Strayer technique) Gastrocnemius > soleus contracture (Silfverskiold test): Strayer + soleus fascial lengthening by striping the aponeurosis leaving muscle intact or gastrocsoleus aponeurotic lengthening (e.g., Baker, Vulpius)
	Nonambulatory child Contracture interfering with bracing or footwear necessary for weight bearing for transfers (GMFCS IV) Contracture interfering with bracing or footwear, or resting of feet on the footplate of wheelchair (GMFCS V) *Note: These apply to any foot deformity in nonambulatory children*	
	If not:	
Equinus: Tendo-Achilles	Fixed equinus contracture involving both gastrocnemius and soleus, seen commonly in hemiplegia	Tendo-Achilles lengthening is the most aggressive method of lengthening the gastrocsoleus complex. This can be done by 2 or 3 hemitenotomy sliding lengthening technique or open z-lengthening
	If not:	
Equino (plano)valgus	Increased hindfoot valgus with collapse of subtalar joint (rocker bottom) and abducted forefoot Poor push off (tendency to crouch) Pain with weight bearing Blistering or callosity over medial prominence of talar head Loss of flexibility: Unbraceable	Lateral column lengthening through the calcaneus, along with plantar flexion osteotomy of first ray. May need lengthening of peroneus brevis; lengthening of gastrocsoleus as needed to address the unmasked equinus after correction of hindfoot valgus Triple C osteotomy: Medial slide osteotomy of calcaneus; opening wedge osteotomy of cuboid: closing wedge osteotomy of medial cuneiform
	If not:	

(continued)

Table 5.18 (continued)

Impairment	Indications for surgery		Procedure
Equino (cavo) varus	To prevent or correct weight bearing on lateral border of the foot which leads to Poor stability in stance Pain and callosity Difficulty with brace and shoe wear Stress fracture of the fourth or fifth metatarsal Poor clearance in swing Flexible hindfoot varus is amenable to tendon transfers Fixed contractures of tibialis posterior require lengthening Hindfoot varus driven by the presence of plantar flexion of the first ray (confirmed by the Coleman block test)		Split tibialis anterior tendon transfer to the cuboid if hindfoot varus is flexible and occurs primarily in swing phase. Split tibialis posterior tendon transfer to the peroneus brevis when the hindfoot varus is flexible but occurs in stance phase as well Requires lengthening of tibialis posterior: Intramuscular tenotomy. Tibialis posterior tendon lengthening may be combined with the split tibialis anterior tendon transfer Plantar fascia release along with extension osteotomy of the base of first metatarsal or medial cuneiform; consider transfer of the peroneus longus to the peroneus brevis. These may be combined with tibialis posterior tendon lengthening All of these may require gastrocsoleus or tendo-Achilles lengthening as needed to address the equinus contracture
	If not:		
UPPERLIMBS			
Shoulder adduction/ internal rotation	Identifiable and improvable functional deficiency Failure to non-surgical methods Severe joint contracture Failure to dressing Constant pain	Functional shoulder	Fractional lengthening of Pectoralis major, Latissimus dorsi and teres major Lengthening of short head biceps and coracobrachialis in severe internal rotation
		Non-functional shoulder	Surgical release of both the subscapularis and pectoralis major muscle insertions (minding the underlying joint capsule) Tenotomies of Pectoralis major, Latissimus dorsi and subscapularis

(continued)

Table 5.18 (continued)

Impairment	Indications for surgery		Procedure
Elbow flexion	Failure to non-surgical methods Severe joint contracture Failure to dressing	Fixed contracture <45°	Fractional lengthening: Release of the lacertus fibrosis Lengthening of the brachialis with two parallel incisions in the brachialis fascia Detachment of the proximal half of the brachioradialis origin from the humerus Z-lengthening of the biceps tendon Phenolization of musculocutaneous nerve
		Fixed contracture >45°	Full elbow flexor release: Division of the lacertus fibrosis, myotomy of the anterior half of the brachialis, detachment of brachioradialis origin from the humerus, Z-lengthening of biceps tendon, and release of anterior elbow capsule
Forearm pronation	Aesthetically pleasure Hygienic limb position More function		Proximal release of flexor digitorum, superficialis flexor digitorum profundus and pronator teres Distal pronator teres and rerouting it around the radius
Wrist flexion	Aesthetic pleasure Hygienic limb position More function	Functional hand	Flexor carpi ulnaris to extensor carpi radialis Brevis tendon transfer Extensor carpi ulnaris to extensor carpi radialis longus tendon transfers (to correct ulnar deviation)
		Non-functional hand	Tenotomy of the extrinsic wrist flexors (flexor carpi radialis, palmaris longus and flexor carpi ulnaris)
Finger flexion	Aesthetic pleasure Hygienic limb position More function	Functional hand	Fractional lengthening of the extrinsic finger flexors (flexor digitorum superficialis and flexor digitorum profundus) Z-lengthening of the flexor carpi radialis and flexor carpi ulnaris
		Non-functional hand	Tenotomy of flexor digitorum superficialis and flexor digitorum profundus Neurectomy of the motor branch of the ulnar nerve

(continued)

Table 5.18 (continued)

Impairment	Indications for surgery	Procedure
Thumb in palm	Aesthetic pleasure Hygienic limb position More function	Superficialis to profundus transfer, Wrist flexor tenotomy, FPL Z-lengthening, Ulnar motor nerve branch transection
	Severe metacarpophalangeal hyperextension and joint instability	+ wrist arthrodesis Thumb metacarpo-phalangeal arthrodesis *Note: variable outcomes*
Swan neck deformity	Aesthetic pleasure Hygienic limb position More function	FDS slip tenodesis Volar tenodesis of lateral band Extensor digitorum communis side to side coaptation
SPINE		
Scoliosis Kyphosis Kyphoscoliosis	Preventing curve progression Achieving a balanced spine Improving the functional quality of life Cobb angle >50° Significant curves resulting in functional or physiological disturbance Increase the respiration capacity Relieve pain	Modern pedicle screw fixation Segmental spinal instrumentation Posterior column wedge osteotomy with opening of anterior column *Note: Combined anterior and posterior surgical approach is recommended for improving the curve and preventing pseudoarthrosis*

frequently paired with pelvic osteotomies—such as the Dega or Salter techniques—to reshape the acetabulum in children with acetabular dysplasia or subluxation [100, 101]. Single-Event Multi-Level Surgery (SEMLS) combines multiple soft tissue and bony corrections during one operative session under a single anesthesia. This approach is typically reserved for ambulatory children with complex multi-planar deformities and aims to achieve efficient, comprehensive alignment correction while minimizing cumulative surgical trauma [35].

Neurological interventions, particularly Selective Dorsal Rhizotomy (SDR), offer an alternative or complementary approach to musculoskeletal surgeries. SDR involves selectively cutting sensory nerve rootlets, usually from L2 to S1, to reduce spasticity in the lower limbs. It is particularly suitable for children with spastic diplegia who have good underlying strength and clear functional goals. When performed early, SDR can reduce spasticity long-term and potentially lessen the future need for orthopedic interventions. Though not a first-line option for all patients, SDR remains a valuable part of comprehensive spasticity management in eligible candidates [73, 102].

Fusion procedures are typically considered in adolescents or adults with CP, particularly when dynamic joint function is no longer a priority and other surgical options have failed. Ankle arthrodesis is recommended for painful, rigid valgus, or varus deformities that have not responded to conservative or corrective procedures. Similarly, subtalar arthrodesis is used to manage severe hindfoot deformities, particularly valgus or varus deviations that interfere with standing or ambulation. These interventions aim to stabilize the foot and reduce pain, improving quality of life and functional mobility in later stages of life [48, 103].

Upper limb surgeries in children with CP primarily aim to enhance functional hand use, improve hygiene, and facilitate caregiving. These procedures yield the best outcomes in individuals who demonstrate some voluntary control of the upper limb and are motivated to achieve functional improvement. Proper candidate selection is essential, as active participation in rehabilitation significantly influences long-term results [104].

Tendon transfers are central to upper limb surgical management, redirecting muscle forces to restore more functional movement. For example, transferring the pronator teres to the extensor carpi radialis brevis helps restore forearm supination, while transferring the brachioradialis to the flexor pollicis longus re-establishes thumb flexion, essential for grasp and pinch. A common and effective procedure for correcting wrist flexion deformity is transferring the flexor carpi ulnaris to the extensor carpi radialis brevis, which improves wrist extension and positioning. Additionally, Z-lengthening and selective tendon transfers are used to balance finger flexor and extensor forces, allowing better hand opening and closing [105, 106].

For children with flexion contractures affecting the wrist or fingers, surgical lengthening of muscles such as the flexor carpi radialis or flexor digitorum superficialis can significantly improve hand extension and grasping ability. Correction of thumb-in-palm deformity—a common issue in CP—typically involves releasing the adductor pollicis and the first dorsal interosseous muscle to improve thumb abduction and opposition, contributing to better hand function [78, 104].

In cases of severe or fixed wrist deformities, especially in older children, wrist arthrodesis may be performed to stabilize the joint in a functional position and support effective grasp. Bony procedures, such as ulnar shortening or radial lengthening, are less commonly indicated but may be necessary to correct longstanding forearm malalignments, such as radial head dislocation. Lastly, in select cases with focal upper limb spasticity, targeted neurectomy of specific motor nerves may be performed to reduce muscle tone and improve movement control [52, 107].

Spinal deformities, particularly scoliosis, are common in individuals with CP, especially those classified as GMFCS levels IV and V who lack independent ambulation. The primary surgical intervention is Posterior Spinal Fusion (PSF), typically extending from the upper thoracic spine (T2–T3) to the sacrum or ilium. This procedure aims to halt curve progression, improve sitting balance, reduce discomfort, and facilitate caregiving. Given the high risk of complications, preoperative optimization—particularly nutritional and pulmonary status—is crucial. In younger children under 10 with severe early-onset scoliosis, growth-friendly techniques such as traditional growing rods or magnetically controlled growing rods (MCGR) are preferred to manage curvature while allowing spinal growth before final fusion [47, 48].

In cases where pelvic obliquity is present, distal fixation using iliac screws or S2-alar-iliac screws helps maintain spinal alignment and stability. Although rarely performed in CP patients, vertebral column resection (VCR) may be considered for the most severe and rigid spinal curves that are unresponsive to standard fusion techniques. Due to its complexity and high complication rate, VCR is regarded as a last-resort option when all other methods are insufficient for achieving spinal correction [108, 109].

The surgical indications for patients with CP are outlined in Table 5.18.

5.13.4.1 Multidisciplinary Care

In the multidisciplinary management of children with cerebral palsy (CP), orthopedic specialists play a pivotal role in identifying and correcting musculoskeletal deformities, including contractures, joint subluxations, scoliosis, and gait abnormalities. Timely surgical interventions, when integrated with comprehensive physiotherapy and occupational therapy, can prevent long-term complications such as joint degeneration, pain, and functional decline [110]. Effective coordination between orthopedic surgeons and other members of the care team—including neurologists, physiotherapists, occupational therapists, speech-language pathologists, and rehabilitation specialists—is essential for preoperative assessment, postoperative rehabilitation, and ongoing monitoring of functional progress [111]. Furthermore, consistent communication allows adjustments to individualized care plans, ensures adherence to therapeutic regimens, and facilitates early recognition of complications or regression in motor function. This collaborative approach not only optimizes surgical outcomes but also significantly enhances overall quality of life and participation in daily activities for children with CP [112].

5.13.4.2 Parent and Caregiver Support

Parents and caregivers are central to the effective long-term management of children with cerebral palsy, as they are responsible for implementing daily rehabilitation exercises, monitoring therapy adherence, and reporting functional changes to the care team. Structured education and training programs empower caregivers to participate actively in clinical decision-making, including understanding surgical options, anticipated outcomes, and rehabilitation goals [111]. Psychological and social support interventions, such as counseling, peer support groups, and stress management resources, are crucial to reduce caregiver burden, improve coping strategies, and enhance overall family well-being [113]. Moreover, clear, timely, and transparent communication from the healthcare team regarding procedural details, postoperative expectations, and potential complications allows caregivers to provide more effective home-based care, ultimately improving the child's functional outcomes and satisfaction with care [114]. Integrating families into the multidisciplinary care process ensures that interventions are consistent across settings, promotes continuity of care, and reinforces the importance of collaboration between healthcare providers and caregivers.

5.14 Conclusion

Managing cerebral palsy requires a comprehensive, multidisciplinary approach, with orthopedic evaluation and treatment playing a central role in improving function and quality of life. This chapter aimed to provide a structured and practical framework for orthopedic assessment of CP patients, incorporating detailed guidance on classification, clinical examination, and diagnostic work-up. By organizing the approach into step-by-step components and supplementing it with visual aids, checklists, and algorithms, we have sought to create a user-friendly reference for clinicians. Recognizing the heterogeneity among CP patients, individualized evaluation and treatment planning are essential. We hope this chapter serves as a valuable guide for healthcare providers, ensuring that no critical aspect is overlooked in the orthopedic care of individuals with CP and ultimately contributing to more effective and holistic patient management.

References

1. Richards CL, Malouin F. Cerebral palsy: definition, assessment and rehabilitation. Handb Clin Neurol. 2013;111:183–95.
2. Pakula AT, Braun KVN, Yeargin-Allsopp M. Cerebral palsy: classification and epidemiology. Phys Med Rehabil Clin. 2009;20(3):425–52.
3. Palmer FB. Strategies for the early diagnosis of cerebral palsy. J Pediatr. 2004;145(2):S8–S11.
4. Rethlefsen SA, Ryan DD, Kay RM. Classification systems in cerebral palsy. Orthop Clin. 2010;41(4):457–67.
5. Sankar C, Mundkur N. Cerebral palsy-definition, classification, etiology and early diagnosis. Indian J Pediatr. 2005;72:865–8.
6. Ahl LE, et al. Functional therapy for children with cerebral palsy: an ecological approach. Dev Med Child Neurol. 2005;47(9):613–9.
7. Sadowska M, Sarecka-Hujar B, Kopyta I. Cerebral palsy: current opinions on definition, epidemiology, risk factors, classification and treatment options. Neuropsychiatr Dis Treat. 2020;16:1505–18.
8. Jones MW, et al. Cerebral palsy: introduction and diagnosis (part I). J Pediatr Health Care. 2007;21(3):146–52.
9. Panteliadis C, Panteliadis P, Vassilyadi F. Hallmarks in the history of cerebral palsy: from antiquity to mid-20th century. Brain Dev. 2013;35(4):285–92.
10. Bartlett DJ, Palisano RJ. A multivariate model of determinants of motor change for children with cerebral palsy. Phys Ther. 2000;80(6):598–614.
11. Barrett RS, Lichtwark GA. Gross muscle morphology and structure in spastic cerebral palsy: a systematic review. Dev Med Child Neurol. 2010;52(9):794–804.
12. Lin J-P. The cerebral palsies: a physiological approach. J Neurol Neurosurg Psychiatry. 2003;74(suppl 1):i23–9.
13. Vitrikas K, Dalton H, Breish D. Cerebral palsy: an overview. Am Fam Physician. 2020;101(4):213–20.
14. Te Velde A, et al. Early diagnosis and classification of cerebral palsy: an historical perspective and barriers to an early diagnosis. J Clin Med. 2019;8(10):1599.
15. Cantero MJP, et al. Comprehensive approach to children with cerebral palsy. An Pediatr (Engl Ed). 2021;95(4):276.e1–e11.
16. Trabacca A, et al. Multidisciplinary rehabilitation for patients with cerebral palsy: improving long-term care. J Multidiscip Healthc. 2016;9:455–62.

17. Gowda VK. Recent advances in cerebral palsy. Karnataka Paediatr J. 2020;35(1):4–18.
18. Deon LL, Gaebler-Spira D. Assessment and treatment of movement disorders in children with cerebral palsy. Orthop Clin. 2010;41(4):507–17.
19. Damiano DL. Activity, activity, activity: rethinking our physical therapy approach to cerebral palsy. Phys Ther. 2006;86(11):1534–40.
20. Huysentruyt K, et al. Nutritional red flags in children with cerebral palsy. Clin Nutr. 2020;39(2):548–53.
21. Rodda J, Graham H. Classification of gait patterns in spastic hemiplegia and spastic diplegia: a basis for a management algorithm. Eur J Neurol. 2001;8:98–108.
22. Chang FM, et al. The role of gait analysis in treating gait abnormalities in cerebral palsy. Orthop Clin. 2010;41(4):489–506.
23. Sharan D. Orthopedic surgery in cerebral palsy: instructional course lecture. Indian J Orthop. 2017;51(3):240–55.
24. Vargus-Adams JN, Martin LK. Measuring what matters in cerebral palsy: a breadth of important domains and outcome measures. Arch Phys Med Rehabil. 2009;90(12):2089–95.
25. Novacheck TF, Trost JP, Sohrweide S. Examination of the child with cerebral palsy. Orthop Clin. 2010;41(4):469–88.
26. Huser A, Mo M, Hosseinzadeh P. Hip surveillance in children with cerebral palsy. Orthop Clin. 2018;49(2):181–90.
27. Campbell R, et al. Orthopaedic management of knee joint impairment in cerebral palsy: a systematic review and meta-analysis. Gait Posture. 2020;80:347–60.
28. Ganjwala D, Shah H. Management of the knee problems in spastic cerebral palsy. Indian J Orthop. 2019;53:53–62.
29. Sebastian D, Chovvath R, Malladi R. The sitting active and prone passive lag test: an inter-rater reliability study. J Bodyw Mov Ther. 2014;18(2):204–9.
30. Gage JR, Novacheck TF. An update on the treatment of gait problems in cerebral palsy. J Pediatr Orthop B. 2001;10(4):265–74.
31. Davids JR, Holland WC, Sutherland DH. Significance of the confusion test in cerebral palsy. J Pediatr Orthop. 1993;13(6):717–21.
32. Foran IM, et al. Impact of Coleman block test on adult hindfoot alignment assessed by clinical examination, radiography, and weight-bearing computed tomography. Foot Ankle Orthop. 2020;5(3):2473011420933264.
33. Larkins LW, Baker RT, Baker JG. Physical examination of the ankle: a review of the original orthopedic special test description and scientific validity of common tests for ankle examination. Arch Rehabil Res Clin Transl. 2020;2(3):100072.
34. Sarathy K, Doshi C, Aroojis A. Clinical examination of children with cerebral palsy. Indian J Orthop. 2019;53:35–44.
35. Theologis T. Lever arm dysfunction in cerebral palsy gait. J Child Orthop. 2013;7(5):379–82.
36. Armand S, Decoulon G, Bonnefoy-Mazure A. Gait analysis in children with cerebral palsy. EFORT Open Rev. 2016;1(12):448.
37. Read HS, et al. Edinburgh visual gait score for use in cerebral palsy. J Pediatr Orthop. 2003;23(3):296–301.
38. Dobson F, et al. Gait classification in children with cerebral palsy: a systematic review. Gait Posture. 2007;25(1):140–52.
39. Britner PA, et al. Stress and coping: a comparison of self-report measures of functioning in families of young children with cerebral palsy or no medical diagnosis. J Child Fam Stud. 2003;12(3):335.
40. Palisano RJ, et al. Content validity of the expanded and revised gross motor function classification system. Dev Med Child Neurol. 2008;50(10):744–50.
41. Makki D, Duodu J, Nixon M. Prevalence and pattern of upper limb involvement in cerebral palsy. J Child Orthop. 2014;8(3):215–9.
42. Shierk A, Lake A, Haas T. Review of therapeutic interventions for the upper limb classified by manual ability in children with cerebral palsy. Semin Plast Surg. 2016;30:14. Thieme Medical Publishers.

43. Eliasson A-C, et al. The manual ability classification system (MACS) for children with cerebral palsy: scale development and evidence of validity and reliability. Dev Med Child Neurol. 2006;48(7):549–54.
44. Arnould C, et al. ABILHAND-kids: a measure of manual ability in children with cerebral palsy. Neurology. 2004;63(6):1045–52.
45. Chan G, Miller F. Assessment and treatment of children with cerebral palsy. Orthop Clin. 2014;45(3):313–25.
46. Cloake T, Gardner A. The management of scoliosis in children with cerebral palsy: a review. J Spine Surg. 2016;2(4):299.
47. Yaman O, Dalbayrak S. Kyphosis and review of the literature. Turk Neurosurg. 2014;24(4):455–65.
48. Howard J, Sees J, Shrader MW. Management of spinal deformity in cerebral palsy. JPOSNA®. 2019;1(1):8.
49. Saether R, et al. Clinical tools to assess balance in children and adults with cerebral palsy: a systematic review. Dev Med Child Neurol. 2013;55(11):988–99.
50. Park S-D, Yu S-H. The effects of abdominal draw-in maneuver and core exercise on abdominal muscle thickness and Oswestry disability index in subjects with chronic low back pain. J Exerc Rehabil. 2013;9(2):286.
51. Fowler EG, et al. Selective Control Assessment of the Lower Extremity (SCALE): development, validation, and interrater reliability of a clinical tool for patients with cerebral palsy. Dev Med Child Neurol. 2009;51(8):607–14.
52. Berker AN, Yalçın MS. Cerebral palsy: orthopedic aspects and rehabilitation. Pediatr Clin N Am. 2008;55(5):1209–25.
53. Kuiper MJ, et al. The Burke-Fahn-Marsden dystonia rating scale is age-dependent in healthy children. Mov Disord Clin Pract. 2016;3(6):580–6.
54. Das SP, Ganesh GS. Evidence-based approach to physical therapy in cerebral palsy. Indian J Orthop. 2019;53:20–34.
55. Heyrman L, et al. A clinical tool to measure trunk control in children with cerebral palsy: the trunk control measurement scale. Res Dev Disabil. 2011;32(6):2624–35.
56. Piscitelli D, et al. Measurement properties of the gross motor function classification system, gross motor function classification system-expanded & revised, manual ability classification system, and communication function classification system in cerebral palsy: a systematic review with meta-analysis. Dev Med Child Neurol. 2021;63(11):1251–61.
57. Pirpiris M, Graham HK. Uptime in children with cerebral palsy. J Pediatr Orthop. 2004;24(5):521–8.
58. Kleiner AFR, et al. Timed up and go evaluation with wearable devices: validation in Parkinson's disease. J Bodyw Mov Ther. 2018;22(2):390–5.
59. Schroeder KM, Heydemann JA, Beauvais DH. Musculoskeletal imaging in cerebral palsy. Phys Med Rehabil Clin. 2020;31(1):39–56.
60. Battisti N, et al. Prevention of hip dislocation in severe cerebral palsy (GMFCS III-IV-V): an interdisciplinary and multi-professional care pathway for clinical best practice implementation. Eur J Phys Rehabil Med. 2023;59(6):714.
61. Wellenberg RHH, et al. Assessment of foot deformities in individuals with cerebral palsy using weight-bearing CT. Skeletal Radiol. 2023;52(7):1313–20.
62. Jin S, et al. Comparative analysis of physical examination, CT scan, and three-dimensional gait analysis in evaluating lower extremity torsion deformities in children with cerebral palsy. Med Sci Monit. 2023;29:e940948.
63. Kim HY, et al. Correlation of the torsion values measured by rotational profile, kinematics, and CT study in CP patients. Gait Posture. 2017;57:241–5.
64. Teixeira FB, et al. Correlation between physical examination and three-dimensional gait analysis in the assessment of rotational abnormalities in children with cerebral palsy. Einstein (Sao Paulo). 2018;16(1):eAO4247.
65. Givon U. Management of the spastic hip in cerebral palsy. Curr Opin Pediatr. 2017;29(1):65–9.

66. Horber V, et al. The role of neuroimaging and genetic analysis in the diagnosis of children with cerebral palsy. Front Neurol. 2020;11:628075.
67. Robinson MN, et al. Magnetic resonance imaging findings in a population-based cohort of children with cerebral palsy. Dev Med Child Neurol. 2009;51(1):39–45.
68. Himmelmann K, et al. MRI classification system (MRICS) for children with cerebral palsy: development, reliability, and recommendations. Dev Med Child Neurol. 2017;59(1):57–64.
69. Chen CL, et al. Anthropometric and fitness variables associated with bone mineral density and broadband ultrasound attenuation in ambulatory children with cerebral palsy. J Child Neurol. 2011;26(5):552–9.
70. Liu W, et al. Reliability and validity of assessing lower-limb muscle architecture of patients with cerebral palsy (CP) using ultrasound: a systematic review. J Clin Ultrasound. 2023;51(7):1212–22.
71. Paul S, et al. A review on recent advances of cerebral palsy. Oxidative Med Cell Longev. 2022;2022(1):2622310.
72. Pham T-T, et al. Ultrasound imaging of hip displacement in children with cerebral palsy. Ultrasound Med Biol. 2023;49(9):1960–9.
73. Alliance NG. Cerebral palsy in under 25s: assessment and management: full guideline. National Institute for Health and Care Excellence; 2017.
74. Rasmussen HM, et al. The Danish cerebral palsy follow-up program. Clin Epidemiol. 2016;8:457–60.
75. Jahan I, et al. Epidemiology of cerebral palsy in low-and middle-income countries: preliminary findings from an international multi-centre cerebral palsy register. Dev Med Child Neurol. 2021;63(11):1327–36.
76. Ismail A, et al. The economic burden and determinant factors of parents/caregivers of children with cerebral palsy in Malaysia: a mixed methods study. Int J Environ Res Public Health. 2022;19(1):475.
77. Sazlina Kamaralzaman TCY, Mohamed S, Toran H, Satari N, Abdullah N. The economic burden of families of children with cerebral palsy in Malaysia. Mal J Public Health Med. 2018;1:156–65.
78. Telléus A, et al. Orthopedic surgical procedures in 3,305 children and young adults with cerebral palsy: a register-based cohort study. Acta Orthop. 2022;93:472–7.
79. Naaz F, et al. Psychosocial and economic burden on families of children with cerebral palsy: a correlation with locomotor severity. Cureus. 2025;17(1):e76794.
80. Garvey MA, et al. Cerebral palsy: new approaches to therapy. Curr Neurol Neurosci Rep. 2007;7(2):147–55.
81. Darrah J, et al. Context therapy: a new intervention approach for children with cerebral palsy. Dev Med Child Neurol. 2011;53(7):615–20.
82. Aisen ML, et al. Cerebral palsy: clinical care and neurological rehabilitation. Lancet Neurol. 2011;10(9):844–52.
83. Novak I, et al. State of the evidence traffic lights 2019: systematic review of interventions for preventing and treating children with cerebral palsy. Curr Neurol Neurosci Rep. 2020;20:1–21.
84. Chin EM, et al. Principles of medical and surgical treatment of cerebral palsy. Neurol Clin. 2020;38(2):397–416.
85. Betancourt JP, et al. Impact of ankle-foot orthosis on gait efficiency in ambulatory children with cerebral palsy: a systematic review and meta-analysis. Am J Phys Med Rehabil. 2019;98(9):759–70.
86. Multani I, et al. Botulinum toxin in the management of children with cerebral palsy. Paediatr Drugs. 2019;21(4):261–81.
87. Kaya Keles CS, Ates F. Botulinum toxin intervention in cerebral palsy-induced spasticity management: projected and contradictory effects on skeletal muscles. Toxins (Basel). 2022;14(11):772.

88. Sozbilen MC, Evren Sahin K. Long-term efficacy and safety of repeated botulinum toxin a applications based on function and anesthesia type in children with cerebral palsy. J Orthop. 2022;29:22–7.
89. Mirska A, et al. Effectiveness of multiple botulinum toxin sessions and the duration of effects in spasticity therapy in children with cerebral palsy. Childs Nerv Syst. 2019;35(1):141–7.
90. Mirska A, et al. Use of botulinum toxin in the treatment of ankle plantar flexor spasticity in children with cerebral palsy. J Pediatr Orthop B. 2014;23(6):517–22.
91. Klein C, Gouron R, Barbier V. Effects of botulinum toxin injections in the upper limbs of children with cerebral palsy: a systematic review of the literature. Orthop Traumatol Surg Res. 2024;110(3):103578.
92. Druschel C, et al. Off label use of botulinum toxin in children under two years of age: a systematic review. Toxins (Basel). 2013;5(1):60–72.
93. Yang H, et al. Safety and efficacy of botulinum toxin type a in children with spastic cerebral palsy aged <2 years: a systematic review. J Child Neurol. 2023;38(6–7):454–65.
94. Ostojic K, Paget SP, Morrow AM. Management of pain in children and adolescents with cerebral palsy: a systematic review. Dev Med Child Neurol. 2019;61(3):315–21.
95. Thomas JL, et al. ACFAS scoring scale user guide. J Foot Ankle Surg. 2005;44(5):316–35.
96. Van Heest AE, House JH, Cariello C. Upper extremity surgical treatment of cerebral palsy. J Hand Surg Am. 1999;24(2):323–30.
97. Tranchida GV, Van Heest A. Preferred options and evidence for upper limb surgery for spasticity in cerebral palsy, stroke, and brain injury. J Hand Surg Eur Vol. 2020;45(1):34–42.
98. Narayanan UG. Lower limb deformity in neuromuscular disorders: pathophysiology, assessment, goals, and principles of management. In: Pediatric lower limb deformities: principles and techniques of management. Cham: Springer International Publishing; 2016. p. 267–96.
99. Hochstetter-Owen J, Stott S, Williams SA. The efficacy of split tibial tendon transfers on functional gait outcomes for children and youth with cerebral palsy and spastic equinovarus foot deformities. Bone Jt Open. 2023;4(5):283–98.
100. Boyer ER, et al. Long-term functional outcomes after an external femoral derotation osteotomy in individuals with cerebral palsy. Gait Posture. 2021;87:184–91.
101. Chen K, et al. Periacetabular osteotomy with or without femoral osteotomy for the treatment of hip subluxation in children and young adults with cerebral palsy. BMC Musculoskelet Disord. 2022;23(1):809.
102. Sharma P, Gupta M, Kalra R. Recent advancements in interventions for cerebral palsy–a review. J Neurorestoratology. 2023;11(3):100071.
103. DiFazio RL, et al. Health-related quality of life and caregiver burden after hip reconstruction and spinal fusion in children with spastic cerebral palsy. Dev Med Child Neurol. 2022;64(1):80–7.
104. Boyd R, Morris M, Graham H. Management of upper limb dysfunction in children with cerebral palsy: a systematic review. Eur J Neurol. 2001;8:150–66.
105. Tonkin M. Tendon transfers in cerebral palsy: art or science? J Hand Surg Eur Vol. 2024;49:390–5. SAGE Publications Sage: London.
106. Lieber RL, Theologis T. Muscle-tendon unit in children with cerebral palsy. Dev Med Child Neurol. 2021;63(8):908–13.
107. Tawonsawatruk T, et al. Comparison of outcome between operative treatment and constraint-induced movement therapy for forearm and wrist deformities in cerebral palsy. A randomized controlled trial. Hand Surg Rehabil. 2022;41(2):258–64.
108. Yen W, Gartenberg A, Cho W. Pelvic obliquity associated with neuromuscular scoliosis in cerebral palsy: cause and treatment. Spine Deform. 2021;9:1259–65.
109. Li Y, et al. Pelvic fixation is not always necessary in children with cerebral palsy scoliosis treated with growth-friendly instrumentation. Spine Deform. 2022;10(4):925–32.
110. Graham B, et al. The American Academy of Orthopaedic surgeons evidence-based clinical practice guideline on: management of carpal tunnel syndrome. J Bone Joint Surg Am. 2016;98(20):1750–4.

111. Novak I, et al. A systematic review of interventions for children with cerebral palsy: state of the evidence. Dev Med Child Neurol. 2013;55(10):885–910.
112. Trionfo A, et al. A multidisciplinary perioperative care coordination pathway for hip and spine reconstruction in non-ambulatory patients with cerebral palsy. JPOSNA®. 2022;4(4):585.
113. Raina P, et al. The health and well-being of caregivers of children with cerebral palsy. Pediatrics. 2005;115(6):e626–36.
114. King S, et al. Family-centered service for children with cerebral palsy and their families: a review of the literature. Semin Pediatr Neurol. 2004;11(1):78–86.

Physical Therapy and Rehabilitation Approaches

6

Fatemeh Azizi and Nastaran Maghbouli

6.1 Case Vignette

Case Mina, 6 years old, right-sided weakness from cerebral palsy.

Mina's mother says, "She just wants to keep up at recess." Together they choose three everyday goals: (1) put on and zip her jacket by herself, (2) climb the playground ladder without help, and (3) run with her class for a short distance without stopping.

What the Team Does They build a simple, home-and-school practice plan using short daily "bursts" (10–15 min). For 4 weeks, Mina wears a soft mitt on her stronger hand at set times so she's nudged to use her weaker hand during play and dressing. Next, the focus shifts to two-hand tasks—opening lunch boxes, building blocks, and playing ball games. Walking, steps, and playground routes are practiced in real places she uses every day. Parents get a one-page plan and brief coaching calls.

What Changes After 8 weeks, Mina can zip her jacket, climb the ladder with a light touch for balance, and join tag at recess instead of watching. Her teacher notices she's moving faster and taking part more confidently.

F. Azizi
Center for Orthopedic Trans-Disciplinary Applied Research, Tehran University of Medical Sciences, Tehran, Iran

N. Maghbouli (✉)
Department of Physical Medicine and Rehabilitation, School of Medicine, Shariati Hospital, Tehran University of Medical Sciences, Tehran, Iran
e-mail: nmaghbouli@sina.tums.ac.ir

A. Presedo et al. (eds.), *Enhancing Quality of Life in Patients with Cerebral Palsy*, https://doi.org/10.1007/978-3-032-20967-2_6

6.2 Introduction

Cerebral palsy (CP) is a complex, heterogeneous condition that impacts movement, muscle tone, and posture, affecting approximately two to three in every 1000 live births. It is characterized as a group of permanent disorders leading to activity limitations, caused by non-progressive disturbances in the developing fetal or immature brain [1, 2]. An important distinction is that while the original neuropathological lesion stays unchanged and does not worsen over time, the clinical symptoms and secondary complications can progress, impacting functional abilities in different ways. Motor impairments are frequently associated with various related issues, including sensory, perceptual, cognitive, communicative, and behavioral disturbances, as well as epilepsy and secondary musculoskeletal problems [3].

Spasticity, characterized by stiff muscles and accounting for approximately 80% of cases, is the most common motor disorder. Other clinical phenotypes include dyskinesia, ataxia, and mixed presentations. These classifications are further refined by the limbs affected, such as spastic hemiplegia, diplegia, or quadriplegia [4]. These impairments, along with a significant presence of musculoskeletal and neuropathic pain, can interrupt balance, gait, coordination, communication, and activities of daily living (ADL), and even lead to structural deformities such as scoliosis, joint subluxations, or dislocations [5].

A common treatment approach for CP includes rehabilitation, such as physical therapy (PT), occupational therapy (OT), and other specialized therapies that target speech, hearing, and developmental challenges. The primary goal of PT and OT is to enhance gross motor function, mobility, balance, and gait, while also preventing secondary musculoskeletal issues, such as contractures and deformities [6].

By synthesizing current research and clinical guidelines, this chapter aims to serve as a practical and authoritative guide for a multidisciplinary audience, emphasizing the vital role of physical therapy and rehabilitation in helping individuals with CP reach their full potential.

6.3 Functional Classification Systems: A Universal Language for Assessment

Functional classification systems for CP, such as the Gross Motor Function Classification System (GMFCS), the Manual Ability Classification System (MACS), the Eating and Drinking Ability Classification System (EDACS), and the Communication Function Classification System (CFCS), are intentionally designed to assess "usual performance" based on the International Classification of Functioning, Disability, and Health (ICF). This focus means they are not just a measure of a neurological deficit but a dynamic assessment that considers the significant and multifaceted influence of environmental and personal factors, such as energy demands, social preferences, motivation, and the physical setting. This holistic perspective is key to a multidisciplinary approach, recognizing that a person's functional abilities stem from complex interactions between impairments and their environment [7].

6.3.1 The Gross Motor Function Classification System (GMFCS)

The GMFCS-E&R (expanded and revised version) is a five-level ordinal system, where Level I signifies the highest level of gross motor function (walking without limitations) and Level V signifies the most severe limitations (transported in a manual wheelchair). The system is uniquely structured with five age bands: under 2, 2–4, 4–6, 6–12, and 12–18 years. These age-specific descriptions are crucial because they reflect the developmental progression of motor skills and the evolving nature of mobility in different life stages. Detailed descriptions for each level and age band are provided in Table 6.1 [8].

Table 6.1 GMFCS-E&R levels by age-band: a summary of functional abilities [8]

GMFCS level	Under 2 years	2–4 years	4–6 years	6–12 years	12–18 years
Level I	Moves in/out of sitting, crawls on hands/knees, pulls to stand. Walks between 18 and 24 months	Sits, moves, and walks without assistive devices. Can transition from sitting to standing and walk indoors/ outdoors	Gets in/out of chairs without support. Walks indoors/ outdoors, climbs stairs. Emerging ability to run/ jump	Walks at home, school, outdoors. Climbs stairs without a railing. Runs/ jumps but with limited speed, balance, and coordination	Walks in all settings, including curbs and stairs without a railing. Runs and jumps, though may have limited speed, balance, or coordination
Level II	Maintains floor sitting with hands for support. Creeps on stomach or crawls on hands/knees. May pull to stand	Sits independently on the floor. Crawls on hands/knees. Can pull to stand. Walks short distances with a hand-held device or adult assistance	Sits independently. Walks on stable surfaces without a device. Uses a railing for stairs. Has difficulty with uneven terrain	Walks in most settings but may need a railing for stairs. Experiences difficulty with long distances, inclines, and crowded areas. Has minimal ability to run/ jump	Walks in most settings. Uses a hand-held device or wheelchair for long distances. Can manage stairs with a railing. Limited balance/ coordination

(continued)

Table 6.1 (continued)

GMFCS level	Under 2 years	2–4 years	4–6 years	6–12 years	12–18 years
Level III	Sits with lower back support. Rolls and creeps forward on stomach	Sits with trunk support. Can crawl or pull to stand. Walks short distances with a hand-held device	Sits in a chair with trunk support. Moves in/out of a chair with assistance. Walks with a hand-held device on level surfaces. Uses a wheelchair for long distances	Walks indoors with a hand-held device. Uses wheeled mobility for long distances in the community. May use a railing for stairs with supervision	Walks with a hand-held device for most settings, but uses a manual or powered wheelchair for longer distances. Can manage stairs with a railing
Level IV	Has head control but needs trunk support for sitting. Can roll to supine and prone	Sits when placed but needs hands for support. Requires adaptive equipment for sitting/standing. Self-mobility is limited to rolling or crawling for short distances	Requires trunk support for sitting. Self-mobility is limited. May use powered mobility or be transported in a manual wheelchair	At home, uses a manual wheelchair or may walk short distances with assistance. Uses a manual or powered wheelchair for all community settings. Requires assistance for transfers	Uses wheeled mobility in most settings, often a manual or powered wheelchair. Requires physical assistance from one or two people for transfers
Level V	Physical impairments limit voluntary movement. Unable to maintain antigravity head/trunk control. Requires assistance to roll	Severe limitations in all areas of motor function. Requires assistance for all mobility and is often transported. Needs adaptive equipment for sitting/standing, which does not fully compensate for limitations	Severe limitations in voluntary movement. Requires assistance in all areas of mobility. Transported in a manual wheelchair	Transported in a manual wheelchair in all settings. Has limited ability to control arm/leg movement and maintain head/trunk upright. Requires complete physical assistance for transfers	Transported in a manual wheelchair in all settings. Requires complete physical assistance for transfers. Limited ability to control head and trunk movements

6.3.2 Manual Ability Classification System (MACS)

The Manual Ability Classification System (MACS) was developed to provide a dedicated tool for assessing hand function, analogous to the GMFCS. It is a five-level system for children aged 4–18 years that classifies how a child uses their hands to manipulate objects in daily activities, with a specific focus on the collaborative use of both hands. A version for younger children, the Mini-MACS, has also been developed for ages 1–4 years. Like the GMFCS, MACS focuses on "typical manual performance" in everyday life, rather than on a child's best possible performance in a controlled test situation. The classification considers a child's ability to handle age-appropriate objects for tasks such as eating, dressing, playing, drawing, or writing (Table 6.2) [9, 10].

An important clinical finding is the high correlation between GMFCS and MACS levels. This strong relationship demonstrates that the underlying neurological injury in CP often results in a complex cascade of effects that simultaneously impact both gross and fine motor skills. This interconnectedness highlights the need for a comprehensive, multi-domain assessment. Clinicians assessing a child's mobility should also consider their manual abilities, and vice versa [7].

Table 6.2 Most commonly used functional classification systems

Level	GMFCS	MACS	CFCS
I	Walks without support or any limitations	Moves and handles objects without limitations	Can effectively and independently communicate as both a sender and a receiver with most people in most environments
II	Walks with some difficulties, may use assistive devices. Limited ability for running and jumping	Handling objects is somewhat challenging, resulting in reduced speed and quality of achievement	Can independently communicate as a sender and receiver, but at a slower pace
III	Walks with an assistive device and uses a wheelchair for long distances	Needs help with managing, preparing, and handling objects	Communication is usually effective with familiar partners but not with unfamiliar ones
IV	They may need powered mobility and walk short distances with the help of assistive devices	Limited ability to handle simple and easily manageable objects	Communication is inconsistent even with familiar partners
V	They need the help of a caregiver to be transported by wheelchairs	Severe limitations in performing tasks and unable to handle objects	They are seldom able to communicate effectively, even with familiar partners

6.3.3 Communication Function Classification System (CFCS)

The Communication Function Classification System (CFCS) is a five-level system that classifies the effectiveness of an individual's everyday communication performance. It was developed as a complementary tool to the GMFCS and MACS, providing a comprehensive functional profile. The CFCS is unique in its focus on the effectiveness of communication between a "sender" and a "receiver," taking into account the familiarity of the communication partner. The CFCS considers all modes of communication, including speech, gestures, facial expressions, and augmentative and alternative communication (AAC) devices [11]. The descriptions for each level can be found in Table 6.2.

6.4 Principles of Physiotherapy and Rehabilitation Approaches

Cerebral palsy (CP) is a complex condition characterized by permanent motor and postural disorders caused by non-progressive disturbances in the developing brain. Motor impairments often come with a wide range of related issues, such as problems with sensation, perception, cognition, and communication, along with secondary musculoskeletal complications. Managing CP requires a tailored, multidisciplinary approach, with physical therapy (PT) and occupational therapy (OT) playing a crucial and integral role within this framework [12].

In recent decades, the paradigm of physiotherapy for children with CP has undergone a fundamental transformation. The field has shifted away from purely passive, therapist-driven models toward an active, goal-directed, and family-centered approach. This evolution is driven by a deeper understanding of the neurological and physiological mechanisms that govern motor learning and skill acquisition in the developing brain. Family involvement is now considered an essential component of the management plan, with their input playing a crucial role in setting therapeutic goals and guiding the intervention [13].

Occupational therapy (OT) is a key discipline that addresses a child's functional abilities, fine motor skills (e.g., writing and drawing), self-care (e.g., feeding, dressing, grooming), cognition and perception, and overall participation in daily activities. The occupational therapist's role is to help children overcome physical and cognitive impairments that make everyday tasks difficult and to teach them how to adapt their environment and use assistive devices to achieve greater independence [14].

6.4.1 Neuroplasticity and Motor Learning

Neuroplasticity is the brain's innate ability to reorganize itself by forming new neural connections in response to experiences, learning, and injury. This capacity for adaptation is the central biological mechanism that makes rehabilitation for CP possible. The immature, developing brain possesses a significantly higher degree of plasticity, which makes early and intensive intervention critical for achieving the best possible outcomes. The fundamental goal of therapy is to exploit this adaptive capacity by encouraging healthy brain regions to take over functions that were compromised by the initial brain injury. The more a new, correct movement is practiced, the stronger and more efficient the corresponding neural pathways become, eventually supplanting the maladaptive movement patterns that may have been established over time [15].

Motor learning is defined as the acquisition of new motor skills through structured, repetitive practice. This framework provides the practical application of neuroplasticity principles in a clinical setting. Key components of a motor-learning approach include [16]:

- *Goal-Directed, Task-Specific Practice*: Interventions are designed to focus on specific, functionally relevant tasks from a child's daily life, such as walking, dressing, or playing. The core idea is that through high-repetition practice of a challenging task, the new motor pattern becomes more deeply ingrained in the nervous system [13].
- *Novelty and Challenge*: To effectively activate and create new neural pathways, the tasks must be novel and sufficiently challenging to keep the child engaged and motivated.
- *Family and Environment Integration*: The most effective motor-learning approaches are implemented within the context of the child's natural environment and through spontaneous play, with the therapist acting as a guide in the interaction between the child and their family. This strategy is crucial for facilitating the transfer of newly acquired skills from the controlled clinical setting to the dynamic, unstructured environments of the home and community [16].

6.4.2 International Clinical Practice Guideline

A comprehensive international clinical practice guideline published in 2022 [17] synthesized the best available evidence to guide interventions aimed at improving physical function in children and young people with cerebral palsy. The guideline places strong emphasis on setting functional, client-centered goals and tailoring interventions to individual needs, preferences, and contexts. It is structured in two parts: first, a set of Good Practice Recommendations (Fig. 6.1) that provide foundational principles for all interventions, and second, Evidence-Based Practice Recommendations (Fig. 6.2) that address specific functional domains such as mobility, upper limb function, self-care, and participation. Together, these recommendations highlight the importance of family engagement, adequate practice intensity, and the integration of therapy into everyday environments. Figures 6.1 and 6.2 summarize the key recommendations, offering clinicians and rehabilitation teams a concise reference for implementing effective, evidence-informed interventions in practice.

Key Recommendations from Jackman et al. (2022) Guideline

	Recommendation	Key Points / Practical Implications
	Good Practice Principles	**These are foundational best-practice guidelines, regardless of specific intervention types.**
1	Client-chosen goals	The child's or family's preferences drive goal setting; goals must be functional, measurable, achievable, and documented.
2	Identify barriers / limiting factors	Observe what is preventing goal achievement (skills, environmental, personal) before planning intervention.
3	Direct targeting of child's chosen goals	Use active practice; break tasks as needed, then move to whole-task; minimize hands-on aid; encourage child problem-solving and clinician feedback.
4	Make the intervention enjoyable & motivating	Monitor child's distress; adapt intervention to match interest, ability, preferences to maintain motivation.
5	Practice in home / community / realistic environments	Real-life context increases carry-over; when not possible, simulate; provide written/visual home-practice instructions.
6	Parent-delivered / family involvement	Provide coaching, structured home programs, ongoing review; support families in autonomy and task-specific practice.
7	Shared decision-making (child/family throughout)	Clinicians present up-to-date evidence; tailor content & timing by child/family preference, age, ability; resources and feasibility considered.
8	Sufficient dose of practice	Plan enough practice (face-to-face + home) depending on goal complexity, context; ensure frequency/intensity are adequate to achieve functional goals.
9	Multidisciplinary / team approach	Use team (child, family, relevant professionals) to set goals and intervention regimens; avoids overburden, improves coordination.

Fig. 6.1 Good practice principles

Evidence-Based Practice Recommendations for Interventions
(adapted and summarized from Jackman et al., 2022)

Domain	Recommended Interventions	Key Details / Practical Notes	Strength of Recommendation & Certainty of Evidence
Mobility (GMFCS I–IV)	• Mobility training using a goal-directed approach in real-life contexts	• Strong evidence that no intervention leads to functional decline (walking, musculoskeletal health). • Mobility training should be embedded in daily activities.	Strong recommendation (high certainty of harm from no intervention)
Walking speed & endurance	• Overground walking practice (with/without walker) • Treadmill training (GMFCS I–III) • HABIT-ILE (GMFCS I–IV)	• Overground training = moderate certainty of benefit • Treadmill = lower certainty, useful adjunct • HABIT-ILE can support endurance across GMFCS I–IV	Conditional; Moderate certainty (overground), Low certainty (treadmill, HABIT-ILE)
Gross motor function & balance	• Goal-directed training (GMFCS I–III) • HABIT-ILE (GMFCS I–IV) • Context-focused therapy (altering environment) or child-focused therapy (altering child factors)	• Choice should consider age, ability, family preference, tolerance for adjunct therapies.	Conditional; Low to moderate certainty
Hand Use / Upper Limb Function (MACS I–IV)	• Goal-directed, task-specific approaches	• Always preferable over impairment-focused approaches.	Conditional recommendation (low certainty)
Unilateral CP	• CIMT (Constraint-Induced Movement Therapy) (MACS I–III) • Bimanual training / HABIT (MACS I–III) • CO-OP, HABIT-ILE (MACS I–IV)	• CIMT: strong evidence, especially for improving functional goals. • Bimanual/HABIT: moderate evidence. • CO-OP and HABIT-ILE: promising but lower certainty.	Strong recommendation for CIMT (high certainty); Strong for bimanual (moderate certainty); Conditional for CO-OP, HABIT-ILE (low certainty)
Bilateral CP	• HABIT / HABIT-ILE (MACS I–III) • CO-OP (MACS I–IV)	• Effective for bilateral functional goals but with lower evidence strength.	Conditional (low certainty)
MACS IV (severe)	• Goal-directed focus plus environmental adaptation & assistive technology	• Equipment can maximize independence when hand function is limited.	Conditional (low certainty)
Self-Care (all motor types)	• Goal-directed, task-specific training • Adaptive equipment to promote independence	• Strong evidence that no intervention causes decline. • Adaptive equipment especially recommended for GMFCS IV–V to improve safety and reduce caregiver burden.	Strong recommendation (high certainty of harm from no intervention)
Skills development	• Goal-directed training • CO-OP • HABIT (GMFCS I–IV) • HABIT-ILE (GMFCS I–IV, suggested)	• Goal-directed, CO-OP, HABIT = moderate certainty. • HABIT-ILE = lower certainty.	Conditional (moderate for goal-directed & HABIT, low for CO-OP & HABIT-ILE)
Leisure & Participation	• Combine goal-directed approaches (CO-OP, goal-directed training, HABIT-ILE for GMFCS I–IV; goal-directed training for GMFCS V) • Focus on overcoming environmental, personal, and social barriers	• Evidence is limited, but participation is key to quality of life. • Most families would choose these approaches.	Conditional recommendation (low certainty)

Fig. 6.2 Evidence-based practice recommendations for interventions

6.4.3 The Evidence-Based "Traffic Light" Framework

To guide clinical decision-making, interventions for cerebral palsy can be classified according to the "State of the Evidence Traffic Lights 2019" review, which organizes therapeutic approaches based on the strength of the evidence from randomized controlled trials and meta-analyses [18, 19]. This framework provides a clear, evidence-based guide for clinicians and families, moving treatment decisions away from anecdote and toward a more rigorous, scientific foundation [19]. Green light interventions are supported with strong evidence for their effectiveness. Yellow light

State of the evidence traffic lights
(adapted and summarized from Novak et al., 2020)

Target of treatment	Green Intervention: *Aim*	Yellow Intervention: *Aim*	Red Intervention: *Aim*
Motor Interventions	• Action observation training: *Hand function* • Bimanual training: *Hand function* • Constraint-induced movement therapy (CIMT): *Hand function, activity and participation* • Goal directed training: *Hand function, gross motor* • Mobility training: *Walking speed* • Treadmill training: *Walking speed, endurance, gross motor* • Partial body weight support treadmill training: *Walking speed* • Occupational therapy post BoNT-A: *Goal achievement* • Task specific training: *Gross motor* • Physical activity: *Walking, fitness, participation, quality of life* • Hippotherapy: *Balance, symmetry*	• Electrical stimulation: *Gait parameters, muscle strength* • Hydrotherapy: *Gross motor* • Taping: *Gross motor, hand function* • Transcranial direct current stimulation: *Walking, mobility, balance, hand function* • Virtual reality (VR) serious gaming: *Hand function, walking* • Suit therapy: *Gross motor* • Vojta: *Gross motor* • Massage: *Gross motor* • Acupuncture: *Gross motor* • Hippotherapy stimulation: *Gross motor, hand function* • Ankle foot orthotics (AFO): *Walking speed, gross motor, stride length, kinematics*	• Craniosacral therapy: *Gross motor* • Hyperbaric oxygen: *Gross motor* • Neurodevelopmental therapy in the original passive format (NDT): *Gross motor* • Sensory integration: *Motor skills*
Tone management	• BoNT-A, ITB, SDR: *Spasticity*	• Dantrolene, Tizanidine, Alcohol: *Spasticity* • BoNT-A, Gabapentin, ITB: *Dystonia, pain management* • NDT, Acupuncture, Hippotherapy: *Spasticity*	
Contracture and alignment	• BoNT-A + Casting, Serial casting alone: *Passive range* • Active strength training: *Strength* • Goal-directed training: *Function regain* • Hip surveillance practices: *Preventing displacement*	• Passive stretching, orthotics, upper limb casting: *Passive range* • Single-event multi-level surgery (SEMLS): *Ankle/ knee passive range* • Biofeedback: *Active range* • SDR: *Prevent hip displacement* • Ankle robotics: *Ankle passive range* • BoNT-A + electrical stimulation: *Passive range, preventing hip displacement* • Whole body vibration: *Passive range*	• NDT: *Preventing contracture*
Cognitive interventions	• Communication devices: *Communication*	• GAME intervention: *Motor training, environmental enrichment, and coaching* • Cognitive orientation to occupational performance (CO-OP): *Problem solving, real life tasks, self care* • Play therapy, Assistive technology robotics: *Play, coping, cognition*	

Fig. 6.3 State of the evidence traffic lights

interventions show promise but require more research to establish their effectiveness conclusively. Red light interventions are not recommended, either due to ineffectiveness or being harmful [18]. The lists of interventions, their classifications, and aims are described in Fig. 6.3.

6.4.4 Individualized Goal Setting, Assessment, and Intervention Selection

Effective physiotherapy for children with cerebral palsy begins with a comprehensive, individualized approach to assessment and goal setting. Assessment serves as the foundation upon which clinicians develop tailored interventions, monitor progress, and make informed decisions about treatment strategies. This process extends beyond a simple diagnosis to include the evaluation of a child's motor abilities, communication skills, and overall quality of life [20].

6.4.4.1 Collaborative Goal Setting

A core tenet of modern pediatric rehabilitation is the collaborative process of goal setting, which ensures that therapy is aligned with the child's and family's priorities to foster motivation and enhance outcomes. The role of caregivers is essential, as they are instrumental in identifying and prioritizing meaningful therapeutic goals that align with the child's daily life demands. Research indicates that when caregiver-selected goals are closely aligned with a child's inherent motor capacities, they can positively affect functional outcomes [21]. Common goal domains include:

- *Self-Care*: The most frequently selected goal, including tasks such as dressing (e.g., buttoning shirts, zipping jackets) and eating (e.g., holding a cup, using cutlery).
- *Leisure*: Activities such as arts, crafts, and computer play.
- *Productivity*: Tasks that are more common as children get older, such as academic responsibilities.

6.4.4.2 Key Assessment Tools

A systematic and standardized approach to assessment is crucial for accurately characterizing a child's condition and tracking changes over time. This allows for the selection of the most appropriate intervention and for objective measurement of progress. These tools are comprehensively discussed and compared in the chapter "Pain and Spasticity Management." Yet, the most commonly used and key assessment tools include:

- *Gross Motor Function Classification System (GMFCS)*. A five-level system used to classify a child's ambulatory capacity (Sect. 3.3).
- *Gross Motor Function Measure (GMFM)*: An assessment tool that evaluates a child's ability to complete motor functions such as sitting, standing, and walking [22].
- *Manual Ability Classification System (MACS)*: A classification tool that assesses a child's ability to handle objects during daily activities (Sect. 3.2).
- *Spasticity Tests*: Specific tests like the Modified Ashworth Scale and the Tardieu Scale measure resistance to passive movement at different velocities to quantify muscle tone [23].
- *Pediatric Evaluation of Disability Inventory (PEDI)*: A tool that measures a child's self-care, social function, and mobility [24].

The selection of a specific intervention should be a data-driven process, guided by a child's personalized goals and the best available evidence. Motor rehabilitation interventions must be adapted to the specific topography of a child's symptoms (e.g., hemiplegia, diplegia), their ambulatory capacity, and their age.

6.5 Upper Limb and Hand Function Interventions

Upper limb dysfunction is a significant challenge in children with CP, often affecting their independence, participation, and overall quality of life. Two of the most studied and evidence-based interventions for improving upper limb function are Constraint-Induced Movement Therapy (CIMT) and Hand-Arm Bimanual Intensive Training (HABIT).

6.5.1 Constraint-Induced Movement Therapy (CIMT)

CIMT is a "Green light" evidence-based rehabilitation strategy primarily used for children with hemiplegic CP (strong recommendation and high certainty of evidence) [17, 18]. Its core principle is to overcome the "learned non-use" of the more affected limb by restricting the use of the less affected, stronger limb. This forced-use paradigm compels the child to use their impaired hand for daily activities, which, through high-repetition practice, promotes neuroplastic changes in the brain. The therapy is often delivered in an intensive block, with children wearing a constraint such as a mitt or sling for a significant portion of their waking hours for several weeks [25]. Key components include:

- *Massed Practice*: Repetitive, high-intensity training of the impaired hand.
- *Shaping*: Gradually increasing the difficulty of a motor task to facilitate skill acquisition.
- *Behavioral Techniques*: Including logbooks and problem-solving to ensure adherence and transfer of skills to the home environment [26].

The original CIMT protocol, often referred to as "classic CIMT," was highly intensive. It typically involved a full-arm cast on the unimpaired limb for 21 consecutive days, combined with 6 h of daily training, for a total dose of 126 h. While effective in improving the quality and amount of use of the impaired limb, this model was resource-intensive and often presented significant compliance challenges for children and their families. Reported adverse events included frustration, refusal of the constraint, and reversible skin irritations [27].

Modified CIMT (mCIMT) protocols were developed to address limitations and improve feasibility. These models include shorter daily sessions (about 3 h), less restrictive devices like a mitt or splint, and a program lasting several weeks, totaling around 60 h. Home-based mCIMT, often caregiver-led and supervised online, offers similar benefits, is more cost-effective, and reduces commuting stress [25, 28].

6.5.2 Hand-Arm Bimanual Intensive Training (HABIT)

HABIT is a "Green Light" intervention designed to improve the coordinated use of both arms (low certainty of evidence) [17, 18]. Developed as an alternative to CIMT, it is based on motor-learning theory and neuroplasticity, but without the physical constraint of the less-affected hand. Instead, it uses structured, play-based activities that require the simultaneous use of both hands. The therapy is delivered intensively, often in a camp-like setting over a 2-week period, with sessions lasting several hours a day.

Evidence supports HABIT's effectiveness in enhancing functional independence and coordination. When compared to CIMT, bimanual therapy can lead to more meaningful improvements in the attainment of functional goals and the coordination of two-handed activities. A variant, HABIT-ILE, integrates intensive upper and lower extremity training for children with bilateral CP, with evidence showing significant improvements in both upper and lower limb functionality [29].

6.5.3 Neurodevelopmental Therapy (NDT)

Neuro-Developmental Treatment (NDT), originally developed by Dr. Karel Bobath, is a multi-faceted, interactive practice model widely used by a multidisciplinary team of clinicians, including physical therapists and occupational therapists [30]. It is applied to address challenges with movement and muscle control. At its core, NDT focuses on the dynamic engagement of the patient, using continuous evaluation and modification based on a comprehensive analysis of movement. The primary objective is to achieve long-term, positive neuroplastic changes that lead to greater functional independence and fuller participation in daily life [31].

This intervention has a nuanced evidence profile. The original, passive form of NDT, which involves passively guided movements and manual stretching, is considered a "Red Light" intervention, as it is seen as an ineffective approach for improving function because it does not require the child to actively engage in problem-solving or activate their motor circuitry [18].

6.6 Lower Limb and Gait Interventions

Physical therapy for the lower extremities aims to improve balance, mobility, and gait efficiency. Interventions range from non-invasive stretching techniques to the use of advanced technologies.

6.6.1 Hand–Arm Bimanual Intensive Therapy Including Lower Extremity (HABIT-ILE)

HABIT-ILE extends classic bimanual intensive training by deliberately integrating trunk and lower-limb practice alongside upper-limb tasks, using high-dose, task-specific, play-based sessions (needs 90 h in 10 days to show efficacy). It is feasible for patients with GMFCS levels I–IV who are older than 4 years (conditional recommendation and low certainty of evidence) [17, 32].

6.6.2 Task-Specific Training (TST)

TST is a "Green Light" approach for both upper and lower extremities that focuses on practicing specific, functional tasks with high repetition and intensity (low certainty of evidence) [17, 18]. For lower extremities, TST programs can be designed to improve walking, balance, and other gross motor skills. The training is highly personalized, focusing on tasks that are relevant and meaningful to the child's daily life, such as walking on a balance beam or climbing stairs. A key aspect is the integration of motor-learning strategies, including repetition and positive feedback, to help the child find effective solutions for their motor problems [33].

A systematic review found that TST could be a recommended component of an intervention program to improve balance performance in children with CP, provided that it is accompanied by consistent use of repetitive practice, feedback, and task modulation strategies. However, the overall evidence for TST to improve gross motor function is limited due to poor study methodology and heterogeneity of interventions [33, 34].

6.6.3 Serial Casting

Serial casting is a non-invasive, "Green Light" intervention used to address spasticity-related contractures and loss of range of motion, most commonly at the ankle (equinus deformity), but also at the knee or wrist (strong recommendation for contracture reduction, and low certainty of evidence for improving gross motor) [17, 18]. It involves the application of a series of progressively adjusted casts, made from fiberglass and/or plaster, to gently stretch the muscle over time. Each cast is worn for approximately 1 week, and the process continues for several weeks until the desired range is achieved.

Serial casting is considered an effective method to reduce hypertonicity and improve passive range of motion (PROM), especially for dorsiflexion (DF) in equinus deformity. It can also help improve gait and may delay or even prevent the need for surgical interventions like tendon lengthening. The procedure is often used in conjunction with Botulinum toxin A injections to achieve and maintain muscle length and reduce tone [35].

6.6.4 Orthotic Interventions

An orthosis is more than just supportive equipment; it is a biomechanical device specifically designed to apply forces to the human body to modify movement, correct alignment, and enhance posture. A key principle in orthotic design is the effective management of pressure and force distribution. The most commonly prescribed types are ankle-foot orthoses (AFO), floor reaction orthosis (FRO), dynamic AFO (DAFO), and posterior leaf spring (PLS) or hinged AFO (HAFO) [36].

Ankle-foot orthoses (AFOs) are the most widely prescribed orthotic device for children with CP ("Yellow light" label, with conditional recommendation for walking speed and gross motor function, and high certainty of evidence for improving ankle kinematics and stride length) [17, 18]. Their primary functions include improving gait efficiency, maintaining or increasing joint range of motion (ROM), and preventing the development of muscle contractures. The effectiveness of an AFO is highly dependent on its specific design, which is selected to address the patient's unique biomechanical needs. Solid AFOs, which are rigid and allow no ankle motion, provide maximum stability and are effective in controlling varus/valgus deformities. They are particularly useful for enabling proper heel strike and toe clearance, providing a secure base of support for walking. In contrast, hinged or dynamic AFOs (DAFOs) incorporate a hinge that allows for controlled ankle movement, facilitating a more natural gait and assisting with foot clearance during the swing phase. The posterior leaf spring AFO (PLSO), a more flexible design, is ideal for mild spastic equinus as it allows for passive ankle dorsiflexion while walking. A ground reaction AFO (GRAFO) is designed to manage crouch gait by applying a strong anterior force to the tibia, promoting knee extension during the stance phase and thereby preventing excessive knee flexion. These varied designs underscore the precision required in orthotic prescription to match the device's biomechanics to the patient's specific gait pathology [36, 37].

6.6.5 Strength Training

The evidence for strength training has a "Green light" for lower limb muscle strength improvements, and a "Yellow light" for gross motor, upper limb strength, and functional outcomes. Also, "active strength training" has "Green light" evidence for managing contracture and alignment [18]. This type of intervention varies widely in its implementation and the caregivers' experiences, which can lead to different study results. Still, it has been shown that strength training can improve balance and gait speed, without increasing spasticity in GMFCS classes of I, II, and III. Examples of exercises include isotonic, isometric, and isokinetic training, pelvic bridging, supine bridging, twisting with a medicine ball, leg press, seated knee extensions with weighted machines, heel lift, squats, jumping and hopping, balance training with a BOSU ball, walking on ramps, stairs, and steps, etc. [38, 39].

6.6.6 Robot-Assisted Therapy

Robot-assisted gait training (RAGT), using devices like the Lokomat (Hocoma; Zurich, Switzerland), is a "Yellow Light" intervention for gait rehabilitation (low certainty of evidence) [17, 18]. These devices provide a controlled environment for high-intensity, repetitive gait training, which is less physically demanding on the therapist. The Lokomat, for instance, uses a body weight support (BWS) harness and robotic orthoses to assist a child in walking on a treadmill [40].

While some studies have reported positive effects, such as improved walking speed and physical fitness, the evidence for RAGT in pediatrics is considered weak and inconsistent, and no clear guidelines exist for training protocols. Despite this, RAGT can be a motivating and engaging therapy for children, especially when combined with virtual reality games. It is currently recommended as an integration to usual rehabilitation, not a replacement [41].

6.7 Emerging and Adjunctive Interventions

In addition to core discipline-specific approaches, new technologies and traditional modalities are used to augment therapy.

6.7.1 Virtual Reality (VR) Therapy

VR is a "Yellow Light" intervention that uses computer technology to create an interactive and motivating environment for therapy (moderate certainty of evidence for improving hand function) [17, 18]. By simulating real-world scenarios in a safe setting, VR promotes motor learning through repetition and multisensory feedback. Studies suggest that VR can significantly improve balance, motor function, and daily living skills, although evidence for upper limb function is mixed. The gamified nature of VR can increase a child's motivation and the frequency of practice, which is crucial for neuroplastic change [42, 43].

6.7.2 Sensory Integration Therapy

Sensory Integration Therapy (SIT) is a specialized occupational therapy that targets how a child's nervous system processes sensory input from their environment. It involves play-based exercises aimed at enhancing sensory processing by engaging with visual, olfactory, tactile, auditory, gustatory, and vestibular stimuli. The core idea of Sensory Integration therapy is to help children respond appropriately to everyday stimuli by offering controlled sensory experiences. This approach is based on neuroplasticity, which seeks to modify the nervous system through experience. Occupational therapists collaborate with children to address issues such as over-responsiveness (avoidance, fear), under-responsiveness (passivity, withdrawal), or sensory seeking behaviors (impulsivity, risk-taking) [44].

Therapy sessions are designed as playful activities within a "sensory-rich" environment that often includes equipment like swings, trampolines, and balance beams to provide vestibular, proprioceptive, and tactile input. The therapist guides the child toward sensory experiences that challenge them to develop an appropriate adaptive response [44, 45].

The evidence for Sensory Integration therapy, particularly in terms of motor outcomes in cerebral palsy, is mixed. The "State of the Evidence Traffic Lights" framework classifies Sensory Integration as a "Red Light" intervention when used for motor goals, meaning it is not recommended due to a lack of evidence for its effectiveness in improving motor function and performance [18, 45].

6.7.3 Hippotherapy

Hippotherapy is a specialized medical intervention in which the therapist utilizes the controlled, rhythmic movement of a horse to achieve specific, individualized treatment goals. In this context, the horse functions as a "live" treatment tool, providing dynamic, three-dimensional sensory and motor input that is manipulated by the clinician to influence neuromotor, sensory, and cognitive systems. The focus remains squarely on the patient's therapeutic response to the horse's movement, with the therapist constantly adjusting variables such as the horse's gait, speed, and direction, as well as the patient's position, to achieve the desired outcomes [46, 47].

The therapeutic efficacy of hippotherapy is rooted in a unique combination of biomechanical and neurophysiological principles. At its core, the therapy is predicated on the fact that the rhythmic, variable, and multidirectional movement of a horse's gait provides a powerful source of motor and sensory input. This continuous, dynamic stimulus repetitively challenges the rider's balance and postural control, requiring the patient to make constant, subtle adjustments to maintain an upright position. These adaptations are not voluntary but are reflexive, stimulating the patient's vestibular and proprioceptive systems, which are fundamental for balance, coordination, and motor planning [48, 49].

In the traffic light approach, this therapeutic intervention has "Green light" evidence for improving balance and symmetry, and "Yellow light" evidence for gross motor and hand function improvements (strong recommendation with high certainty of evidence) [17, 18].

6.8 Speech and Language Rehabilitation

Speech and language impairments represent a significant challenge for individuals with cerebral palsy (CP), profoundly affecting their ability to communicate, interact socially, and participate in daily life. The prevalence of these difficulties varies widely across studies, a discrepancy that highlights a lack of a universal classification and measurement standard in the field. Estimates suggest that up to 75% of children with CP may have some form of speech or language disorder, while a more focused systematic review estimates that approximately 20% of children with CP experience severe communication impairment, classifying them as non-verbal [50, 51] (Find more details about this rehabilitative approach in the chapter "Speech and Language Therapy for Cerebral Palsy").

6.8.1 Functional Classification Systems

Standardized classification tools are increasingly vital for consistent evaluation, clinical communication, and research. Two key examples are the Communication Function Classification System (CFCS) and the Eating and Drinking Ability Classification System (EDACS).

The CFCS is a tool that classifies an individual's everyday communication effectiveness into one of five levels, with Level I representing an independent and effective communicator and Level V representing a person who is seldom able to communicate effectively (see Sect. 3.3) [11].

The EDACS is a clinical tool that assesses a person's functional capacity to eat and drink. It uses five levels, from complete independence to requiring full assistance, and accounts for factors such as motor control, posture, and the need for food texture modifications for safe intake. The shift toward using these functional classification systems and other standardized tools represents a change in the field, recognizing that a child's true communication and swallowing ability are about their real-world participation, not just isolated clinical metrics [52].

6.8.2 Evidence-Based Therapeutic and Rehabilitative Approaches

Modern speech and language interventions for cerebral palsy are increasingly grounded in principles of neuroplasticity and motor learning (PML). These principles—including task repetition, practice intensity, and salience—suggest that adherence to specific guidelines can improve motor speech outcomes. This focus on intensive, well-structured practice is a direct response to the understanding that dysarthria is a motor programming deficit, not a simple weakness, and therefore requires a systematic approach to retraining the neural pathways involved in speech [53].

Several motor speech interventions have been developed to improve speech intelligibility in children with CP. Lee Silverman Voice Treatment (LSVT LOUD), an intensive protocol originally designed for individuals with Parkinson's disease, has shown promise in children with CP by focusing on increasing vocal loudness. Another program, the Speech Systems Approach, focuses on breath support and speech rate to improve overall intelligibility [54].

Given the shared musculature for eating, swallowing, and speaking, oral motor therapy is an essential component of rehabilitation. Oral Motor and Swallowing Therapy (OMT) encompasses a range of exercises, including tongue push-ups, lip puckering, and jaw movements, designed to enhance the strength, coordination, and function of the oral musculature. Research, including a randomized controlled trial, has shown that OMT is effective in improving feeding and swallowing functions. The study demonstrated significant improvements in mandible mobility, tongue retraction, and a notable reduction in the frequency of drooling. These findings indicate that OMT can directly enhance a child's ability to eat and drink safely, thereby improving their nutritional status and overall health [55].

For children with severe speech impairments, Augmentative and Alternative Communication (AAC) is not a supplemental tool but a vital, often primary, communication strategy. AAC encompasses a wide range of methods, from unaided techniques such as gestures, facial expressions, and sign language to aided systems that utilize external equipment. Aided AAC can range from low-tech options, such as communication boards with pictures, to high-tech solutions, including tablets with speech-generating apps and specialized speech-generating devices [56].

6.9 Parent and Caregiver Support

The principles of modern rehabilitation, endorsed by leading international guidelines, place the family at the center of care, acknowledging their constant and enduring presence in the child's life. The international clinical practice guideline (ICPG) on interventions to improve physical function for CP explicitly recommends that therapeutic plans include "support to empower families" and integrate "child/family preferences" to achieve functional goals [17]. High-quality evidence shows that family-centered service (FCS)—where care is organized around family priorities, shared decision-making, and respect for family expertise—improves parent psychosocial outcomes, service satisfaction, and care processes, and also is associated with better adherence to therapy plans [57]. The ICPG guideline explicitly embeds these principles, recommending client-chosen goals, parent-delivered practice at home, and care in real-life contexts (i.e., home and community) to maximize carryover and participation. The ICPG emphasizes structured home practice, written/visual instructions, and ongoing review, with the team helping families problem-solving barriers (time, motivation, equipment) [17].

In practice, a strong caregiver-support pathway includes: (1) collaborative goal setting (child/family priorities first), (2) co-designed home programs with achievable daily "micro-doses," (3) routine check-ins (in-person or telehealth) to adjust tasks and troubleshoot, (4) caregiver wellbeing screening and referrals (e.g., mental health, social services, respite), and (5) peer connections and practical navigation of equipment, funding, and school/community inclusion (Table 6.3) [57, 58].

Table 6.3 Parent-facing home program: what to emphasize

Goals	"Green-light" parent actions	Adjuncts to consider (conditions apply)	Avoid/Not recommended
Mobility & endurance	Daily goal-directed walking/transfer practice; real-life routes; simple step-counts or timers	Treadmill, VR, biofeedback when motivating/access available; AFOs if indicated and tolerated	Robot-led gait where the device does most of the work; suit therapy
Upper limb/ hand use	CIMT (unilateral) or bimanual/HABIT (structured play tasks); integrate into ADLs	Action observation, CO-OP, VR, hand splints (night) as adjuncts; Botox + intensive practice when spasticity limits function	Stand-alone impairment-only drills without task linkage
Self-care & participation	Whole-task practice (dressing, feeding, grooming) in real contexts; adaptive equipment to boost independence and reduce burden	Hydrotherapy/hippotherapy (plus land carry-over), taping for short-term alignment during task practice	Equipment without training; programs that ignore family routines

6.10 Guide for the Multidisciplinary Team

Effective CP services are built around a coordinated multidisciplinary team (MDT). Current guidance emphasizes four areas: (1) family-centered, goal-directed care; (2) ICF-based assessment using common classification systems; (3) evidence-based intervention pathways with planned dose and home practice; and (4) structured surveillance for preventable complications (hips, respiratory, nutrition/dysphagia), with clear escalation to advanced therapies [17, 59].

1. Team & process: MDTs typically include developmental pediatrics/physiatry, neurology, orthopedics, PT, OT, speech-language pathologist (SLP), psychology, social work, dietetics, nursing, orthotics/assistive tech, and (where available) gait analysis. Care is organized around client-chosen goals and whole-task practice in real-life contexts, with parents as decision-makers and dose-drivers (structured home programs) [17]. The UK NICE guidance further operationalizes shared decisions, timely access to equipment, and embedding therapy in daily routines [60].
2. Assessment framework: Use the ICF (activity/participation focus; environmental facilitators/barriers) and CP classification systems to align the team: GMFCS (gross motor), MACS (manual ability), CFCS (communication), and EDACS/ Mini-EDACS (eating & drinking) [61, 62]. These tools improve common language, risk stratification (e.g., aspiration risk at EDACS III–V), and outcome selection [11].
3. Evidence-based interventions: The 2021 international guideline prioritizes goal-directed, task-specific training across domains (mobility, upper limb, self-care, participation) and specifies where evidence is strong vs conditional (e.g., CIMT/

bimanual therapy strong; treadmill/VR conditional). Pair this with the Traffic Lights 2019 synthesis to grade "green/yellow" priorities for the plan families can act on at home [17].

4. Surveillance & safety nets: MDTs should embed hip surveillance (schedule by GMFCS, clinical + radiographic intervals) to prevent displacement and follow spasticity pathways (PT/OT foundations; orthoses; focal chemodenervation; ITB; SDR) with mandatory post-procedure therapy dosing [63]. Add respiratory and sialorrhea care pathways where indicated, and screen routinely for nutrition/dysphagia using EDACS and SLP assessment [64].
5. Implementation & transition: Use care-pathway tools and fidelity checklists to standardize delivery and dose; recent work has produced practical fidelity instruments for the 2021 guideline. Plan transition to adult services early; audits highlight gaps without structured MDT handover [65].

6.11 Conclusion

The field of physical therapy and rehabilitation for cerebral palsy has advanced into an evidence-based, integrated practice. It now utilizes core principles, modalities, and assistive technology that extend beyond motor treatments, centered on a motor-learning framework that emphasizes active, purposeful practice within a family-centered, transdisciplinary care model. This optimistic approach aims to shift from symptom management to improving independence, health, and quality of life for individuals with CP. While higher-level evidence and inclusive research remain challenges, the shift to a collaborative, science-based practice offers a promising way forward.

References

1. Rosenbaum P, Paneth N, Leviton A, Goldstein M, Bax M, Damiano D, et al. A report: the definition and classification of cerebral palsy April 2006. Dev Med Child Neurol Suppl. 2007;109(Suppl 109):8–14.
2. Vitrikas K, Dalton H, Breish D. Cerebral palsy: an overview. Am Fam Physician. 2020;101(4):213–20.
3. Patel DR, Neelakantan M, Pandher K, Merrick J. Cerebral palsy in children: a clinical overview. Trans Pediatr. 2020;9(Suppl 1):S125.
4. Centers for Disease Control and Prevention. Cerebral palsy. Updated 17 Mar 2025. Available from: https://www.cdc.gov/cerebral-palsy/about/index.html.
5. Wahyuni LK. Multisystem compensations and consequences in spastic quadriplegic cerebral palsy children. Front Neurol. 2023;13:1076316.
6. Trabacca A, Vespino T, Di Liddo A, Russo L. Multidisciplinary rehabilitation for patients with cerebral palsy: improving long-term care. J Multidiscip Healthc. 2016;9:455–62.
7. Compagnone E, Maniglio J, Camposeo S, Vespino T, Losito L, De Rinaldis M, et al. Functional classifications for cerebral palsy: correlations between the gross motor function classification system (GMFCS), the manual ability classification system (MACS) and the communication function classification system (CFCS). Res Dev Disabil. 2014;35(11):2651–7.

8. Palisano R, Rosenbaum P, Bartlett D, Livingston M, Walter S, Russell D. GMFCS-E&R. CanChild Centre for Childhood Disability Research, McMaster University. 2007;200(7).
9. Eliasson A-C, Krumlinde-Sundholm L, Rösblad B, Beckung E, Arner M, Öhrvall A-M, Rosenbaum P. The manual ability classification system (MACS) for children with cerebral palsy: scale development and evidence of validity and reliability. Dev Med Child Neurol. 2006;48(7):549–54.
10. Eliasson A-C, Ullenhag A, Wahlström U, Krumlinde-Sundholm L. Mini-MACS: development of the manual ability classification system for children younger than 4 years of age with signs of cerebral palsy. Dev Med Child Neurol. 2017;59(1):72–8.
11. Hidecker MJC, Paneth N, Rosenbaum PL, Kent RD, Lillie J, Eulenberg JB, et al. Developing and validating the communication function classification system for individuals with cerebral palsy. Dev Med Child Neurol. 2011;53(8):704–10.
12. Anttila H, Autti-Rämö I, Suoranta J, Mäkelä M, Malmivaara A. Effectiveness of physical therapy interventions for children with cerebral palsy: a systematic review. BMC Pediatr. 2008;8(1):14.
13. Foscan M, Luparia A, Molteni F, Bianchi E, Gandelli S, Pagliano E, Fedrizzi E. Development of a play-based motor learning approach (a.MO.GIOCO) in children with bilateral cerebral palsy: theoretical framework and intervention methodology. Children. 2024;11(1):127.
14. Steultjens EM, Dekker J, Bouter LM, van de Nes JC, Lambregts BL, van den Ende CH. Occupational therapy for children with cerebral palsy: a systematic review. Clin Rehabil. 2004;18(1):1–14.
15. Kachmar O, Kozyavkina N, Kushnir A, Kozyavkina O. Neuroplasticity in rehabilitation of children with cerebral palsy. Int Neurol J. 2025;21(1):52–9.
16. Bar-Haim S, Harries N, Nammourah I, Oraibi S, Malhees W, Loeppky J, et al. Effectiveness of motor learning coaching in children with cerebral palsy: a randomized controlled trial. Clin Rehabil. 2010;24(11):1009–20.
17. Jackman M, Sakzewski L, Morgan C, Boyd RN, Brennan SE, Langdon K, et al. Interventions to improve physical function for children and young people with cerebral palsy: international clinical practice guideline. Dev Med Child Neurol. 2022;64(5):536–49.
18. Novak I, Morgan C, Fahey M, Finch-Edmondson M, Galea C, Hines A, et al. State of the evidence traffic lights 2019: systematic review of interventions for preventing and treating children with cerebral palsy. Curr Neurol Neurosci Rep. 2020;20(2):3.
19. Alonso-Coello P, Schünemann HJ, Moberg J, Brignardello-Petersen R, Akl EA, Davoli M, et al. GRADE evidence to decision (EtD) frameworks: a systematic and transparent approach to making well informed healthcare choices. 1: introduction. BMJ. 2016;353:i2016.
20. Javvaji CK, Vagha JD, Meshram RJ, Taksande A. Assessment scales in cerebral palsy: a comprehensive review of tools and applications. Cureus. 2023;15(10):e47939.
21. Hwang Y, Kwon JY. Personalized goal setting and predictors of functional gains following constraint-induced movement therapy in preschool-aged children with unilateral cerebral palsy. PLoS One. 2025;20(8):e0329002.
22. Ko J, Kim M. Reliability and responsiveness of the gross motor function measure-88 in children with cerebral palsy. Phys Ther. 2013;93(3):393–400.
23. Yoo M, Ahn JH, Rha D-w, Park ES. Reliability of the modified Ashworth and modified Tardieu scales with standardized movement speeds in children with spastic cerebral palsy. Children. 2022;9(6):827.
24. Shore BJ, Allar BG, Miller PE, Matheney TH, Snyder BD, Fragala-Pinkham M. Measuring the reliability and construct validity of the pediatric evaluation of disability inventory–computer adaptive test (PEDI-CAT) in children with cerebral palsy. Arch Phys Med Rehabil. 2019;100(1):45–51.
25. Tanabe H, Tanabe H, Okuda S, Mikawa T, Sakurai Y, Takata Y. Evaluation of effectiveness of modified pediatric constraint-induced movement therapy performed on children with cerebral palsy by a home-treatment program. Am J Med. 2025;10(1)
26. Jamali AR, Amini M. The effects of constraint-induced movement therapy on functions of cerebral palsy children. Iran J Child Neurol. 2018;12(4):16–27.

27. Morris D, Taub E, Mark V. Constraint-induced movement therapy: characterizing the intervention protocol. Eura Medicophys. 2006;42(3):257.
28. Boyd RN, Ziviani J, Sakzewski L, Miller L, Bowden J, Cunnington R, et al. COMBIT: protocol of a randomised comparison trial of COMbined modified constraint induced movement therapy and bimanual intensive training with distributed model of standard upper limb rehabilitation in children with congenital hemiplegia. BMC Neurol. 2013;13:68.
29. Qu YL, Harun D, Chai SC, Ebner-Karestinos D, Araneda R, Zanudin A. Effectiveness of hand-arm bimanual intensive therapy including lower extremities in the rehabilitation of children with cerebral palsy: a systematic review protocol. BMJ Open. 2025;15(3):e091062.
30. Zanon MA, Porfírio GJ, Riera R, Martimbianco ALC. Neurodevelopmental treatment approaches for children with cerebral palsy. Cochrane Database Syst Rev. 2015;2015(11):CD011937.
31. Zanon MA, Pacheco RL, Latorraca COC, Martimbianco ALC, Pachito DV, Riera R. Neurodevelopmental treatment (Bobath) for children with cerebral palsy: a systematic review. J Child Neurol. 2019;34(11):679–86.
32. Carton de Tournai A, Herman E, Ebner-Karestinos D, Gathy E, Araneda R, Renders A, et al. Hand-arm bimanual intensive therapy including lower extremities in infants with unilateral cerebral palsy: a randomized clinical trial. JAMA Netw Open. 2024;7(11):e2445133.
33. Toovey R, Bernie C, Harvey AR, McGinley JL, Spittle AJ. Task-specific gross motor skills training for ambulant school-aged children with cerebral palsy: a systematic review. BMJ Paediatr Open. 2017;1(1):e000078.
34. Karnadipa T, Xin W, Pickering D, Carrier J. Effectiveness of task-specific training for improving balance performance in children with cerebral palsy (CP): a narrative systematic review. Physiother Q. 2024;32(1):15–24.
35. Milne N, Miao M, Beattie E. The effects of serial casting on lower limb function for children with cerebral palsy: a systematic review with meta-analysis. BMC Pediatr. 2020;20(1):324.
36. Aboutorabi A, Arazpour M, Ahmadi Bani M, Saeedi H, Head JS. Efficacy of ankle foot orthoses types on walking in children with cerebral palsy: a systematic review. Ann Phys Rehabil Med. 2017;60(6):393–402.
37. Morris C, Bowers R, Ross K, Stevens P, Phillips D. Orthotic management of cerebral palsy: recommendations from a consensus conference. NeuroRehabilitation. 2011;28:37–46.
38. Liang X, Zhujiang T, Guojun Y, Jianguo C, Jinggang W, Qing L, Turong C. Effectiveness of exercise interventions for children with cerebral palsy: a systematic review and meta-analysis of randomized controlled trials. J Rehabil Med. 2020;53(4):2733.
39. Merino-Andrés J, García de Mateos-López A, Damiano DL, Sánchez-Sierra A. Effect of muscle strength training in children and adolescents with spastic cerebral palsy: a systematic review and meta-analysis. Clin Rehabil. 2022;36(1):4–14.
40. Nam KY, Kim HJ, Kwon BS, Park J-W, Lee HJ, Yoo A. Robot-assisted gait training (Lokomat) improves walking function and activity in people with spinal cord injury: a systematic review. J Neuroeng Rehabil. 2017;14(1):24.
41. Cherni Y, Ziane C. A narrative review on robotic-assisted gait training in children and adolescents with cerebral palsy: training parameters, choice of settings, and perspectives. Disabilities. 2022;2(2):293–303.
42. Komariah M, Amirah S, Abdurrahman MF, Handimulya MFS, Platini H, Maulana S, et al. Effectivity of virtual reality to improve balance, motor function, activities of daily living, and upper limb function in children with cerebral palsy: a systematic review and meta-analysis. Ther Clin Risk Manag. 2024;20:95–109.
43. Michaud B, Cherni Y, Begon M, Girardin-Vignola G, Roussel P, editors. A serious game for gait rehabilitation with the Lokomat. In: 2017 International conference on virtual rehabilitation (ICVR), 19–22 June 2017
44. Warutkar VB, Kovela RK, Warutkar V. Review of sensory integration therapy for children with cerebral palsy. Cureus. 2022;14(10):e30714.
45. Kantor J, Hlaváčková L, Du J, Dvořáková P, Svobodová Z, Karasová K, Kantorová L. The effects of ayres sensory integration and related sensory based interventions in children with cerebral palsy: a scoping review. Children. 2022;9(4):483.

46. Hays A, Meera B, Caitlin Peters B, Erdman E, Fields B. Hippotherapy practice and safety patterns for adult clients in the United States. Hum Anim Interact. 2025;13(1):0003.
47. Du Plessis N, Uys K, Buys T. Hippotherapy concepts: a scoping review to inform transdisciplinary practice guidelines. Scand J Occup Ther. 2023;30:1424–40.
48. Assis G, Schlichting T, Mateus B, Lemos A, Santos A. Physical therapy with hippotherapy compared to physical therapy alone in children with cerebral palsy: systematic review and meta-analysis. Dev Med Child Neurol. 2021;64:156–61.
49. Koca TT, Ataseven H. What is hippotherapy? The indications and effectiveness of hippotherapy. N Clin Istanb. 2015;2(3):247–52.
50. Andersen G, Mjøen TR, Vik T. Prevalence of speech problems and the use of augmentative and alternative communication in children with cerebral palsy: a registry-based study in Norway. Perspect Augment Altern Commun. 2010;19(1):12–20.
51. Hustad KC, Oakes A, Allison K. Variability and diagnostic accuracy of speech intelligibility scores in children. J Speech Lang Hear Res. 2015;58(6):1695–707.
52. Calderone A, Militi D, Cardile D, Corallo F, Calabrò RS, Militi A. Swallowing disorders in cerebral palsy: a systematic review of oropharyngeal dysphagia, nutritional impact, and health risks. Ital J Pediatr. 2025;51(1):57.
53. Korkalainen M, McCabe P, Smidt A, Morgan C. Motor speech interventions for children with cerebral palsy: a systematic review. J Speech Lang Hear Res. 2023;66:110–25.
54. Pennington L, Rauch R, Smith J, Brittain K. Views of children with cerebral palsy and their parents on the effectiveness and acceptability of intensive speech therapy. Disabil Rehabil. 2020;42(20):2935–43.
55. Sığan SN, Uzunhan TA, Aydınlı N, Eraslan E, Ekici B, Çalışkan M. Effects of oral motor therapy in children with cerebral palsy. Ann Indian Acad Neurol. 2013;16(3):342–6.
56. Hustad KC, Miles LK. Alignment between augmentative and alternative communication needs and school-based speech-language services provided to young children with cerebral palsy. Early Child Serv. 2010;4(3):129–40.
57. King S, Teplicky R, King G, Rosenbaum P. Family-centered service for children with cerebral palsy and their families: a review of the literature. Semin Pediatr Neurol. 2004;11(1):78–86.
58. Kuhlthau KA, Bloom S, Van Cleave J, Knapp AA, Romm D, Klatka K, et al. Evidence for family-centered care for children with special health care needs: a systematic review. Acad Pediatr. 2011;11(2):136–43.e8.
59. NICE Guideline. Cerebral palsy in under 25s: assessment and management. 25 Jan 2017. Available from: https://www.nice.org.uk/guidance/ng62/chapter/Recommendations#multidisciplinary-care.
60. Clinical Guideline. Spasticity in under 19s: management. 25 July 2012 [updated 29 Nov 2016]. Available from: https://www.nice.org.uk/guidance/cg145/chapter/Recommendations?utm_source=chatgpt.com.
61. Bykova KM, Frank U, Girolami GL. Eating and drinking ability classification system to detect aspiration risk in children with cerebral palsy: a validation study. Eur J Pediatr. 2023;182(7):3365–73.
62. International Classification of Functioning, Disability and Health (ICF). 2018. Available from: https://www.who.int/standards/classifications/international-classification-of-functioning-disability-and-health?utm_source=chatgpt.com.
63. Shrader MW, Wimberly L, Thompson R. Hip surveillance in children with cerebral palsy. J Am Acad Orthop Surg. 2019;27(20):760–8.
64. Blackmore AM, Gibson N, Cooper MS, Langdon K, Moshovis L, Wilson AC. Interventions for management of respiratory disease in young people with cerebral palsy: a systematic review. Child Care Health Dev. 2019;45(5):754–71.
65. Jackman M, Thorley M, Toovey R, Burgess A, Blatch-Williams R, Sakzewski L, et al. Implementing clinical practice guidelines for improving function in cerebral palsy: development of a Fidelity tool. Pediatr Phys Ther. 2025;37(1):4–13.

Assistive Devices, Orthotics, and Bracing 7

Kaveh Same

7.1 Introduction

A 17-month-old girl was presented to a healthcare facility in London with her parents complaining of delayed motor skills in their child. The girl could crawl but was unable to stand or step independently. A diagnosis of cerebral palsy was suspected, which was ultimately confirmed 3 months later. The disease presented with bilateral spasticity primarily affecting the lower limbs. Several orthoses were prescribed for her during a 10-month treatment period, and her physical and motor functions were assessed several times during this period. Using an ankle-foot orthosis and footwear combination, aided by a walker frame, she was able to develop the ability to walk independently, and significant improvements were observed in her gait speed and other assessed parameters [1].

7.1.1 Background

Use of external devices to prevent certain deformity developments or make functional improvements has a long history in medicine. Explaining the importance of using leather-based material as in-shoe supports, Durlacher, a chiropodist from England, is considered to have provided one of the first descriptions of a foot orthosis [2]. Used with increasing frequency and variety through time, orthoses have since been made from a broad range of synthetic and natural materials [3], each more suited for a different condition and body region.

K. Same (✉)
Michael Ogon Laboratory for Orthopaedic Research, Orthopaedic Hospital Speising, Vienna, Austria

Doctoral Programme MedUni Vienna, Medical University of Vienna, Vienna, Austria
e-mail: kaveh.same@oss.at

A. Presedo et al. (eds.), *Enhancing Quality of Life in Patients with Cerebral Palsy*, https://doi.org/10.1007/978-3-032-20967-2_7

A disease with severe potential impact on the patient's physical ability and movement, cerebral palsy (CP) can directly contribute to the development of a wide range of deformities throughout the child's life, even further impacting their function and well-being. A systematic review of qualitative studies assessed the perspectives of children with CP about themselves, concluding that the extent of their physical disabilities has a profound impact on their view of themselves, partly due to its effect on their social inclusion and participation [4]. Focusing on a somewhat different but related subject, Feldner et al. conducted a qualitative study to assess stakeholder priorities (in this case, chiefly the patients with CP) with regard to supportive mobility devices. As expected, the majority of responses emphasized the need for such devices to be able to answer the users' needs [5]. These findings point to the potential of supportive devices to improve the patients' lives and make significant boosts to their physical activity and social participation, if designed and used properly and according to the users' needs. Going one step further, orthoses have the ability not only to correct deformities and improve function but also to prevent many deformity formations, making them a non-invasive and cost-effective form of intervention in many cases.

The following sections will aim to first establish a basic understanding of such devices' different types and functions, and then to take a closer look at their specific examples, as well as their uses and effects.

7.1.2 Definitions and Principles of Function

7.1.2.1 Orthoses

Orthoses design and application revolve around the simple idea of using externally attached devices to prevent, manage, or even correct deformities. Over time, numerous designs have been developed for various deformities and conditions, spanning all parts of the human body and incorporating a myriad of working principles and structural materials. In his 1995 review of orthoses and prostheses, Hailey describes three main functions through which orthoses can affect treatment [6]:

- Controlling movements of the musculoskeletal system
- Compensating for absent functions
- Correcting deformities

Believing an accurate prescription of the right orthosis to hinge on a correct identification of the nature and details of the patient's impairment, Schnell et al. note the exact *diagnosis* to be of less importance when it comes to determination of the orthosis type and specification [7].

As a condition that mostly affects the physical abilities of the patient and makes them especially prone to the development of deformities, the use of different orthoses has been a cornerstone of treatment in individuals with CP. In the following sections, the most frequently used examples of such orthoses will be discussed along with their use cases and potential benefits.

7.1.2.2 Assistive Devices

Assistive devices (ADs) include a wide range of instruments designed to help individuals with their daily tasks. ADs can be differentiated from orthoses as they are used to compensate for their users' disability and to enhance their physical performance in a certain task, ultimately allowing them more independence in their daily life. On the other hand, orthoses mainly function as a means of deformity correction or prevention. Common examples of ADs include the following:

- Wheelchairs and Walkers
- Adapted Seating Systems
- Portable Ramps
- Adapted Beds and Seating Positions
- Bathing and Toileting Aids
- Communication Devices
- Others

7.1.3 Use and Efficacy Assessment

Even the best orthosis is only effective if used properly and continuously. Therefore, having the ability to accurately assess patient adherence to the treatment and their proper use of the prescribed orthosis is crucial in determining the device's effectiveness. Traditionally, this has been achieved via patient-reported, subjective accounts of their use of the device. However, in a systematic review on the subject, Devanand et al., arguing the importance of objective assessments due to unreliability and overestimation of patient-reported use of orthoses, investigated the objective methods of orthotic device usage in patients. Based on their findings, the use of electronic sensors was the main way by which patient compliance was tracked and monitored. Temperature sensors, pressure sensors, accelerometers, a step counter, or a combination of them were used by different studies to allow an objective assessment of the orthosis use and patient compliance. Single-sensor monitoring was expectedly found to be less accurate than multi-sensor solutions, while the latter could potentially lead to more bulky designs with more wires, itself a big hindrance to their frequent use. Overall, while the obtained data through the implementation of sensors were found to be valuable for clinical judgment of the prescribed treatment, nearly all the devices used in the included studies were reported to be more suited for research rather than everyday use by the patient due to their unrefined designs, warranting the need for refined, more *consumer-friendly* designs if they are to be employed in large scale [8].

Despite their shortcomings, and while their augmentation with other means of use assessment seems to be the way forward, as of now, patient-reported, subjective accounts of their use of the orthoses and their satisfaction with them remain the main method of patient compliance evaluation. While simple, unstructured interviews between patients and their healthcare provider are the most prevalent form of obtaining such accounts, Bettoni et al. summarized the existing questionnaires for evaluation of patient satisfaction with limb orthoses. Based on their results, four questionnaires were found to be sufficiently validated to warrant their use. Of the four, two were designed for general orthotic use [9]:

- Quebec User Evaluation of Satisfaction with Assistive Technology 2.0 (QUEST 2.0): A usually self-administered 12-item questionnaire that assesses the device, as well as the *service* (i.e., device's setup, repair service, and follow-up quality). Each item is answered using a 5-point scale, from "not satisfied at all" to "very satisfied" for each. Developed through rigorous item reduction and validation, the questionnaire exhibits moderate to high internal consistency and test–retest reliability [10].
- Client Satisfaction with Device (CSD) module of the Orthotics and Prosthetics Users' Survey (OPUS): The original CSD was a self-administered questionnaire, including 10–11 items, rated on a 4-point Likert scale from "strongly disagree" to "strongly agree" to assess aspects like device fit, comfort, durability, ease of use, pleasant appearance, and manageability of weight and repairs. A later refined version uses eight items, validated via Rasch analysis for psychometric consistency, with a score range from 8 to 32 [11].

Finally, advances in curriculum and teaching methods in the last 50 years have transformed the science of orthotics, training professionals who not only are capable of designing more advanced and functional devices but are also experts in proper device prescription, patient education, and follow-up, ultimately leading to increased patient satisfaction and improved adherence to the chosen treatment [12].

7.2 A Closer Look: Orthoses and Braces

Motor impairments frequently present in cerebral palsy include muscle weakness, spasticity and contracture, poor selective control, and difficulties with balance. Orthoses and braces are prescribed for many children with CP to maintain joint range, influence biomechanics during movement, and prevent secondary deformities. They are often used together with physiotherapy, strength training, or botulinum toxin injections rather than as stand-alone treatments. The evidence base is still evolving; most trials are small and heterogeneous, so clinicians must apply principles of biomechanics and individual assessment when prescribing devices.

The sections below summarize major orthoses used in the upper limb, lower limb, and spine of children with CP. Furthermore, they provide historical context, biomechanical principles, prescription guidelines, evidence of effectiveness, and practical considerations.

7.2.1 Upper Limb

Static Wrist/Hand Orthoses

Static wrist-hand orthoses (sometimes called resting splints) immobilize the wrist and hand in a neutral or extended position. They were first made from plaster or metal in the early twentieth century; modern devices use thermoplastics and Velcro straps. They are typically worn at night to provide a prolonged low-load stretch. The Swedish Cerebral Palsy Follow-Up Program (CPUP) upper-limb orthosis guide notes that these splints aim to provide a sustained stretch, maintain or increase range of motion, and prevent abnormal postures [13]. Static splints should not replace therapy; rather, they are an adjunct to exercises and should be reviewed regularly.

Evidence for static hand splints is limited. In a cross-over study by Krumlinde-Sundholm and colleagues, discontinuing overnight splint use for 3 months led to a significant reduction in passive wrist and thumb range of motion; resuming splints increased or maintained range. A pragmatic, multi-center randomized controlled trial comparing rigid wrist-hand orthoses plus usual care with usual care alone found modest improvements in passive wrist extension at 6 and 12 months (mean difference 13°–21°), but results beyond 18 months were inconclusive [14]. The trial was stopped early due to insufficient recruitment, illustrating the difficulty of conducting long-term orthotic studies.

Dynamic Wrist-Hand Orthoses

Dynamic or functional wrist-hand orthoses include devices such as spring-assisted exoskeletons (e.g., SaeboFlex) or hinged splints that allow controlled movement. They attempt to augment active grasping and releasing by storing energy in springs and releasing it to assist wrist extension. Evidence in CP is sparse. A 2019 randomized controlled trial in children with CP or brain injury investigated the immediate effect of a functional wrist orthosis; manual dexterity (box-and-block test) did not differ between orthotic and non-orthotic conditions, suggesting that wearing the device alone does not improve immediate hand function [15]. The authors recommended combining orthoses with task-specific training.

Dynamic Elastomeric Fabric Orthoses (Gloves and Garments)

Dynamic elastomeric fabric orthoses (DEFOs) are elastic Lycra® garments or gloves that provide gentle compression and resistance. They were introduced in the 1990s and marketed under names such as *DMOrthotics*. The mild compression is thought to enhance proprioception, support muscles, and influence alignment. Several studies have described improvements in sitting balance, grasping, and self-feeding in children wearing Lycra garments and gloves [16, 17]. These garments may therefore provide immediate improvement in proximal stability and hand function when combined with therapy.

7.2.2 Lower Limb

Ankle-Foot Orthoses (AFOs)

AFOs are the most frequently prescribed orthoses for children with CP. Early AFOs were leather-and-metal "calipers"; modern designs are molded from polypropylene or carbon fiber. The *plantar-flexor–knee extension couple* is critical for walking, and appropriate AFO prescription aims to optimize this relationship [18]. AFOs vary by stiffness, trim lines, and joint design. Key types include:

- *Solid AFO (SAFO)*—rigid plastic that restricts ankle motion to provide maximum stability.
- *Dynamic or hinged AFO (HAFO/DAFO)*—includes an articulated ankle joint that allows dorsiflexion but limits plantarflexion; dynamic AFOs have flexible trim lines to allow some sagittal-plane motion.
- *Posterior leaf spring AFO (PLS)*—has a narrow posterior ankle section acting like a leaf spring to assist dorsiflexion and push-off.
- *Ground-reaction AFO (GRAFO or Floor-reaction AFO)*—extends higher on the anterior tibia; by restricting dorsiflexion, it shifts the ground reaction force anterior to the knee to promote knee extension; used in crouch gait.

The scoping review by Ricardo and colleagues summarized the design and function of these AFOs: solid AFOs limit ankle motion for stability; dynamic AFOs allow sagittal movement; hinged AFOs permit dorsiflexion but prevent plantarflexion; PLS AFOs have a posterior trim line to act as a leaf spring; and ground-reaction AFOs use an anterior shell to promote knee extension [19]. AFOs should be prescribed according to gait pattern (e.g., true equinus, jump, apparent equinus, crouch), muscle strength, and range of motion and should be used with appropriate footwear.

Prescription guidelines emphasize adjusting the ankle angle to match the knee-extended dorsiflexion range and using footwear modifications to optimize alignment [18]. Allowing dorsiflexion (e.g., with a hinged AFO) may aid functional activities like stair climbing but may risk midfoot collapse when the gastrocsoleus complex is tight, so selection must balance motion and stability. Research summarized in the same guideline found strong evidence that posterior AFOs improve temporospatial gait parameters (stride length > cadence > speed) and moderate evidence for improved gross motor function. Evidence for improvements in balance, daily activities, or energy cost is limited [18].

A 2024 systematic review of lower-limb orthoses included 11 randomized trials. Highlights from the review include:

- *Dynamic AFO vs adjustable dynamic response AFO*—improved step length and hip extension; parents preferred the dynamic AFO because it was lighter.
- *Ground-reaction AFO vs solid AFO*—improved balance and temporal-spatial parameters in children with diplegia.
- *TheraTogs + ground-reaction AFO vs rehabilitation alone*—combination therapy improved gait more than either intervention alone.

- *Neuromuscular taping + AFO vs AFO alone*—both improved velocity and step length; no significant difference.
- *AFO vs day/night AFO*—no difference between day-use alone versus day-plus night-use.

Overall, AFOs consistently improved gait parameters and sometimes balance or gross motor function, but evidence quality was low, and trials were small. The scoping review concluded that AFO use results in better walking speed, stride length, cadence, and joint range of motion and makes the gait of children with CP more similar to that of typically developing children [19].

Knee-Ankle-Foot Orthosis (KAFO)

KAFOs extend proximally to the thigh and include knee joints that lock in extension. They were traditionally used for polio and severe lower-limb weakness; in CP, they are occasionally prescribed to prevent equinus or crouch deformities. A randomized controlled trial studied a KAFO with a dynamic ankle power unit and fixed knee worn every other night for 1 year; 28 children with spastic CP were randomized. The trial found no significant difference in passive dorsiflexion or gait parameters between the KAFO and control groups and reported poor tolerance due to discomfort. The authors concluded that a KAFO with a fixed knee and dynamic ankle does not prevent equinus and has limited acceptability [20].

Hip Abduction Orthoses and Hip Braces

Hip displacement is a common problem in non-ambulatory children with CP. Hip abduction orthoses aim to maintain the femoral head within the acetabulum by keeping the hips abducted. Devices include underwear-type hip abduction orthoses (Cosa Active) and novel hip braces with adjustable abduction settings.

A randomized clinical trial in 66 non-ambulatory children (GMFCS IV–V) investigated a novel hip brace worn ≥12 h/day for 12 months. The brace group showed a decrease in the Reimers migration index (MI) at 6 months (mean −8.7 percentage points) and 12 months (−12.7 points), whereas MI increased in the control group; quality-of-life scores also improved [21]. The authors concluded that the brace effectively prevented progression of hip displacement and improved caregiver-perceived quality of life.

Dynamic Elastomeric Fabric Orthoses for the Lower Body

Lycra suits covering the pelvis and legs provide compression and proprioceptive input. A 2024 randomized trial compared dynamic elastomeric fabric orthoses (DEFO) for the lower body versus physiotherapy alone; only stride length and pelvic tilt improved in the DEFO group [22]. Earlier case reports have shown that TheraTogs, combined with conventional therapy, improved gait and gross motor function. Evidence remains limited, but such suits may benefit children with spastic diplegia or hemiplegia when used alongside therapy.

7.2.3 Spine and Torso

Thoracolumbosacral Orthosis (TLSO) and Scoliosis Braces

Scoliosis is common in children with CP, especially those who are non-ambulatory. Rigid thoracolumbosacral orthoses (TLSOs), such as the Boston brace, aim to prevent curve progression and improve sitting posture. Evidence in CP is scarce. A 2025 systematic review analyzed eight studies (six retrospective and two prospective) and concluded that bracing provides temporary improvements in Cobb angle and quality of life, but the benefits disappear when the brace is removed; long-term effectiveness is limited, and many children ultimately require surgery [23]. Braces seem most effective in younger children (<15 years) and can reduce pain and improve posture while worn.

Customized seating systems have also been used. A study comparing a *body shape-molded inner system* (BSMIS) with conventional seats found that the BSMIS significantly reduced Cobb angle and pelvic obliquity in children with non-fixed scoliosis [24]. The system is individually molded to the child's body and integrated into a wheelchair, providing passive postural support without the rigidity of a brace.

Dynamic Trunk Orthoses (Vest-Type DEFO)

Dynamic elastomeric fabric vests offer a flexible alternative to rigid TLSOs. In a single-blind randomized controlled trial, 24 children with GMFCS III–IV were randomized to a DEFO vest worn for 2 h versus 6 h during therapy or to a control group. Both DEFO groups showed greater improvements in the Sitting Assessment Scale than the control group, and the improvements were similar whether the vest was worn for 2 h or 6 h (Giray). The trial also found immediate improvements in sitting balance and gross manual dexterity when the vest was donned. Another trial focusing on lower body DEFO reported improved stride length and frontal plane pelvic tilt [22]. DEFO vests thus appear to enhance trunk control, but long-term evidence is limited.

The details of common brace types and orthoses, along with their use cases and advantages/limitations, are further summarized in Table 7.1.

Table 7.1 Common brace and orthosis types in cerebral palsy

Orthosis	Principles of action	Prescription guidelines and clinical indications	Adjustments/ Customization	Benefits and limitations in CP
Upper limb				
Static wrist/hand orthosis (resting splint)	Provides prolonged, low-load stretch to wrist/fingers, maintains joints in functional alignment and reduces muscle stiffness	Typically worn at night; indicated for children with spastic hemiplegia or diplegia who lack active wrist extension or have risk of contracture. Should be combined with therapy and regular stretching	Splints are custom-molded from thermoplastic; straps and padding can be adjusted as the child grows. Some orthoses include thumb or finger components	Can maintain joint range and slow contracture progression. However, evidence of functional benefit is limited; compliance may be poor because night wear can disturb sleep; should not replace active therapy
Dynamic wrist-hand orthosis	Hinged or spring-loaded splints assist finger and wrist extension to facilitate functional tasks	Used during therapy sessions to practice grasping/releasing or to stretch wrist flexors; not generally worn full-time	Adjustable spring tension allows grading of assistance; custom fit to hand size	Provides dynamic assistance and may support task-specific training but may hinder sensory feedback. Limited pediatric evidence and relatively bulky devices reduce everyday use
Dynamic elastomeric fabric orthosis (glove or vest)	Provides compression, resistance and sensory feedback to improve proprioception, promote muscle activation and align limbs	Gloves are used for hemiplegic upper limbs to enhance hand opening; vests and suits used to improve trunk and shoulder stability. Usually worn during waking hours alongside physiotherapy	Garments are custom-sized; panels and straps provide targeted compression; can be adjusted as child grows	Offers immediate improvements in proximal stability and hand function and may be well-tolerated. Evidence is based mainly on small case studies and short-term trials; benefits depend on concurrent therapy and may diminish when garment is removed

(continued)

Table 7.1 (continued)

Orthosis	Principles of action	Prescription guidelines and clinical indications	Adjustments/ Customization	Benefits and limitations in CP
Lower limb				
Solid AFO (SAFO)	Prevents ankle motion in all planes; provides stable base, controls equinus and subtalar alignment	Indicated for children with spasticity causing true equinus or ankle instability; used to reduce plantar flexor contracture and improve knee extension	Custom molding; footplate length and ankle angle adjusted. Worn with supportive footwear; can be paired with wedges to set tibial inclination	Provides maximal stability and reduces energy cost; may restrict ankle motion needed for stair climbing or running. Risk of midfoot collapse if dorsiflexion allowed with tight gastroc-soleus
Dynamic/hinged AFO (DAFO/HAFO)	Flexible trim lines or hinges allow sagittal-plane ankle motion while controlling frontal plane; maintain alignment but permit dorsiflexion	Prescribed when some ankle motion is desirable (e.g., jump gait, knee hyperextension) or for children needing more dynamic balance	Dorsiflexion stops or plantarflexion straps can be adjusted; footplates may extend under toes or stop at metatarsal heads	Allow more natural gait and easier stair climbing; require careful tuning to avoid excessive dorsiflexion leading to crouch; provide less mediolateral control than solid AFOs
Posterior leaf spring AFO (PLS)	Stores energy during stance and releases it during swing to assist foot clearance; minimal medial–lateral control	Suitable for mild foot drop or apparent equinus; not for severe spasticity	Posterior trim line thickness controls stiffness; footplate length adjusted	Lightweight and allows near-normal ankle motion; limited support for spastic equinus or mediolateral instability
Ground-reaction AFO (GRAFO/floor-reaction AFO)	Restricts dorsiflexion so that ground reaction force moves anterior to knee, promoting knee extension in crouch gait	Used for crouch gait or quadriceps weakness; angle set in slight plantarflexion	Height and ankle angle adjusted; combination with therapy and gait training is essential	Helps correct crouch gait and reduces knee flexion moment; may cause discomfort at anterior tibia; restricted dorsiflexion can make sit-to-stand difficult
Knee-ankle-foot orthosis (KAFO)	Maintains knee extension and controls ankle; dynamic ankle hinges can provide stretching	Prescribed to prevent equinus or crouch in children unable to control knee. Typically worn at night due to bulk	Angle of ankle and knee lock customized; heavy and difficult to don	May stretch tight muscles but cumbersome and poorly tolerated; not recommended for routine prevention of equinus

Hip abduction orthosis/hip brace	Maintain hips in abduction to reduce femoral head migration	Indicated for non-ambulatory children with GMFCS IV–V or those at risk of hip displacement. Worn ≥12 h/day	Adjustable abduction angle; custom sizes; can be integrated into underwear	Effective for preventing hip migration and improving caregiver satisfaction; compliance may be challenging due to bulk or hygiene issues; may restrict static sitting
Dynamic elastomeric fabric suit	Provide compression and proprioceptive feedback to pelvis and limbs; improve pelvic stability	Used for spastic diplegia, hemiplegia or hypotonia; worn during therapy sessions; often combined with AFOs	Custom-fit garments with adjustable straps; can be layered for additional resistance	May enhance proximal stability and encourage correct movement patterns; evidence is limited, and effect may diminish once removed; can be warm to wear
Spine and torso				
Thoracolumbosacral orthosis (TLSO)/ scoliosis brace	Applies three-point pressure to correct spinal curvature and maintain trunk alignment	Indicated for progressive scoliosis (Cobb angle <40°–50°) in children with sufficient growth remaining. Worn up to 23 h/day; typically removed for bathing and therapy	Custom-molded to torso; periodic adjustments needed as child grows	May slow curve progression and reduce pain while worn; compliance can be poor; long-term correction is limited, and many children eventually require spinal surgery
Body shape-molded inner system (custom seating)	Provides molded support to trunk and pelvis, reducing spinal curvature and pelvic obliquity in non-fixed scoliosis	Used for non-ambulatory children with flexible scoliosis; integrated into wheelchair seating	Custom plaster or foam molding; adjustable cushions; replaced as child grows	Improves sitting posture without restricting breathing; not suitable for fixed or severe curves; requires specialized fabrication
Dynamic trunk DEFO (vest)	Provides elastic compression and proprioceptive feedback to enhance trunk stability and postural control; does not physically correct curve	Prescribed for children with poor trunk control or mild scoliosis; worn during therapy and daily activities for 2–6 h/day	Vests are made of stretch fabric with targeted panels; adjustability in straps; replaced as child grows	Comfortable and allows movement; improves proximal stability; evidence is short-term and does not address scoliosis progression; may be expensive

7.3 A Closer Look: Assistive Devices

Including a wide range of aids and instruments, ADs are designed to assist individuals with their daily tasks. While most ADs may be primarily aimed at improving the user's *mobility*, they can also be used to assist with *self-care* and *social functions* of the individual. In a study in Norway, Østensjø et al. investigated the impact of ADs and other environmental modifications on care and activities of children with CP [25]. Including 95 children, a total of 1075 devices or life-modifications were assessed. Roughly 9% were recorded not to be in regular use, with the reasons for non-use classified into four main categories:

- Minimal need of the device or improper device prescription: Eating utensils were often reported to be *not-needed*, while bathing and toilet instruments were frequently unsuitable for the child's conditions.
- Unrealistic device time demands: Transfer devices were sometimes seen as less time-efficient than lifting the child.
- Mismatch between living conditions/habits and the device: Inability to use transportation aids in the bathroom, or due to limits in available space.
- Insufficient education and training for effective use of the device: Powered mobility devices or communication aids sometimes proved hard to use due to a lack of proper training.

Overall, the use of ADs increased with the severity of physical movement disability, and their use was predominantly for movement assistance. Significant reductions in the children's need for caregiver assistance were also observed in mobility. The same was true for caregiver-rated improvements in the child's function, where once again the most prominent improvements were reported to be present in mobility [25].

In another study on 130 individuals with CP, the same team assessed the use and benefits of different Ads [26]. Of the included children, 78 reported using Ads (excluding orthoses) in their daily living. While no significant differences were observed between AD use or non-use, and gender or age, there was a marked difference across different levels of physical ability, with higher degrees of motor disability expectedly resulting in higher AD utilization. Among AD users, no difference was observed between age groups (12–35, 36–59, and 60–81 months), though use of Ads for mobility was lower in the first age group compared with the rest (possibly a direct effect of their lower age), while being the most widely reported reason for AD use overall. As for the exact type of ADs used, adapted seating Ads were the most frequent among those aiding with *positioning*, while special bicycles and walking aids were the two most common types of ADs used for *mobility*, and bathing aids were the most commonly used in *self-care*. The result details are summarized in Table 7.2 [26].

Aiming to assess the subjective benefits of ADs from their intended users firsthand, Huang et al. conducted a qualitative study, asking children with CP about their experiences regarding AD use in school [27]. A total of 44 participants were included in the study, including 15 children, 15 mothers, and 14 teachers. Overall, the results showed a high AD use in the school setting. Extracted from their

Table 7.2 Number of children using/not using the different types of ADs, n = 130. Reproduced from Moen et al. 2024, licensed under CC-BY 4.0

Type and number of ADs in use	Using ADs n (%)	Not using ADs n (%)
Positioning (n = 95)		
Adapted chair/seating	54 (41.5)	76 (58.5)
Standing frame	41 (31.5)	89 (68.5)
Mobility (n = 150)		
Adapted bicycle	44 (33.8)	86 (66.2)
Walking aid	34 (26.2)	96 (73.8)
Special need pushchair	32 (24.6)	98 (75.4)
Manual wheelchair	27 (20.8)	103 (79.2)
Powered mobility device	13 (10.0)	117 (90.0)
Self-care (n = 48)		
Bathing aid	19 (14.6)	111 (85.4)
Toileting aid	18 (13.8)	112 (86.2)
Adapted bed	7 (5.4)	123 (94.6)
Eating utensil	4 (3.1)	126 (96.9)
Training, stimulation and play (n = 16)		
Training device	10 (7.7)	120 (92.3)
Device for play/stimulation	6 (4.6)	124 (95.4)
Environmental modifications (n = 21)		
Ramp	7 (5.4)	123 (94.6)
Automatic door opener	6 (4.6)	124 (95.4)
Lifting aid or hoist	5 (3.8)	125 (96.2)
Threshold eliminator	3 (2.3)	127 (97.7)

interview results, researchers identified the following four main reasons for children's willingness to utilize their ADs in school:

- ADs are viewed as a means of allowing them to overcome their limitations and compensate for their physical disabilities.
- School is viewed as a formal institution with its distinct rules and expectations, and ADs are a way for the children to be able to stand up to those expectations.
- AD use is believed to be rewarding as it allows them to take part in and achieve higher degrees of participation in their favorite activities.
- Their other peers are, for the most part, accepting of their use of ADs, making it easier for them to also accept them in their daily lives.

However, negative sentiments and attitudes toward AD use were still observed among students, as some mentioned instances of mockery or bullying from other students when they used their ADs. As for teachers and mothers, teachers had a positive view of AD use by the children with CP and believed their use to be beneficial to the children's participation and inclusion. They also believed school to be particularly suitable for children to learn how to use such devices, as it provided a formal, yet safe environment for that purpose. Mothers also had a positive opinion about ADs and emphasized their role to allow their children to overcome their physical limitations [27].

7.4 Emerging Technologies

7.4.1 3D Scan and Print

Large-scale adoption of 3D scanners and printers (Fig. 7.1) has revolutionized the field of industrial design in the last two decades. Such scanners usually function by using lasers to create a computerized model of an object, calculating its geometry based on the reflection time of the emitted beams. 3D printing, on the other hand, works by depositing a thin layer of a material upon each pass of the print head, allowing for very fine control over the final shape of the object being printed. The exact method of material deposition, as well as the type of material used, varies significantly based on the exact printing technology and the expected properties of the product. Using the two alongside one another, the entire process of creating a three-dimensional, digital model of a physical object, doing necessary manipulations via computer, and producing a physical prototype of the final product can be done in less than a day, and with very little manufacturing cost. Largely tailor-made for each individual, orthosis design and manufacturing can benefit immensely from these technologies, allowing for more precise designs and accurate builds based on the patient's size, body morphology, and needs.

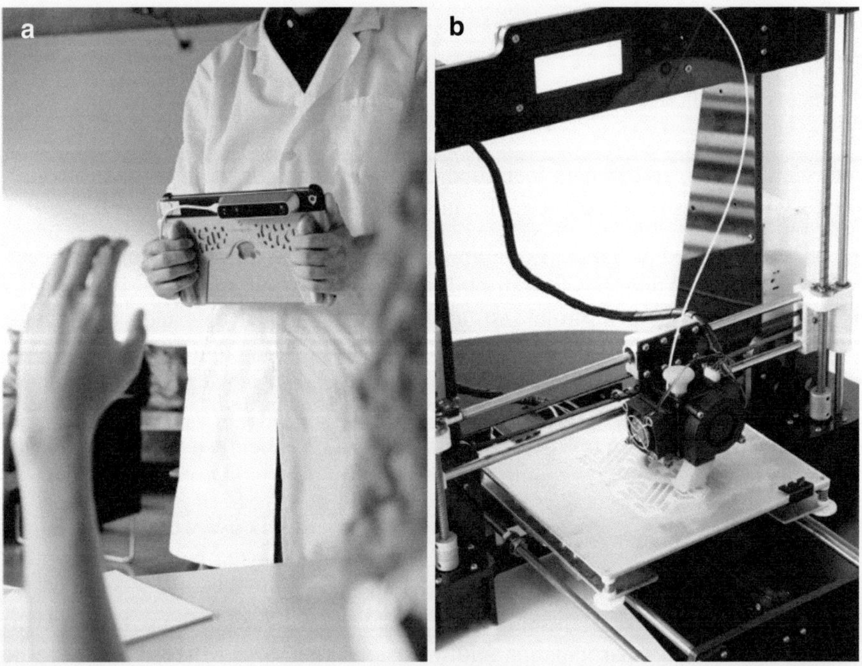

Fig. 7.1 (**a**) A 3D scanner attached to a tablet, used to create a digital model of someone's hand. (**b**) A 3D printer. Printing bed and nozzle are clearly shown. (Photos by Tom Claes and NEW DATA SERVICES on Unsplash (unsplash.com), respectively)

Aiming to produce a better-fitting brace for treating hip subluxation in CP children, Kim et al. used a 3D scanner to create a digital model of 19 subjects, which was later used to produce a custom-designed brace. Objective efficacy of the brace, as well as patient comfort and pain, were measured, and results were found to be satisfactory, with patients reporting significant improvements in their comfort and pain levels upon spending more time wearing the brace [28]. Though comparisons with conventional methods of size measurement were not performed in the study, the results can be used as a proof of concept, showcasing the potential benefits of 3D scan utilization in brace and orthosis design.

Recognizing the limited availability of upper extremity orthoses for CP patients with hand involvement, Ragni et al. employed 3D printing to produce customized, low-cost, forearm thumb opponens and dynamic upper extremity orthoses to be used during the patients' physical therapy sessions. The device proved to have a significant effect as all participants showed improvements in functional scores upon several therapy sessions [29]. In another example, Thorsen and colleagues fabricated an assistive device used to help with cutlery holding via 3D printing. The study emphasizes the benefits of being able to do rapid iterations and fine customizations to optimize the final product for each patient's needs and measurements [30].

7.4.2 Robotic Solutions

In contrast with conventional, passive orthoses, robotic exoskeletons are not only theoretically capable of providing the same passive support to prevent contractures and help with deformity correction but also, having active motors inside, provide active assistance to the wearer during voluntary muscle movements, decreasing the movement's burden on the individual. Although their use has been relatively common in recent years as part of robotic-assisted gait training (RAGT) setups [31], acting as wired and stationary active supports [32, 33], several studies have proposed the use of wireless and more streamlined versions as standalone, assistive devices in children with CP (Fig. 7.2). In their systematic review on the subject, Hunt et al. investigated the effectiveness of such wireless robotic exoskeletons, including 13 studies and several types of exoskeletons in their review. They concluded that their use was accompanied by improvements in knee and hip extension and other parameters, as well as a reduction in the metabolic cost of walking for the individual [34].

7.4.3 Artificial Intelligence

The post-COVID world has witnessed a revolution in both the availability and the power of AI tools such as machine-learning (ML) and deep-learning (DL) models, and therefore, it is no surprise to see their use attempted in the field of orthotics as well. Choo et al. tried to provide an overview of the current status and possible use cases of the technology in this field, in their systematic review on the subject.

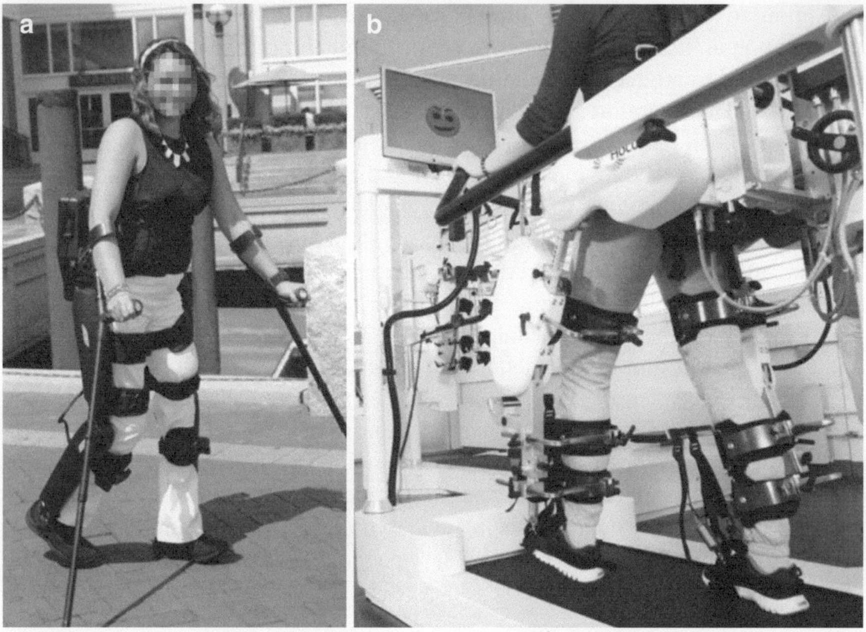

Fig. 7.2 (**a**) A wireless robotic exoskeleton, used as a walking assistance device. (**b**) Wired exoskeleton, as part of an RAGT setup. (Reprinted in part from Wang et al. [31])

Including 13 studies on the use of ML in prosthetics and orthotics, their findings suggested that although this technology has not yet been implemented in the clinic, several studies have used AI tools for various purposes. In particular, their results showed that ML was used to predict the need for an orthosis and to monitor movements in real-time while wearing the orthosis [35]. Future research will provide insight into the true power and applications of AI in orthotics. ML and DL are especially useful for leveraging big data banks, processing existing data in new ways, and arriving at solutions previously overlooked or out of reach through conventional analytical methods. In the near future, AI use may show real benefits in areas such as patient selection, training, and even orthosis design.

7.5 Recommendations

7.5.1 For Parents and Caregivers

- *Promote consistent orthosis and device use*: Ensure that prescribed orthoses and assistive devices (ADs) are used as directed to maximize functional gains and prevent deformities.
- *Participate in training and education*: Seek guidance from therapists and orthotists on proper use, maintenance, and troubleshooting of devices.
- *Monitor comfort and adherence*: Report discomfort, redness, or fitting issues promptly to healthcare providers.

- *Encourage participation and independence*: Support children in using ADs and orthoses in daily and social activities to improve confidence and inclusion.
- *Advocate for emotional support*: Address potential stigma or bullying in social settings related to device use.
- *Engage in follow-up and reassessment*: Regularly attend review appointments to ensure the devices remain appropriate as the child grows or their condition evolves.

7.5.2 For Healthcare Professionals and Policy Makers

- *Ensure individualized prescriptions*: Base orthotic and assistive device selection on functional assessment, gait analysis, and family goals.
- *Integrate objective monitoring tools*: Encourage the use of multi-sensor systems for adherence tracking where feasible.
- *Provide structured caregiver education programs*: Standardize training for families on proper device use and maintenance.
- *Invest in innovation*: Support research and clinical implementation of 3D printing, robotics, and AI to improve customization, comfort, and accessibility.
- *Improve accessibility and funding*: Develop policies to subsidize orthoses and ADs for low-income families to ensure equitable access.
- *Encourage multidisciplinary clinics*: Facilitate collaboration among orthotists, physiotherapists, physicians, and engineers in pediatric rehabilitation services.

7.5.3 For Interdisciplinary Teams

- *Adopt a patient-centered approach*: Collaborate closely with families to align device design and therapy goals with the child's daily life.
- *Combine interventions*: Use orthoses and ADs alongside physiotherapy, strength training, and occupational therapy for optimal outcomes.
- *Share data across disciplines*: Implement digital platforms to document progress, adherence, and adjustments.
- *Support translational research*: Collaborate with engineers and data scientists to advance the use of AI, robotics, and 3D printing in orthotic development.
- *Focus on long-term follow-up*: Regularly reassess the child's motor development, comfort, and device fit over time.

7.6 Conclusions

Cerebral palsy remains one of the most common causes of motor impairment in children, often resulting in lifelong challenges in movement, posture, and social participation. The effective use of orthoses and assistive devices can significantly enhance mobility, independence, and quality of life when prescribed and managed appropriately. However, their success depends not only on the design and function of the devices but also on the collaborative involvement of caregivers, healthcare providers, and interdisciplinary teams.

For caregivers, understanding and adhering to prescribed treatment regimens, maintaining open communication with professionals, and fostering positive attitudes toward device use are crucial. Healthcare professionals and policymakers must ensure access to individualized, evidence-based interventions, develop educational resources, and encourage the integration of emerging technologies such as 3D printing, robotic exoskeletons, and AI-based monitoring systems. Meanwhile, interdisciplinary collaboration ensures that each child receives holistic and continuous care—combining biomechanical expertise with psychosocial and developmental support.

Future directions in pediatric orthotics and assistive technology should emphasize personalization, comfort, and cost-effectiveness while promoting inclusive participation in daily life. Continuous innovation, patient-centered design, and caregiver empowerment form the cornerstone of progress in this field. By bridging clinical expertise with technological advancement and family engagement, society can help children with cerebral palsy reach their fullest functional potential and enjoy improved autonomy and social inclusion.

References

1. Young J, Jackson S. Improved motor function in a pre-ambulatory child with spastic bilateral cerebral palsy, using a custom rigid ankle-foot orthosis-footwear combination: a case report. Prosthetics Orthot Int. 2019;43(4):453–8.
2. Peter C. The running shoe book. Mountain View: Anderson World Inc.; 1980.
3. Khan MN, Jacobs BC, Ashbaugh S. Considerations in footwear and orthotics. Prim Care. 2013;40(4):1001–12.
4. Lindsay S. Child and youth experiences and perspectives of cerebral palsy: a qualitative systematic review. Child Care Health Dev. 2016;42(2):153–75.
5. Feldner HA, et al. Supportive mobility devices across the lifespan in cerebral palsy: a modified Delphi study to establish stakeholder research priorities. Disabil Rehabil Assist Technol. 2024;19(4):1739–47.
6. Hailey DM. Orthoses and prostheses. Int J Technol Assess Health Care. 1995;11(2):214–34.
7. Schnell MD, Bowker J, Bunch W. The orthotist. In: Orthopedic rehabilitation. New York: Churchill Livingstone; 1982. p. 103–35.
8. Devanand DB, Kedgley AE. Objective methods of monitoring usage of orthotic devices for the extremities: a systematic review. Sensors. 2023;23(17):7420.
9. Bettoni E, et al. A systematic review of questionnaires to assess patient satisfaction with limb orthoses. Prosthetics Orthot Int. 2016;40(2):158–69.
10. Demers L, Weiss-Lambrou R, Ska B. Quebec user evaluation of satisfaction with assistive technology version 2.0. Webster: The Institute for Matching Persons and Technology; 2000.
11. Jarl GM, Heinemann AW, Norling Hermansson LM. Validity evidence for a modified version of the orthotics and prosthetics users' survey. Disabil Rehabil Assist Technol. 2012;7(6):469–78.
12. Spaulding SE, et al. Education in prosthetic and orthotic training: looking back 50 years and moving forward. Prosthetics Orthot Int. 2020;44(6):416–26.
13. CPUP. [cited Sept 2025]. Available from: https://cpup.se.

14. Imms C, et al. Implications of providing wrist-hand orthoses for children with cerebral palsy: evidence from a randomised controlled trial. Disabil Rehabil. 2023;45(12):2046–56.
15. Jackman M, Novak I, Lannin N. Effectiveness of hand splints in children with cerebral palsy: a systematic review with meta-analysis. Dev Med Child Neurol. 2014;56(2):138–47.
16. Grandi A, et al. Listening to the patient as a possible route to cost-effective rehabilitation: a case report. J Med Case Rep. 2012;6(1):19.
17. Knox V. The use of Lycra garments in children with cerebral palsy: a report of a descriptive clinical trial. Br J Occup Ther. 2003;66(2):71–7.
18. Wright E, DiBello SA. Principles of ankle-foot orthosis prescription in ambulatory bilateral cerebral palsy. Phys Med Rehabil Clin. 2020;31(1):69–89.
19. Ricardo D, et al. Effects of ankle foot orthoses on the gait patterns in children with spastic bilateral cerebral palsy: a scoping review. Children. 2021;8(10):903.
20. Maas J, et al. A randomized controlled trial studying efficacy and tolerance of a knee-ankle-foot orthosis used to prevent equinus in children with spastic cerebral palsy. Clin Rehabil. 2014;28(10):1025–38.
21. Kim BR, et al. Efficacy of a hip brace for hip displacement in children with cerebral palsy: a randomized clinical trial. JAMA Netw Open. 2022;5(11):e2240383.
22. Bezgin S, et al. Effects of dynamic elastomeric fabric orthoses in children with cerebral palsy: a single-blind randomized controlled trial. Prosthetics Orthot Int. 2025;49(2):220–7.
23. Merkelbach N, Pauw A, van Campenhout A. Bracing for scoliosis in children with cerebral palsy-a systematic review. J Child Orthop. 2025;19(5):405–15.
24. Suh YJ, et al. Attenuation of spinal curvature and pelvic obliquity by body shape molded inner system in cerebral palsy with non-fixed scoliosis. J Korean Acad Rehabil Med. 2011;35(35):259–64.
25. Ostensjø S, Carlberg EB, Vøllestad NK. The use and impact of assistive devices and other environmental modifications on everyday activities and care in young children with cerebral palsy. Disabil Rehabil. 2005;27(14):849–61.
26. Moen RD, Østensjø S. Understanding the use and benefits of assistive devices among young children with cerebral palsy and their families in Norway: a cross-sectional population-based registry study. Disabil Rehabil Assist Technol. 2024;19(4):1454–62.
27. Huang IC, Sugden D, Beveridge S. Assistive devices and cerebral palsy: the use of assistive devices at school by children with cerebral palsy. Child Care Health Dev. 2009;35(5):698–708.
28. Kim JM, et al. Application of 3D scanner to measure physical size and improvement of hip brace manufacturing technology in severe cerebral palsy patients. Sci Rep. 2023;13(1):20691.
29. Ragni LB, et al. Design and use of a 3D-printed dynamic upper extremity orthosis for children with cerebral palsy and severe upper extremity involvement: a pilot study. Am J Occup Ther. 2023;77(4):7704205060.
30. Thorsen R, et al. A parametric 3D printed assistive device for people with cerebral palsy—assessment of outcomes and comparison with a commercial counterpart. Assist Technol. 2024;36(1):16–21.
31. Wang T, et al. A review on the rehabilitation exoskeletons for the lower limbs of the elderly and the disabled. Electronics. 2022;11(3):388.
32. Lefmann S, Russo R, Hillier S. The effectiveness of robotic-assisted gait training for paediatric gait disorders: systematic review. J Neuroeng Rehabil. 2017;14(1):1.
33. Bayón C, et al. Robotic therapies for children with cerebral palsy: a systematic review. Transl Biomed. 2016;7:44.
34. Hunt M, et al. Effectiveness of robotic exoskeletons for improving gait in children with cerebral palsy: a systematic review. Gait Posture. 2022;98:343–54.
35. Choo YJ, Chang MC. Use of machine learning in the field of prosthetics and orthotics: a systematic narrative review. Prosthetics Orthot Int. 2023;47(3):226–40.

8 Speech and Language Pathology Perspective on Cerebral Palsy: Clinical Features and Management Strategies

Seyyedeh Maryam Khoddami, Zahra Soleymani, Toktam Maleki Shahmahmood, and Mohamadreza Afshar

8.1 Case Report

The Story of Communicative Challenges in a Child with Cerebral Palsy

Hana was a 5-year-old girl diagnosed with spastic cerebral palsy (CP), primarily affecting muscle tone and motor control in both lower limbs, mildly involving the upper limbs and moderately involving oral–motor mechanisms. She was delivered at term but experienced hypoxia caused by a prolonged and complicated labor. She had significant challenges with feeding from birth. Feeding her was a tribble and burden experience for her mother because of repeated occurrences of vomiting, cough and choking, and prolonged feeding times (up to 45 min). Poor lip seal and decreased tongue lateralization, resulted in difficulties with sucking and chewing solid foods. She required modified diet and caregiver assistance during all meals to ensure safe swallowing. Although he began to utter her first words at the expected time, her speech was unintelligible and characterized by imprecise articulation, reduced

(continued)

S. M. Khoddami (✉) · Z. Soleymani · M. Afshar
Department of Speech Therapy, School of Rehabilitation, Tehran University of Medical Sciences, Tehran, Iran
e-mail: khoddami@tums.ac.ir

T. M. Shahmahmood
Department of Speech Therapy, Faculty of Paramedical Sciences and Rehabilitation, Mashhad University of Medical Sciences, Mashhad, Iran

A. Presedo et al. (eds.), *Enhancing Quality of Life in Patients with Cerebral Palsy*, https://doi.org/10.1007/978-3-032-20967-2_8

speech rate, poor breath support, and strained and struggled voice. Though, receptive and expressive language skills were relatively preserved, she predominantly used gestures, facial expressions, and simple vocalizations to communicate, especially in social situations. Communication barriers that stem from speech characteristics had restricted her ability to engage with peers, participate in group activities, and express feelings, which contributes to social isolation and frustration, as well as decreased self-esteem and emotional well-being. Her overall quality of life (QoL) was impacted by these challenges, underscoring the need for multidisciplinary interventions including speech therapy, occupational therapy, and caregiver support.

8.2 Communication

Human beings need to communicate with others to live and develop. Communication is vital for social interaction. Verbal and non-verbal communication are the two types of communication. Verbal communication includes speaking and listening. Acquiring verbal communication skills in early ages of life is essential for learning to write and read in the school ages. In a longitudinal study, it has been found that lexical definition and word retrieval skills which are related to semantic skills, predicted second-grade reading comprehension; also, phonological awareness abilities in preschool predicted single-word reading at first and second grades [1]. Nonverbal communication consists of body language, hand gestures, eye contact, and facial expressions. During face-to-face interaction, vocal (language and paralanguage) and visible activities are synchronized to convey the meaning [2].

When speakers and listeners achieve a shared understanding about an issue, communication becomes effective. This requires a combination of skills such as linguistic and social-cognitive skills. Speakers convey their communicative goals through the “semantic” meaning of their idea. By considering socio-cultural contexts and pragmatic principles, they use language to achieve specific communicative aims [3]. Children’s communicative development is deeply influenced by the interplay of language, cognitive, and motor skills. Motor skills development enables children to explore their environment and interact with others [4]. The emergence of concepts and first words is closely linked, highlighting the critical role of cognitive skills in early language development. Conversely, language development also significantly shapes a child’s cognitive achievements [5].

From early childhood, motor skills play a significant role in the development of communication. The first signs of communication in children include turning their heads toward their caregivers in response to their names and raising their arms to signal a desire to be picked up. From 8 months, children’s first communicative acts are shaped through showing and giving objects. Parents and caregivers often mirror these gestures, fostering early interactions. These gestures serve as precursors to the pointing gesture, a milestone in development [6]. Research suggests that gestures are at the cutting edge of early language development, providing a simple yet effective way for toddlers to convey complex information before they acquire the necessary verbal skills [7]. As children grow, motor skills continue to play a vital role, particularly in speech production, which relies on the coordination of multiple motor functions.

In children with CP, motor, intellectual, and sensory impairments are the factors that contribute to communication difficulties [8]. The hallmark symptom of CP is difficulty with movement, muscle tone and muscle control which frequently includes oral-motor dysfunction. It is found that oral sensorimotor stimulation can enhance oral-motor performance in these children [9]. Given the well-established interdependence of language, motor skills, and perception, children with CP often face challenges in both communication and cognition. The following section discusses these challenges in greater details.

8.2.1 Communication in Children with Cerebral Palsy

Children with CP may experience a range of speech and language disorders including complete inability to speak (anarthria), speech motor impairment paired with language comprehension difficulties, and, speech motor impairment with typical language comprehension. Research indicates that the severity of motor impairment in children with CP, correlates with reduced use of communication functions [10]. Based on the International Classification of Functioning, Disability and Health for Children and Youth (ICF-CY) framework, which emphasize on different levels of activity, participation, and environmental factors [11], speech and language pathologists (SLPs) play a vital role in improving communication functions for children with CP with different profiles of problems. Communication functions are different ways that are used to reach specific aims or achieve requirements in every day interaction. Language, vocalizations, initiations, requests, comments, protests are the examples of communication functions [12].

Children with communication disorders often rely on unconventional signals to interact. It is important for families and teachers to recognize and appropriately respond to these signals. Responsive caregivers play a pivotal role in fostering cognitive and communication skills in these children [13]. Establishing a shared understanding between caregivers (parents or teachers) and specialists about the communication challenges faced by children with CP helps caregivers to recognize their communication attempts to communicate and respond effectively, thereby reducing frustration [14].

With the aim of creating a shared language for caregivers and healthcare professionals, several user-friendly scales have been developed to measure communication skills in children with CP. These scales, which can be used by caregivers or healthcare personnel, help them to become familiar with the different levels of communication in a child with CP. One such tool is the communication function classification system which categorizes everyday communication functions of an individual with CP into 1–5 levels in accordance with success of communication. Categorization of levels is based on the child's skills to send and receive message, knowing his audience and situation (familiar and unfamiliar), and the frequency of message exchanges. It integrates ICF factors (activity, participation, and environment) to determine levels:

Level 1: The child communicates successfully and independently in most settings.
Level 5: The child rarely communicates, even with familiar people.

The other levels represent varying degrees of communication difficulties with familiar and unfamiliar people across different environments. This system has been translated into multiple languages, including Farsi [14]. Communication difficulties significantly impact children's family, social, and educational lives, making intervention essential. To enhance communication skills and foster independence in social interactions, children with CP are often referred to speech and language pathology (SLP) services. SLPs, also called speech therapists assess, diagnose and treat these communication disorders. Given the wide variability in communication disorders, there is no single comprehensive approach to treat all children with CP. These children typically require extensive healthcare support, including long-term speech and language therapy, while the treatment approaches are also individualized based on the child's profile of problem and needs [8]. Depending on the characteristics of the child's specific communication challenges, therapy may focus on developing natural receptive and expressive language abilities or implementing augmentative and alternative communication (AAC) systems when needed. AAC systems are methods that are used to enhance speech (augmentative communication) or substitute it totally once individuals with CP are unable to speak (alternative communication) [15].

In AAC systems, specific codes and symbols are used to facilitate chatting and communication for individuals with CP. These tools enable children with CP who have speech or motor difficulties to communicate effectively, express their needs, and involve in social interactions. The use of such coded communication within AAC improves their ability to take part in conversations and daily life activities. It is worth noting that the partners of these individuals should also know how to use AAC. A wide range of AAC methods should be available for the individual with communication difficulties including unaided AAC (e.g., gestures, signs), low- tech AAC systems (e.g., communication boards), high- tech AAC systems (e.g., speech-generating devices), and communication apps. Applying AAC enhance communication competence in individual with communication needs that is essential for QoL [16].

8.3 Cognition in Children with Cerebral Palsy

Children with CP may experience global cognitive impairments, as reflected in their intellectual quotient (IQ) scores, or they may exhibit deficits limited to specific cognitive domains [17]. Approximately 23–44% of children with CP have an IQ score below 70, indicating intellectual disability. However, some children with CP achieve IQ scores above 120, demonstrating that high cognitive functioning is possible in this population [18, 19]. A significant proportion of children with CP experiences cognitive impairments, which are influenced by both motor and sensory impairments. Research demonstrates that the severity and extent of motor impairments—particularly the number of limbs affected—significantly influences cognitive abilities. Greater limbs involvement in motor impairment is associated with more pronounced cognitive deficits [19]. Epilepsy is common among children with CP, affecting approximately 20–40% of this population. When epilepsy is present, cognitive impairment tends to be more severe [18].

Visual perception impairments occur in 40–50% of children with CP. These impairments affect critical skills such as shapes and spatial relationships discrimination, motion processing, and figure-ground perception, all of which are essential for daily living activities and academic performance [20]. Given the importance of visual perception in this area, addressing such impairments is crucial for improving the QoL and functional independence of children with CP [21].

8.4 Academic Performance in Children with Cerebral Palsy

School-aged children with CP often experience delays in academic development. Intellectual disabilities affect approximately half of all children with CP, significantly impacting their academic performance. Even children with CP who have a normal IQ face academic challenge, as their performance in reading, spelling, and mathematics tasks tends to fall below their age-matched peers [21]. Several cognitive measures related to language, reading, and math that, play a critical role in completing these tasks. For example, reading requires the ability to decode written words into phonemes (phonological awareness), phonological working memory is closely tied to language processing, and mathematical reasoning depends on symbolic comparison and visuospatial working memory [22]. Additionally, researches highlight a relationship between communicative performances and intellectual functions [23].

In children with CP, those with more severe speech impairments have more restricted communication abilities. A child with unintelligible speech cannot effectively convey messages to the listeners, which limits his/her participation in various settings. Given the strong link between communication skills, intellectual functioning and social development in school-aged children with CP, conducting screening tests—and comprehensive assessments when necessary—is essential. Early diagnosis and intervention by SLPs can enhance communication skills and help prevent future social and academic challenges.

8.5 Speech Disorders in Cerebral Palsy

Speech production is a goal-directed process requiring precise timing and accurate coordination of various speech muscles and subsystems, including the jaw, lips, tongue, velum, vocal folds, and respiratory system [24]. The impairment of speech subsystems in individuals with CP may result from a poor connection between motor commands and the perceptual consequences of speech movements [25]. Speech disorder is a broad term that constitute the core problems in the profile of disorders such as dysarthria and apraxia of speech [26], each of them reflects a specific level of impairment in the speech chain, requiring highly targeted intervention strategies [27].

Dysarthria is a motor speech disorder that affects speech subsystems including respiration, phonation, resonance, articulation, and prosody [28]. Although the presentation of dysarthria in individuals with CP can vary considerably, in most cases, all speech subsystems are affected by the motor control impairments [29]. Phonological delay is when a child's speech sound development is slower than expected, using error patterns that younger children typically outgrow (for example, in English, 'stopping' like saying/doo/for/zoo/) [30]. In phonological disorder, children may exhibit unusual error patterns, such as 'denasalization' (e.g., saying/doze/for/nose/), not seen in typical development [31, 32]. Childhood apraxia of speech (CAS) influences a child's capability to articulate speech sounds and syllables in the correct sequence, as well as to pronounce words and sentences with precision and appropriate speech rhythm [33]. In a sample of preschool children diagnosed with CP, 82% showed some types of speech disorder or delay. More specifically, 78% had dysarthria, 54% faced delays or disorders in articulation, 43% dealt with phonological delays or disorders, and 17% exhibited characteristics of CAS [27]. Although people with CP vary widely in their speech characteristics, the vast majority exhibit reduced speech intelligibility [34].

8.6 Speech Intelligibility in Cerebral Palsy

Speech intelligibility refers to the degree to which a listener can understand a speaker's message [35]. In children with CP, intelligibility is often significantly reduced compared to their typically developing peers due to speech impairments that impact all speech subsystems [36]. A study by Mei et al. (2020), which assessed 84 children with CP, found that speech intelligibility was reduced to some extent in all cases, and the lowest intelligibility was observed in those displaying concurrent symptom of dysarthria and features of CAS [27]. Although articulation therapy can occasionally improve the precision of individual sounds, it usually must be paired with more comprehensive motor strategies in individual with CP because multiple speech subsystems are affected. Sakash et al. (2020) suggested that using a slow speech strategy may be especially beneficial for CP children with moderate to severe speech intelligibility deficits, particularly those who can produce longer utterances [37].

Similarly, research on adults with CP reveals a similar pattern. Sholderle et al. (2016) discovered that most adults with CP experienced moderate to severe speech disorders, characterized by imprecise articulation, along with respiratory and prosodic features, which were identified as significant indicators of speech intelligibility [38]. Decreased speech intelligibility may expose individuals with CP to the risk of social isolation and a diminished QoL due to difficulties in verbally expressing their thoughts and experiences [39, 40].

8.7 Respiration for Speech Production

Respiratory system is one of the main subsystems of speech which supplies necessary power for voice production [41]. Respiration for speech, which is also called speech breathing, can be described as all mechanic respiratory events for inhalation before speaking and also generation and keeping subglottal air pressure during speech production [42]. For speech breathing, the vocal folds are closes at midline to build up subglottal air pressure. When the air pressure moves the vocal folds apart, the vibrational source of phonation is created [43–45]. No prolonged phonation can be produced without this airflow. Also, the effective interaction between the subglottal air pressure and airflow rate passing through the vocal folds determines the vocal characteristics of the produced signal [43–49]. This process is precisely controlled and its patterns are not adult-like until 10 years of age in individuals who are typically developing [50, 51]. Moreover, balance between respiratory subsystem and the two others voice subsystems including phonatory and resonatory is essential for healthy voice production from a physiological perspective [41].

8.7.1 Respiration for Speech in Cerebral Palsy

It has been realized for a long time that both children and adults with CP have breathing problems [42]. Breathing problems have been reported as the second most common problem of the speech mechanism in individuals with CP [52]. Speech breathing impairments which are occurred due to deficit in motor control in individuals with CP, causing various difficulties for speech production.

However, there is a small number of studies that have demonstrated speech breathing is different between children with CP and typically developing children [50, 53–55]. Some of these research studies support this hypothesis that children with CP utilize an inefficient strategy for speech breathing. Indeed, they heavily rely on active muscle forces during speech production [54, 55] even though respiratory muscles lack strength in this population [56]. This pattern may not be seen in those children with CP who have no speech motor involvement [50]. Children with CP often have several respiratory problems including shallow breathing, inefficient exhalation, and poor coordination between breathing and phonation. Shallow breathing limits the respiratory power of speech production resulting in weak voice, short utterances, and difficulty with producing longer phrases and sentences [42]. Inefficient exhalation and poor coordination between breathing and phonation are related to each other. Coordination of breathing and phonation refers to appropriate control and timing between breathing and phonation. This respiratory feature which is essential for producing healthy voice primarily affects lung volume measures [50]. If coordination of breathing and phonation is impaired, exhalatory breathing is not sufficient for speech production, leading to speaking on a diminished air supply or on residual air. So, phonation may be effortful and vocal folds may be vibrated slowly and irregularly which results in in low pitched, monotone, breathy, and harsh voice as well as frequent pitch breaks [57]. On the other hand, if exhalation is inefficient, coordination of breathing and phonation will be difficult [58].

Additionally, children with CP show speech breathing problems because of muscular problems and inefficient valving function in the vocal tract [59–61]. Muscular problems due to dysarthria such as weakness or spasticity in the respiratory system can impact breathing control by reduced chest wall mobility [59]. Uncoordinated movements of the chest wall are also more likely common in children with CP [61] which leads to inefficient speech production. Several researches indicated respiratory muscle activity is increased during speech production in children with CP compared to typically developing peers [50, 54, 55]. Also, inefficient valving that can be observed in several parts of the vocal tract such as larynx, velopharynx, and orofacial articulators may lead to air wastage during speech breathing [60].

It should be noted that respiratory problems may be variable depending on type of dysarthria. For instance, shallow breathing as well as forced and uncontrolled exhalations can be frequently observed in spastic CP, whereas individuals with athetoid CP may exhibit irregular breathing patterns [62, 63]. It has also been stated that individuals with athetoid CP show more severe speech and breathing problems compared to the other types [64, 65]. Meanwhile, there are individual variations in speech breathing in children with CP [42]. Furthermore, speech tasks can impact speech production and speech breathing in both groups of children with CP and their typically developing peers [50]. This finding supports the concept that respiratory subsystem is an excellent way to illustrate interaction between the speech motor and cognitive–linguistic systems during speech production [50]. It is suggested that understanding how the respiratory system adjusts during various speech tasks will be helpful to design effective interventions in children with CP, particularly those managements that target speech breathing impairment [50, 66].

The respiratory problems may cause various speech characteristics including difficulties with loudness control, monotone voice, pitch break, and reduced stress. These problems may also create slow speech rate, reduced utterance length, imprecise articulation, and consequently reduced speech intelligibility [57, 58, 67, 68]. All of these speech characteristics are common among individuals with CP.

SLPs can play a crucial role in the management of speech breathing problems in individuals with CP. Different methods have been suggested to improve respiratory functions in children with CP, such as strengthening respiratory muscles, respiratory muscle training, inhibiting muscle tone, swimming, treadmill walking, cycle ergometer training, and ergonomic approach which most of them were provided in the field of physical therapy [53, 69–76]. Interestingly, one study showed that singing therapy can improve peak flow measure in adults with CP [77]. However, there are no evidence-based interventions that directly target speech breathing by SLPs in children with CP [50]. It has been confirmed that there is a connection between nonspeech breathing and speech breathing [42, 64, 78, 79]; it means that working on nonspeech breathing may lead to improved speech.

For the management of speech breathing, it is firstly recommended to evaluate speech breathing. A four-parameter framework has been suggested for the assessment of speech breathing, consisting of alveolar pressure, lung volume, airflow, and chest wall shape during speech [42]. As mentioned earlier, muscle weakness and incoordination are two main factors contributing speech breathing problems in children with CP [42]. Therefore, treatment strategies should address these two factors in children with CP. At first, body positioning is used to manage postural difficulties and reduce abnormal muscle activity. It can also be addressed simultaneously with the other two factors [42]. Therefore, it is recommended for SLPs to optimizing body positioning, focus on controlling respiratory effort, and coordinating respiration and phonation to facilitate efficient breathing [42, 80–82]. The SLPs can enhance breath support through strengthening inspiratory and expiratory muscles, training diaphragmatic breathing, and strengthening laryngeal muscle [69, 83–85]. The other objective which is the improvement of coordination of respiration and phonation [86], can be achieved by some speech strategies such as speaking at a comfortable rate and appropriate phrasing based on the clinical experiences. Some speech strategies such as speaking at a comfortable rate and appropriate phrasing may be useful to improve coordination between respiration and phonation. Also, it is possible for patients to produce louder voice and clearer speech [58]. Since speech production results from the interactive relationship of subsystems of voice production, it is expected that speech intelligibility improves by increased control of breathing for speech [80, 82, 87].

It is recommended for the SLPs to use an evidence-based practice model for the working on speech breathing. It is also suggested that individual variabilities be addressed when selecting a treatment strategy. Effective strategies may be tailored for each child considering individual variabilities [42]. Type of dysarthria is another main factor which should be considered. For example, it is not clear whether expiratory muscle strengthening would be helpful for children with spastic or athetoid CP, unlike those with hypotonia. However, in spastic CP, combination of strengthening tasks with relaxation techniques is useful [42].

Overall, little evidence is available regarding the management of speech breathing in individuals with CP. There is a critical need to understand the nature of speech breathing as well as to design treatment studies targeting speech breathing in this population [42].

8.8 Phonation in Speech Production

Speech production results from coordination between three subsystems including phonatory, respiratory, and resonatory. The phonatory subsystem which is known as source of voice production refers to the laryngeal structures, particularly true vocal folds. The voice signal is produced by vibration of the true vocal folds by interaction with respiratory system and then is modified in the vocal tract. The voice signal represents several features including loudness, pitch, quality, and flexibility of the voice. These vocal parameters can be evaluated by auditory-perceptual voice assessment—golden standard—and acoustic analysis. Voice is the element that carries speech and makes the acoustic signal to be heard easily. The voice production considers as a powerful tool for communication in humans. The speakers can express their intents, emotions, and feelings by the altered vocal features [88–90].

8.8.1 Voice Disorders in Cerebral Palsy

Voice disorders refer to any abnormal differences in loudness, pitch, quality, or flexibility of the voice compared with peers with similar demographic characteristics, cultural background, and even geographic location [88–90]. In the general population, the prevalence of voice disorders is estimated to range between 3% and 10% [91], whereas in children the prevalence is reported from 1.4% to 6.7% [92, 93]. Although the exact prevalence of voice disorders in CP has not been recognized, CP is known as one of the primary disorder etiologies for such disorders [41]. Therefore, the prevalence of voice disorders in this population is expected to be higher compared to general population. Individuals with CP present with a variety of voice problems. In children with CP, the ability to control vocal loudness is often reduced and vocal quality is frequently altered [57, 67, 94–99]. Reported vocal quality changes include strain/struggle, harshness, creaky voice, wet hoarseness/gurgly voice, and both hypo- or hyper-nasality. Other common voice characteristics are fluctuations in pitch and loudness, reduced pitch and loudness flexibility, and a slower rate of speech [38, 95, 100, 101]. Based on the findings of a recent study, children with CP often demonstrate a constricted and creaky voice quality because of lower spectral tilt and increased noise which reflects reduced overall voice quality [94]. Identifying voice problems in this population is crucial, and some studies have focused on measuring acoustic features to facilitate the early diagnosis of dysarthria in children with CP [102, 103]. It is supposed that similar voice characteristics are still present in adulthood among individuals with CP [95, 104].

The nature and severity of voice problems vary widely among individuals with CP. Dysarthria is common in this population, and voice problems in CP are categorized as "neurologic voice disorders". These often occur in combination with other motor speech disorders, including respiratory, articulatory, resonatory, and prosodic impairments. The type and range of voice problems largely depends on the underlying dysarthria [91, 105–109]. To illustrate, flaccid dysarthria is typically associated with reduced loudness, breathy voice, and diplophonia as well as hypernasality and nasal air emission. In contrast, spastic dysarthria is characterized by a strained, rough, and hyper nasal voice quality with low pitch, slow speech rate, and monoprosody [41]. The severity of voice problems generally parallels the severity of dysarthria; mild dysarthria is associated with milder voice problems, whereas severe dysarthria leads to more severe voice problems. Therefore, it is not surprising that variant type and extent of voice disorders are observed in individuals with CP. Interestingly, the voice quality of children with CP is often inconsistent and may fluctuate even within a single sentence [98]. Voice quality can also vary depending on the speech tasks. For instance, poorer quality has been reported during the production of sustained vowels- particularly low vowels such as/a/- compared to high vowels such as/i/ [94]. Furthermore, children with CP show greater impairments in loudness and breath support during longer utterances compared to single-word productions, likely due to the increased demands on speech motor control [110, 111]. These reports and other similar findings demonstrate the potential of connected speech for identifying the speech difficulties in CP [112].

Despite these findings, many aspects of vocal folds function in CP still remain unclear and results across studies are inconsistent. For example, spectrographic findings have shown that the acoustic signal in children with CP is noisier and less stable rather than in typically developing peers [99], while acoustic measures of voice stability had no significant differences [102]. Given the limited and inconsistent evidence, the underlying causes of voice quality differences in CP are not fully understood [94]. However, two main etiological factors have been proposed: (1) motor control deficits of the laryngeal subsystem and/or (2) impaired coordination between the laryngeal and respiratory subsystems [94].

The voice problems described above significantly affect communication in individuals with CP. Additionally, these problems restrict social interactions and participation, particularly when the impairments are severe. Reduced opportunities for social interaction, in turn, negatively impact the QoL of in children and adults with CP [113]. Considering the critical role of voice problems in communication and social participation as well as the QoL, the importance of providing speech therapy services to improve voice problems in CP is evident.

As CP is a primary neurological disorder, the management of associated voice problems requires a combination of appropriate medical, surgical, educational, and rehabilitative interventions. The SLPs, who are directly responsible for the evaluation and management of voice disorders, typically work as part of an interdisciplinary team [41]. Within this framework, SLPs provide educational and rehabilitative interventions commonly referred to as voice therapy or vocal rehabilitation. The primary aim of voice therapy is to restore the best possible voice quality, taking into account individual needs, social participation, and activities of daily living [114].

Voice therapy is generally classified into indirect and direct interventions. Indirect voice therapy, often referred to as hygienic voice therapy, focuses on identifying, eliminating, or modifying behavioral factors that contribute to voice problems—such as shouting, screaming, excessive throat clearing, habitual coughing, or poor hydration [41]. Indirect voice therapy is typically the first step in intervention, particularly for reducing compensatory vocal behaviors that have become habituated due to underlying conditions such as CP. Although direct evidence is lacking for hygienic voice therapy in individuals with CP, it is generally assumed that indirect voice therapy may also be beneficial, especially for those exhibiting vocal misuse or phonotraumatic behaviors. In direct voice therapy, vocal characteristics are generally targeted through direct manipulation [41, 115]. There are several evidence-based direct voice therapy techniques that are well-established in voice therapy [41, 115–127]. Based on their theoretical principles, it appears reasonable to assume that many of these techniques could also benefit for children and adults with CP, although further research is required.

Among the various techniques of direct voice therapy, Lee Silverman Voice Treatment (LSVT LOUD) is the only direct voice therapy method with published evidence supporting its effectiveness for vocal improvement in both children and adults with CP [104, 110, 128–131]. The LSVT is originally developed by Dr. Lorraine Ramig for individuals with Parkinson disease. It is an intensive voice therapy program primarily designed to increase vocal loudness by improving vocal fold adduction. The standard protocol includes 16 one-hour sessions, delivered four times per week for 4 weeks by a certified SLP [126, 127, 132–135].

Although LSVT was firstly developed for Parkinson's disease, its effectiveness has been demonstrated in other neurological conditions, including CP [110, 128–131]. Parents of children with CP have reported immediate improvements in vocal loudness following LSVT LOUD [110, 129]. Neuroimaging evidence also suggests that LSVT LOUD enhances the integrity of white matter speech networks in children with motor speech disorders, including CP [136]. Beyond vocal loudness, the method has been shown to improve speech intelligibility, communication effectiveness, and QoL [130, 137]. Interestingly, it has also been associated with reductions in drooling in children with CP [138].

To explore more detailed aspects of the implementation of LSVT LOUD, the researchers found while treatment intensity (dose) is necessary, it may not be sufficient for all patients. In other words, weak responders may require longer treatment durations, better-timed intervention phases, or enhanced motivation to engage in daily communication [128]. A scoping review in 2024 concluded that the majority of included studies provided promising results for LSVT LOUD in children with CP. This review concludes that LSVT LOUD improves voice and speech skills effectively in children with CP. So that, parents of these children would recommend LSVT LOUD to other parents. However, this review highlighted the need for larger, well-designed clinical trials. Also, it declared that SLPs and other clinicians need to carefully follow LSVT LOUD outcomes in children with CP [139].

Fewer studies have investigated the effectiveness of LSVT LOUD in adults with CP. Evidence includes a case study on a 36-year-old female with severe spastic dysarthria and a group study on 16 adults with CP comparing in-person versus tele practice-based LSVT LOUD. Both studies reported significant improvements in target vocal measures even across tele practice model [104, 131]. Nonetheless, given the limited evidences, future research is essential. Overall, LSVT LOUD appears particularly useful for individuals with CP who exhibit reduced loudness, respiratory weakness, or impaired coordination of the respiratory and phonatory systems [101, 110].

Because individuals with CP are often able to manipulate vocal loudness to some extent, increasing loudness has become a central focus of many evidence-based interventions such as LSVT LOUD in this population. It is hypothesized that louder speech promotes positive changes in both articulatory and laryngeal subsystems, thereby improving overall speech production [130]. Acoustic analyses indicate that decreased noise and increased acoustic energy in higher harmonics and formants in louder speech may lead to better speech intelligibility in these children [140]. Another treatment with a focus on vocal loudness in children with CP aimed to improve vocal characteristics include the "Subsystem Approach" [80–82, 104, 141–144].

The "Subsystem Approach" is an intensive intervention (16–18 sessions over 4–6 weeks) based on the motor learning principles. In this approach, all processes involved in speech production are addressed. This intervention targets respiratory effort and coordination of exhalation with phonation, because these processes are essential for the producing a healthy and strong vocal signal [141, 142, 145, 146]. To increase respiratory effort and coordinate of exhalation and phonation, the subjects are taught to maintain sufficient breath support for producing loud and clear words and to breathe at appropriate points in phrases. In addition to respiration and phonation, the approach addresses prosody (pitch, loudness, timing), nasality, articulation, and speech rate [141, 142, 145, 146] whereases LSVT LOUD only focuses on both respiration and phonation. Additionally, in the "Subsystem Approach," only those children who have weak voice are encouraged to produce loud voice; However, those who are not able to change vocal loudness appropriately across a phrase are encouraged to maintain respiratory effort by using a "nice and easy" voice [100].

Consequently, there is no evidence about the effectiveness of other direct voice therapy techniques except for LSVT LOUD in individuals with CP. Therefore, SLPs should consider cautious of conducting direct voice therapy methods for this population. It is recommended that SLPs carefully monitor outcomes of other voice therapy techniques with no research evidence on a case-by-case basis. Furthermore, more research is urgently needed to validate effectiveness of voice therapy techniques for this population. It should be noted that since most of the voice therapy techniques require patient education and cooperation, they may not be applicable for those individuals with CP who have cognitive impairments or severe physical limitations. Additionally, using voice therapy in the form of tele practice is another useful and practical solution for individuals with CP who have reduced mobility. However, it should be noted that tele practice is not suitable for those with severe motor or cognitive impairments [131].

8.9 Resonance in Speech Production

The resonatory subsystem refers to the several parts of vocal tract from the true vocal folds up to lips. It involves the supraglottal space, pharynx, oral, and nasal cavities. The primary sound produced by vocal fold vibration should be reinforced and modified in the vocal tract. If the sound is not resonated in the vocal tract reveals a voice lacking any ring. Such a voice is totally unrecognizable as human voice. Resonance is influenced by size and shape of the vocal tract and altered by movements of the speech articulators. Also, the function of the velopharyngeal (VP) valve contributes resonance features. Therefore, the vocal tract as a filter plays an essential role to creating the perceptual features of voice, including pitch, loudness, nasality, and quality [41].

Most of the speech sounds are resonated in the oral cavity (oral sounds) while in, few sounds such as/m/,/n/, and /ŋ/ (nasal sounds) are resonated in the nasal cavity. For normal production of oral speech sounds, the VP valve must completely be closed to prevent air passing from the nasal cavity [147]. During oral sounds production, if the nasal cavity is not closed off, the oral speech sounds are nasalized [58]. Range of movement and the ability to provide an adequate closure at the VP valve are necessary components for producing oral speech sounds. Additionally, speed and timing of movements are other important factors which will impact airflow and resonance [148, 149]. However, in nasal speech sounds, the VP valve is open and airflow is passed into the nasal cavity, leading to nasal quality [58, 147]. Normal structure and function of the VP mechanism are necessary for normal speech production [41, 147].

8.9.1 Resonance Problems in Cerebral Palsy

In individuals with CP, dysarthria affects all subsystems of speech production including resonatory along with other subsystems [58]. Consequently, resonance problems can be observed associated with other speech production involvements in CP. Resonance problems are referred to as velopharyngeal dysfunction (VPD). The VPD is a general term refers to several dysfunctions in the VP valve including VP insufficiency, VP incompetency, and/or VP mislearning. The VP insufficiency is a type of VPD associated with structural abnormality such as cleft palate whereas VP mislearning is an isolated articulation disorder or a compensatory articulation disorder in which nasal or pharyngeal sounds are substituted with oral sounds. However, VP incompetency results from neuromotor disorders where no structural impairment is available in the VP valve [150]. The latter is frequent in dysarthria including CP, leading to hypernasality voice quality because of weak or slow movement of the soft palate. In this condition, the nasal passage may not be fully closed during speech. Additionally, nasal emission can be observed in this condition [41, 150]. Interestingly, a research study has been reported that both hyper nasality and hyponsality as resonance problems in children with CP, mostly with mild severity [27].

Resonance features can be evaluated by several non-instrumental and instrumental tools. Non-instrumental evaluations represent perceptual methods done by a SLP to assess hypernasality, hyponasality, nasal emission, and articulatory errors across different speech samples. There are several instruments for the assessment of resonance including nasometer, videofluroscopy, and nasopharyngoscopy. The nasometer measures acoustic energy of the oral and nasal cavities during the speech production and data is interpreted by SLPs. The videofluroscopy assesses the closure of VP during speech and the results are interpreted by both radiologists and SLPs. Observation of the vocal tract is performed using the nasopharyngoscopy which is conducted by SLPs. Both SLPs and surgeons interpret the nasopharyngoscopic videos [147, 150].

There are several interventions for the management of VP impairments in dysarthria including prosthetic, surgical, and behavioral interventions. Palatal lifts, nasal or nasopharyngeal obturators, and palatal desensitization along with palatal lifts are all considered prosthetic interventions [151]. Research studies demonstrated decreased hypernasality associated with improvement in articulation, speech intelligibility, and respiratory support for speech following palatal lifting in individuals with dysarthria [152, 153]. Prosthetic intervention has a long history for improving speech function in dysarthria; however, it would not be recommended for all dysarthric individuals. To be more exact, there are some indicators of candidacy that have been reported for prosthetic interventions. The most critical indicator is the soft palate weakness, preventing of the VP closure during speech. Furthermore, there are other speech and nonspeech candidacy indicators. Speech indicators involve pharyngeal wall movement, appropriate oral articulation, and sufficient respiratory support for speech. Also, those patients who have a relatively stable clinical course are good candidates for prosthetic interventions. Nonspeech indicators include intact swallowing, normal cognition, and manual skills associated with the desire to communicate through speech [151–153]. Since the great range of candidacy indicators and high prevalence of VP impairment in dysarthric individuals, prosthetic intervention would not be an appropriate clinical option for the majority of dysarthric speakers. For these cases who are poor candidates for prosthetic interventions, behavioral intervention and AAC are recommended [151].

Surgical intervention involves pharyngeal flap surgery, pharyngeal implants, and Teflon injections [151]. The benefits of surgical intervention are less than prosthetic interventions and is a subject of controversy for children with CP [154, 155]. Overall, there is a lack of sufficient evidence is available to recommend surgical intervention for individuals with dysarthria. Therefore, surgical intervention is only considered in conditions where other interventions have failed or are ineffective [151].

In general, behavioral interventions refer to motor exercises to raise the soft palate and close off the nasal cavities [156]. These exercises include modifying the pattern of speaking, resistance exercises with continuous positive airway pressure, and biofeedback techniques. There are several methods for modifying the pattern of speaking such as producing speech with increased effort, producing speech with a slower rate as well as clear speech [156–159]. The resistance exercises strengthen the VP closure muscles by requiring them to work against a resistance force [160, 161]. In techniques of biofeedback, various feedbacks can be provided to help patients to decrease hypernasality and nasal airflow during speech efforts [162]. These interventions generally are appropriate for those individuals who can compensate VP impairment during several speech tasks used to evaluate stimulability [151, 163]. Behavioral exercises have been introduced in textbooks for the management of nasality, however, there is currently no sufficient evidence to evaluate the effectiveness of them.

Consequently, among several interventions suggested for the VP impairments in dysarthria, the palatal lift has been recommended for individuals with CP. However, it is only recommended for selected cases and it is not widely used for individuals with CP [8]. Further studies are needed to evaluate the effectiveness of various interventions in dysarthria, particularly for individuals with CP.

8.10 Prosody for Speech Production and Communication

Prosody, the non-verbal aspects of speech, refers to the patterns of intonation, stress, and rhythm in connected speech. These patterns reflect significant changes in pitch, loudness, duration, and pause across words, phrases, and sentences which depend on respiratory and laryngeal control [58, 164–166]. Variations in these perceptual characteristics are represented through variations in acoustic parameters such as fundamental frequency, intensity, and duration [167, 168]. Although prosody of speech refers to the non-verbal aspects of speech, it highly impacts speech intelligibility and naturalness [166, 167, 169–172]. Additionally, prosody has a variety of communicative and linguistic functions. It also plays various social and psychological roles [173]. To illustrate, prosody is utilized for conveying meaning, highlighting prominent information, as well as marking sentence modality [173–182]. Therefore, prosody helps the speakers to express their emotional and attitudinal states and aids listeners to interpret information more effectively [173]. Consequently, prosodic components are essential for efficient communication [183]. Development of prosodic skills starts from childhood and continues throughout adolescence [184–190]. Successful acquisition of prosodic skills is closely associated with cognitive, emotional, and physical development [184–186].

8.10.1 Prosodic Problems in Cerebral Palsy

Prosodic problems are another aspect of neurological motor speech disorders in dysarthria, which are created by limited motor control over the speech production system [106, 166, 191]. Prosodic impairments are considered one of the earliest cues of dysarthric speech [192, 193]. Due to high prevalence of prosodic impairments in dysarthria, prosody-based measures have been introduced as a useful tool for the assessment of dysarthria, particularly with a better classification of mild dysarthria [192–194].

Given that CP is a common cause of motor speech disorders, prosodic impairments are also prevalent in this population [169]. These problems can be documented by perceptual and acoustic evaluations [167, 168]. Common prosodic challenges in individuals with CP include reduced or accelerated speech rate, rhythmic disturbances, and difficulties with sentence stress and accent. Some individuals with CP show monopitch and monoloudness while other individuals indicate exaggerated prosody [106, 169, 170, 174, 191, 195–198]. Impaired prosody affects the intelligibility and naturalness of speech [166, 167, 169–172, 199]. Due to the critical role of prosody on communication; prosodic impairments can also significantly impact effectiveness of communication [173, 183].

According to the literature, individuals with CP may have different problems with modulation acoustic parameters like intensity, fundamental frequency, and duration to indicate prosodic features such as stress, intonation, rhythm, and speech rate [57, 168, 173, 199–201]. For instance, if children with CP are not able to manipulate acoustic parameters to mark stress, this issue affects their ability to highlight important words and makes some challenges in daily interactions [202]. Some prosodic differences have been reported between individuals with CP and healthy speakers. However, the results of the studies were contradictory. According to some studies, children and adults with dysarthria due to CP rely more on increased intensity to mark sentential stress compared to control group while in, duration associated with reduced pitch and loudness variations was the strategy of speakers with CP in another research [168, 203, 204]. Moreover, adults with CP convey lexical stress differently compared to control speakers with more reliance on duration than other prosodic cues. This difference was greater for second-syllable stressed words rather than first-syllable stressed words [205]. Overall, it can be concluded that compensatory mechanisms for producing prosodic features are different in individuals with dysarthria from healthy peers when the pitch variations are difficult for them, frequently with reliance on the intensity and/or duration-related features [165].

In contrast, there are multiple studies that failed to find prosodic differences between speakers with CP and healthy peers. Several studies which have investigated intonation patterns in children with CP showed that children with moderate to severe CP are able to use intonation reliably in communication with their caregivers [206, 207]. Also, several studies declared although individuals with CP have restricted pitch and loudness range and apply different method to mark stress rather than healthy speakers, they can successfully convey contrastive stress [57, 173, 200, 201]. Adults with CP can control prosodic features despite severely impaired control on segmental features, particularly during production of isolated vowels and short phrases with interrogative versus imperative tone. Interestingly, adults with CP who utilized AAC because of severe dysarthria were able to consistently control duration and also to control pitches in production of the sustained vowel, showing potential ability to rely on phonatory control [200]. A study revealed that adults with CP are able to utilize contrastive stress but they increased intensity greater than the control group. This finding may represent a compensatory physiological strategy to show contrastive stress in individuals with CP [201]. Consequently, some aspects of prosodic skills may remain intact or show little differences in CP.

As mentioned above, there are several research studies tried to explore prosodic features in children and adults with CP. However, interventional studies in this field are limited. Intonation is one prosodic feature that has been addressed in interventional studies in CP [142, 183]. Although intonation is known as variations in pitch, intervention strategies can be applied without directly focusing on this aspect. Expanding the subject, pitch is controlled using complex interaction between laryngeal muscles, subglottal air pressure, and aerodynamic forces. Therefore, those interventions targeting both phonation and breathing could effectively lead to intonation variations. One of the intervention approaches takes this strategy is the "Subsystem Approach" [142, 183]. Moreover, considering the relationship of pitch and loudness, it might be expected that changes in pitch control results from those interventions targeting loudness such as LSVT LOUD. This conclusion has been verified in a study on children with spastic CP in 2012 [110].

The findings which demonstrated the relation between prosody and speech intelligibility, suggest that working on prosody may be valuable in improving speech intelligibility in children with CP [199]. Also, it is expected that the management of prosodic impairments enhance communication effectively. In order to boost functional communication in CP, it is suggested that future interventions leverage the prosodic differences of individuals with CP compared to healthy peers [168]. The research studies which demonstrated prosodic differences between speakers with CP and healthy peers emphasize that intervention can be personalized, and SLPs can target these prosodic features and their acoustic correlates for further evaluation [165]. Limited evidence-based interventions targeting prosody in CP highlight the significant need for future investigations.

8.11 Oropharyngeal Dysphagia in Cerebral Palsy

Swallowing is a complex and coordinated process in which food, liquids, or saliva transported from the mouth to the stomach. This process occurs in three distinct stages including oral, pharyngeal, and esophageal phases. Oral phase encompasses of voluntary movements of oral muscles, where the bolus is prepared and propelled backward into the throat. Pharyngeal phase triggered involuntary by entering the bolus into the throat. This stage ensures safe passage by closing off the airway and directing the substance into the esophagus. Esophageal phase involves rhythmic involuntary muscle contractions in the esophagus to push the material down into the stomach [208].

Oropharyngeal dysphagia (OPD), as the most common swallowing disorder in neurologic condition, is a disruption of oral and pharyngeal phase of swallowing function, encompassing difficulties with the ingestion and handling of solids or liquids from the oral cavity into the esophagus [209]. This common complication in individuals with CP contributes substantially to raised risk of infections, morbidity, decreased participation, and reduced well-being and QoL [210–212]. Recent researches indicate that OPD is highly prevalent among individuals with CP across the lifespan, with rates reaching approximately 85–99% in those with the most severe impairments, particularly in pediatric populations [210].

In CP, OPD results from a mix of compromised voluntary and involuntary motor function in the orofacial, pharyngeal, and respiratory muscles, along with irregular muscle tone (either hypertonia or hypotonia). Additional factors include oral–sensorimotor impairments, lack of coordination, and reduced ability to regulate the timing and the force of movements essential for safe swallowing. Other contributing factors are dental malocclusion, poor posture, contractures (which negatively affect head and trunk stability and oral mechanics) which worsen swallowing efficiency in persons with CP. Additionally, Other factors that also can impact swallowing efficiency in this population are drooling, associated comorbidities (e.g., intellectual disability, epilepsy, gastroesophageal reflux disorder, and behavioral feeding problems [213–215].

Large observational studies and recent systematic reviews report that clinically significant feeding and swallowing problems occur in approximately 40–99% of children and adults with CP, with wide variation depending on case ascertainment and severity [210].

Swallowing dysfunction in individuals with CP often impacts all phases of swallowing including oral preparatory, oral transit, and pharyngeal phases. During the oral phase, poor lip closure, insufficient bolus preparation, trouble clearing food from a spoon, challenges with drinking from a cup or bottle, difficulty chewing, and slowed oral transit are common. In the pharyngeal phase, delays in swallow triggering, pharyngeal residue, and the penetration or aspiration of material into the airway may occur. Additionally, compromised airway protection due to an ineffective cough and silent or overt aspiration is frequently observed. Clinical indicators like excessive drooling, difficulties with self-feeding, extended meal durations, and recurrent chest infections are often common clinical signs that frequently coexist. The severity and combination of these symptoms vary among individuals and tend to be more pronounced in those with greater motor impairment [214, 216, 217]. Table 8.1 provides an overview of swallowing problems, their underlying physiological mechanisms and potential outcomes in individuals with CP, as documented

Table 8.1 Summary of swallowing problems, physiological causes, and potential consequences in CP

Phase	Typical clinical signs	Probable physiological causes	Potential consequences
Oral preparatory / Oral transit	Poor lip closure Food loss during eating Drooling Prolonged/inefficient chewing Delayed/inefficient bolus formation Oral residue post-swallowing Prolonged mealtimes Increase or persistence of primitive oral reflexes (e.g., tongue thrust, bite reflex)	Orofacial hypotonia/ hypertonia Weak or reduced movement of the oral structures (lips, cheeks, tongue, jaw) Impaired tongue coordination Reduced oral sensation Dental malocclusion Poor jaw stability	Reduced intake malnutrition Prolonged feeding time Aspiration of secretions Refusal to eat Boring feeding time for caregivers Reduced QoL
Pharyngeal (including swallow initiation)	Delayed swallow initiation Multiple swallows Throat clearing Wet breathing Wet hoarseness/gurgly voice Coughing during/after meals Gagging Chocking Recurrent chest infections Difficulty managing secretions	Delayed pharyngeal reflex Incoordination of pharyngeal muscles Reduced pharyngeal sensation Impaired velopharyngeal closure	Penetration/ aspiration (overt or silent) Pneumonia Stressful feeding time for caregivers Refusal to eat Reduced QoL

(continued)

Table 8.1 (continued)

Phase	Typical clinical signs	Probable physiological causes	Potential consequences
Pharyngeal (airway protection/ respiratory-swallow coordination)	Silent aspiration (no cough) Reduce protective reflexes Inefficient cough Regurgitations and vomiting Recurrent lower respiratory tract infections Whizzing, stridor or breathing difficulties during feeding Fremitus (rattly chest) High respiratory rate Eye tearing Color change	Poor laryngeal elevation/ closure Impaired cough strength Impaired sensation Discoordination of breathing and swallowing Reduced pulmonary reserve	Aspiration pneumonia Chronic lung disease Hospitalization Increased mortality risk
Gastroesophageal reflux-related feeding problems	Regurgitation Vomiting Feeding refusal Irritability during/after feeds	Gastroesophageal reflux disorder Impaired gastric emptying Positioning issues	Esophagitis Aspiration Feeding aversion Poor weight gain

Adopted from Benfer et al. [214, 216, 217], Wilson et al. [218], Ahmed et al. [219], Guare et al. [220] and Arvedson et al. [208]
CP cerebral palsy, *Qol* quality of life

in studies using clinical observations, instrumental evaluations or caregiver reports [208, 214, 216–220].

Although much of the research on dysphagia centers on children, many individuals continue to experience swallowing difficulties well into adolescence and adulthood. Neonatal and Early feeding challenges in infancy such as poor suck–swallow–breathe coordination) often serve as indicators of later swallowing impairment. However, outcomes vary widely; some children show improvement with age and targeted intervention, as evidenced by the decline of OPD prevalence from 79.7% at 18–24 months to 43.5% in preschool-aged children [210]. Others, however, face ongoing or worsening difficulties [210, 221]. The severity and persistence of dysphagia, as well as poorer overall outcomes, are most strongly linked to the degree of gross motor impairment [214, 217]. For instance, instability in the pelvis and trunk can compromise head and neck positioning, hindering controlled oropharyngeal movements needed to regulate food flow and protect the airway [208, 210]. Limited upper limb mobility further exacerbates challenges with self-feeding [222]. Additionally, severe speech impairments and intellectual disabilities are also associated with more pronounced feeding dysfunction and greater caregiver burden [210]. The presence of gastroesophageal reflux disease also increases the risk of aspiration, feeding aversion, and adverse health outcomes related to swallowing problems.

Caregivers and healthcare providers should conduct regular evaluations to monitor feeding challenges, track nutritional status and growth, document caregiver-reported feeding behaviors, as well as any signs of OPD obtain caregiver reports of feeding behaviors and observe any sign of OPD [223, 224]. If screening indicates a risk of dysphagia, a comprehensive multidisciplinary assessment should be initiated. This evaluation should involve specialists including SLPs, gastroenterologists, nutritionists, respiratory physicians or physiotherapists, occupational therapists, dentists, and neurologists. The assessment should cover medical history and current medications, nutritional and hydration status, oral-motor and feeding skills, oral sensory processing issues, posture and positioning during feeding and swallowing safety [208]. Instrumental assessment like video-fluoroscopic swallow study (VFSS) or fiberoptic endoscopic evaluation of swallowing (FEES) are highly sensitive for detecting silent aspiration. These tools help identify the underlying physiological impairments affecting swallowing and guide targeted intervention [208, 224]. Clinical or instrumental dysphagia assessment should be always coupled with evaluation of nutritional status (e.g., weight and growth metrics) and respiratory screening (e.g., chest X-ray if indicated, pulmonary function tests when possible). In cases of recurrent infections, aspiration-related pneumonia should be considered a potential cause [208]. A thorough evaluation must also examine the patient's mealtime routines, behaviors, utensil use, food textures, and caregiver skills [225]. Mealtimes are not only essential for nutrition but also serve as critical social interactions. Mealtime challenges can restrict participation, increase caregiver stress and burden, and reduce opportunities for social engagement. So, to plan a feasible intervention program, decision-making about the intervention should be family-centered and reflect family priorities and simultaneously, balance safety, nutrition, oral intake enjoyment, participation, and QoL [225, 226]. Table 8.2 summarizes key intervention principles and practical techniques supported by research [208, 224, 226–232].

Regular multidisciplinary meetings are critical for delivering care for swallowing difficulties of individuals with CP. These meetings should involve neurologists or developmental pediatricians to oversee neurological diagnoses; SLPs to address swallowing mechanics and oral-motor function); dietitians to customize nutritional plans and food textures; psychologists to provide psychosocial support; and importantly, caregivers to ensure practical implementation at home [228, 232]. This collaborative approach facilitates personalized goal-setting, consistent intervention strategies across settings, and ongoing progress monitoring. For example, if a VFSS reveals pharyngeal-phase impairments, the team can implement targeted interventions: The SLPs design oral sensory-motor therapeutic exercises and compensatory techniques, the dietitian adjusts food, and liquid consistencies for safety. Also, caregivers are trained in optimal feeding positions and compensatory strategies to support safe swallowing and adequate nutrition at home [229, 232]. The importance of caregiver training becomes even more evident when, the results of studies show that feeding recommendations for children with CP were widely provided to caregivers; however, there is no consistent follow-up to ensure actual implementation. So, without structured training and periodic monitoring, these guidelines may fail to integrate effectively into daily routines [226].

Table 8.2 Practical techniques for improvement of swallowing and feeding function in individuals with CP

Intervention	Goal	Techniques
Direct or task-specific swallowing therapy method	Reducing physiological disorders that underlie problems at oral or pharyngeal phases of swallowing Increasing the neuromuscular strength and control	*Repetitive oral sensorimotor stimulation*
		Swallowing maneuvers such as effortful swallow, Mendelsohn maneuver, bolus control drills, when the patient can cooperate and motor patterns permit
		Using from motor learning principles: distributed practice, variable contexts, and feedback
Indirect method	Improving feeding and swallowing safety and independence through compensatory strategy training	*Optimize positioning and postural support:* Correcting head, trunk and pelvis alignment to improve airway protection, oral control, breathing function and the function of digestive system Using from adaptive seating that helps positioning the hips-knees- ankles at 90-degree angles and supporting the neutral head and neck alignment Small position changes depending on the nature of the swallowing impairment such as chin tuck, slight trunk flexion or head and neck extension can be effective in improving the swallow safety in some patient
		Individualized texture and consistency *modifications based on the age and skills of the patient* to reduce aspiration risk and improve bolus control. Issues that must be considered: Energy-dense textures to meet nutritional needs. Dehydration and constipation when using thicker fluids. Response to children's cue for feeding. Exposure to novel foods and textures, as soon as possible.
		Altering the sensory stimulation of blouse: serving a cold, warmed up, aerated or flavored bites
		Altering the rate of presentation: Increasing the intervals between bite Using slower-flowing cups/bottles Training the caregivers to be responsive to the patient's cues of readiness for the next bite Self-feeding training which decreases the rate of feeding
		Environmental changes: Train caregivers in safe feeding techniques and fatigue management Providing a quiet environment to enhance concentration on swallowing during meal time
		Adapted feeding equipment: Cups, spoons, …
		Protheses such as palatal lift that could be used for velopharyngeal incompetency
		Tube feeding when oral intake is unsafe or insufficient

Adopted from Arvedson et al. [208], Steele et al. [224], Maggioni and Araújo [226], Taylor et al. [227], Kuperminc et al. [228], Erasmus et al. [229], Kamal et al. [230], Parr et al. [231], Momora et al. [232]
CP cerebral palsy

For patients facing limited access to healthcare due to mobility challenges, transportation issues, or geographic distance tele-practice combined with occasional in-person visits offers a viable alternative to observe mealtimes, evaluate feeding and swallowing and training the caregivers [224, 233].

8.12 Drooling in Cerebral Palsy

Drooling or sialorrhea refers to the unintentional spillage of saliva from the mouth beyond the margin of the lips, on the face or clothing. Drooling which is also known as anterior drooling is a symptom that is evident in 10–40% of children with CP [234]. Higher prevalence rates and persistence into adulthood can occur in children with more severe sensory-motor impairments and comorbid intellectual disabilities [235, 236]. Anterior drooling is visible; however, saliva can also spill posteriorly. Posterior drooling may occur simultaneously, or independently of, anterior drooling and can lead to saliva spilling into the hypopharynx and eventually larynx, potentially resulting in chronic aspiration and its consequences, such as pulmonary infections [237].

Drooling is a multifactorial condition. In patients with neurologic disorders including CP, it most often arises from impaired oral motor control and diminished oral sensation and awareness. Impaired oral motor control can cause drooling by several factors including incomplete lip seal, reduced tongue control, weak oral suction, and decreased cheek and perioral musculature coordination Additionally, reduced spontaneous or volitional swallow frequency and ineffective bolus transport/clearance can result in drooling. Other factors include a forward-flexed head posture due to poor trunk, neck and head control, and certain medications that increase hypersalivation or worsen saliva control [238].

Managing drooling is very important because saliva can soil clothing, toys, books, furniture, and electronic devices as well as produce unpleasant odors. It also contributes to dehydration and persistent irritation of the facial skin and interfere with chewing and speech. In cases with posterior drooling, this condition may be associated with dysphagia and respiratory complications [237]. Beyond these physical effects, from a psychosocial standpoint, deficient oral secretion control is associated with reduced self-esteem and impaired community participation, representing a substantial component of disease burden. Due to the increased care time, caregiver stress, healthcare financial costs, and social isolation probability, it negatively impacts the QoL of caregivers [208, 235]. Drooling has been reported as the primary concern and the most significant problem observed to caregivers [235].

Clinical assessment as the prerequisite of intervention, should be performed multidisciplinary, by SLPs, pediatric neurologists or physiatrists, otolaryngologists, gastroenterologists, dentists, occupational therapists, and parents or caregivers. In this multidisciplinary approach, different factors of this complex problem should take into account, including:

1. The severity, frequency, and the pattern of drooling;
2. Related physical and functional complications:
   - Impaired oral-motor function in drinking, chewing, swallowing or speech;
   - Skin irritation and drooling-related dermatitis or infections;
   - Malocclusion, dental caries, or gingivitis;
   - Inability or difficulty in maintaining postural stability;
   - Increased risk of pneumonia aspiration when it associated with swallowing impairment;
   - Dehydration risk, when the oral intake is reduced due to swallowing problems;
   - Postural issues.
3. Social effects (e.g., stigma, reduced participation), and how these interpersonal consequences intersect with daily care demands and costs;
4. Impact on the QoL and well-being of the affected individual and his/her caregivers.

While many drooling treatments have been reported in the literature, ranging from highly invasive procedures such as salivary gland excision to less invasive strategies like behavioral modification, it seems that they suffer from significant limitations including inconsistent methodologies, insufficient evidence across different intervention types, lack of procedural detail, lack of evidence related to effectiveness and safety of interventions and a shortage of long-term outcome data [235, 239]. Choosing a treatment from the range of options depends on individual factors (e.g., age, drooling severity, neurological or cognitive condition, comorbidities, aspiration risk) as well as family preferences. Consequently, no single approach fits all patients [208, 240]. Noninvasive interventions, such as oral sensory-motor or behavioral interventions, could be often used in patients with a mild or moderate severity, and more invasive methods, such as pharmacotherapy and surgery, are often suitable for more severe cases. As a general rule, treatment can be focused on noninvasive and reversible methods first, and if these methods are ineffective, can be intensified after considering the benefits and risks. Table 8.3 represents the treatment options that can be used for drooling intervention, based on literature [239, 241–245]. Complete elimination of drooling may be unrealistic goal in some patients; so, focus on meaningful reduction that improve hygiene, social participation and reduce caregiver burden may be ideal [245].

Table 8.3 Treatment options for Drooling

Interventional options			Efficacy
Nonpharmacologic/ conservative management	*Oro-motor therapy and behavioral approaches (provided by SLPs)*	Oral motor exercises and stimulations	Evidences are controversial; benefits are greater for mild or moderate drooling and when used intensively by skilled SLPs; less effects are reported in severe cases.
		Functional practice and cueing to increase swallow frequency	
		Purposeful swallow training	
		Kinesio-taping	
		Postural management (chin tuck, head support, seating systems)	
		Adaptive equipment (straws, cups) to improve swallow dynamics	
		Behavioral strategies including cueing, biofeedback (surface electromyography), and caregiver training for consistent prompting and structured routines	
	Oral and dental management	Treat mouth breathing, excessive drooling secondary to teething or oral disease.	
		Dental alignment or prostheses rarely used; routine oral hygiene to prevent skin and dental complications	
	Environmental/ adaptive	Clothing protectors Absorbent bibs Frequent face wiping	Reduce social and skin problems but not underlying cause.
Pharmacologic treatments	*Anticholinergic/ sublingual medications*	Glycopyrrolate	Reduce secretion but have some systemic side effects such as dry mouth, urinary retention, constipation, blurred vision, and cognitive effects that may limit their use.
		Scopolamine	
		Atropine	
		Trihexyphenidyl and other antimuscarinics	
	Botulinum toxin injections into the salivary glands		Reduce saliva production for several months (commonly 3–6 months); decrease drooling severity and caregiver burden. However, it has some side effects and risks including the swallowing difficulty, thickened secretions, and local pain.

(continued)

Table 8.3 (continued)

Interventional options		Efficacy
Surgical (for sever cases; usually after 4 years age)	Submandibular duct relocation	Effective for anterior drooling; unsuitable for patients with posterior pooling
	Submandibular gland excision (with or without parotid duct ligation)	Reduces saliva production; accompanied with risks including dry mouth, dental caries, risk of aspiration in an unsafe swallow, failure/ recurrence, and surgical morbidity.
	Parotid duct ligation/ parotidectomy	

Adopted from Walshe et al. [239], Hughes et al. [241], Yellepeddi et al. [242], Van der Burg et al. [243], Erasmus et al. [244], Riva et al. [245]
SLPs speech and language pathologists

8.13 How Oro-Motor and Communication Impairments Affect Quality of Life

QoL is a comprehensive and multifaceted concept that encompasses various dimensions, including physical health, emotional well-being, social engagement, independence, and more. The World Health Organization defines QoL as an individual's perception of their position in life, considering the cultural context in which they exist, along with their goals, expectations, standards, and concerns [246]. In healthcare, we often focus on health-related quality of life (HRQoL), which refers to how a specific health condition affects an individual [247]. In practice, assessing QoL in individuals with CP typically involves using questionnaires designed for children or adolescents, such as Cerebral Palsy Quality of Life (CP-QoL) [248], Child Health Questionnaire (CHQ) [249], KIDSCREEN [250], and Quality of Life Instrument for Young adults (YAQoL) [251], or more general scales like Pediatric Quality of Life Inventory (PedsQoL) [252, 253] and 36-Item Short Form Health Survey (SF-36) [254, 255]. These tools gather information from adolescents and adults with CP, as well as children with CP or their parents, covering various aspects such as physical functioning, communication, social interactions, emotions, and family life.

Speech is widely regarded as a crucial component of QoL. For instance, research conducted by Dickinson et al. (2007) revealed that children with CP who experienced any form of speech impairment scored significantly lower in the "relationship with parents" domain of a QoL survey [250]. Additionally, qualitative research involving adolescents with CP emphasized communication as a fundamental domain of QoL, with both adolescents and their parents underscoring its importance to overall well-being [256]. When speech is unclear, speakers may be misunderstood, may struggle to take turns in conversations, or may even refrain from speaking altogether [250, 257]. A child with limited verbal communication skills may find it difficult to engage with peers, may be misunderstood in class, or may be left out of group activities [258]. Likewise, when a child with CP has impaired speech or gestures, parents may struggle to interpret their communicative attempts, leading to interaction breakdowns and fewer reciprocal, meaningful conversations [259].

Communication barriers significantly limit employment and social participation for adults with CP. According to Quality Statement 5 of the NICE Shared Decision-Making standard, communication difficulties can impede participation in social, familial, and economic activities [260]. An individual who faces challenges in being understood may be less likely to express themselves, cultivate relationships, or advocate for their own needs. This struggle can ultimately reduce their independence and overall satisfaction with life. While some studies indicate that adults with CP reported a level of well-being comparable to the population norms [261–263], those with unresolved speech difficulties frequently express higher levels of frustration and social anxiety. In a study examining non-ambulatory young people with CP, challenges in understanding parents/guardian were identified as a significant predictor of lower overall QoL [264]. This suggests that, even among individuals with severe impairments, communication proficiency influences QoL more profoundly than physical limitations.

In conclusion, the overall well-being of individual with CP is affected by many elements, such as mobility, pain, cognitive ability, and the environment; nonetheless, communication stands out as a vital component. A child who can express thoughts clearly is more likely to engage in family and peer activities, which can boost self-esteem. Conversely, CP people with speech difficulties often become withdrawn or reliant on others for support. Given that QoL is inherently subjective, it is important to note that two children with similar physical limitations may experience varying levels of life satisfaction. Nonetheless, evidence indicates that improving speech intelligibility can be beneficial for communication and potentially for social participation [265].

8.14 Speech Therapy and Quality of Life

The primary goal of speech therapy for individuals with CP is to enhance speech intelligibility, thus improving their overall QoL [266]. Research on speech motor interventions indicates that targeted treatment can lead to significant improvements in speech intelligibility scores. For instance, Pennington and her colleagues implemented an intensive 6-week program focusing on respiratory support, phonation, and speech rate for children and adolescents with dysarthria. The studies reported that, on average, participants showed marked improvement in speech intelligibility for both familiar and unfamiliar listeners, with these gains sustained at follow-up assessments conducted at 6 and 12 weeks [142, 143]. Additionally, strategies such as deliberately slowing speech [267], voice amplification [129], and multi-cue treatments involving both expanded articulatory range and vocal intensity [268–270] have been identified as effective in enhancing speech intelligibility in individuals with CP. This evidence suggests that even persistent speech impairments in individuals with CP can be effectively ameliorated [271].

Oro-pharyngeal dysphagia and excessive drooling as common symptoms in individuals with CP, leading to risks of aspiration, malnutrition, and social isolation [272]. Evidence shows that tailored interventions, such as oral-motor exercises and behavioral strategies, enhance swallowing safety, reduce drooling severity, and promote better nutritional intake. These improvements directly correlate with increased participation in social activities, reduced hospitalizations, and lower stress for families [273, 274]. By addressing these challenges, speech therapy not only supports physical health but also fosters dignity and social inclusion for individuals with CP.

When a child gains the ability to express his/her needs—whether verbally through AAC devices— and engage more effectively with others after therapy, following treatment, it is often reduces likely to diminish feelings of frustration and feelings of isolation. However, comprehensive studies directly linking treatment to QoL outcomes are limited. Most intervention studies focus on measuring speech intelligibility or acoustic performance. In practice, enhancements in QoL are often most evident through qualitative observations, as both parents and patients frequently express increased happiness and confidence after finding successful communication strategies. Furthermore, AAC serves as a crucial intervention when speech output is insufficient. Researchers recommend AAC when functional speech is lacking [275–277]. Users of AAC technologies, ranging from communication boards to advanced speech-generating devices, often experience greater independence and social inclusion, which in turn is likely to enhance their QoL. For instance, clinical experience suggests that a nonverbal adult who learns to use a speech device can begin articulate their opinions, thereby alleviating feelings of helplessness [278].

8.15 Conclusion

In summary, extensive research across various age groups indicates that speech and language disorders as well as swallowing disorders in individuals with CP significantly impact multiple aspects of QoL. Both children and adults with more intelligible speech tend to enjoy better social interactions and report higher ratings of life satisfaction. Well-structured and evidenced- based interventions should incorporate speech therapy delivered by SLPs as a fundamental component of a comprehensive approach that addresses both physical health and psychosocial needs. Providing timely and tailored speech therapy services or the use of AAC can significantly enhance the QoL for individuals with CP and their families. Medical and rehabilitation team should establish realistic yet optimistic goals, as even modest progress (such as consistent use of simple words or improved breath control) can significantly impact communication success. Future studies are recommended to better understand communication problems in CP and establish evidenced- based interventions. The prevailing message in the literature is unequivocal: communication is essential. Any initiative that empowers individuals with CP to express themselves more effectively can enhance their overall life satisfaction, boost self-confidence, and improve social participation.

8.16 Guide for Multidisciplinary Teams

8.16.1 Refer to SLP Services Early

The early identification of speech and language delays/disorders is vital. It is essential to collaborate closely with SLPs and refer children with CP for speech/language assessments as soon as possible. Early intervention can significantly enhance communication outcomes, ultimately improving the QoL for individuals with CP and their families.

8.16.2 Take a Collaborative Approach

A multidisciplinary team, comprising SLPs, occupational therapists, physical therapists, and other relevant specialists such as neurologists and orthopedists, should collaboratively manage these patients. The goals and methods of communication for individuals with CP should be determined during team meetings, incorporating the direct input from the SLPs and integrated into the patient's overall intervention plan.

8.16.3 Recognize the Range of Communication Needs

The range of speech and communication challenges in individuals with CP can vary widely, ranging from mild articulation difficulties to very limited verbal output. It is important to remember that restricted verbal expression does not necessarily indicate a lack of cognitive ability. Be open to exploring alternative communication methods, including AAC systems, such as communication boards and speech-generating devices. This encourages individuals with CP and their families to utilize these supportive tools.

8.16.4 Use an Evidence-Based Practice Model

To work on different speech, communication, and swallowing problems in individuals with CP, select evidence-based intervention programs, while simultaneously address individual variabilities. Please, pay attention that effective strategies for one patient may be ineffective for the others. It should be noted that evidences of therapeutic studies in CP are limited and conflicting. so, future researches with sufficient sample size are needed.

8.16.5 Keep in Mind the Importance of Systematic Caregiver Training and Monitoring

Providing recommendations to caregivers alone cannot guarantee their effective integration into daily routines. Structured training to caregivers and periodic monitoring could be helpful in this regard.

8.17 Parent/Caregiver Support

8.17.1 Work Together with Your SLPs

Participate in regular speech therapy sessions to significantly improve communication skills for individuals with CP. These sessions can also provide you useful strategies for improving communication at home.

8.17.2 Support All Forms of Communication

Recognize that individuals with CP may have limited verbal abilities but can express themselves through various means, including sounds, gestures, facial expressions, and body postures. It is essential to pay close attention to these signals and respond warmly and encouragingly. Positive reinforcement can greatly enhance their motivation to communicate. Additionally, some individuals may benefit from alternative or AAC systems, such as communication boards or speech-generating devices. Consult with your SLPs to explore the most suitable options.

8.17.3 Foster a Supportive Communication Environment

Incorporate speech and language exercises into your daily routines, allowing the person with CP to engage in everyday activities. Encourage their participation in group events and family gatherings, creating opportunities for communication in a supportive and inclusive environment.

8.17.4 Utilize Tele-Practice If You Facing Limited Access to Healthcare

Tele-practice combined with occasional clinical could be served as alternative method for delivering speech, language and swallowing therapy, especially in underserved areas.

8.17.5 Focus on Meaningful Reduction in Obvious Problems

Complete elimination of speech, communication, and swallowing problems may be unrealistic goal in some patients; so, focus on meaningful reduction that improve abilities and social participation and reduce caregiver burden may be ideal.

References

1. Roth FP, Speece DL, Cooper DH. A longitudinal analysis of the connection between oral language and early reading. J Educ Res. 2002;95:259–72.
2. Poyatos F. Language and nonverbal systems in the structure of face-to-face interaction. Lang Commun. 1983;3:129–40.
3. Schell V, Sabbagh M. Theory of mind and communication: developmental perspectives. In: Bar-On A, Ravid D, Dattner E, editors. Handbook of communication disorders: theoretical, empirical, and applied linguistic perspectives. De Gruyter; 2018.
4. Hofsten CV. Action, the foundation for cognitive development. Scand J Psychol. 2009;50:617–23.
5. Gopnik A, Meltzoff AN. Relations between semantic and cognitive development in the one-word stage: the specificity hypothesis. Child Dev. 1986;57:1040–53.
6. Guevara I, Rodriguez C. Developing communication through objects: ostensive gestures as the first gestures in children's development. Dev Rev. 2023;68:101076.
7. Özçalışkan Ş, Goldin-Meadow S. Gesture is at the cutting edge of early language development. Cognition. 2005;96:B101–B13.
8. Pennington L, Goldbart J, Marshall J. Speech and language therapy to improve the communication skills of children with cerebral palsy. Cochrane Database Syst Rev. 2004;2:CD003466.
9. Baghbadorani MK, Soleymani Z, Dadgar H, Salehi M. The effect of oral sensorimotor stimulations on feeding performance in children with spastic cerebral palsy. Acta Med Iran. 2014;52:899–904.
10. Zhang JY, Oskoui M, Shevell M. A population-based study of communication impairment in cerebral palsy. J Child Neurol. 2015;30:277–84.
11. Organization WH. International classification of functioning, disability, and health: Children & Youth Version: ICF-CY. Geneva: World Health Organization; 2007.
12. Paul R. Language disorders from infancy through adolescence: assessment & intervention. Elsevier Health Sciences; 2007.
13. Ingber S, Most T. Parental involvement in early intervention for children with hearing loss. In: Bar-On A, Ravid D, Dattner E, editors. Handbook of communication disorders: theoretical, empirical, and applied linguistic perspectives. De Gruyter; 2018.
14. Soleymani Z, Joveini G, Baghestani AR. The communication function classification system: cultural adaptation, validity, and reliability of the Farsi version for patients with cerebral palsy. Pediatr Neurol. 2015;52:333–7.
15. Saturno CE, Ramirez ARG, Conte MJ, Farhat M, Piucco EC. An augmentative and alternative communication tool for children and adolescents with cerebral palsy. Behav Inform Technol. 2015;34:632–45.
16. Light J, McNaughton D. Communicative competence for individuals who require augmentative and alternative communication: a new definition for a new era of communication? Taylor & Francis; 2014. p. 1–18.
17. Stadskleiv K. Cognitive functioning in children with cerebral palsy. Dev Med Child Neurol. 2020;62:283–9.

18. Odding E, Roebroeck ME, Stam HJ. The epidemiology of cerebral palsy: incidence, impairments and risk factors. Disabil Rehabil. 2006;28:183–91.
19. Stadskleiv K, Jahnsen R, Andersen GL, von Tetzchner S. Neuropsychological profiles of children with cerebral palsy. Dev Neurorehabil. 2018;21:108–20.
20. Ego A, Lidzba K, Brovedani P, Belmonti V, Gonzalez-Monge S, Boudia B, et al. Visual–perceptual impairment in children with cerebral palsy: a systematic review. Dev Med Child Neurol. 2015;57:46–51.
21. Wotherspoon J, Whittingham K, Sheffield J, Boyd R. Cognition and learning difficulties in a representative sample of school-aged children with cerebral palsy. Res Dev Disabil. 2023;138:104504.
22. Archibald LM, Cardy JO, Ansari D, Olino T, Joanisse MF. The consistency and cognitive predictors of children's oral language, reading, and math learning profiles. Learn Individ Differ. 2019;70:130–41.
23. Koopmans C, Sakash A, Soriano J, Long HL, Hustad KC. Functional communication abilities in youth with cerebral palsy: association with impairment profiles and school-based therapy goals. Lang Speech Hear Serv Sch. 2022;53:88–103.
24. Green JR, Moore CA, Higashikawa M, Steeve RW. The physiologic development of speech motor control: lip and jaw coordination. J Speech Lang Hear Res. 2000;43:239–55.
25. Hoon AH Jr, Stashinko EE, Nagae LM, Lin DD, Keller J, Bastian A, et al. Sensory and motor deficits in children with cerebral palsy born preterm correlate with diffusion tensor imaging abnormalities in thalamocortical pathways. Dev Med Child Neurol. 2009;51:697–704.
26. Dodd B, Morgan AT. Intervention case studies of child speech impairment. J & R Press; 2017.
27. Mei C, Reilly S, Bickerton M, Mensah F, Turner S, Kumaranayagam D, et al. Speech in children with cerebral palsy. Dev Med Child Neurol. 2020;62:1374–82.
28. Duffy JR. Motor speech disorders: substrates, differential diagnosis, and management. Elsevier Health Sciences; 2012.
29. Kuschmann A, van Brenk F, editors. Acoustic characterization of dysarthria in children with cerebral palsy: exploring age-related effects. In: 19th international congress of phonetic sciences. Melbourne, Australia, 2019.
30. Dodd B. Differential diagnosis and treatment of children with speech disorder. Wiley; 2013.
31. Preston JL, Hull M, Edwards ML. Preschool speech error patterns predict articulation and phonological awareness outcomes in children with histories of speech sound disorders. Am J Speech Lang Pathol. 2013;22:173–84.
32. Dodd B. Differentiating speech delay from disorder: does it matter? Top Lang Disord. 2011;31:96–111.
33. Morgan AT, Murray E, Liegeois FJ. Interventions for childhood apraxia of speech. Cochrane Database Syst Rev. 2018;5:CD006278.
34. Allison KM, Hustad KC. Data-driven classification of dysarthria profiles in children with cerebral palsy. J Speech Lang Hear Res. 2018;61:2837–53.
35. Bauman-Waengler J, Garcia D. Phonological treatment of speech sound disorders in children: a practical guide. San Diego: Plural Publishing; 2018.
36. Hustad KC, Schueler B, Schultz L, DuHadway C. Intelligibility of 4-year-old children with and without cerebral palsy. J Speech Lang Hear Res. 2012;55:1177–89.
37. Sakash A, Mahr TJ, Natzke PE, Hustad KC. Effects of rate manipulation on intelligibility in children with cerebral palsy. Am J Speech Lang Pathol. 2020;29:127–41.
38. Schölderle T, Staiger A, Lampe R, Strecker K, Ziegler W. Dysarthria in adults with cerebral palsy: clinical presentation and impacts on communication. J Speech Lang Hear Res. 2016;59:216–29.
39. Colver A, Rapp M, Eisemann N, Ehlinger V, Thyen U, Dickinson HO, et al. Self-reported quality of life of adolescents with cerebral palsy: a cross-sectional and longitudinal analysis. Lancet. 2015;385(9969):705–16.
40. Fauconnier J, Dickinson HO, Beckung E, Marcelli M, McManus V, Michelsen SI, et al. Participation in life situations of 8-12 year old children with cerebral palsy: cross sectional European study. BMJ. 2009;338:b1458.

41. Stemple JC, Roy N, Klaben BK. Clinical voice pathology: theory and management. 6th ed. San Diego: Plural Publishing; 2018.
42. Solomon NP, Charron S. Speech breathing in able-bodied children and children with cerebral palsy: a review of the literature and implications for clinical intervention. Am J Speech Lang Pathol. 1998;7:61–78.
43. Noordzij JP, Ossoff RH. Anatomy and physiology of the larynx. Otolaryngol Clin N Am. 2006;39:1–10.
44. Hixon TJ. Respiratory function in speech and song. (No Title). 1987.
45. Titze IR. Principles of voice production. Englewood Cliffs: Prentice-Hall; 1994.
46. Scherer R. Physiology of phonation: a review of basic mechanics. In: Ford CN, Bless DM, editors. Phonosurgery: assessment and surgical management of voice disorders. New York: Raven Press; 1991. p. 77–94.
47. Scherer RC. Laryngeal function during phonation. In: Rubin JS, Sataloff RT, Korovin GS, editors. Diagnosis and treatment of voice disorders. 2nd ed. Clifton Park: Delmar Learning; 2003. p. 87–106.
48. Gauffin J, Sundberg J. Spectral correlates of glottal voice source waveform characteristics. J Speech Lang Hear Res. 1989;32:556–65.
49. Davis PJ, Bartlett DJ, Luschei ES. Coordination of the respiratory and laryngeal systems in breathing and vocalization. J Acoust Soc Am. 1997;102:1838–45.
50. Kovacs S, Darling-White M. A descriptive study of speech breathing in children with cerebral palsy during two types of connected speech tasks. J Speech Lang Hear Res. 2022;65:4557–76.
51. Hoit JD, Hixon TJ, Watson PJ, Morgan WJ. Speech breathing in children and adolescents. J Speech Lang Hear Res. 1990;33:51–69.
52. Wolfe WG. A comprehensive evaluation of fifty cases of cerebral palsy. J Speech Hear Disord. 1950;15:234–51.
53. Redstone F. The effects of seating position on the respiratory patterns of preschoolers with cerebral palsy. Int J Rehabil Res. 2004;27:283–8.
54. Clair-Auger JM, Gan LS, Norton JA, Boliek CA. Simultaneous measurement of breathing kinematics and surface electromyography of chest wall muscles during maximum performance and speech tasks in children: methodological considerations. Folia Phoniatr Logop. 2016;67:202–11.
55. Edgson MR, Tucker BV, Archibald ED, A. Boliek C. Neuromuscular and biomechanical adjustments of the speech mechanism during modulation of vocal loudness in children with cerebral palsy and dysarthria. Neurocase. 2021;27:30–8.
56. Wang H-Y, Chen C-C, Hsiao S-F. Relationships between respiratory muscle strength and daily living function in children with cerebral palsy. Res Dev Disabil. 2012;33:1176–82.
57. Patel R. Acoustic characteristics of the question-statement contrast in severe dysarthria due to cerebral palsy. J Speech Lang Hear Res. 2003;46:1401–15.
58. Pennington L. Speech and communication in cerebral palsy. Eastern J Med. 2012;17:171.
59. Ersöz M, Selçuk B, Gündüz R, Kurtaran A, Akyüz M. Decreased chest mobility in children with spastic cerebral palsy. Turk J Pediatr. 2006;48:344–50.
60. Hardy JC. Suggestions for physiological research in dysarthria. Cortex. 1967;3:128–56.
61. Hull HC, Bryngelson B. A study of the respiration of fourteen spastic paralysis cases during silence and speech*. Speech Monogr. 1941;8:114–21.
62. Clement M, Twitchell TE. Dysarthria in cerebral palsy. J Speech Hear Disord. 1959;24:118–22.
63. Hoberman SE, Hoberman M. Speech Habilitation in cerebral palsy. J Speech Hear Disord. 1960;25:111–23.
64. Blumberg ML. Respiration and speech in the cerebral palsied child. Am J Dis Child. 1955;89:48–53.
65. Palmer MF. Speech therapy in cerebral palsy. J Pediatr. 1952;40:514–24.
66. Huber JE, Stathopoulos ET. Speech breathing across the life span and in disease. In: The handbook of speech production. Wiley; 2015. p. 11–33.

67. Workinger MS. Perceptual analysis of the dysarthrias in children with athetoid and spastic cerebral palsy. In: Dysarthria and apraxia of speech: perspectives on management. Baltimore: Paul H. Brookes; 1991.
68. Haas E, Ziegler W, Schölderle T. Developmental courses in childhood dysarthria: longitudinal analyses of auditory-perceptual parameters. J Speech Lang Hear Res. 2021;64:1421–35.
69. Rothman JG. Effects of respiratory exercises on the vital capacity and forced expiratory volume in children with cerebral palsy. Phys Ther. 1978;58:421–5.
70. Hutzler Y, Chacham A, Bergman U, Szeinberg A. Effects of a movement and swimming program on vital capacity and water orientation skills of children with cerebral palsy. Develop Med Child Neurol. 1998;40:176–81.
71. Maltais D, Bar-Or O, Pierrynowski M, Galea V. Repeated treadmill walks affect physiologic responses in children with cerebral palsy. Med Sci Sports Exerc. 2003;35:1653–61.
72. Nsenga AL, Shephard RJ, Ahmaidi S. Aerobic training in children with cerebral palsy. Int J Sports Med. 2013;34:533–7.
73. Shin H-K, Byeon E-J, Kim SH. Effects of seat surface inclination on respiration and speech production in children with spastic cerebral palsy. J Physiol Anthropol. 2015;34:17.
74. Keles MN, Elbasan B, Apaydin U, Aribas Z, Bakirtas A, Kokturk N. Effects of inspiratory muscle training in children with cerebral palsy: a randomized controlled trial. Braz J Phys Ther. 2018;22:493–501.
75. Lee HY, Cha YJ, Kim K. The effect of feedback respiratory training on pulmonary function of children with cerebral palsy: a randomized controlled preliminary report. Clin Rehabil. 2014;28:965–71.
76. Nwaobi OM, Smith PD. Effect of adaptive seating on pulmonary function of children with cerebral palsy. Develop Med Child Neurol. 1986;28:351–4.
77. Pingel J, Andersen CT, Raffalt P, Kowalczyk C. Singing therapy improving peak flow, speech and eating abilities in adults with cerebral palsy. Open J Therapy Rehabil. 2022;10:158–78.
78. Robin D, Solomon N, Moon J, Folkins J. Nonspeech assessment of the speech production mechanism. In: Clinical management of sensorimotor speech disorders. Thieme; 1997. p. 49–62.
79. Hull HC. A study of the respiration of fourteen spastic paralysis cases during silence and speech. Minneapolis: University of Minnesota; 1939.
80. Love RJ. Childhood motor speech disability. Merrill; 1992.
81. Hodge M, Wellman L. Management of dysarthria in children. Clinical management of motor speech disorders in childhood. New York: Thieme; 1999. p. 209–80.
82. Strand EA, editor. Treatment of motor speech disorders in children. Seminars in speech and language. New York: Thieme Medical Publishers; 1995.
83. Jones EI, Hardy JC, Shipton HW. Development of electrical stimulation in modifying respiratory patterns of children with cerebral palsy. J Speech Hear Disord. 1963;28:230–8.
84. Cerny F, Panzarella K, Stathopoulos E. Expiratory muscle conditioning in hypotonic children with low vocal intensity levels. J Med Speech Lang Pathol. 1997;5:141–52.
85. Cerny F, Loeffler R, Stull A, Burton H. Does abdominal muscle training improve expiratory muscle strength or endurance. Med Sci Sports Exerc. 1990;22:S53.
86. Netsell R, Hixon T. Inspiratory checking in therapy for individuals with speech breathing dysfunction. ASHA. 1992;34:152.
87. Yorkston KM. Management of motor speech disorders in children and adults. Pro-Ed; 1999.
88. Aronson AE. Clinical voice disorders: an interdisciplinary approach. New York: Thieme; 1985.
89. Mathieson L. Greene and Mathieson's the voice and its disorders. Wiley; 2001.
90. Boone DR. The voice and voice therapy. Boston: Allyn & Bacon; 2010.
91. Rubin JS, Sataloff RT, Korovin GS. Diagnosis and treatment of voice disorders. Clifton Park: Delmar Learning; 2003.
92. Duff MC, Proctor A, Yairi E. Prevalence of voice disorders in African American and European American preschoolers. J Voice. 2004;18:348–53.

93. Bhattacharyya N. The prevalence of pediatric voice and swallowing problems in the United States. Laryngoscope. 2015;125:746–50.
94. Nip IS, Garellek M. Voice quality of children with cerebral palsy. J Speech Lang Hear Res. 2021;64:3051–9.
95. Nordberg A, Miniscalco C, Lohmander A. Consonant production and overall speech characteristics in school-aged children with cerebral palsy and speech impairment. Int J Speech Lang Pathol. 2014;16:386–95.
96. Nip IS, Arias CR, Morita K, Richardson H. Initial observations of lingual movement characteristics of children with cerebral palsy. J Speech Lang Hear Res. 2017;60:1780–90.
97. Patel R. Prosodic control in severe dysarthria. J Speech Lang Hear Res. 2002;45:858–70.
98. Allison KM, Hustad KC. Impact of sentence length and phonetic complexity on intelligibility of 5-year-old children with cerebral palsy. Int J Speech Lang Pathol. 2014;16:396–407.
99. Hanson HM, Stevens KN, Kuo H-KJ, Chen MY, Slifka J. Towards models of phonation. J Phon. 2001;29:451–80.
100. Pennington L, Lombardo E, Steen N, Miller N. Acoustic changes in the speech of children with cerebral palsy following an intensive program of dysarthria therapy. Int J Lang Commun Disord. 2018;53:182–95.
101. Ansel BM, Kent RD. Acoustic-phonetic contrasts and intelligibility in the dysarthria associated with mixed cerebral palsy. J Speech Lang Hear Res. 1992;35:296–308.
102. Lee J, Hustad KC, Weismer G. Predicting speech intelligibility with a multiple speech subsystems approach in children with cerebral palsy. J Speech Lang Hear Res. 2014;57:1666–78.
103. Allison KM, Hustad KC. Acoustic predictors of pediatric dysarthria in cerebral palsy. J Speech Lang Hear Res. 2018;61:462–78.
104. Moya-Galé G, Galgano J, Ferrone C, Chang YM, Ramig LA. LSVT LOUD® applied to an adult with cerebral palsy: acoustic findings. Commun Disord Q. 2022;43:119–27.
105. Verdolini K, Abbott KV, Rosen CA, Branski RC, Andrews ML, American Speech-Language-Hearing Association. Special Interest Division 3 V, et al. Classification manual for voice disorders-I. New Jersey: Lawrence Erlbaum; 2006.
106. Darley F, Aronson A, Brown J. Motor speech disorders. Philadelphia: WB Saunders; 1975.
107. Duffy J. Motor Speech Disorders. St. Louis: Mosby; 1995.
108. Sudarsky L, Feudo P, Zubick H. Vocal aberrations in dysarthria. In: Fried M, editor. The larynx: a multidisciplinary approach. Boston: Little, Brown; 1988. p. 179–90.
109. Griffiths C, Bough ID Jr. Neurologic diseases and their effect on voice. J Voice. 1989;3:148–56.
110. Fox CM, Boliek CA. Intensive voice treatment (LSVT LOUD) for children with spastic cerebral palsy and dysarthria. J Speech Lang Hear Res. 2012;55:930–45.
111. Levy ES, Ramig L, Camarata S. The effects of two speech interventions on speech function in pediatric dysarthria. J Med Speech Lang Pathol. 2013;20:82–7.
112. van Brenk F, Kuschmann A, editors. Acoustic markers of dysarthria in children with cerebral palsy: comparison of speech tasks. Boston: Annual ASHA Convention; 2018.
113. Schölderle T, Staiger A, Schumacher B, Ziegler W. The impact of dysarthria on laypersons' attitudes towards adults with cerebral palsy. Folia Phoniatr Logop. 2019;71:309–20.
114. Colton RH, Casper JK, Leonard R. Understanding voice problems: a physiological perspective for diagnosis and treatment. Philadelphia: Wolters Kluwer Health/Lippincott Williams & Wilkins; 2011.
115. Sapienza C, Hoffman B. Voice disorders. 4th ed. San Diego: Plural Publishing; 2020.
116. Dromey C, Nissen SL, Roy N, Merrill RM. Articulatory changes following treatment of muscle tension dysphonia: preliminary acoustic evidence. J Speech Lang Hear Res. 2008;51:196–208.
117. Roy N, Bless DM, Heisey D, Ford CN. Manual circumlaryngeal therapy for functionaldysphonia: an evaluation of short-and long-term treatment outcomes. J Voice. 1997;11:321–31.
118. Sabol JW, Lee L, Stemple JC. The value of vocal function exercises in the practice regimen of singers. J Voice. 1995;9:27–36.
119. Stemple JC, Lee L, D'Amico B, Pickup B. Efficacy of vocal function exercises as a method of improving voice production. J Voice. 1994;8:271–8.

120. Verdolini K, Druker DG, Palmer PM, Samawi H. Laryngeal adduction in resonant voice. J Voice. 1998;12:315–27.
121. Yiu EM-L, Lo MC, Barrett EA. A systematic review of resonant voice therapy. Int J Speech Lang Pathol. 2017;19:17–29.
122. Kotby M, El-Sady S, Basiouny S, Abou-Rass Y, Hegazi M. Efficacy of the accent method of voice therapy. J Voice. 1991;5:316–20.
123. Bassiouny S. Efficacy of the accent method of voice therapy. Folia Phoniatr Logop. 1998;50:146–64.
124. Kotby MN, Fex B. The accent method: behavior readjustment voice therapy. Logoped Phoniatr Vocol. 1998;23:39–43.
125. Verdolini-Marston K, Burke MK, Lessac A, Glaze L, Caldwell E. Preliminary study of two methods of treatment for laryngeal nodules. J Voice. 1995;9:74–85.
126. Ramig LO, Countryman S, Thompson LL, Horii Y. Comparison of two forms of intensive speech treatment for Parkinson disease. J Speech Lang Hear Res. 1995;38:1232–51.
127. Ramig LO, Sapir S, Fox C, Countryman S. Changes in vocal loudness following intensive voice treatment (LSVT®) in individuals with Parkinson's disease: a comparison with untreated patients and normal age-matched controls. Movement Disord. 2001;16:79–83.
128. Boliek CA, Fox CM. Individual and environmental contributions to treatment outcomes following a neuroplasticity-principled speech treatment (LSVT LOUD) in children with dysarthria secondary to cerebral palsy: a case study review. Int J Speech Lang Pathol. 2014;16:372–85.
129. Boliek CA, Fox CM. Therapeutic effects of intensive voice treatment (LSVT LOUD®) for children with spastic cerebral palsy and dysarthria: a phase I treatment validation study. Int J Speech Lang Pathol. 2017;19:601–15.
130. Langlois C, Tucker BV, Sawatzky AN, Reed A, Boliek CA. Effects of an intensive voice treatment on articulatory function and speech intelligibility in children with motor speech disorders: a phase one study. J Commun Disord. 2020;86:106003.
131. Kim KM, Park SA, Hwang SH, Park A, Kim HH, Hwang J, et al. Efficacy of in-person and telepractice-based extended Lee Silverman voice treatment LOUD® on dysarthria and dysphagia in adults with cerebral palsy. Digital Health. 2025;11:20552076251315296.
132. Yuan F, Guo X, Wei X, Xie F, Zheng J, Huang Y, et al. Lee Silverman voice treatment for dysarthria in patients with Parkinson's disease: a systematic review and meta-analysis. Eur J Neurol. 2020;27:1957–70.
133. Sapir S, Ramig LO, Spielman JL, Fox C. Formant centralization ratio: a proposal for a new acoustic measure of dysarthric speech. J Speech Lang Hear Res. 2010;53:114.
134. Saffarian A, Shavaki YA, Shahidi GA, Hadavi S, Jafari Z. Lee Silverman voice treatment (LSVT) mitigates voice difficulties in mild Parkinson's disease. Med J Islam Repub Iran. 2019;33:5.
135. Constantinescu G, Theodoros D, Russell T, Ward E, Wilson S, Wootton R. Treating disordered speech and voice in Parkinson's disease online: a randomized controlled non-inferiority trial. Int J Lang Commun Disord. 2011;46:1–16.
136. Reed A, Cummine J, Bakhtiari R, Fox CM, Boliek CA. Changes in white matter integrity following intensive voice treatment (LSVT LOUD®) in children with cerebral palsy and motor speech disorders. Dev Neurosci. 2017;39:460–71.
137. Spielman J, Mahler L, Halpern A, Gilley P, Klepitskaya O, Ramig L. Intensive voice treatment (LSVT® LOUD) for Parkinson's disease following deep brain stimulation of the subthalamic nucleus. J Commun Disord. 2011;44:688–700.
138. McInerney M, Imms C, Carding PN, Reddihough DS. Evaluation of an intensive voice treatment to reduce anterior drooling in children with cerebral palsy: protocol for a concurrent multiple-baseline, single case experimental design study. Contemp Clin Trials Commun. 2021;24:100872.
139. Papadopoulos A, Voniati L, Ziavra N, Tafiadis D. The effectiveness of Lee Silverman voice treatment (LSVT LOUD) on children's speech and voice: a scoping review. Brain Sci. 2024;14:937.

140. Nip IS. Articulatory and vocal fold movement patterns during loud speech in children with cerebral palsy. J Speech Lang Hear Res. 2024;67:477–93.
141. Pennington L, Smallman C, Farrier F. Intensive dysarthria therapy for older children with cerebral palsy: findings from six cases. Child Lang Teach Ther. 2006;22:255–73.
142. Pennington L, Miller N, Robson S, Steen N. Intensive speech and language therapy for older children with cerebral palsy: a systems approach. Dev Med Child Neurol. 2010;52:337–44.
143. Pennington L, Roelant E, Thompson V, Robson S, Steen N, Miller N. Intensive dysarthria therapy for younger children with cerebral palsy. Dev Med Child Neurol. 2013;55:464–71.
144. Miller N, Pennington L, Robson S, Roelant E, Steen N, Lombardo E. Changes in voice quality after speech-language therapy intervention in older children with cerebral palsy. Folia Phoniatr Logop. 2014;65:200–7.
145. Fox C, Bolieck C, Namdaran N, Nickerson C, Gardner B, Piccott C, et al., editors. Intensive voice treatment (LSVT (R) LOUD) for children with spastic cerebral palsy. Movement disorders. Hoboken: Wiley-Liss Div John Wiley & Sons; 2008.
146. Robson S, Eftychiou E, Couteur J, Pennington L, Miller N, Steen N, editors. Associations between speech intelligibility of children with cerebral palsy and the loudness and clarity of their voice. Royal College of Speech and Language Therapists Conference; 2008.
147. Howard S, Lohmander A, Howard S. Cleft palate speech: assessment and intervention. Wiley Online Library; 2011.
148. Dotevall H, Ejnell H, Bake B. Nasal airflow patterns during the velopharyngeal closing phase in speech in children with and without cleft palate. Cleft Palate Craniofac J. 2001;38:358–73.
149. Warren DW, Dalston RM, Mayo R. Hypernasality in the presence of "adequate" velopharyngeal closure. Cleft Palate Craniofac J. 1993;30:150–4.
150. Kummer AW. Cleft palate and craniofacial conditions: a comprehensive guide to clinical management. Burlington: Jones & Bartlett Learning; 2018.
151. Spencer K, Beukelman D. Evidence-based practice guidelines for dysarthria: management of velopharyngeal function. J Med Speech Lang Pathol. 2001;9:257–74.
152. Bedwinek AP, O'Brien RL. A patient selection profile for the use of speech prostheses in adult dysarthria. J Commun Disord. 1985;18:169–82.
153. La Velle WE, Hardy JC. Palatal lift prostheses for treatment of palatopharyngeal incompetence. J Prosthet Dent. 1979;42:308–15.
154. Hardy JC, Rembolt RR, Spriestersbach DC, Jayapathy B. Surgical management of palatal paresis and speech problems in cerebral palsy: a preliminary report. J Speech Hear Disord. 1961;26:320–5.
155. Lotz WK, Netsell R. Velopharyngeal management for a child with dysarthria and cerebral palsy. In: Recent advances in clinical dysarthria. Boston: College Hill; 1989. p. 139–44.
156. Yorkston KM. Management of motor speech discorders in children and adults. Bethesda: National Library of Medicine; 2010.
157. Liss J. Direct training of velopharyngeal musculature. J Med Speech Lang Pathol. 1994;2:243–51.
158. Yorkston KM, Beukelman DR. Ataxic dysarthria: treatment sequences based on intelligibility and prosodic considerations. J Speech Hear Disord. 1981;46:398–404.
159. Picheny MA, Durlach NI, Braida LD. Speaking clearly for the hard of hearing I: intelligibility differences between clear and conversational speech. J Speech Lang Hear Res. 1985;28:96–103.
160. Kuehn D, Wachtel J. CPAP therapy for treating hypernasality following closed head injury. In: Till JA, Yorkston KM, Beukelman DR, editors. Motor speech disorders: advances in assessment and treatment. Baltimore: Paul H. Brookes Publishing; 1994.
161. Kuehn DP. The development of a new technique for treating hypernasality: CPAP. Am J Speech Lang Pathol. 1997;6:5–8.
162. Rosenbek JC, LaPointe LL. The dysarthrias: description, diagnosis, and treatment. In: Johns D, editor. Clinical management of neurogenic communication disorders. Boston: Little Brown; 1985. p. 97–152.

163. Netsell R, Rosenbek J. Treating the dysarthrias. Speech and language evaluation in neurology: adult disorders. New York: Grune & Stratton; 1985.
164. Brown K. Encyclopedia of language and linguistics. London: Elsevier; 2005.
165. Mendoza Ramos V, Lowit A, Van den Steen L, Kairuz Hernandez-Diaz HA, Hernandez-Diaz Huici ME, De Bodt M, et al. Acoustic identification of sentence accent in speakers with dysarthria: cross-population validation and severity related patterns. Brain Sci. 2021;11:1344.
166. Darley FL, Aronson AE, Brown JR. Differential diagnostic patterns of dysarthria. J Speech Hear Res. 1969;12:246–69.
167. Patel R. Assessment of prosody. In: Lowit A, Kent RD, editors. Assessment of motor speech disorders. San Diego: Plural Publishing; 2010. p. 75–95.
168. Kuschmann A, Lowit A. Sentence stress in children with dysarthria and cerebral palsy. Int J Speech Lang Pathol. 2019;21:336–46.
169. Kent RD, Rosenbek JC. Prosodic disturbance and neurologic lesion. Brain Lang. 1982;15:259–91.
170. Yorkston KM, Beukelman DR, Minifie F, Sapir S. Assessment of stress patterning. In: The dysarthria: physiology, acoustics, perception, management. Boston: College-Hill Press; 1984. p. 131–62.
171. De Bodt MS, Huici MEH-D, Van De Heyning PH. Intelligibility as a linear combination of dimensions in dysarthric speech. J Commun Disord. 2002;35:283–92.
172. Falk TH, Chan W-Y, Shein F. Characterization of atypical vocal source excitation, temporal dynamics and prosody for objective measurement of dysarthric word intelligibility. Speech Comm. 2012;54:622–31.
173. Patel R, Campellone P. Acoustic and perceptual cues to contrastive stress in dysarthria. J Speech Lang Hear Res. 2009;52:206–22.
174. Peppé SJ. Why is prosody in speech-language pathology so difficult? Int J Speech Lang Pathol. 2009;11:258–71.
175. Sluijter AM, Van Heuven VJ. Spectral balance as an acoustic correlate of linguistic stress. J Acoust Soc Am. 1996;100:2471–85.
176. Sluijter AM, Van Heuven VJ, editors. Acoustic correlates of linguistic stress and accent in Dutch and American English. Proceeding of Fourth International Conference on Spoken Language Processing ICSLP'96. IEEE; 1996.
177. Cutler A. Stress and accent in language production and understanding. In: Gibbon D, Richter H, editors. Intonation, accent and rhythm: studies in discourse phonology. Berlin, New York: de Gruyter; 1984. p. 77–90.
178. Rietveld T, Van Heuven VJ. Algemene Fonetiek (3e geheel herziene druk). Bussum: Coutinho; 2009.
179. Thies T, Mücke D, Lowit A, Kalbe E, Steffen J, Barbe MT. Prominence marking in parkinsonian speech and its correlation with motor performance and cognitive abilities. Neuropsychologia. 2020;137:107306.
180. Eady SJ, Cooper WE. Speech intonation and focus location in matched statements and questions. J Acoust Soc Am. 1986;80:402–15.
181. Baltaxe CA. Use of contrastive stress in normal, aphasic, and autistic children. J Speech Lang Hear Res. 1984;27:97–105.
182. Cutler A, Dahan D, Van Donselaar W. Prosody in the comprehension of spoken language: a literature review. Lang Speech. 1997;40:141–201.
183. Kuschmann A, Miller N, Lowit A, Pennington L. Intonation patterns in older children with cerebral palsy before and after speech intervention. Int J Speech Lang Pathol. 2017;19:370–80.
184. Baltaxe CA, Simmons JQ III. Prosodic development in normal and autistic children. In: Communication problems in autism. Boston: Springer; 1985. p. 95–125.
185. Samuelsson C. Prosody in Swedish children with language impairment. Perceptual, acoustic and interaction aspects published doctoral dissertation. Lund: Lund University; 2004.
186. Snow D. Regression and reorganization of intonation between 6 and 23 months. Child Dev. 2006;77:281–96.

187. Atkinson-King K. Children's acquisition of phonological stress contrasts. Dissertation Abstracts International, section a the humanities and social sciences. 1973;34.
188. Stathopoulos ET, Sapienza CM. Developmental changes in laryngeal and respiratory function with variations in sound pressure level. J Speech Lang Hear Res. 1997;40:595–614.
189. Tingley BM, Allen GD. Development of speech timing control in children. Child Dev. 1975;46:186–94.
190. Wells B, Peppé S, Goulandris N. Intonation development from five to thirteen. J Child Lang. 2004;31:749–78.
191. Darley FL, Aronson AE, Brown JR. Clusters of deviant speech dimensions in the dysarthrias. J Speech Hear Res. 1969;12:462–96.
192. Hernandez A, Kim S, Chung M. Prosody-based measures for automatic severity assessment of dysarthric speech. Appl Sci. 2020;10:6999.
193. Rusz J, Cmejla R, Ruzickova H, Ruzicka E. Quantitative acoustic measurements for characterization of speech and voice disorders in early untreated Parkinson's disease. J Acoust Soc Am. 2011;129:350–67.
194. Bocklet T, Nöth E, Stemmer G, Ruzickova H, Rusz J, editors. Detection of persons with Parkinson's disease by acoustic, vocal, and prosodic analysis. 2011 IEEE workshop on automatic speech recognition & understanding. Waikoloa: IEEE; 2011.
195. Rosenbek JC, LaPointe LL. The dysarthrias: description, diagnosis, and treatment. In: Johns DF, editor. Clinical management of neurogenic communicative disorders. 2nd ed. Boston: Little Brown; 1985. p. 97–152.
196. Duffy JR. Motor speech disorders: substrates, differential diagnosis, and management. St. Louis: Elsevier; 2019.
197. Lowit A, Kuschmann A, MacLeod JM, Schaeffler F, Mennen I. Sentence stress in ataxic dysarthria: a perceptual and acoustic study. J Med Speech Lang Pathol. 2010;18:77–82.
198. Lowit A, Kuschmann A, Kavanagh K. Phonological markers of sentence stress in ataxic dysarthria and their relationship to perceptual cues. J Commun Disord. 2014,50.8–18.
199. Patel R, Hustad KC, Connaghan KP, Furr W. Relationship between prosody and intelligibility in children with dysarthria. J Med Speech Lang Pathol. 2012;20:17.
200. Patel R. Phonatory control in adults with cerebral palsy and severe dysarthria. Augment Altern Commun. 2002;18(1):2–10.
201. Patel R. The acoustics of contrastive prosody in adults with cerebral palsy. J Med Speech Lang Pathol. 2004;12:189–94.
202. Kuschmann A, Lowit A. Pausing and sentence stress in children with dysarthria due to cerebral palsy. Folia Phoniatr Logop. 2021;73:298–307.
203. Le Dorze G, Ouellet L, Ryalls J. Intonation and speech rate in dysarthric speech. J Commun Disord. 1994;27:1–18.
204. Patel R. Prosodic control in severe dysarthria: preserved ability to mark the question-statement contrast. J Speech Lang Hearing Res. 2002;45:858–70.
205. Kim H, Hasegawa-Johnson M, Perlman A, editors. Acoustic cues to lexical stress in spastic dysarthria. Proceedings of speech prosody. 2010.
206. Patel R, Salata A. Using computer games to mediate caregiver-child communication for children with severe dysarthria. J Med Speech Lang Pathol. 2006;14:279–85.
207. Whitehill TL, Patel R, Lai JF. Use of prosody by children with severe dysarthria: a Cantonese extension study. J Med Speech Lang Pathol. 2008;16:293–300.
208. Arvedson JC, Brodsky L, Lefton-Greif MA. Pediatric swallowing and feeding: assessment and management. San Diego: Plural Publishing; 2019.
209. Zuckerman M, Wang S, Kaneoka A, Coster WJ, Leonard R, Langmore SE, et al. Conceptualizing adult dysphagia in the United States within the international classification of functioning, disability and health (ICF). Arch Phys Med Rehabil. 2024;105:1008–18.
210. Calderone A, Militi D, Cardile D, Corallo F, Calabrò RS, Militi A. Swallowing disorders in cerebral palsy: a systematic review of oropharyngeal dysphagia, nutritional impact, and health risks. Ital J Pediatr. 2025;51:1–47.

211. Foster BA, Lane JE, Massey E, Noelck M, Green S, Austin JP. The impact of malnutrition on hospitalized children with cerebral palsy. Hosp Pediatr. 2020;10:1087–95.
212. Yi YG, Oh B-M, Seo HG, Shin H-I, Bang MS. Dysphagia-related quality of life in adults with cerebral palsy on full oral diet without enteral nutrition. Dysphagia. 2019;34:201–9.
213. Menezes EC, Santos FAH, Alves FL. Cerebral palsy dysphagia: a systematic review. Revista CEFAC. 2017;19:565–74.
214. Benfer KA, Weir KA, Bell KL, Ware RS, Davies PS, Boyd RN. Oropharyngeal dysphagia in preschool children with cerebral palsy: oral phase impairments. Res Dev Disabil. 2014;35:3469–81.
215. Vianna CIO, Suzuki HS. Cerebral palsy: analysis of swallowing patterns before and after speech therapy intervention. Revista CEFAC. 2011;13:790–800.
216. Benfer KA, Weir KA, Bell KL, Ware RS, Davies PS, Boyd RN. Clinical signs suggestive of pharyngeal dysphagia in preschool children with cerebral palsy. Res Dev Disabil. 2015;38:192–201.
217. Benfer KA, Weir KA, Bell KL, Ware RS, Davies PSW, Boyd RN. Oropharyngeal dysphagia and cerebral palsy. Pediatrics. 2017;140:e20170731.
218. Wilson EM, Hustad KC. Early feeding abilities in children with cerebral palsy: a parental report study. J Med Speech Lang Pathol. 2009;nihpa57357
219. Ahmed YA-ER, Ahmed HA-EK, Aldin MRI, Aladawy MAE, Amin YBS. Gastrointestinal disorders in children with cerebral palsy. Int J Health Sci. 2022;6:4068–77.
220. Guare RO, Ferreira MC, Leite MF, Rodrigues JA, Lussi A, Santos MT. Dental erosion and salivary flow rate in cerebral palsy individuals with gastroesophageal reflux. J Oral Pathol Med. 2012;41:367–71.
221. Rajati F, Ahmadi N, Naghibzadeh ZA-S, Kazeminia M. The global prevalence of oropharyngeal dysphagia in different populations: a systematic review and meta-analysis. J Transl Med. 2022;20:175.
222. Morris SE, Klein MD. Pre-feeding skills: a comprehensive resource for mealtime development. San Antonio: Tsb/Harcourt; 2000.
223. Rabaey PA, Barlow K, Jama H, Lehr V. Investigation of assessment tools in the area of pediatric feeding evaluation: a mixed-methods study. Am J Occup Ther. 2023;77:7704205110.
224. Steele CM, Bayley MT, Bohn MK, Higgins V, Peladeau-Pigeon M, Kulasingam V. Reference values for videofluoroscopic measures of swallowing: an update. J Speech Lang Hear Res. 2023;66:3804–24.
225. Lee WS, Tee CW, Tan AG, Wong SY, Chew KS, Cheang HK, et al. Parental concern of feeding difficulty predicts poor growth status in their child. Pediatr Neonatol. 2019;60:676–83.
226. Maggioni L, Araújo CMT. Guidelines and practices on feeding children with cerebral palsy. J Human Growth Dev. 2020;30:65–74.
227. Taylor C, Kong AC, Foster J, Badawi N, Novak I. Caregivers' feeding experiences and support of their child with cerebral palsy. J Child Fam Stud. 2022;31:819–30.
228. Kuperminc M, Gottrand F, Samson-Fang L, Arvedson J, Bell K, Craig G, et al. Nutritional management of children with cerebral palsy: a practical guide. Eur J Clin Nutr. 2013;67:S21–S3.
229. Erasmus CE, van Hulst K, Rotteveel JJ, Willemsen MA, Jongerius PH. Clinical practice: swallowing problems in cerebral palsy. Eur J Pediatr. 2012;171:409–14.
230. Kamal S, Kamaralzaman S, Sharma S, Jaafar NH, Chern PM, Hassan NI, et al. A review of food texture modification among individuals with cerebral palsy: the challenges among cerebral palsy families. Nutrients. 2022;14:5241.
231. Parr J, Pennington L, Taylor H, Craig D, Morris C, McConachie H, et al. Parent-delivered interventions used at home to improve eating, drinking and swallowing in children with neurodisability: the FEEDS mixed-methods study. Health Technol Assess (Winchester, England). 2021;25:1.
232. Momora A, Gołda-Bąk M, Więch P. The role of the therapeutic team in the assessment of nutritional status of children with cerebral palsy. Nurs Interdiscip Healthc. 2023:195.

233. Kantarcigil C, Sheppard JJ, Gordon AM, Friel KM, Malandraki GA. A telehealth approach to conducting clinical swallowing evaluations in children with cerebral palsy. Res Dev Disabil. 2016;55:207–17.
234. Speyer R, Cordier R, Kim JH, Cocks N, Michou E, Wilkes-Gillan S. Prevalence of drooling, swallowing, and feeding problems in cerebral palsy across the lifespan: a systematic review and meta-analyses. Dev Med Child Neurol. 2019;61:1249–58.
235. Crysdale WS, McCann C, Roske L, Joseph M, Semenuk D, Chait P. Saliva control issues in the neurologically challenged: a 30 year experience in team management. Int J Pediatr Otorhinolaryngol. 2006;70:519–27.
236. Novak I, Morgan C, Adde L, Blackman J, Boyd RN, Brunstrom-Hernandez J, et al. Early, accurate diagnosis and early intervention in cerebral palsy: advances in diagnosis and treatment. JAMA Pediatr. 2017;171:897–907.
237. Dias BLS, Fernandes AR, Maia Filho HS. Sialorrhea in children with cerebral palsy. J Pediatr. 2016;92:549–58.
238. Reddihough DS, Johnson H. Assessment and management of saliva control problems in children and adults with neurological impairment. J Dev Phys Disabil. 1999;11:17–24.
239. Walshe M, Smith M, Pennington L. Interventions for drooling in children with cerebral palsy. Cochrane Database Syst Rev. 2012;11:CD008624.
240. Montgomery J, McCusker S, Lang K, Grosse S, Mace A, Lumley R, et al. Managing children with sialorrhoea (drooling): experience from the first 301 children in our saliva control clinic. Int J Pediatr Otorhinolaryngol. 2016;85:33–9.
241. Hughes A, van Hulst K, van der Burg J, Parr J, Pennington L, Reddihough D, et al. Evidence-informed management of sialorrhea in children and youth with cerebral palsy. Oral motor performance in children with neurodevelopmental disabilities-about dysphagia and drooling Nijmegen. Radboud Repository. 2019:99–120.
242. Yellepeddi VK, Race JA, Mcfarland MM, Constance JE, Fanaeian E, Murphy NA. Effectiveness of atropine in managing sialorrhea: A systematic review and meta-analysis. Int J Clin Pharmacol Ther. 2024;62:267.
243. Van der Burg JJ, Jongerius PH, Van Hulst K, Van Limbeek J, Rotteveel JJ. Drooling in children with cerebral palsy: effect of salivary flow reduction on daily life and care. Dev Med Child Neurol. 2006;48:103–7.
244. Erasmus CE, Van Hulst K, Rotteveel LJ, Jongerius PH, Van Den Hoogen FJ, Roeleveld N, et al. Drooling in cerebral palsy: hypersalivation or dysfunctional oral motor control? Dev Med Child Neurol. 2009;51:454–9.
245. Riva A, Amadori E, Vari MS, Spalice A, Belcastro V, Viri M, et al. Impact and management of drooling in children with neurological disorders: an Italian Delphi consensus. Ital J Pediatr. 2022;48:118.
246. Group W. The World Health Organization quality of life assessment (WHOQOL): position paper from the World Health Organization. Soc Sci Med. 1995;41:1403–9.
247. de Wit M, Hajos T. Health-related quality of life. In: Gellman MD, Turner JR, editors. Encyclopedia of behavioral medicine. New York: Springer; 2013. p. 929–31.
248. Calley A, Williams S, Reid S, Blair E, Valentine J, Girdler S, et al. A comparison of activity, participation and quality of life in children with and without spastic diplegia cerebral palsy. Disabil Rehabil. 2012;34:1306–10.
249. Bjornson KF, Belza B, Kartin D, Logsdon RG, McLaughlin J. Self-reported health status and quality of life in youth with cerebral palsy and typically developing youth. Arch Phys Med Rehabil. 2008;89:121–7.
250. Dickinson HO, Parkinson KN, Ravens-Sieberer U, Schirripa G, Thyen U, Arnaud C, et al. Self-reported quality of life of 8–12-year-old children with cerebral palsy: a cross-sectional European study. Lancet. 2007;369:2171–8.
251. Jiang B, Walstab J, Reid SM, Davis E, Reddihough D. Quality of life in young adults with cerebral palsy. Disabil Health J. 2016;9:673–81.
252. Du RY, McGrath C, Yiu CK, King NM. Health-and oral health-related quality of life among preschool children with cerebral palsy. Qual Life Res. 2010;19:1367–71.

253. Russo RN, Goodwin EJ, Miller MD, Haan EA, Connell TM, Crotty M. Self-esteem, self-concept, and quality of life in children with hemiplegic cerebral palsy. J Pediatr. 2008;153:473–7. e2
254. Jahnsen R, Villien L, Stanghelle JK, Holm I. Fatigue in adults with cerebral palsy in Norway compared with the general population. Dev Med Child Neurol. 2003;45:296–303.
255. van der Slot W, Nieuwenhuijsen C, van den Berg-Emons RJ, Wensink-Boonstra AE, Stam HJ, Roebroeck M, et al. Participation and health-related quality of life in adults with spastic bilateral cerebral palsy and the role of self-efficacy. J Rehabil Med. 2010;42:528–35.
256. Davis E, Shelly A, Waters E, Mackinnon A, Reddihough D, Boyd R, et al. Quality of life of adolescents with cerebral palsy: perspectives of adolescents and parents. Dev Med Child Neurol. 2009;51(3):193–9.
257. Dang VM, Colver A, Dickinson HO, Marcelli M, Michelsen SI, Parkes J, et al. Predictors of participation of adolescents with cerebral palsy: a European multi-centre longitudinal study. Res Dev Disabil. 2015;36:551–64.
258. van der Wilt F, van der Veen C, van Kruistum C, van Oers B. Language abilities and peer rejection in kindergarten: a mediation analysis. Early Educ Dev. 2020;31:269–83.
259. Pennington L, McConachie H. Interaction between children with cerebral palsy and their mothers: the effects of speech intelligibility. Int J Lang Commun Disord. 2001;36:371–93.
260. Excellence NIfHaC. Shared decision making: quality standard [QS191]. 2022.
261. Jacobson DN, Löwing K, Tedroff K. Health-related quality of life, pain, and fatigue in young adults with cerebral palsy. Dev Med Child Neurol. 2020;62:372–8.
262. Hergenröder H, Blank R. Subjective well-being and satisfaction with life in adults with spastic cerebral palsy: a pilot study of a randomized sample. Dev Med Child Neurol. 2009;51:389–96.
263. Pagliano E, Casalino T, Mazzanti S, Bianchi E, Fazzi E, Picciolini O, et al. Being adults with cerebral palsy: results of a multicenter Italian study on quality of life and participation. Neurol Sci. 2021;42:4543–50.
264. Kolman SE, Glanzman AM, Prosser L, Spiegel DA, Baldwin KD. Factors that predict overall health and quality of life in non-ambulatory individuals with cerebral palsy. Iowa Orthop J. 2018;38:147.
265. Pennington L, Cunningham S, Hiu S, Khattab G, Ryan V. The impact of the speech systems approach on intelligibility for children with cerebral palsy: a secondary analysis. Efficacy Mech Eval. 2023;10:1–94.
266. Workinger MS. Cerebral palsy resource guide for speech-language pathologists. Clifton Park: Thomson Delmar Learning; 2005.
267. McAuliffe MJ, Fletcher AR, Kerr SE, O'Beirne GA, Anderson T. Effect of dysarthria type, speaking condition, and listener age on speech intelligibility. Am J Speech Lang Pathol. 2017;26:113–23.
268. Levy ES, Chang YM, Ancelle JA, McAuliffe MJ. Acoustic and perceptual consequences of speech cues for children with dysarthria. J Speech Lang Hear Res. 2017;60:1766–79.
269. Levy ES, Chang YM, Hwang K, McAuliffe MJ. Perceptual and acoustic effects of dual-focus speech treatment in children with dysarthria. J Speech Lang Hear Res. 2021;64:2301–16.
270. Moya-Galé G, Keller B, Escorial S, Levy ES. Speech treatment effects on narrative intelligibility in French-speaking children with dysarthria. J Speech Lang Hear Res. 2021;64:2154–68.
271. Mokhlesin M, Ebadi A, Yadegari F, Ghoreishi ZS. Translation and psychometric properties of the Persian version of the feeding/swallowing impact survey in Iranian mothers. Folia Phoniatr Logop. 2024;76:22–9.
272. Benfer KA, Weir KA, Bell KL, Ware RS, Davies PS, Boyd RN. Oropharyngeal dysphagia and cerebral palsy. Pediatrics. 2017;140:e20170731.

273. Le Roux R. Caregivers? Perceptions of caregiver burden, quality of life and support needs in caring for a child with cerebral palsy with feeding and/or swallowing difficulties within the context of the Western Cape, South Africa. 2023.
274. Smith R, Bryant L, Hemsley B. Dysphagia and quality of life, participation, and inclusion experiences and outcomes for adults and children with dysphagia: a scoping review. Perspectives. 2022;7:181–96.
275. Avagyan A, Mkrtchyan H, Shafa FA, Mathew JA, Petrosyan T. Effectiveness and determinant variables of augmentative and alternative communication interventions in cerebral palsy patients with communication deficit: a systematic review. Codas. 2021;33:e20200244.
276. Cockerill H, Elbourne D, Allen E, Scrutton D, Will E, McNee A, et al. Speech, communication and use of augmentative communication in young people with cerebral palsy: the SH & PE population study. Child Care Health Dev. 2014;40:149–57.
277. McFadd ED, Hustad KC. Communication modes and functions in children with cerebral palsy. J Speech Lang Hear Res. 2020;63:1776–92.
278. Parrott LC. Communication participation of adult aided communicators with cerebral palsy; a discourse analytic approach. Exeter: University of Exeter; 2014.

Nutrition Therapy in Cerebral Palsy

9

Asieh Mansour and Sayed Mahmoud Sajjadi-Jazi

Scenario

A 14-year-old male with spastic quadriplegic cerebral palsy (CP), classified as Gross Motor Function Classification System (GMFCS) level IV, was referred to the nutrition clinic with a 4-month history of progressively worsening feeding difficulties accompanied by unintentional weight loss of approximately 8 lbs. Caregivers reported prolonged mealtimes, frequent coughing and choking during meals, and difficulty tolerating both solid and some pureed foods.

A multidisciplinary evaluation, including consultation with a gastroenterologist, was conducted. Videofluoroscopic swallow study demonstrated significant oropharyngeal dysphagia, characterized by a delayed swallowing reflex, poor bolus clearance, and mild esophageal residue. No structural obstruction was identified.

9.1 Introduction

CP is the most common cause of physical disability in childhood, and its consequences extend beyond motor impairments to profoundly affect growth and nutrition. Across diverse global contexts, children and adults with CP consistently

A. Mansour
Endocrinology and Metabolism Research Center, Endocrinology and Metabolism Clinical Sciences Institute, Tehran University of Medical Sciences, Tehran, Iran
e-mail: amansour@tums.ac.ir

S. M. Sajjadi-Jazi (✉)
Endocrinology and Metabolism Research Center, Endocrinology and Metabolism Clinical Sciences Institute, Tehran University of Medical Sciences, Tehran, Iran

Department of Endocrinology, Shariati Hospital, School of Medicine, Tehran University of Medical Sciences, Tehran, Iran
e-mail: m_sajadi@tums.ac.ir

A. Presedo et al. (eds.), *Enhancing Quality of Life in Patients with Cerebral Palsy*, https://doi.org/10.1007/978-3-032-20967-2_9

present with a high burden of malnutrition, encompassing both undernutrition and overnutrition. Wang et al. reported high rates of malnutrition among children with CP in China, with stunting at 42.4%, underweight at 12.7%, thinness at 21.5%, and overweight/obesity at 18.5%. Thinness predominated in older children (12–18 years), while overweight/obesity was more common in younger children (2–12 years) and closely linked to functional impairment severity [1]. Consistent findings from population-based studies in Nepal and Uganda further reveal that children at higher GMFCS levels exhibit significantly increased odds of stunting and impaired longitudinal growth relative to peers without CP [2, 3].

Undernutrition remains a critical challenge in CP; however, overweight and obesity are increasingly reported among individuals with milder motor impairments [1, 4]. Hospital-based surveillance in Vietnam confirmed that both severe motor disability and poor socioeconomic status were major predictors of undernutrition [5].

Bioimpedance analysis has revealed excess body fat not captured by conventional anthropometry, underscoring the risk of hidden overnutrition [4]. A European study further demonstrated poor agreement between caregiver or clinician perceptions and objective nutritional assessments, reinforcing the need for standardized screening tools [6]. At the same time, evidence shows that standard pediatric growth charts can overestimate malnutrition in CP. Araújo et al. (2013) found that while 51% of children were classified as underweight using Centers for Disease Control and Prevention (CDC) references, only 10% met this criterion with CP-specific curves. Poor growth was also strongly associated with complications such as dysphagia, constipation, and recurrent respiratory infections, suggesting that CP-specific growth charts may provide a more accurate picture of nutritional vulnerability [7].

Reflecting these complexities, nutritional assessment and management in CP have also evolved. A recent narrative review emphasized a shift away from reliance on single measures, such as body mass index (BMI), which is often inaccurate in this population, towards a multidimensional approach using multiple anthropometric indicators. Newly standardized tools, including the Subjective Global Nutrition Assessment (SGNA) and the Eating and Drinking Ability Classification System (EDACS), are now being adopted to provide a more comprehensive evaluation of nutritional status and feeding ability [8].

9.2 Feeding and Swallowing Difficulties (Dysphagia)

Feeding difficulties are central contributors to poor nutrition in CP. Dysphagia is highly prevalent among people with CP, with estimates varying based on the population studied and assessment methods used [9]. Costa et al. (2021) reported that all children in a Spanish special needs school presented with oropharyngeal dysphagia, with 90.6% showing impaired swallowing safety, strongly associated with malnutrition, dehydration, and poor oral health [10]. In children with severe, generalized CP, the prevalence of dysphagia can be as high as 99% [11].

A prospective study of children with swallowing disorders, the majority of whom had congenital brain damage, found that 82.5% exhibited symptoms of dysphagia [12]. Among adults, nearly one-third experienced clinically significant swallowing impairments, with body weight decreasing in tandem with worsening eating and drinking ability [13]. While a systematic review found the pooled prevalence for feeding and swallowing problems exceeds 50%, data on these issues, including drooling, remains limited for the adult population [9].

Children with CP have a markedly lower dysphagia limit than typically developing peers; even those at EDACS level I swallow only ~7 mL per bolus, one-third the typical 22 mL [14]. Dysphagia prevalence strongly correlates with motor impairment (GMFCS), rising from 16.3% in level I to 97.9% in level V, with all children at level V experiencing feeding difficulties [9]. Importantly, swallowing deficits are not limited to severe cases, highlighting the necessity of universal screening across all GMFCS levels [15, 16].

9.3 Types of Feeding and Swallowing Problems

Swallowing and feeding problems in CP are multifaceted and stem from impaired oral sensorimotor function. These issues can manifest in any phase of the swallowing process.

Oral Phase Impaired lip and tongue control, chewing, and bolus formation cause spillage, drooling, and inefficient, energy-intensive eating [16].

Pharyngeal Phase Pharyngeal phase impairments are prevalent in children with CP and significantly increase the risk of aspiration. Clinical signs of aspiration affect up to 68% of preschool-aged children, with frequency rising in parallel with motor impairment severity. Common manifestations include coughing, choking, wet or "gurgly" voice, multiple swallows per bolus, and respiratory distress. Silent aspiration, airway entry of food or liquid without obvious symptoms, is particularly concerning, representing a substantial proportion of aspiration events in CP and necessitating instrumental assessment for accurate diagnosis [17].

Feeding Behaviors and Prolonged Mealtimes Children with CP often experience feeding disorders that extend beyond swallowing mechanics. Mealtimes are frequently prolonged, often exceeding 30 min, which is considered a red flag. Caregivers commonly report that feeding is tiring and stressful for both themselves and the child [18]. Prolonged feeding can induce fatigue, resulting in incomplete nutrient intake. In adults with CP consuming a full oral diet, those with meal durations exceeding 45 min had significantly lower BMI compared to individuals who completed meals in under 15 min [19].

9.4 Practical Strategies and Interventions

9.4.1 Optimizing Oral Intake

Making food safer to swallow must also ensure adequate nutrition and support the social aspects of eating. Because texture-modified diets are often lower in energy and nutrients, they increase the risk of malnutrition [20]. Strategies such as enriching foods with protein powder, butter, oils, or infant cereals can boost nutrient density without adding volume [20, 21]. Hypercaloric or high-protein supplements and formulas may also be used to meet requirements. Research shows that shaped, nutrient-enriched texture-modified diets can significantly improve energy and protein intake, leading to weight gain [20].

The unappetizing appearance of texture-modified food is a primary reason for refusal, which can lead to caregiver stress and a reduced quality of life [22]. To combat this, several food design strategies can be employed. Serving different food components separately on a plate, rather than mixed together, improves visual appeal. Furthermore, using food moulds to reshape pureed food into its original form (e.g., a carrot shape for pureed carrots) can significantly improve satisfaction, with studies showing a 15% increase in food intake and favorable effects on both energy and protein consumption. Advanced techniques like molecular gastronomy (spherification, gelification) and 3D food printing also offer promising ways to enhance the visual appeal of meals. Flavor is another critical aspect, as texture-modified foods often have a reduced profile due to dilution with liquids and less chewing. The use of natural flavors like garlic, pepper, and herbs can increase food intake and help overcome the "food monotony" that caregivers report when children become bored with repetitive meals [21].

Beyond sensory appeal, textural safety is paramount, as excessively thick foods can become dangerously sticky, heightening aspiration risk. The International Dysphagia Diet Standardisation Initiative (IDDSI) Spoon Tilt Test, applied to foods at Levels 4 (pureed/extremely thick) and 5 (Minced and Moist), evaluates food adhesiveness and cohesiveness by assessing whether a full spoonful holds its shape yet slides off easily when tilted or turned sideways, leaving only a thin, transparent film on the spoon. A sample failing this test due to excessive stickiness indicates a choking and aspiration hazard [23]. Using this method, seven puree samples, potato, rice, pumpkin, taro, chestnut, black fungus, and snow fungus, were classified as too sticky, with excessive residue remaining on the spoon. The study highlighted that both adhesiveness and cohesiveness critically determine perceived stickiness, emphasizing the need for careful formulation of high-starch or high-polysaccharide foods to ensure safe swallowing [24].

9.4.2 Positioning for Feeding

Optimal positioning is a cornerstone of safe and efficient feeding for children with CP, requiring an upright, stable posture with the head aligned over the trunk, a slight chin tuck, and 90-degree flexion at the hips, knees, and ankles. This specific alignment facilitates effective swallowing, significantly reducing the risk of aspiration and diminishing oral leakage [25]. Proper positioning, often achieved with adaptive seating, not only improves oral-motor skills and mealtime efficiency [26] but also enhances the child's mood and willingness to cooperate during meals and reduces caregiver stress during the feeding process [27]. An individualized assessment by a multidisciplinary team is crucial to determine the most beneficial posture [28], as an erect position is often best for pharyngeal phase difficulties, while a semi-reclined posture may help with oral phase challenges [26].

9.4.3 Adaptive Equipment and Utensils

The use of specialized spoons or cups can help control bolus size and placement. However, many caregivers continue to use inappropriate utensils like bottles, which can be detrimental to orofacial development and swallowing safety [18].

9.5 Gastrointestinal Issues in CP

9.5.1 Gastroesophageal Reflux Disease (GERD) and Nutrition

GERD, a condition defined by complications from the chronic backflow of stomach contents into the esophagus, affects an estimated 15–77% of children with CP and shares a complex, bidirectional relationship with their nutritional status [29]. One study of children with CP who presented with gastrointestinal symptoms found that 66% had GERD confirmed by biopsies [30]. Factors inherent to CP, such as chronic supine positioning, scoliosis, increased abdominal pressure from spasticity, and anticonvulsant medications, contribute to GERD, which in turn can lead to significant complications like poor weight gain, feeding aversion, and respiratory issues [29]. GERD impairs nutrition through multiple pathways: reflux-induced esophagitis causes pain, irritability, back-arching, and food refusal, while recurrent regurgitation and vomiting lead to direct nutrient loss [30, 31]. Furthermore, reflux-related discomfort can exacerbate dysphagia, further limiting oral intake [29], and GERD symptoms may mimic neurobehavioral events such as seizures, increasing the risk of misdiagnosis [31].

For children with severe swallowing disorders, nasogastric tubes (NGTs) provide short-term feeding for less than 2 months, while gastrostomy tubes (G-tubes) are used for long-term nutritional support. While G-tubes can improve weight gain, they carry a significant risk of causing or worsening GERD. One study found that six out of ten children without prior GERD developed it after the procedure [30].

Management requires a comprehensive approach, beginning with nutritional strategies such as thickening feeds with pectin, avoiding trigger foods like caffeine and fatty items, and implementing postural adjustments. If initial methods fail, acid-suppressing proton pump inhibitors (PPIs) are used. For severe, treatment-resistant cases, Nissen fundoplication surgery is an option but carries a higher complication rate in children with neurologic impairments [29].

9.5.2 Constipation and Dehydration

Constipation is a prevalent and burdensome gastrointestinal issue for children with CP, frequently linked to both low fluid and fiber intake [10]. Studies have shown that children with functional constipation consume less total water and have higher urinary osmolality compared to their peers, indicating a state of hypohydration. In fact, an association has been found between total water intake below the dietary reference intake (DRI) recommendations and functional constipation, particularly in boys [32]. This inadequate fluid intake is a significant concern for children with CP, as feeding difficulties and oromotor dysfunction can directly impair their ability to stay hydrated, leading to dehydration [33]. Dehydration not only contributes to constipation by increasing water reabsorption from the fecal mass, which hardens stools, but it also has wider health implications [10]. In schoolchildren, hypohydration can cause detrimental changes in cognitive performance, mood, motor skills, and memory [34]. Therefore, ensuring adequate fluid intake is a critical nutritional strategy in the management of CP, not only to alleviate constipation but also to support overall cognitive and physical well-being [10].

9.6 Resting Energy Expenditure (REE) in CP

REE represents the energy required to sustain vital physiological functions at rest, excluding the energy expended for physical activity and food processing. As a major component of total energy expenditure (TEE), REE is essential for determining nutritional requirements. However, accurate estimation of energy needs in children with CP is challenging due to altered body composition, reduced physical activity, abnormal muscle tone, and frequently diminished dietary intake [35, 36]. Compared with typically developing peers, children and adolescents with CP generally exhibit lower energy requirements, with reductions proportional to the severity of gross motor impairment. For instance, wheelchair-bound individuals may require only 60–70% of the energy intake recommended for healthy children [37]. One study reported a 46% reduction in REE compared to estimated caloric needs of healthy controls [38]. REE assessment in CP primarily relies on two methods: indirect calorimetry, the gold standard, whose clinical utility is limited by cost and specialized expertise, and prediction equations, which are more accessible but exhibit poor accuracy [39]. Notably, commonly used predictive formulas tend to overestimate REE in children with CP, increasing the risk of overnutrition [35].

Intensive nutritional support can have a significant impact on REE in children with CP. One study found that 4 weeks of intensive nutritional support produced a significant increase in energy expenditure in children with CP [39]. This suggests that REE can be normalized if children with CP receive adequate energy intake [40].

9.7 Key Nutrients and Dietary Considerations

9.7.1 Caloric Needs and Protein

Children with neurological impairment, such as CP, generally require the same protein intake as their unaffected peers, as recommended by the DRIs [41]. However, increased protein intake is warranted in specific clinical contexts. Severely undernourished children with CP may benefit from a protein intake of 2.0–2.4 g/kg/day to support catch-up growth [37, 41, 42]. Increased protein intake is also recommended for patients with decubitus ulcers (pressure ulcers) [41].

For tube-fed children on very low-calorie diets, using high-protein formulas or supplements can help meet their nutritional needs [41]. Protein plays a crucial role not only in supporting growth and lean tissue development but also in repairing body tissues and aiding recovery from malnutrition [37]. In a study by Anker–van der Wel et al., protein intake was assessed in 19 children with spastic CP (mean age 11). Although the average total intake (62.1 g/day) met recommendations, only the dinner meal consistently provided ≥25 g of protein, the level considered necessary for muscle maintenance. The primary protein sources were dairy, meat, poultry, and bread. The authors suggest redistributing protein intake more evenly across breakfast and lunch to better support muscle growth and function [43].

A recent retrospective study demonstrated that supplementing diets with high-calorie whole protein or peptide formulas significantly improved malnutrition and enhanced gross motor function development in children with CP [44]. Furthermore, a randomized controlled trial in undernourished children with CP demonstrated that a high-calorie formula produced superior weight gain, improved weight-for-age z-scores, and greater Gross Motor Function Measure (GMFM) improvements over 6 months compared to a professionally planned Chinese diet, with comparable safety and higher rates of nutritional normalization [45].

9.7.2 Fats

In individuals with CP who require nutritional support through increased dietary fat intake, careful assessment of energy requirements is essential. Among the most reliable predictors of energy requirements are a person's lean (fat-free) mass and ambulatory status, because standard predictive equations frequently overestimate needs, particularly in those who are non-ambulatory or severely impaired. To enhance caloric density without substantially increasing food volume, dietary enrichment should focus on integrating healthy fats (such as oils, avocado, nut butters, cream, and full-fat dairy) rather than relying solely on greater carbohydrate intake [42]. Preference should be given to unsaturated fats, while saturated fat intake ought to be restricted to about 10% or less of total energy intake to minimize cardiovascular and metabolic risk [46]. In cases where epilepsy co-occurs, ketogenic or medium-chain triglyceride (MCT)-rich fat-heavy diets should be used only under specialist supervision, with frequent monitoring of growth, lipid status, and overall health [42].

9.7.3 Micronutrients of Concern

9.7.3.1 Vitamin D Deficiency and Bone Health

Studies have consistently shown a high prevalence of vitamin D deficiency among children with CP. A meta-analysis including 430 children with CP demonstrated a pooled prevalence of deficiency of 42.18% [47]. Other studies have reported even higher rates, with one observing deficiency in 32% and insufficiency in 61% of children with CP [48]. Reported prevalence of vitamin D deficiency and insufficiency varies due to inconsistent definitions. Cutoffs for insufficiency range from 12 to 30 ng/mL, while deficiency is defined between <10 and <20 ng/mL across studies. These differing thresholds significantly affect prevalence estimates [47].

Several factors contribute to the elevated prevalence of vitamin D deficiency in children with CP. Limited mobility, particularly among non-ambulatory individuals, often restricts outdoor activity and subsequently reduces exposure to sunlight, the primary source of endogenous vitamin D synthesis [48]. Feeding difficulties are common in children with CP due to oral motor dysfunction, which can lead to inadequate intake of dietary vitamin D and calcium [48]. Epilepsy, a common comorbidity, also plays a role; enzyme-inducing antiepileptic drugs (AEDs) such as carbamazepine and phenytoin accelerate vitamin D metabolism, lowering circulating levels [48, 49]. The severity of motor impairment, as measured by the GMFCS, is often linked to lower vitamin D levels [50]. Some studies have observed a negative correlation between age and vitamin D levels, with older children being more prone to deficiency. This may be due to reduced outdoor activity with increasing age [49].

Low vitamin D levels in children with CP are associated with multiple adverse health outcomes. Deficiency is a major contributor to reduced bone mineral density, predisposing to osteopenia, osteoporosis, and fracture risk, even after minor trauma. Prolonged and severe deficiency may also result in rickets, characterized by impaired bone mineralization [49, 51]. Beyond skeletal effects, vitamin D deficiency has been linked to reduced muscle strength, impaired balance, and poorer coordination, further exacerbating motor limitations in CP [52]. Emerging evidence suggests a link between vitamin D deficiency and an increased risk of cardiometabolic issues, such as high triglyceride levels, in children with CP [53].

Addressing vitamin D deficiency is a critical component of comprehensive care for children with CP. Supplementation has consistently been shown to raise serum vitamin D levels effectively, with studies demonstrating benefits across a range of regimens, from single high-dose administration to daily supplementation, without significant adverse effects such as hypercalcemia [54]. While the recommended daily intake for healthy children is 600 IU, children with CP often require higher doses, typically 800–1000 IU/day, to achieve sufficiency [51]. Given the high risk, routine measurement of 25-hydroxyvitamin D levels is recommended for children with CP to allow for early detection and treatment of deficiency [49].

9.7.3.2 Iron Deficiency and Anemia

Studies across different countries show a high prevalence of anemia and iron deficiency among children with CP, ranging from latent iron deficiency to clinically significant anemia [55–57]. The risk is multifactorial, with primary contributors including dysphagia and inadequate dietary intake, further exacerbated by greater motor impairment (higher GMFCS levels) [58] and malnutrition, especially underweight status [56]. Regular monitoring of iron status, particularly serum ferritin as an early marker of iron deficiency, is recommended [55]. In cases of deficiency, iron supplementation may be necessary [58]. One study found that lactoferrin was an effective and superior oral iron replacement therapy compared to iron hydroxide polymaltose complex for treating iron deficiency anemia in children with CP, with fewer side effects [59].

9.8 Summary and Conclusions

Children with CP face a disproportionately high risk of malnutrition, largely due to oromotor dysfunction, feeding difficulties, gastroesophageal reflux, and constipation [54, 60]. In response, nutrition interventions typically begin with caregiver training in optimal positioning and feeding techniques, which can markedly improve feeding efficiency and safety even if measurable improvements in nutritional status take longer to manifest [61]. When safe oral intake is insufficient, transitioning to modified food textures and, if necessary, to enteral feeding methods is often required to ensure sufficient caloric and nutrient delivery [20, 37].

Among dietary strategies, high-calorie and high-protein formulations have consistently outperformed standard diets, yielding greater weight gain, improved biochemical markers of nutrition, and enhanced gross motor function [44, 45]. Beyond energy enrichment, growing attention has turned to "neurotrophic" supplementation with nutrients such as docosahexaenoic acid, choline, uridine-5-monophosphate, polyunsaturated fatty acids, specific amino acids (e.g., arginine), and probiotics. Some studies suggest potential benefits for motor, cognitive, and language outcomes [62, 63]. However, systematic reviews caution that the overall quality of evidence remains weak: many studies suffer from methodological limitations (small sample sizes, high bias risk, shorter follow-ups) [54]. Thus, a holistic, individualized approach guided by clinical monitoring and adapted to each child's needs is the most prudent path forward until more rigorous trials are available.

References

1. Wang F, Cai Q, Shi W, Jiang H, Li N, Ma D, et al. A cross-sectional survey of growth and nutritional status in children with cerebral palsy in West China. Pediatr Neurol. 2016;58:90–7.
2. Jahan I, Muhit M, Al Imam MH, Ghose R, Chhetri AB, Badawi N, et al. Nutritional status of children with cerebral palsy in Gorkha, Nepal: findings from the Nepal cerebral palsy register. Nutrients. 2021;13:2537.

3. Hamid Namaganda L, Andrews C, Wabwire-Mangen F, Peterson S, Forssberg H, Kakooza-Mwesige A. Nutritional status and growth of children and adolescents with and without cerebral palsy in eastern Uganda: a longitudinal comparative analysis. PLoS Global Public Health. 2023;3:e0001241.
4. de Zabarte Fernández JMM, Arnal IR, Segura JLP, Romero RG, Martínez GR. Nutritional status of a population with moderate-severe cerebral palsy: beyond the weight. Anales de Pediatría (English Edition). 2020;92:192–9.
5. Karim T, Jahan I, Dossetor R, Giang NTH, Van Anh NT, Dung TQ, et al. Nutritional status of children with cerebral palsy—findings from prospective hospital-based surveillance in Vietnam indicate a need for action. Nutrients. 2019;11:2132.
6. Fogarasi A, Fazzi E, Smorenburg AR, Mazurkiewicz-Beldzinska M, Dinopoulos A, Pobiecka A, et al. The PURPLE N study: objective and perceived nutritional status in children and adolescents with cerebral palsy. Disabil Rehabil. 2022;44:6668–75.
7. Araújo LA, Silva LR. Anthropometric assessment of patients with cerebral palsy: which curves are more appropriate? J Pediatr. 2013;89:307–14.
8. Oftedal S, McCormack S, Stevenson R, Benfer K, Boyd RN, Bell K. The evolution of nutrition management in children with severe neurological impairment with a focus on cerebral palsy. J Hum Nutr Diet. 2025;38:e13277.
9. Speyer R, Cordier R, Kim JH, Cocks N, Michou E, Wilkes-Gillan S. Prevalence of drooling, swallowing, and feeding problems in cerebral palsy across the lifespan: a systematic review and meta-analyses. Dev Med Child Neurol. 2019;61:1249–58.
10. Costa A, Martin A, Arreola V, Riera SA, Pizarro A, Carol C, et al. Assessment of swallowing disorders, nutritional and hydration status, and oral hygiene in students with severe neurological disabilities including cerebral palsy. Nutrients. 2021;13:2413.
11. Calis EA, Veugelers R, Sheppard JJ, Tibboel D, Evenhuis HM, Penning C. Dysphagia in children with severe generalized cerebral palsy and intellectual disability. Dev Med Child Neurol. 2008;50:625–30.
12. Caramico-Favero DCO, Guedes ZCF, MORAIS MBd. Food intake, nutritional status and gastrointestinal symptoms in children with cerebral palsy. Arq Gastroenterol. 2018;55:352–7.
13. McAllister A, Sjöstrand E, Rodby-Bousquet E. Eating and drinking ability and nutritional status in adults with cerebral palsy. Dev Med Child Neurol. 2022;64:1017–24.
14. Schepers FV, van Hulst K, Spek B, Erasmus CE, van den Engel-Hoek L. Dysphagia limit in children with cerebral palsy aged 4 to 12 years. Dev Med Child Neurol. 2022;64:253–8.
15. Ron AG, Toboso RG, Gascón MB, De Santos M, Vecino R, Pinedo AB. Nutritional status and prevalence of dysphagia in cerebral palsy: usefulness of the eating and drinking ability classification system scale and correlation with the degree of motor impairment according to the gross motor function classification system. Neurología (English Edition). 2023;38:35–40.
16. Arvedson J. Feeding children with cerebral palsy and swallowing difficulties. Eur J Clin Nutr. 2013;67:S9–S12.
17. Benfer KA, Weir KA, Bell KL, Ware RS, Davies PS, Boyd RN. Clinical signs suggestive of pharyngeal dysphagia in preschool children with cerebral palsy. Res Dev Disabil. 2015;38:192–201.
18. Maggioni L, Araújo CMT. Guidelines and practices on feeding children with cerebral palsy. J Human Growth Dev. 2020;30(1):65–74.
19. Yi YG, Oh B-M, Seo HG, Shin H-I, Bang MS. Dysphagia-related quality of life in adults with cerebral palsy on full oral diet without enteral nutrition. Dysphagia. 2019;34:201–9.
20. Silva DC, Cunha M, Santana A, Alves AM, Santos MP. Nutritional interventions in children and adolescents with cerebral palsy: systematic review. Rev Paul Pediatr. 2023;42:e2022107.
21. Smith R, Bryant L, Reddacliff C, Hemsley B. A review of the impact of food design on the mealtimes of people with swallowing disability who require texture-modified food. Int J Food Design. 2022;7:7–28.
22. Kamal S, Hamzaid NH, Kamaralzaman S, Sharma S, Jaafar NH, Chern PM, et al. A qualitative study on feeding experiences among caregivers of children with cerebral palsy requiring food texture modification. Available at SSRN 4857162.

23. Cichero JA, Lam P, Steele CM, Hanson B, Chen J, Dantas RO, et al. Development of international terminology and definitions for texture-modified foods and thickened fluids used in dysphagia management: the IDDSI framework. Dysphagia. 2017;32:293–314.
24. Wong MC, Chan KM, Wong TT, Tang HW, Chung HY, Kwan HS. Quantitative textural and rheological data on different levels of texture-modified food and thickened liquids classified using the international dysphagia diet standardisation initiative (IDDSI) guideline. Foods. 2023;12:3765.
25. Rauf W, Sarmad S, Khan I, Jawad M. Effect of position on gross motor function and spasticity in spastic cerebral palsy children. J Pak Med Assoc. 2021;71:801–5.
26. Snider L, Majnemer A, Darsaklis V. Feeding interventions for children with cerebral palsy: a review of the evidence. Phys Occup Ther Pediatr. 2011;31:58–77.
27. Mlinda S, Leyna G, Massawe A. The effect of a practical nutrition education programme on feeding skills of caregivers of children with cerebral palsy at Muhimbili National Hospital, in Tanzania. Child Care Health Dev. 2018;44:452–61.
28. Vuković M, Todorović J. Eating and swallowing disorders in children with cerebral palsy. Med Pregl. 2021;74:200–4.
29. Fernando T, Goldman RD. Management of gastroesophageal reflux disease in pediatric patients with cerebral palsy. Can Fam Physician. 2019;65:796–8.
30. Asgarshirazi M, Farokhzadeh-Soltani M, Keihanidost Z, Shariat M. Evaluation of feeding disorders including gastro-esophageal reflux and oropharyngeal dysfunction in children with cerebral palsy. J Family Reprod Health. 2017;11:197.
31. Bayram AK, Canpolat M, Karacabey N, Gumus H, Kumandas S, Doğanay S, et al. Misdiagnosis of gastroesophageal reflux disease as epileptic seizures in children. Brain Dev. 2016;38:274–9.
32. Boilesen SN, Dias FC, Tahan S, Melli LC, de Morais MB. Fluid intake and urinary osmolality in pediatric patients with functional constipation. Eur J Nutr. 2021;60:4647–55.
33. Usman H. Frequency of feeding problems in children with cerebral palsy. J Islamabad Med Dental College. 2017;6:31–4.
34. Baron S, Courbebaisse M, Lepicard EM, Friedlander G. Assessment of hydration status in a large population. Br J Nutr. 2015;113:147–58.
35. Penagini F, Borsani B, Bosetti A, Mameli C, Dilillo D, Ramponi G, et al. Resting energy expenditure in children with cerebral palsy: accuracy of available prediction formulae and development of a population-specific formula. Clin Nutr ESPEN. 2018;25:44–9.
36. Borsani B, Biganzoli G, Penagini F, Bosetti A, Pendezza E, Perico V, et al. Resting energy expenditure in children and adolescents with cerebral palsy: accuracy of available prediction formulas and development of population-specific methods. Front Pediatr. 2023;11:1097152.
37. Bell K, Samson-Fang L. Nutritional management of children with cerebral palsy. Eur J Clin Nutr. 2013;67:S13–S6.
38. Gale R, Namestnic J, Singer P, Kagan I. Caloric requirements of patients with brain impairment and cerebral palsy who are dependent on chronic ventilation. J Parenter Enter Nutr. 2017;41:1366–70.
39. García-Contreras AA, Vásquez-Garibay EM, Romero-Velarde E, Ibarra-Gutiérrez AI, Troyo-Sanromán R. Energy expenditure in children with cerebral palsy and moderate/severe malnutrition during nutritional recovery. Nutr Hosp. 2015;31:2062–9.
40. Arrowsmith FE, Allen JR, Gaskin KJ, Somerville H, Birdsall J, Barzi F, et al. Nutritional rehabilitation increases the resting energy expenditure of malnourished children with severe cerebral palsy. Dev Med Child Neurol. 2012;54:170–5.
41. Romano C, Van Wynckel M, Hulst J, Broekaert I, Bronsky J, Dall'Oglio L, et al. European Society for Paediatric Gastroenterology, Hepatology and nutrition guidelines for the evaluation and treatment of gastrointestinal and nutritional complications in children with neurological impairment. J Pediatr Gastroenterol Nutr. 2017;65:242–64.
42. Tufail T, Ain HBU, Mahwish NS, Ijaz A, Ikram A, et al. Intake of high-calorie diet and phytonutrients: a new paradigm to treat cerebral palsy in children. eFood. 2025;6:e70042.

43. Anker–van der Wel I, Smorenburg AR, de Roos NM, Verschuren O. Dose, timing, and source of protein intake of young people with spastic cerebral palsy. Disabil Rehabil. 2020;42:2192–7.
44. Cai X, Qin Y, Liu C, Xie L, Zhu J. High-calorie, whole protein/peptide nutritional formulations for children with cerebral palsy: a retrospective clinical study. Am J Transl Res. 2024;16:3171.
45. Zhao Y, He L, Peng T, Liu L, Zhou H, Xu Y, et al. Nutritional status and function after high-calorie formula vs. Chinese food intervention in undernourished children with cerebral palsy. Front Nutr. 2022;9:960763.
46. Brown MC, Marciniak CM, Garrett AM, Gaebler-Spira DJ. Diet quality in adults with cerebral palsy: a modifiable risk factor for cardiovascular disease prevention. Dev Med Child Neurol. 2021;63:1221–8.
47. Alenazi KA, Alanezi AA. Prevalence of vitamin D deficiency in children with cerebral palsy: a meta-analysis. Pediatr Neurol. 2024;159:56–61.
48. Manohar S, Gangadaran RP. Vitamin D status in children with cerebral palsy. Int J Contemp Pediatr. 2017;4:615–9.
49. Toopchizadeh V, Barzegar M, Masoumi S, Jahanjoo F. Prevalence of vitamin D deficiency and associated risk factors in cerebral palsy a study in north-west of Iran. Iranian J Child Neurol. 2018;12:25.
50. Tosun A, Erisen Karaca S, Unuvar T, Yurekli Y, Yenisey C, Omurlu IK. Bone mineral density and vitamin D status in children with epilepsy, cerebral palsy, and cerebral palsy with epilepsy. Childs Nerv Syst. 2017;33:153–8.
51. Alenazi KA. Vitamin D deficiency in children with cerebral palsy: a narrative review of epidemiology, contributing factors, clinical consequences and interventions. Saudi J Biol Sci. 2022;29:2007–13.
52. Kumar R, Kumar G, Runu R, Gupta AK, Sharma DK, Shekhar R. Vitamin D status in children with cerebral palsy: a tertiary care center study. Int J Health Sci. 2022;6:11438–45.
53. Barja S, Le Roy C, Sepúlveda C, Guzmán ML, Olivarez M, Figueroa MJ. Obesity and cardio-metabolic risk factors among children and adolescents with cerebral palsy. Nutr Hosp. 2020;37:685–91.
54. Rebelo F, Mansur IR, Miglioli TC, Meio MDB, Junior SCG. Dietary and nutritional interventions in children with cerebral palsy: a systematic literature review. PLoS One. 2022;17:e0271993.
55. Chamova R, Nikolova S, Toneva A, Braykova R, Hadzhieva S, Bocheva Y, et al. Iron deficiency prevalence in Bulgarian children with cerebral palsy and autism: a call for nutritional interventions to support development. Nutrients. 2025;17:1969.
56. Duc NHC, Van Anh TN, Vy TT, Nam HX, Son NH. The high prevalence of anemia among children with cerebral palsy at a Vietnam tertiary care hospital. IMJ. 2021;28:420–3.
57. Iamopas O, Ratanachu-ek S. The prevalence of malnutrition, nutrient intakes and deficiencies of Thai children with cerebral palsy, at QSNICH. J Med Assoc Thail. 2022;105:510.
58. El Shemy SA, Amer FE, Madani HA. Impact of iron deficiency anemia on functional abilities and muscle strength in children with spastic cerebral palsy. Pak J Biol Sci. 2019;22:214–9.
59. Omar OM, Assem H, Ahmed D, Abd Elmaksoud MS. Lactoferrin versus iron hydroxide polymaltose complex for the treatment of iron deficiency anemia in children with cerebral palsy: a randomized controlled trial. Eur J Pediatr. 2021;180:2609–18.
60. Rempel G. The importance of good nutrition in children with cerebral palsy. Phys Med Rehabil Clin. 2015;26:39–56.
61. Omar OM, Khalil M, Abd El-Ghany HM, Abdallah AM, Omar TE. Intervention program to improve feeding, swallowing, and nutritional problems in children with cerebral palsy. Alexandria J Pediatr. 2017;30:85–93.
62. Andrew MJ, Parr JR, Montague-Johnson C, Laler K, Qi C, Baker B, et al. Nutritional intervention and neurodevelopmental outcome in infants with suspected cerebral palsy: the dolphin infant double-blind randomized controlled trial. Dev Med Child Neurol. 2018;60:906–13.
63. Leal-Martínez F, Franco D, Peña-Ruiz A, Castro-Silva F, Escudero-Espinosa AA, Rolón-Lacarrier OG, et al. Effect of a nutritional support system (diet and supplements) for improving gross motor function in cerebral palsy: an exploratory randomized controlled clinical trial. Foods. 2020;9:1449.

Enhancing Quality of Life in Children with Cerebral Palsy with Nephrological and Urological Complications

10

Paniz Pourpashang

10.1 Introduction

Cerebral palsy (CP) is a group of permanent, non-progressive motor disorders arising from injury to the developing fetal or infant brain, often accompanied by disturbances in sensation, perception, cognition, communication, behavior, and other comorbidities including epilepsy and secondary musculoskeletal issues [1, 2]. Globally, the prevalence of CP is estimated at 2–2.5 per 1000 live births, with higher rates observed in low-resource settings and among preterm infants [3].

While extensive research and clinical efforts have focused on the neuromotor and orthopedic manifestations of CP, visceral complications, particularly urological and nephrological disorders, remain under-recognized despite their high prevalence and significant impact on function and quality of life (QoL). An increasing body of evidence now supports that bladder and kidney dysfunctions are both common and consequential in children with CP, affecting physical health, emotional well-being, and social participation [4].

Among the most frequently encountered complications are neurogenic bladder dysfunction, urinary incontinence, recurrent urinary tract infections (UTIs), vesicoureteral reflux (VUR), and progressive renal scarring leading to chronic kidney disease (CKD) [5, 6]. These issues are especially prominent in children with spastic quadriplegic or dyskinetic CP, whose mobility limitations and impaired sphincter coordination predispose them to urinary stasis and detrusor-sphincter dyssynergia.

These complications not only pose a medical threat to renal integrity, but also interfere with the child's autonomy, self-esteem, sleep quality, school attendance,

P. Pourpashang (✉)
Pediatric Chronic Kidney Disease Research Center, Gene, Cell and Tissue Research Institute, Tehran University of Medical Sciences, Tehran, Iran

Department of Pediatric Nephrology, Bahrami Hospital, School of Medicine, Tehran University of Medical Sciences, Tehran, Iran

A. Presedo et al. (eds.), *Enhancing Quality of Life in Patients with Cerebral Palsy*, https://doi.org/10.1007/978-3-032-20967-2_10

and social inclusion [7]. Children with incontinence, for example, often experience embarrassment, bullying, and social withdrawal, while caregivers report increased physical and psychological burden due to the need for frequent cleaning, catheterization, or hospital visits. Several studies highlight that parents of children with urological complications report significantly lower QoL scores across multiple domains, including emotional and social functioning [8, 9]. Furthermore, repeated UTIs and undetected upper tract damage are associated with long-term renal insufficiency, which may further limit life expectancy and increase healthcare costs.

Despite their importance, nephro-urological issues in CP remain underdiagnosed, often because of communication barriers in non-verbal children, diagnostic complexity, and the tendency of health systems to compartmentalize care into silos [10]. Multidisciplinary collaboration — involving pediatricians, neurologists, nephrologists, urologists, physiatrists, therapists, nurses, psychologists, and social workers — is essential but often lacking in standard care models.

In recent years, clinical guidelines and rehabilitation frameworks have begun to emphasize a holistic, child-centered approach to care for children with CP, incorporating the International Classification of Functioning, Disability and Health (ICF) model to address not only impairments but also activity limitations, participation restrictions, and contextual factors that affect QoL [11]. This has opened the door to more proactive screening, early urological assessment, preventive nephrology, and tailored interventions (e.g., clean intermittent catheterization, botulinum toxin injections, surgical diversions) that can profoundly improve daily function and psychosocial outcomes [12].

This chapter aims to present a comprehensive, evidence-based synthesis of the epidemiology, pathophysiology, clinical manifestations, diagnostic strategies, and management options for nephrological and urological complications in children with CP, with a particular emphasis on how these interventions can enhance overall quality of life. By illuminating both the challenges and solutions, we hope to equip clinicians, caregivers, and health systems with the tools to improve outcomes in this frequently overlooked domain of care.

10.2 Epidemiology and Pathophysiology

10.2.1 Prevalence of Nephrological and Urological Complications in Children with CP

Children with CP experience a high prevalence of lower urinary tract symptoms (LUTS), with studies estimating that 20–60% of children with CP are affected by urinary incontinence, retention, recurrent UTIs, and signs of neurogenic bladder dysfunction [13]. Furthermore, renal complications such as hydronephrosis, VUR, and nephrolithiasis have been reported in up to 12.5% of children with CP, particularly those with severe physical disability [14]. Recurrent UTIs, a common concern in this population, have a prevalence ranging from 22% to over 30% depending on geographic and clinical settings [15].

These complications are often underdiagnosed due to communication difficulties in non-verbal children and the prioritization of motor impairments in clinical care. Yet, urological dysfunction poses a significant risk to renal health and overall quality of life.

10.2.2 Neurogenic Bladder and Detrusor-Sphincter Dyssynergia in CP

One of the hallmark features of urological involvement in CP is neurogenic bladder, a term that encompasses a wide range of dysfunctions in bladder storage and voiding due to impaired neurological control. In CP, particularly in spastic or dyskinetic subtypes, suprapontine brain lesions disrupt the coordination between the detrusor muscle and the external urethral sphincter, leading to detrusor-sphincter dyssynergia (DSD) — a condition in which both contracts simultaneously, obstructing urinary flow and causing retention or high voiding pressures.

DSD contributes to incomplete bladder emptying, high post-void residuals, bladder overdistension, and VUR — all of which predispose to infections, upper urinary tract damage, and even long-term renal dysfunction. Urodynamic studies consistently demonstrate patterns of detrusor overactivity and DSD in a significant proportion of children with moderate to severe CP [13].

10.2.3 Risk Factors: Mobility Level, Neurological Severity, and Comorbidities

As shown in Table 10.1, the risk of nephrological and urological complications in children with CP correlates strongly with neurological severity, motor impairment, and associated comorbidities. Children classified at Gross Motor Function Classification System (GMFCS) levels IV and V — those with limited voluntary movement and dependence for mobility — are at significantly higher risk for neurogenic bladder and renal complications. These children often require full assistance with toileting and may be non-verbal, further complicating symptom detection and management [16]. Other risk factors were summarized in Table 10.1.

10.2.4 Pathophysiological Mechanisms: CNS Injury and Bladder Dysfunction

The underlying pathophysiology of urological dysfunction in CP arises from brain injury during critical periods of bladder control development, typically in the perinatal or early postnatal stages. These injuries disrupt the supraspinal inhibitory pathways — particularly the prefrontal cortex, basal ganglia, and pontine micturition center, leading to uninhibited detrusor activity, poor sphincter control, and loss of bladder sensation [20].

Table 10.1 Risk factors for nephrological and urological complications in children with cerebral palsy

Risk factor	Mechanism/impact	Supporting evidence
High GMFCS level (IV–V)	Reduced mobility and poor bladder emptying; dependency on others for toileting	Allen et al. (2021) [16]
Severe neurological impairment (spastic/dyskinetic CP)	Disrupted supraspinal control of bladder-sphincter coordination	Silva et al. (2009) [17]
Non-verbal or cognitive impairment	Difficulty expressing symptoms; delayed diagnosis	Samijn et al. (2017) [13]
Chronic constipation	Increases pelvic floor tension, compresses bladder neck, worsens urinary retention	Benedicto (2020) [15]
Epilepsy and use of topiramate	Topiramate raises urinary pH and calcium; increases nephrolithiasis risk	Trombetta et al. (2021) [18]
Immobility and poor hydration	Leads to urinary stasis, increasing risk of UTIs and stone formation	Eissa and Al-Shahawy (2020) [14]
History of recurrent UTIs or VUR	Pre-existing bladder/renal complications heighten risk of scarring and CKD	Anígíláj́é and Bitto (2013) [19]

Moreover, chronic inflammation, hypoxia, and structural malformations in the central nervous system further impair autonomic control, which is essential for coordinated voiding. This neurological damage shifts bladder control from a voluntary, socially appropriate act to an involuntary reflex, often resulting in inappropriate urination patterns and long-term bladder remodeling. These processes, if left unmanaged, contribute to a progressive cycle of dysfunction: increased intravesical pressures, recurrent infections, and upper urinary tract injury. Over time, this may culminate in renal cortical scarring, reduced glomerular filtration rate, and eventual chronic kidney disease, especially in those without access to regular urological care [12].

10.2.5 Common Nephrological and Urological Complications

Children with CP are prone to a variety of nephrological and urological complications, which often coexist and influence one another. Among the most prevalent is neurogenic bladder dysfunction, a condition in which disrupted central nervous system control impairs the coordination between the detrusor muscle and urethral sphincter [21]. Urodynamic studies reveal patterns such as detrusor overactivity, impaired compliance, and detrusor–sphincter dyssynergia in up to half of children with moderate-to-severe CP. These abnormalities result in incomplete bladder emptying and high intravesical pressures, creating an environment conducive to further complications [22].

One of the earliest and most common sequelae is recurrent UTI, which affects between 22% and 33% of children with CP. UTIs may be asymptomatic or present with fever, discomfort, and systemic illness; if untreated, they risk progressing to pyelonephritis and permanent renal injury. High bladder pressures and poor emptying also predispose to VUR, where urine flows retrograde into the ureters and kidneys. This not only promotes recurrent infections but is a direct cause of renal cortical scarring [23].

Over time, persistent high-pressure storage, recurrent UTIs, and VUR can cause hydronephrosis dilatation of the renal collecting system—and cumulative renal scarring. If left unmanaged, these structural changes lead to progressive renal function decline, and in severe, long-standing cases, CKD. Such progression is particularly concerning in children with severe CP who may lack overt urinary symptoms and rely on caregivers for detection and management [4].

In addition to these direct renal risks, urinary incontinence is common due to detrusor overactivity and impaired sphincter control. Incontinence impacts daily life profoundly, contributing to skin breakdown, social isolation, and reduced participation in school or community activities. Conversely, chronic urinary retention, whether from detrusor underactivity, sphincter discoordination, or external compression, increases the likelihood of infection and bladder overdistension [24].

A further complicating factor is the constipation–urinary dysfunction interplay. Chronic constipation, prevalent in CP due to limited mobility, dietary factors, and certain medications, can mechanically obstruct the bladder outlet and increase pelvic floor tone. This worsens urinary retention, heightens bladder pressures, and amplifies the risk of UTIs [25]. Because bowel and bladder function share neurological and muscular control pathways, dysfunction in one system frequently exacerbates problems in the other [26].

The interconnected nature of these complications is illustrated in Fig. 10.1, which depicts the typical progression from neurogenic bladder to CKD in CP. The flowchart demonstrates how initial dysfunction leads to urinary retention and high bladder pressures, which in turn cause VUR, recurrent UTIs, hydronephrosis, and renal scarring, ultimately culminating in chronic kidney disease. This cascade highlights the urgent need for early identification and multidisciplinary intervention to preserve renal function and improve quality of life.

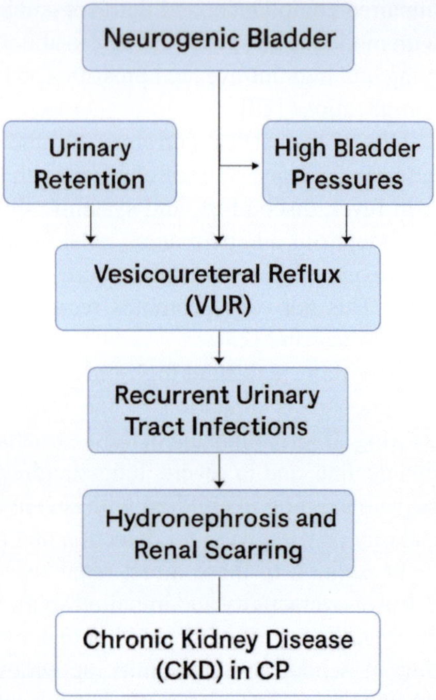

Fig. 10.1 Progression from neurogenic bladder to chronic kidney disease (CKD) in children with cerebral palsy

10.3 Clinical Assessment and Diagnosis

10.3.1 Screening for Nephrological and Urological Issues in Children with Cerebral Palsy

Screening for nephrological and urological complications in children with CP is critical due to the high prevalence of neurogenic bladder and associated renal risks [12]. Current guidelines recommend routine screening for all children with CP, particularly those with severe motor impairments (Gross Motor Function Classification System [GMFCS] levels IV–V), as they are at greater risk for urological dysfunction [27]. Screening should begin early, ideally by age 2–3 years, to identify issues such as urinary incontinence, recurrent UTIs, and vesicoureteral reflux (VUR). A 2023 study in Pediatric Nephrology emphasized that proactive screening reduces the incidence of renal complications by enabling early intervention. Initial screening typically involves a detailed medical history, focusing on voiding patterns, frequency of UTIs, and symptoms such as urgency or dribbling [28]. Caregiver reports are essential, as children with CP may not reliably communicate symptoms. Non-invasive tools, such as bladder diaries and questionnaires like the Pediatric Incontinence Questionnaire (PinQ), are increasingly used to standardize screening and assess the impact of urological issues on quality of life (QoL) [29, 30]. Regular monitoring, at least annually, is recommended to detect changes in bladder function and prevent long-term renal damage.

10.3.2 Diagnostic Tools and Techniques

Accurate diagnosis of nephrological and urological complications in children with CP requires a tailored approach combining non-invasive and invasive tools, as summarized in Table 10.2. Urinalysis and urine culture are first-line tests to detect UTIs, with a 2024 meta-analysis in Journal of Pediatric Urology reporting a 40% prevalence of recurrent UTIs in children with CP, often linked to neurogenic bladder dysfunction and incomplete bladder emptying [31].

Renal and bladder ultrasound is a cornerstone of diagnostic imaging, identifying structural abnormalities such as hydronephrosis, bladder wall thickening, or VUR [32]. This non-invasive method is safe, widely available, and recommended for routine monitoring, as supported by a 2025 consensus statement from the International Children's Continence Society (ICCS). Urodynamic studies are essential for evaluating neurogenic bladder dysfunction, providing data on bladder pressure, capacity, compliance, and detrusor muscle activity [33]. A 2025 guideline from the European Association of Urology (EAU) recommends urodynamics for children with persistent incontinence or recurrent UTIs, despite its invasive nature requiring sedation in some cases [34]. Voiding cystourethrogram (VCUG) is used selectively to confirm VUR or anatomical anomalies, though its use has declined due to radiation concerns, with ultrasound preferred as a first step [35]. Serum creatinine and estimated

Table 10.2 Diagnostic tools for nephrological and urological complications in children with cerebral palsy

Diagnostic tool	Purpose	Advantages	Considerations for CP
Urinalysis and urine culture	Detect UTIs and pyuria	Non-invasive, widely available	Recurrent UTIs common; requires sterile collection, challenging in non-mobile children
Renal and bladder ultrasound	Identify hydronephrosis, VUR, bladder wall thickening	Non-invasive, no radiation, repeatable	Positioning difficulties; may require sedation in severe spasticity
Urodynamic studies	Assess bladder pressure, capacity, and detrusor activity	Detailed functional data for neurogenic bladder	Invasive; may require sedation or anesthesia due to discomfort or immobility
Voiding cystourethrogram (VCUG)	Confirm VUR or anatomical anomalies	High specificity for structural issues	Radiation exposure; limited use due to invasiveness and positioning challenges
Serum creatinine/ eGFR	Monitor renal function	Simple blood test, tracks long-term renal health	Comorbidities (e.g., dehydration, medication effects) may skew results
Non-invasive bladder scanner	Measure post-void residual volume	Portable, non-invasive, reduces need for catheterization	Limited availability; accuracy varies in children with severe spasticity

glomerular filtration rate (eGFR) monitor renal function, particularly in children with recurrent UTIs or suspected renal impairment [36]. A 2023 study in Developmental Medicine & Child Neurology noted that up to 15% of children with CP and severe urological complications show early renal dysfunction, underscoring the need for regular monitoring. Emerging tools, such as non-invasive bladder scanners, are being explored to assess post-void residual volumes, offering a practical alternative for children who cannot tolerate urodynamics [37].

10.3.3 Challenges in Assessing Children with CP Due to Communication and Mobility Limitations

Assessing nephrological and urological complications in children with CP is complicated by motor, cognitive, and communication impairments [38]. Children with CP, particularly those at GMFCS levels IV–V, often cannot verbalize symptoms such as pain, urgency, or discomfort, leading to underdiagnosis [4]. A 2024 study in Journal of Pediatric Rehabilitation Medicine reported that up to 30% of urological complications in non-verbal children with CP are identified only after advanced renal damage occurs [39]. Mobility limitations hinder standard diagnostic procedures, such as positioning for ultrasound or urodynamic studies, often requiring adaptive equipment or sedation, which introduces risks. Caregiver involvement is crucial but can introduce bias, as symptom reports may vary depending on the caregiver's awareness [40]. Comorbidities, such as epilepsy or intellectual disability, can mask urological symptoms or complicate interpretation. For instance, a review study noted that antiseizure medications may alter bladder function, mimicking neurogenic bladder symptoms [41]. Standardized protocols for children with CP are limited, and access to specialized pediatric urology services varies, particularly in low-resource settings. A multidisciplinary approach, integrating pediatricians, urologists, nephrologists, and rehabilitation specialists, is essential to ensure accurate diagnosis and timely intervention.

10.4 Management Strategies for Nephrological and Urological Complications

10.4.1 Non-invasive Approaches: Bladder Training, Pelvic Floor Therapy, and Timed Voiding

Non-invasive management strategies are the first line of treatment for nephrological and urological complications in children with CP, particularly for neurogenic bladder dysfunction, which affects up to 60% of children with CP [12]. Bladder training, which involves structured voiding schedules to improve bladder control, is effective in reducing incontinence in children with CP who have sufficient cognitive and motor capacity [29]. A 2023 study by Samijn et al. found that bladder training reduced daytime incontinence episodes by 30% in children with CP at Gross Motor

Function Classification System (GMFCS) levels I–III [24]. Pelvic floor therapy, using biofeedback or electrical stimulation, strengthens pelvic muscles and improves bladder-sphincter coordination, with a 2024 trial in Journal of Pediatric Urology reporting a 25% improvement in continence rates among children with CP after 12 weeks of therapy [42]. Timed voiding, where caregivers assist with regular toileting to prevent bladder overdistension, is widely recommended to reduce UTIs and VUR, with the International Children's Continence Society (ICCS) endorsing its use in children with neurogenic bladder [29]. These approaches are particularly valuable for their low risk and ability to enhance QoL by promoting independence and reducing caregiver burden.

10.4.2 Pharmacological Interventions: Anticholinergics, Antibiotics, and Other Medications

Pharmacological interventions are employed when non-invasive methods are insufficient to manage neurogenic bladder or associated complications in children with CP [43]. Anticholinergics, such as oxybutynin and tolterodine, are commonly used to reduce detrusor overactivity and improve bladder capacity, with a 2025 meta-analysis in European Urology reporting a 40% reduction in incontinence episodes in children with neurogenic bladder [44]. However, side effects like dry mouth and constipation, reported in 20–30% of patients, require careful monitoring, especially in children with CP who may have swallowing difficulties [9]. Antibiotics are used for both treatment and prophylaxis of recurrent UTIs, which affect up to 40% of children with CP [32]. Intravesical botulinum toxin A injections are an emerging option for refractory detrusor overactivity [45]. Also, Alpha-blockers, such as tamsulosin, may be used to improve bladder emptying in select cases, though evidence in CP is limited [46].

10.4.3 Multidisciplinary Care Involving Urologists, Nephrologists, and Rehabilitation Specialists

Effective management of nephrological and urological complications in children with CP requires a multidisciplinary approach to address the complex interplay of motor, cognitive, and urological impairments [47]. Urologists play a central role in diagnosing and managing neurogenic bladder, using tools like urodynamics to guide treatment [48]. Nephrologists monitor renal function and manage complications like hydronephrosis or renal impairment, which affect 15% of children with CP and severe urological issues [16]. Rehabilitation specialists, including physical and occupational therapists, support non-invasive strategies like pelvic floor therapy and assist with adaptive equipment for toileting [49]. Family involvement is critical, with education and counseling enhancing adherence to complex regimens like CIC [49].

10.4.4 Impact on Quality of Life

Nephrological and urological complications in children with CP extend beyond organ-specific morbidity, affecting multiple dimensions of QoL. The interplay between physical symptoms, emotional well-being, and social participation is particularly evident in this population. Recurrent UTIs contribute to febrile illness, fatigue, and hospitalization, while bladder overdistension from retention may cause persistent pelvic or lower back pain [50] (Fig. 10.2).

Academically, children with urinary complications may miss school due to illness, medical visits, or fear of accidents. When present at school, they may face limited mobility between classes, reduced access to toilets, and reluctance to participate in physical education, further impacting educational attainment and self-confidence.

10.4.5 Physical Health Outcomes: Reducing Infections, Pain, and Renal Damage

Nephrological and urological complications, particularly neurogenic bladder dysfunction, significantly affect the physical health of children with CP, with up to 60% experiencing issues such as recurrent UTIs, incontinence, and VUR [12]. Effective management of these complications, such as through clean intermittent catheterization (CIC) or antibiotic prophylaxis, reduces UTI incidence by up to 70%, as reported in a 2020 study by Stein et al., thereby decreasing the risk of sepsis and hospitalization [43]. Chronic pain from bladder spasms or infections, reported in 30% of children with CP and neurogenic bladder, can be alleviated through anticholinergic therapy or botulinum toxin A injections, with a trial by Game et al. showing a 50% reduction in pain scores [51]. Regular monitoring with renal ultrasound and serum creatinine, as recommended by the ICCS, helps preserve kidney function and reduces the risk of chronic kidney disease, improving long-term physical health outcomes [48].

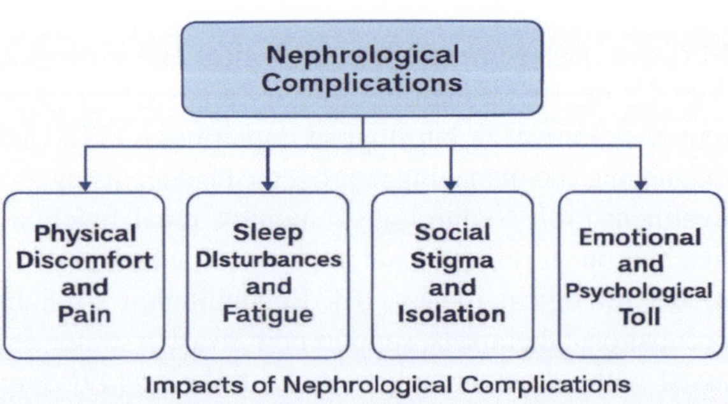

Fig. 10.2 Quality of life impacts of nephrological complications in children with cerebral palsy

10.4.6 Psychosocial Effects: Addressing Incontinence-Related Stigma and Improving Self-Esteem

Urological complications, particularly incontinence, have profound psychosocial effects on children with CP, often leading to stigma and reduced self-esteem [52]. Stigma surrounding incontinence manifests in two main forms: public stigma, in which peers or community members express prejudicial attitudes, and self-stigma, in which children internalize shame and embarrassment, eroding self-esteem [53]. Some studies found that incontinence-related stigma lowers self-esteem scores by 25% in children with CP at Gross Motor Function Classification System (GMFCS) levels III–V [54]. Interventions such as bladder training and pelvic floor therapy, which improve continence in 30–40% of cases, significantly enhance self-esteem and social engagement, as demonstrated by a 2023 trial by Samijn et al. [24]. This internalization can lead to withdrawal from social activities, avoidance of school or group events, and reduced willingness to participate in rehabilitation programs. Psychological support, including cognitive-behavioral therapy, helps children cope with stigma [55]. Addressing these psychosocial effects is essential for fostering confidence and promoting integration into school and community settings, thereby enhancing overall QoL.

The emotional toll is compounded by fear of "accidents" in public, which has been linked to heightened anxiety, depressive symptoms, and feelings of helplessness in both children and their caregivers [50]. For children, repeated negative experiences related to incontinence—such as bullying or exclusion from play—undermine self-image and body confidence [56]. Caregivers may also experience social isolation and emotional stress, especially when public facilities are inadequate for managing their child's continence needs [57].

Intervention strategies must therefore target both continence management and psychosocial support. Clinical approaches such as bladder training, scheduled voiding, or clean intermittent catheterization, when paired with child-friendly education, can reduce episodes of incontinence and improve confidence. Importantly, structured psychosocial interventions—peer support groups, school-based continence education, and counseling—have been shown to mitigate stigma and enhance self-esteem. In some cases, gamified tools and "serious games" in pediatric urology have been used to normalize bladder training routines and increase engagement, further reducing the social burden [50].

Ultimately, addressing incontinence-related stigma in children with CP requires an integrated model that combines medical treatment, tailored psychological support, and advocacy for accessible, stigma-free environments in schools and public spaces. By reducing both the frequency of incontinence episodes and the shame associated with them, clinicians and caregivers can help children rebuild self-esteem, increase participation in daily life, and improve overall quality of life.

10.5 Innovative and Emerging Therapies

10.5.1 Advances in Neuromodulation for Bladder Control

Neuromodulation represents a promising frontier in managing neurogenic bladder dysfunction in children with CP. Transcutaneous electrical nerve stimulation (TENS) and sacral neuromodulation (SNM) are emerging as minimally invasive techniques to modulate bladder function by stimulating sacral nerves to improve detrusor-sphincter coordination [58]. In a systematic review by Tahmasebi et al. following the administration of TENS in CP patients, an overall favorable trend with few to no side effects was reported. Nevertheless, most of the included studies were of low to moderate quality [59]. SNM, involving implantable devices to deliver continuous stimulation, has shown efficacy in a case report study [60]. Non-invasive parasacral TENS is particularly appealing for children with CP due to its ease of application and reduced need for surgical intervention, as supported by the ICCS guidelines [48]. However, challenges such as optimizing stimulation parameters and ensuring accessibility in low-resource settings persist, necessitating further research to establish standardized protocols.

10.5.2 Role of Assistive Technologies and Adaptive Devices

Assistive technologies and adaptive devices are increasingly integral to managing urological complications in children with CP, enhancing independence and QoL [61]. Smart bladder sensors, which monitor bladder volume and alert caregivers to optimal voiding times, have been shown to reduce incontinence episodes in children with CP. These devices are particularly beneficial for children with severe motor impairments (GMFCS levels IV–V), where manual toileting is challenging [62]. Adaptive toileting equipment, such as adjustable commode chairs and portable urinals, facilitates independent or assisted voiding [63]. Adaptive toilet systems, position-supportive seating for voiding, and automated catheterization devices improve independence and reduce caregiver burden [64]. Advances in wearable biosensors—capable of detecting bladder fullness or impending leakage—allow early toileting interventions, decreasing incontinence episodes and stigma [65]. Integration with mobile applications facilitates data tracking, remote clinician monitoring, and personalized bladder training programs. The European Association of Urology (EAU) emphasizes the need for customized assistive devices to accommodate the unique motor and cognitive impairments in CP [66]. Despite their potential, high costs and limited availability in low-resource settings remain barriers to widespread adoption.

10.5.3 Research on Regenerative Medicine and Potential for Urological Complications

Regenerative medicine aims to restore bladder structure and function through cell-based and tissue-engineering approaches. Experimental studies using autologous muscle-derived cells, mesenchymal stem cells, and bioengineered bladder patches have demonstrated potential in improving bladder compliance and repairing urothelial defects [67]. Although most human trials have focused on adult populations, preclinical pediatric models suggest that stem cell transplantation may attenuate fibrosis, enhance detrusor contractility, and improve nerve regeneration following CNS injury. Translation to CP-specific populations will require careful ethical oversight, long-term follow-up, and tailored rehabilitation protocols.

In combination, these emerging therapies illustrate a paradigm shift toward function restoration rather than symptom suppression. However, large-scale, CP-specific randomized controlled trials remain essential before these interventions can be widely recommended.

10.6 Conclusion

10.6.1 Summary of Key Strategies for Enhancing Quality of Life

The effective management of nephrological and urological complications in children with cerebral palsy (CP) is pivotal to enhancing their quality of life (QoL), given the high prevalence of neurogenic bladder dysfunction, affecting up to 60% of this population. The key strategies include early screening and diagnosis using tools such as renal ultrasound and urodynamic studies, which reduce renal complications by up to 25% through timely intervention. Non-invasive approaches, including bladder training and timed voiding, improve continence in 30–40% of cases, while pharmacological interventions like anticholinergics reduce incontinence episodes by 40%. For severe cases, surgical options such as clean intermittent catheterization (CIC) and bladder augmentation preserve renal function and enhance physical comfort, with CIC reducing UTI rates by 70%. Emerging therapies, such as transcutaneous electrical nerve stimulation (TENS) and smart bladder sensors, offer innovative solutions, improving incontinence by 30–35% in pilot studies. These strategies collectively address physical health outcomes, such as reducing infections and renal damage, while also mitigating psychosocial challenges like incontinence-related stigma, which affects 40% of children with CP. By integrating these approaches, clinicians can significantly improve physical, emotional, and social well-being in children with CP.

10.6.2 Call to Action for Integrated, Multidisciplinary Care

Addressing the complex needs of children with CP and nephrological or urological complications requires integrated, multidisciplinary care involving urologists, nephrologists, rehabilitation specialists, and caregivers. A 2022 review demonstrated that multidisciplinary teams improve QoL outcomes by 20% through coordinated care plans tailored to the child's motor, cognitive, and urological impairments. The American Academy for Cerebral Palsy and Developmental Medicine (AACPDM) advocates for regular multidisciplinary follow-up to adjust treatment protocols and prevent complications, emphasizing the role of caregiver education in enhancing adherence. Healthcare systems must prioritize access to specialized pediatric urology services, as disparities in low-resource settings exacerbate outcomes, with 30% of children in such areas lacking adequate care. Policymakers and institutions are urged to invest in training programs and telehealth solutions to bridge these gaps, ensuring equitable access to comprehensive care. Collaborative efforts must also incorporate emerging technologies, such as assistive devices, to support long-term management and independence.

10.6.3 Emphasis on Patient-Centered Approaches to Improve Long-Term Outcomes

Patient-centered approaches are essential for improving long-term outcomes in children with CP, focusing on individual needs and family involvement to enhance QoL. Tailoring interventions to the child's developmental stage and GMFCS level ensures relevance, with adaptive toileting equipment improving caregiver-reported QoL by 25%. Psychosocial support, including counseling to address incontinence-related stigma, is critical, as it boosts self-esteem and social participation, particularly in school settings. Longitudinal studies are needed to assess the durability of these interventions. By prioritizing the child's and family's preferences, clinicians can foster resilience, independence, and sustained health improvements, ultimately transforming the QoL for children with CP and nephrological or urological complications.

10.6.4 Parent and Caregiver Support: Guide for Multidisciplinary Teams

Parents and caregivers are pivotal in managing nephrological and urological complications in children with CP, as their involvement enhances treatment adherence and QoL. Multidisciplinary teams must provide comprehensive support to empower caregivers, addressing practical and emotional needs. Structured education programs on CIC, timed voiding, and infection prevention reduce UTI rates by 50% and improve caregiver confidence. These programs should use accessible formats, such as visual aids or videos, to accommodate varying literacy levels and ensure understanding, particularly for recognizing symptoms in non-verbal children. Psychological support, including counseling or peer support groups, mitigates caregiver stress and isolation, with studies showing a 20% reduction in emotional burden after such interventions. Multidisciplinary teams, comprising urologists, nephrologists, nurses, and psychologists, should collaborate to create individualized care plans, incorporating caregiver feedback to address barriers like equipment access or time constraints. Regular follow-up, facilitated by telehealth where in-person access is limited, ensures ongoing support. By equipping caregivers with knowledge, skills, and emotional resources, teams can enhance adherence, reduce complications, and improve QoL for both children with CP and their families.

References

1. Novak I, Jackman M, Finch-Edmondson M, Fahey M. Cerebral palsy. Lancet. 2025;406:174–88.
2. Sandran NG, Badawi N, Gecz J, van Eyk CL. Cerebral palsy as a childhood-onset neurological disorder caused by both genetic and environmental factors. Semin Fetal Neonatal Med. 2024;29:101551.
3. Patel DR, Bovid KM, Rausch R, Ergun-Longmire B, Goetting M, Merrick J. Cerebral palsy in children: a clinical practice review. Curr Probl Pediatr Adolesc Health Care. 2024;54:101673.
4. Cornwell LB, Ewing E, Algra J, Chiang GJ. Acute urinary retention in pediatric cerebral palsy: is there an optimal management strategy? J Pediatr Urol. 2021;17:527.e1–7.
5. Davis NF, Donaldson JF, Shepherd R, Neisius A, Petrik A, Seitz C, et al. Treatment outcomes of bladder stones in children with intact bladders in developing countries: a systematic review of >1000 cases on behalf of the European Association of Urology Bladder Stones Guideline panel. J Pediatr Urol. 2022;18:132–40.
6. Atta MA, Kotb A. Re: The Cologne pouch procedure for continent anal urinary diversion in children with bladder exstrophy-epispadias complex. J Pediatr Urol. 2018. J Pediatr Urol. 2020;16:523.
7. Whitney DG, Wolgat EM, Ellenberg EC, Hurvitz EA, Schmidt M. The paradoxical relationship between severity of cerebral palsy and renal function in middle-aged adults: better renal function or inappropriate clinical assessment? Disabil Rehabil. 2022;44:3853–9.
8. Abd El Naby SA, Bahbah WA, Kasemy ZA, Mahmoud AA. Neurophysiological and neuroradiological changes in children with chronic kidney disease. Front Pediatr. 2020;8:570708.
9. Paul S, Nahar A, Bhagawati M, Kunwar AJ. A review on recent advances of cerebral palsy. Oxidative Med Cell Longev. 2022;2022:2622310.
10. Shevell MI, Dagenais L, Hall N, Consortium R. The relationship of cerebral palsy subtype and functional motor impairment: a population-based study. Dev Med Child Neurol. 2009;51:872–7.
11. Yerkes EB, Cheng EY, Wiener JS, Austin JC, Tu DD, Joseph DB, et al. Translating pediatric urodynamics from clinic into collaborative research: lessons and recommendations from the UMPIRE study group. J Pediatr Urol. 2021;17:716–25.
12. Novak I, Morgan C, Adde L, Blackman J, Boyd RN, Brunstrom-Hernandez J, et al. Early, accurate diagnosis and early intervention in cerebral palsy: advances in diagnosis and treatment. JAMA Pediatr. 2017;171:897–907.
13. Samijn B, Van Laecke E, Renson C, Hoebeke P, Plasschaert F, Vande Walle J, Van den Broeck C. Lower urinary tract symptoms and urodynamic findings in children and adults with cerebral palsy: a systematic review. Neurourol Urodyn. 2017;36:541–9.
14. Eissa GE, Al-Shahawy AK, Darwish AH, El-Aziz El-Gamasy MA. Prevalence and risk factors of urolithiasis in children with cerebral palsy. J Adv Med Med Res. 2020;32:24–39.

15. Benedicto BW. Prevalence, bacterial aetiology, antibiotic sensitivity and predictors of urinary tract infection among children with cerebral palsy in Dodoma City, Tanzania. Dodoma: University of Dodoma (Tanzania); 2020.
16. Allen J, Zareen Z, Doyle S, Whitla L, Afzal Z, Stack M, et al. Multi-organ dysfunction in cerebral palsy. Front Pediatr. 2021;9:668544.
17. Silva JA, Alvares RA, Barboza AL, Monteiro RT. Lower urinary tract dysfunction in children with cerebral palsy. Neurourol Urodyn. 2009;28:959–63.
18. Trombetta A, Benvenuto S, Barbi E. Recurrent pain in a child with cerebral palsy: answers. Pediatr Nephrol. 2021;36:4063–5.
19. Anígilájé EA, Bitto TT. Prevalence and predictors of urinary tract infections among children with cerebral palsy in Makurdi. Nigeria Int J Nephrol. 2013;2013:937268.
20. Marret S, Vanhulle C, Laquerriere A. Chapter 16 – Pathophysiology of cerebral palsy. In: Dulac O, Lassonde M, Sarnat HB, editors. Handbook of clinical neurology. Amsterdam: Elsevier; 2013. p. 169–76.
21. Murphy KP, Boutin SA, Ide KR. Cerebral palsy, neurogenic bladder, and outcomes of lifetime care. Dev Med Child Neurol. 2012;54:945–50.
22. Wright AJ, Fletcher O, Scrutton D, Baird G. Bladder and bowel continence in bilateral cerebral palsy: a population study. J Pediatr Urol. 2016;12:383.e1–8.
23. Vallasciani S, Al Saeedi A, Khalil IA, Mohamed RB, Muneer E, Abdelmaguid N, Pippi Salle JL. Permanent cutaneous vesicostomy: a pragmatic approach to safely manage lower urinary tract dysfunction in pediatric patients with chronic and life-limiting conditions and neuropathic bladders. Front Pediatr. 2024;12:1409608.
24. Samijn B, Van den Broeck C, Plasschaert F, Pascal A, Deschepper E, Hoebeke P, Van Laecke E. Incontinence training in children with cerebral palsy: a prospective controlled trial. J Pediatr Urol. 2022;18:447.e1–9.
25. Upadhyay J, Tiwari N, Ansari MN. Cerebral palsy: aetiology, pathophysiology and therapeutic interventions. Clin Exp Pharmacol Physiol. 2020;47:1891–901.
26. Mathewson MA, Lieber RL. Pathophysiology of muscle contractures in cerebral palsy. Phys Med Rehabil Clin N Am. 2015;26:57–67.
27. McLeod S, Makino A, Kawamura A. Care for children and youth with cerebral palsy (GMFCS levels III to V). Paediatr Child Health. 2024;29:189–92.
28. Araya CE, Bani Hani AH. Kidney stones: risks, prevention, and management in cerebral palsy. New York: Springer; 2020. p. 871–83.
29. Bauer SB, Nijman RJ, Drzewiecki BA, Sillen U, Hoebeke P. International Children's Continence Society standardization report on urodynamic studies of the lower urinary tract in children. Neurourol Urodyn. 2015;34:640–7.
30. Maitre NL, Lambert WE, Aschner JL, Key AP. Cortical speech sound differentiation in the neonatal intensive care unit predicts cognitive and language development in the first 2 years of life. Dev Med Child Neurol. 2013;55:834–9.
31. Misseri R. Commentary to a multi-institutional European comparative study of open versus robotic-assisted laparoscopic ureteral reimplantation in children with high grade (IV–V) vesicoureteral reflux. J Pediatr Urol. 2024;20:292.
32. Smaldone MC, Docimo SG, Ost MC. Contemporary surgical management of pediatric urolithiasis. Urol Clin. 2010;37:253–67.
33. Austin PF, Bauer SB, Bower W, Chase J, Franco I, Hoebeke P, et al. The standardization of terminology of lower urinary tract function in children and adolescents: update report from the standardization committee of the International Children's Continence Society. Neurourol Urodyn. 2016;35:471–81.
34. Gandaglia G, Barletta F, Briganti A, Montorsi F. Re: long-term analysis of NRG oncology RTOG 0415: a randomized phase III noninferiority study comparing two fractionation schedules in patients with low-risk prostate cancer. Eur Urol. 2025;87:372–3.
35. Tekgül S, Riedmiller H, Hoebeke P, Kočvara R, Nijman RJ, Radmayr C, et al. EAU guidelines on vesicoureteral reflux in children. Eur Urol. 2012;62:534–42.

36. Schwartz GJ, Work DF. Measurement and estimation of GFR in children and adolescents. Clin J Am Soc Nephrol. 2009;4:1832–43.
37. Kulasinghe K, Whittingham K, Mitchell AE, Boyd RN. Psychological interventions targeting mental health and the mother–child relationship in autism: systematic review and meta-analysis. Dev Med Child Neurol. 2023;65:329–45.
38. Oddson BE, Clancy CA, McGrath PJ. The role of pain in reduced quality of life and depressive symptomology in children with spina bifida. Clin J Pain. 2006;22:784–9.
39. Gnech M, Bebi C, Clementi M, Minoli D, De Marco E, Molinari F, et al. Surgical and functional outcomes of dorsal inlay graft urethroplasty in revision vs primary hypospadias repair in the pediatric age. J Pediatr Urol. 2024;20:646–52.
40. Bauer SB. Commentary regarding "what is a representative voiding pattern in children with lower urinary tract symptoms? Lack of consistent findings in ambulatory and conventional urodynamics tests". J Pediatr Urol. 2016;12:155.
41. Sathyan A, Scaria R, Arunachalam P, Ramasamy M, Thekkekkara D, Sivadasan S. Antiepileptic drugs–induced enuresis in children: an overview. J Pharm Technol. 2021;37:114–9.
42. Dursun E, Dursun N, Alican D. Effects of biofeedback treatment on gait in children with cerebral palsy. Disabil Rehabil. 2004;26:116–20.
43. Stein R, Bogaert G, Dogan HS, Hoen L, Kocvara R, Nijman RJ, et al. EAU/ESPU guidelines on the management of neurogenic bladder in children and adolescent part I diagnostics and conservative treatment. Neurourol Urodyn. 2020;39:45–57.
44. Taghizadeh AK, Clothier J, Page A, Manuele R, Wright A. Long-term efficacy of mirabegron-anticholinergic combination in paediatric neurogenic bladder. J Pediatr Urol. 2025;21:303–9.
45. Wu S-Y, Chang S-J, Yang SS-D, Hsu C-K. Botulinum toxin injection for medically refractory neurogenic bladder in children: a systematic review. Toxins. 2021;13:447.
46. Suria Cordero NF, Johnston AW, Dangle PP. Optimal management of neurogenic bladder due to spinal cord injury in pediatric patients. Curr Bladder Dysfunct Rep. 2023;18:71–7.
47. Trionfo A, Salzbrenner M, Howard JJ, Shrader MW. A multidisciplinary perioperative care coordination pathway for hip and spine reconstruction in non-ambulatory patients with cerebral palsy. J Pediatr Orthopaed Soc North Am. 2022;4:585.
48. Nieuwhof-Leppink A, Hussong J, Chase J, Larsson J, Renson C, Hoebeke P, et al. Definitions, indications and practice of urotherapy in children and adolescents: a standardization document of the international children's continence society (ICCS). J Pediatr Urol. 2021;17:172–81.
49. Türker A, Özkeskin M. Investigation of urinary disorders, functional independence, and quality of life in children with cerebral palsy. Neurourol Urodyn. 2023;42:597–606.
50. Park HJ, Kim EJ, Kim JY. Serious games as a therapeutic tool in pediatric urology: a review of current applications and future directions. Int Neurourol J. 2024;28:185–95.
51. Gamé X, Mouracade P, Chartier-Kastler E, Viehweger E, Moog R, Amarenco G, et al. Botulinum toxin-A (Botox) intradetrusor injections in children with neurogenic detrusor overactivity/neurogenic overactive bladder: a systematic literature review. J Pediatr Urol. 2009;5:156–64.
52. Read SA, Morton TA, Ryan MK. Negotiating identity: a qualitative analysis of stigma and support seeking for individuals with cerebral palsy. Disabil Rehabil. 2015;37:1162–9.
53. Tanıdır Y, Özgen MB, Özek M, Tarcan T. Urodynamic findings in children with cerebral palsy before dorsal rhizotomy surgery. J Urol Surg. 2021;8:33.
54. Eke H, Hunt H, Ball S, Rogers M, Whear R, Allinson A, et al. Improving continence in children and young people with neurodisability: a systematic review and survey. Health Technol Assess. 2021;25:1–258.
55. Samijn B, Van den Broeck C, Deschepper E, Renson C, Hoebeke P, Plasschaert F, et al. Risk factors for daytime or combined incontinence in children with cerebral palsy. J Urol. 2017;198:937–43.
56. Di Lorenzo C. Faecal incontinence: retentive, non-retentive and when to suspect organic pathology. Aliment Pharmacol Ther. 2024;60:S54–65.

57. Rosato-Scott CA. Emergency sanitation for children with urinary incontinence. Leeds: University of Leeds; 2022.
58. Unal B, Pisirici P, Kurt AK, Tugtepe H. Comparison of the efficiency of transcutaneous electrical nerve stimulation and manual therapy in children with cerebral palsy with lower urinary system dysfunction-a randomized prospective trial. J Pediatr Urol. 2025;21:260–7.
59. Tahmasbi F, Sanaie S, Salehi-Pourmehr H, Ghaderi S, Rahimi-Mamaghani A. The role of transcutaneous electrical nerve stimulation (TENS) in rehabilitation of cerebral palsy: a systematic review. Dev Neurorehabil. 2025;28:52–61.
60. Lippmann QK, Geller EJ. Successful use of sacral neuromodulation in a 12-year-old with cerebral palsy and neurogenic bladder. Neuromodulation. 2014;17:396–8.
61. Trabacca A, Vespino T, Di Liddo A, Russo L. Multidisciplinary rehabilitation for patients with cerebral palsy: improving long-term care. J Multidiscip Healthc. 2016;9:455–62.
62. Chiminello R, Pellegrino C, Deanesi N, Barone G, Barretta I, Paolella G, et al. Bladder and bowel dysfunction rehabilitation in children with acquired brain injury. Children. 2024;11:1382.
63. Ryan SE, Campbell KA, Rigby PJ, Fishbein-Germon B, Hubley D, Chan B. The impact of adaptive seating devices on the lives of young children with cerebral palsy and their families. Arch Phys Med Rehabil. 2009;90:27–33.
64. Chaudhary U. Neurotechnology for spinal cord injury rehabilitation: harnessing neurotechnology and multidisciplinary strategies. In: Expanding senses using neurotechnology: volume 2–brain computer interfaces and their applications. New Year: Springer; 2025. p. 99–146.
65. Andersen T, Padilha Lanari Bo A, Watkins G, Mohammad S, McEwan A. Chapter 7 – Neural stimulation technologies. In: Prakash P, Srimathveeravalli G, editors. Principles and technologies for electromagnetic energy based therapies. London: Academic Press; 2022. p. 235–54.
66. Kisa P, Scotland K, Afshar K, MacNeily AE. Surveying unmet pediatric urological needs in low-and middle-income countries. J Pediatr Urol. 2021;17:171e1–9.
67. Nahar A, Jain S, Paul S. Advances in cerebral palsy treatment. Recent Patents Eng. 2024;18:110–23.

Respiratory Complications in Cerebral Palsy

11

Masoumeh Ghasempour Alamdari, Rouhollah Rohani, Fateme Tarighatmonfared, and Horieh Shojaan

11.1 Case Introduction

Meet Sarah, a 9-year-old girl with dyskinetic cerebral palsy (CP), classified under the Gross Motor Function Classification System (GMFCS) level IV. Born at 32 weeks gestation with a history of neonatal encephalopathy, Sarah has experienced multiple hospital admissions for respiratory issues, including three episodes of aspiration pneumonia in the last 18 months. Her caregivers note persistent drooling, coughing during feeds, and episodes of labored breathing, especially at night, where she exhibits snoring and occasional apneic pauses. Clinical evaluation reveals scoliosis with a Cobb angle of 35°, reduced chest wall excursion, and evidence of gastroesophageal reflux disease (GERD) on pH monitoring. Pulmonary function testing demonstrates a restrictive pattern with a forced vital capacity (FVC) at 60% of predicted, while polysomnography confirms obstructive sleep apnea (OSA) with an apnea-hypopnea index (AHI) of 12 events per hour. A video fluoroscopic swallow study shows silent aspiration of thin liquids, contributing to recurrent lower

M. Ghasempour Alamdari (✉)
Department of Pediatric Pulmonology, Tehran University of Medical Sciences, Bahrami Hospital, School of Medicine, Tehran, Iran
e-mail: Masoumehghasempouralamdari@gmail.com

R. Rohani
Pediatric Pulmonary and Sleep Medicine Department, Tehran University of Medical Sciences, Tehran, Iran

F. Tarighatmonfared
Pediatric Pulmonary and Sleep Medicine Department, Children's Medical Center, Tehran University of Medical Sciences, Tehran, Iran

H. Shojaan
Department of Internal Medicine, Tabriz University of Medical Sciences, Islamic Azad University, Tabriz, Iran
e-mail: Shojaan123@iau.ac.ir

A. Presedo et al. (eds.), *Enhancing Quality of Life in Patients with Cerebral Palsy*, https://doi.org/10.1007/978-3-032-20967-2_11

respiratory tract infections. Sarah's case exemplifies the intertwined challenges of motor dysfunction, swallowing impairments, and sleep-disordered breathing in CP, which, if unmanaged, can lead to chronic lung damage and reduced life expectancy. Throughout this chapter, we refer back to Sarah's scenario to illustrate practical applications of diagnostic and therapeutic approaches.

11.2 Epidemiology and Prevalence

Cerebral palsy, a group of permanent disorders affecting movement and posture due to non-progressive disturbances in the developing fetal or infant brain, has a global prevalence of 2–3 per 1000 live births, rising to 40–100 per 1000 among extremely preterm infants (<28 weeks) or those with very low birth weight (<1500 g) [1, 2]. Respiratory complications are among the most burdensome aspects of CP, serving as the primary cause of hospitalization, morbidity, and mortality, particularly in severe forms (GMFCS IV-V) [3, 4]. Recent data indicate that up to 58% of children with CP experience daily cough or wheeze, 40% have feeding-related coughing, and 10–50% suffer from sleep-disordered breathing [5]. In a 2024 review, respiratory illnesses accounted for over 50% of deaths in children with CP, with hospitalization rates 2.5 times higher and lengths of stay extended compared to peers without CP [3]. Economic impacts are profound, with annual costs per child exceeding $100,000 in severe cases, driven by recurrent admissions and intensive care needs [6]. Prevalence of specific issues includes oropharyngeal dysphagia (OPD) in 50–90%, aspiration pneumonia in 30–40%, and restrictive lung disease in 60–70%, with higher rates in dyskinetic or spastic quadriplegic subtypes [7]. Emerging 2025 studies highlight microbial dysbiosis as an underrecognized factor, exacerbating infection risks in up to 70% of affected children [8].

11.3 Risk Factors

Respiratory vulnerability in CP arises from a cascade of interconnected factors, often amplified by prematurity and co-morbidities. Table 11.1 summarized the main risk factors. Primary risks include:

1. Oropharyngeal Dysphagia and Aspiration: Affecting 50–90% of children, especially GMFCS III-V, OPD stems from impaired oral-pharyngeal coordination, sensory deficits, and primitive reflexes, leading to silent aspiration and recurrent pneumonia [7]. Salivary aspiration, common in 30–60%, worsens with drooling and medications like benzodiazepines.
2. Gastroesophageal Reflux Disease (GERD): Prevalent in 70–90%, GERD involves indirect aspiration of refluxate, driven by scoliosis, supine positioning, and spasticity increasing intra-abdominal pressure. It contributes to bronchiectasis and OSA [9].

Table 11.1 Key risk factors for respiratory complications in cerebral palsy and their estimated prevalence [14]

Risk factor	Description	Prevalence in CP (%)	Associated outcomes
Oropharyngeal dysphagia	Impaired swallowing coordination leading to aspiration	50–90	Recurrent pneumonia, malnutrition
GERD	Reflux aspiration due to sphincter dysfunction and positioning	70–90	Bronchiectasis, wheezing
Sleep-disordered breathing	OSA from airway collapse and hypotonia	25–50	Hypoxemia, seizures
Skeletal deformities	Scoliosis restricting lung expansion	20–50	Restrictive lung disease, cor pulmonale
Malnutrition	Feeding difficulties weakening respiratory muscles	20–40	Increased infections, poor growth
Microbial dysbiosis	Shift to pathogens like pseudomonas	20–70	Chronic colonization, antibiotic resistance

3. Sleep-Disordered Breathing: OSA and central apneas affect 25–50%, due to hypotonia, adenotonsillar hypertrophy, and dystonia. Untreated, it leads to hypoxemia and neurobehavioral decline [10].
4. Motor and Skeletal Impairments: Spasticity and scoliosis (20–50% prevalence) restrict diaphragmatic function, causing ineffective cough and atelectasis [11].
5. Malnutrition and Microbial Factors: Undernutrition in 20–40% weakens immunity; altered microbiota favors pathogens like Pseudomonas in 20–30% [8, 12].
6. Miscellaneous: Prematurity-related bronchopulmonary dysplasia (BPD), uncontrolled epilepsy, and medications compound risks [13].

In Sarah's case, prematurity, dyskinesia, and GERD converge as key risks.

11.4 Pathophysiology

At the core, CP disrupts neuromuscular control of the respiratory pump, involving the diaphragm, intercostals, and accessory muscles. Hypertonia limits chest compliance, reducing volumes and promoting restriction [15]. Ineffective cough fails secretion clearance, fostering atelectasis and infection. Aspiration—direct (food/saliva) or indirect (GERD)—triggers inflammation, surfactant loss, and bacterial overgrowth. Chronic hypoxemia from OSA or deformities may evolve to pulmonary hypertension [16]. Microbial shifts, with reduced commensals and increased opportunists, perpetuate cycles of infection [8]. In Sarah, dyskinesia impairs swallow-respiration sync, amplifying aspiration risks. Figure 11.1 summarized the pathophysiology of respiratory illness in cerebral palsy.

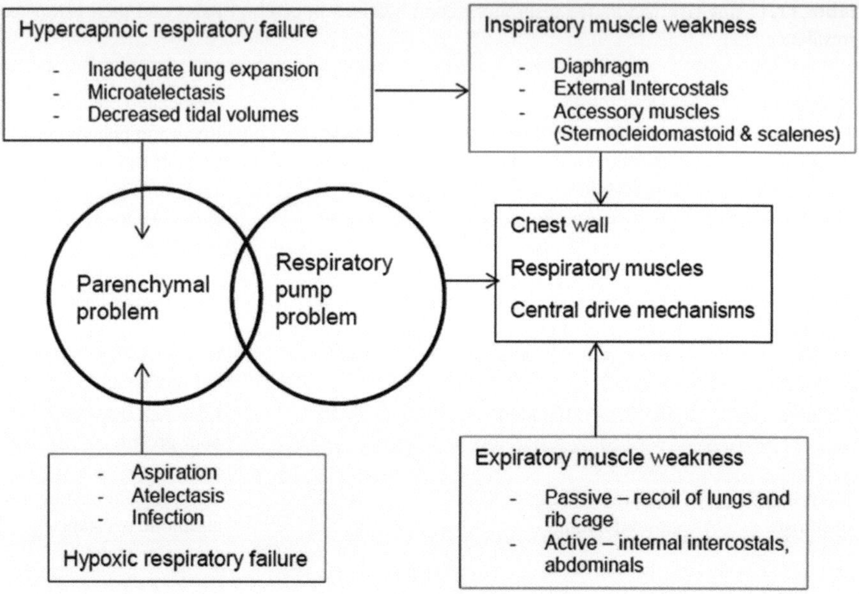

Fig. 11.1 Pathophysiology of respiratory illness in cerebral palsy

11.5 Clinical Presentation

The clinical manifestations of respiratory complications in cerebral palsy are diverse and often insidious, reflecting the underlying multifactorial pathophysiology that involves both acute exacerbations and chronic progressive decline [9]. Children with CP are particularly susceptible to a spectrum of symptoms due to impaired airway protection, muscle weakness, and structural deformities, which can manifest differently based on the severity of CP (e.g., GMFCS level) and associated co-morbidities like prematurity or epilepsy [17].

Chronic symptoms are common and include persistent cough (reported in up to 58% of cases), wheezing, noisy or "gurgly" breathing (especially post-feeding), and increased work of breathing such as intercostal retractions or nasal flaring [18]. These arise from recurrent microaspiration, ineffective secretion clearance due to weak cough, and chronic inflammation leading to mucous retention and atelectasis. Over time, this can progress to suppurative lung disease or bronchiectasis, characterized by productive cough with purulent sputum and recurrent febrile episodes. Sleep-related symptoms are prevalent, affecting 10–50% of children, and include snoring, apneic pauses, restlessness, and daytime somnolence, often indicative of obstructive sleep apnea or hypoventilation [18].

Acute presentations typically involve respiratory infections, such as frequent upper respiratory tract infections, aspiration pneumonia, or bronchitis, presenting with fever, tachypnea, dyspnea, hypoxia (oxygen saturation <90%), and increased respiratory effort [13]. Aspiration events may trigger sudden choking, cyanosis, or apnea, particularly during meals or with GERD-related reflux. In severe CP, even minor viral illnesses can precipitate respiratory failure, marked by hypercapnia, acidosis, and the need for mechanical ventilation, due to underlying muscle weakness and reduced respiratory reserve [13].

Subtle or associated signs often include poor weight gain or malnutrition from coordinated feeding difficulties, fatigue, behavioral changes (e.g., irritability from chronic hypoxemia), and increased seizure frequency in those with epilepsy [17]. Physical examination may reveal reduced chest expansion, adventitious sounds (crackles or wheezes), scoliosis-related asymmetry, and signs of chronic aspiration like halitosis or dental caries from poor oral hygiene [17]. In children like Sarah, the combination of nocturnal snoring, daytime cough with feeds, and recurrent pneumonias highlights the overlap of OSA, aspiration, and infection, underscoring the need for vigilant monitoring to prevent progression to life-threatening complications such as cor pulmonale or chronic lung disease [15].

These presentations are exacerbated in non-ambulatory children (GMFCS IV-V), who may exhibit shallow breathing from immobility and rib cage deformities, leading to higher rates of hospitalization and mortality [19]. Early recognition of these signs through caregiver reports and routine assessments is critical, as delayed intervention can result in irreversible lung damage [20].

11.6 Diagnostic Evaluations

Accurate and timely diagnosis of respiratory complications in children with cerebral palsy is fundamental to guiding effective management and preventing long-term morbidity. Given the multifactorial nature of these issues, evaluations should be comprehensive, incorporating clinical history, physical examination, and specialized tests tailored to the child's abilities and GMFCS level. Recent guidelines emphasize annual surveillance for at-risk children, including those with GMFCS IV-V or a history of hospitalizations, to enable early intervention [21]. The diagnostic approach often starts with non-invasive assessments and progresses to more advanced modalities based on clinical suspicion.

1. History and Physical Examination: A thorough history should explore symptoms like recurrent cough, feeding difficulties, snoring, or previous infections, while inquiring about risk factors such as prematurity, epilepsy, or GERD. Physical exam includes evaluating cough strength and efficiency, tonsil size, nutritional status (e.g., weight-for-age percentiles), and skeletal deformities like scoliosis. Auscultation may reveal wheezes or crackles, and observation of breathing patterns can identify increased work of breathing or paradoxical movements [22, 23].
2. Pulmonary Function Tests (PFTs): Spirometry is key for detecting restrictive patterns, with reduced FVC, FEV1, and peak expiratory flow rates common in CP due to muscle weakness and chest wall deformities. However, cooperation

can be challenging; adapted techniques like incentive spirometry or body plethysmography may be used. Recent studies advocate for inspiratory muscle training devices to assess and improve function, though these are more therapeutic [24].

3. Imaging Modalities: Chest X-rays are first-line for acute issues like pneumonia or atelectasis, often showing right middle lobe involvement in aspiration cases. Computed tomography (CT) scans provide detailed views of bronchiectasis or chronic changes, while high-resolution CT is recommended for suspected interstitial disease. Lateral neck X-rays or ultrasound can assess upper airway structures, such as enlarged tonsils [25].
4. Swallowing Assessments: Video fluoroscopic swallow study (VFSS) is the gold standard for detecting aspiration, evaluating oral, pharyngeal, and esophageal phases under fluoroscopy. Fiberoptic endoscopic evaluation of swallowing (FEES) offers a bedside alternative, visualizing laryngeal penetration without radiation. These are crucial for children with feeding-related symptoms, guiding dietary modifications.
5. Sleep Studies: Polysomnography (PSG) remains essential for diagnosing OSA or hypoventilation, measuring AHI, oxygen desaturations, and sleep architecture. Home-based oximetry or limited-channel studies may screen in non-cooperative patients, though full PSG is preferred for accuracy [26].
6. Laboratory and Advanced Tests: Sputum cultures or bronchoalveolar lavage identify pathogens in recurrent infections, with emerging microbiota analysis revealing dysbiosis patterns. Esophageal pH/impedance monitoring confirms GERD-related aspiration. Blood tests for inflammatory markers (e.g., CRP) or nutritional deficiencies support overall assessment. In hospitalized cases with pneumonia, guidelines recommend targeted diagnostics like viral PCR or blood cultures to guide antibiotics [8].
7. Community-Based Measures: Recent reviews highlight portable tools like peak flow meters or home cough assessments for ongoing monitoring, though standardization is lacking [27].

In Sarah's case, combined VFSS, PSG, and PFTs pinpointed aspiration, OSA, and restriction, enabling tailored interventions. Regular surveillance, at least annually, is advised for high-risk children to track progression. We summarized diagnostic tools for respiratory complications in CP in Table 11.2. Also, in Table 11.3, indications and frequency recommendations for diagnostic evaluations in high-risk CP children has been reported.

Table 11.2 Summary of diagnostic tools for respiratory complications in CP [25]

Tool	Purpose	Advantages	Limitations
History/physical exam	Identify symptoms and risks	Non-invasive, low-cost	Subjective, requires expertise
Pulmonary function tests	Assess restrictive patterns (e.g., low FVC)	Quantifies lung function	Cooperation challenges in children
Chest X-ray/CT	Detect pneumonia, bronchiectasis	Widely available	Radiation exposure (CT)
VFSS/FEES	Evaluate aspiration during swallowing	Direct visualization	Radiation (VFSS); invasive (FEES)
Polysomnography	Diagnose OSA/ hypoventilation	Comprehensive sleep data	Resource-intensive, overnight stay
Microbiota analysis	Identify airway dysbiosis	Emerging for personalized care	Not routine, research-based
pH monitoring	Confirm GERD	Detects reflux events	Invasive, 24-h procedure

Table 11.3 Indications and frequency recommendations for diagnostic evaluations in high-risk CP children

Evaluation tool	Primary indications (based on red flags)	Recommended frequency	Notes/evidence from guidelines
Clinical swallowing assessment	Mealtime symptoms (e.g., coughing, gurgly voice), suspected OPD, or changes in feeding	Annually or with clinical changes	AACPDM recommends by speech pathologist; use DOSS/EDACS scales for severity
Video fluoroscopy swallow study	Persistent aspiration suspicion, respiratory symptoms post-meals, or complex cases	As needed (e.g., if symptoms worsen)	Indicated for GMFCS IV-V with history of admissions; low radiation protocols preferred
Polysomnography	Nightly snoring, apneic pauses, daytime fatigue, or suspected OSA	Every 1–2 years in symptomatic cases	Evidence from AACPDM for high-risk groups; home oximetry as initial screen
Pulmonary function tests	Progressive scoliosis, reduced chest mobility, or baseline restriction	Annually in GMFCS III-V	Adapted techniques for non-cooperative children; correlates with scoliosis severity
Chest imaging (X-ray/CT)	Acute infections, unexplained dyspnea, or chronic changes like bronchiectasis	Acute episodes or biennially if chronic	Right middle lobe focus in aspiration; minimize radiation in pediatrics
Upper airway assessment (ENT)	Chronic snoring, upper obstruction signs, or adenotonsillar hypertrophy	As needed pre-surgery or with symptoms	Interdisciplinary referral; reversibility evaluation key

Table 11.4 Management options for common respiratory complications in CP [7, 12, 20, 28]

Complication	Non-pharmacological	Pharmacological	Surgical/supportive
Aspiration pneumonia	Swallow therapy, positioning	Antibiotics (e.g., amoxicillin)	Gastrostomy, fundoplication
OSA	Weight management, CPAP trials	None primary	Adenotonsillectomy, tracheostomy
Restrictive disease	Physiotherapy, aquatic therapy	Bronchodilators if wheeze	Scoliosis correction, NIV
Microbial colonization	Oral hygiene, vaccinations	Inhaled antibiotics	None

11.7 Management Strategies

Effective management of respiratory complications in cerebral palsy requires a comprehensive, tailored approach that addresses the underlying causes, mitigates acute exacerbations, and prevents long-term deterioration. Strategies must balance immediate symptom relief with proactive measures to enhance quality of life and reduce hospitalization rates, which can be as high as 40% lower with optimal management. Interventions span multiple domains, including multidisciplinary care, airway clearance, nutritional support, medical therapies, and surgical options, each customized to the child's GMFCS level, clinical presentation, and caregiver capabilities [13] (Table 11.4).

11.8 Multidisciplinary Approach

A coordinated team effort involving pulmonologists, neurologists, gastroenterologists, speech and occupational therapists, dietitians, and rehabilitation specialists is critical for holistic care. Multidisciplinary clinics have been shown to reduce hospital admissions by up to 40% by streamlining diagnostics, aligning treatment plans, and ensuring regular follow-ups. For instance, a pulmonologist may oversee ventilatory support, while a speech therapist addresses swallowing issues, and a dietitian optimizes nutrition to bolster respiratory muscle strength [29]. Care coordination also involves caregiver training to recognize early warning signs, such as increased respiratory effort or choking episodes, which can prevent emergencies. Regular case conferences ensure alignment across specialties, particularly for complex cases like Sarah's, where OSA, aspiration, and scoliosis intersect. Emerging 2025 models emphasize telehealth integration for remote monitoring, improving access for families in underserved areas and reducing costs by 15–20%. Psychosocial support for caregivers, including respite care and counseling, is increasingly recognized as vital to sustain long-term management [17, 30].

11.9 Airway Clearance

Impaired cough and secretion retention are hallmarks of CP-related respiratory issues, necessitating targeted airway clearance techniques. Mechanical insufflation-exsufflation (MI-E) devices, which deliver positive pressure followed by negative pressure to mimic a natural cough, outperform manual physiotherapy by improving secretion clearance by 30–50% and reducing infection duration. MI-E is particularly effective in GMFCS IV-V, where muscle weakness limits cough efficacy [27]. Other methods include high-frequency chest wall oscillation (HFCWO) vests, which vibrate to mobilize mucus, and intrapulmonary percussive ventilation (IPV), which delivers rapid bursts of air. Manual techniques, such as chest physiotherapy with postural drainage, remain useful in resource-limited settings but are less effective for severe cases. For Sarah, MI-E could be prioritized to address her recurrent pneumonias, with caregiver training to ensure consistent home use. Positioning strategies, such as elevating the head of the bed to 30°, complement clearance efforts by reducing aspiration risk during sleep. Regular suctioning, using portable devices, is critical during acute episodes or for children with excessive drooling [4].

11.10 Nutritional Support

Oropharyngeal dysphagia and malnutrition, affecting 20–40% of children with CP, significantly exacerbate respiratory complications by weakening respiratory muscles and increasing infection susceptibility. Non-invasive strategies include thickened feeds (using starch or gum-based thickeners) to reduce aspiration risk, guided by swallow study results. Speech therapists may employ sensorimotor interventions, such as oral stimulation or thermal-tactile techniques, to improve swallowing coordination, with studies showing a 25% reduction in aspiration events after 6 months of therapy [20]. For severe OPD, as in Sarah's case, enteral feeding via gastrostomy or jejunostomy tubes ensures adequate caloric intake but requires careful consideration of caregiver burden and complications like tube dislodgement (10–15% incidence). Botulinum toxin injections into salivary glands can reduce drooling and salivary aspiration by 40–60%, offering a temporary (3–6 months) solution. For GERD, lifestyle modifications (e.g., smaller, frequent meals and upright positioning) are first-line, supplemented by prokinetics or proton pump inhibitors, though the latter may increase bacterial aspiration risk. Nutritional plans should target 100–120% of estimated energy needs to account for spasticity-related caloric demands [31].

11.11 Medical Management

Pharmacological interventions address infections, bronchospasm, and ventilatory support needs. For aspiration pneumonia, empiric antibiotics like amoxicillin-clavulanate cover common anaerobes and gram-negative pathogens, with a 7–10-day course recommended. In cases with Pseudomonas colonization, inhaled antibiotics (e.g., tobramycin) reduce recurrence by 30%, particularly in bronchiectasis [32]. Bronchodilators (e.g., albuterol) are trialed for wheezing, though response rates are lower in CP than in asthma (20% vs. 60%). Non-invasive ventilation (NIV), such as bilevel positive airway pressure (BiPAP), is a cornerstone for OSA and hypoventilation, improving AHI by 50–70% and reducing daytime fatigue. However, adherence is challenging due to mask discomfort, with only 60% of children tolerating long-term use. Supplemental oxygen is reserved for persistent hypoxia ($SpO_2 < 90\%$), guided by pulse oximetry [33]. Antiepileptics, like levetiracetam, should be optimized to minimize seizure-related aspiration, but side effects like sedation require monitoring. In Sarah's case, a trial of NIV and targeted antibiotics for her pneumonias would align with her OSA and infection history [34, 35].

11.12 Surgical Interventions

Surgical options are considered when non-invasive measures fail or complications are severe. Adenotonsillectomy is the primary treatment for OSA due to airway obstruction, reducing AHI by 60–80% in eligible cases, though postoperative risks (e.g., bleeding, airway edema) are higher in CP (10–15% complication rate) [36]. Uvulopalatopharyngoplasty is a secondary option for persistent OSA but carries similar risks. For refractory GERD, fundoplication reduces reflux volume but has a 10–20% failure rate in CP due to underlying dysmotility, requiring careful patient selection. Tracheostomy is reserved for chronic respiratory failure or severe airway obstruction, providing a stable airway but increasing caregiver burden and infection risk (20–30% complication rate). Scoliosis correction surgery may improve lung volumes in severe cases (Cobb angle >50°), with studies showing a 10–15% increase in FVC post-intervention, but it requires preoperative PFTs to assess risks. In Sarah's case, adenotonsillectomy may address her OSA, while fundoplication could be considered if GERD persists despite medical management [35, 37].

11.13 Preventive Measures

Vaccinations, hygiene, and monitoring prevent 30% of issues [25]. Pilot programs show action plans reduce admissions.

11.14 Insights for Other Specialists Involved in CP Care

- Neurologists: Optimize seizure control to cut aspiration by 25%; monitor meds for respiratory depression.
- Orthopedists: Preoperative PFTs for scoliosis surgery; strengthen core muscles via referral to prevent hypoventilation.
- Gastroenterologists: Prioritize reflux volume reduction over acid suppression to avoid bacterial risks.
- Rehabilitation: Integrate respiratory therapy (e.g., aquatic) for lung function gains.
- All: Screen microbiota in recurrent cases.

11.15 Key Information for Parents and Caregivers

- Monitor signs like coughing during feeds or snoring; early reporting prevents pneumonia.
- Use upright positioning for meals; thicken liquids if advised.
- Ensure annual vaccinations and dental care to reduce infections.
- Track growth; malnutrition worsens breathing—consult for supplements.
- Learn emergency signs (e.g., blue lips) and have a home plan.
- Join support groups; caregiver education cuts hospitalizations.

Untreated issues shorten life; regular check-ups extend it.

11.16 Conclusion

Respiratory complications in CP, as in Sarah's case, demand proactive, integrated care to enhance outcomes. Future directions include microbiota-targeted therapies and personalized prevention.

References

1. Shengyi Y, Jiayue X, Jing G, Lina W. Increasing prevalence of cerebral palsy among children and adolescents in China 1988–2020: a systematic review and meta-analysis. J Rehabil Med. 2021;53:2798.
2. Ryan JM, Albairami F, Hamilton T, Cope N, Amirmudin NA, Manikandan M, et al. Prevalence and incidence of chronic conditions among adults with cerebral palsy: a systematic review and meta-analysis. Dev Med Child Neurol. 2023;65:1174–89.
3. Spoto G, Accetta AS, Grella M, Di Modica I, Nicotera AG, Di Rosa G. Respiratory comorbidities and complications of cerebral palsy. Dev Neurorehabil. 2024;27:194–203.

4. Peneva P, Pancheva R, Nikolova SP. Unveiling respiratory challenges in cerebral palsy: a comprehensive review. Biomed Rev. 2023;34:121–32.
5. Kana CAN, Deugoue RB, Dongmo FN, Enyama D, Noukeu D, Mah E, et al. Comorbidities in children with cerebral palsy. Pediatr Oncall J. 2022;19:79–85.
6. Marpole RM, Blackmore AM, Wilson AC, Cooper MS, Depiazzi J, Langdon K, et al. Can respiratory hospital admissions in children with cerebral palsy be reduced? A feasibility randomized controlled trial (RESP-ACT). J Pediatr. 2025;287:114755.
7. Calderone A, Militi D, Cardile D, Corallo F, Calabrò RS, Militi A. Swallowing disorders in cerebral palsy: a systematic review of oropharyngeal dysphagia, nutritional impact, and health risks. Ital J Pediatr. 2025;51:57.
8. Peneva P, Pancheva R, Nikolova SP. Respiratory microbiota and health risks in children with cerebral palsy: a narrative review. Children (Basel). 2025;12:358.
9. Amer AR, Sobeih AA, Hekal HH. Respiratory complications in children with cerebral palsy. Benha Med J. 2024;41:233–45.
10. Gozal D. Sleep and breathing in children with cerebral palsy: it's complicated….! J Pediatr (English Edition). 2025;101:101434.
11. Novak I, Jackman M, Finch-Edmondson M, Fahey M. Cerebral palsy. Lancet. 2025;406:174–88.
12. Apostolou G, Cooper MS, Antolovich G, Vandeleur M, Frayman KB. The management of Pseudomonas aeruginosa respiratory infection in children with cerebral palsy: a narrative review. Pediatr Pulmonol. 2024;59:3170–7.
13. Marpole R, Blackmore AM, Gibson N, Cooper MS, Langdon K, Wilson AC. Evaluation and management of respiratory illness in children with cerebral palsy. Front Pediatr. 2020;8:333.
14. Abd Elmagid DS, Magdy H. Evaluation of risk factors for cerebral palsy. Egyptian J Neurol Psychiat Neurosurg. 2021;57:13.
15. Dias BLS, de Lima FM. Respiratory system impairments in children with cerebral palsy: outpatient surveillance, diagnosis, and treatment. Med Res Arch. 2021;9:2594.
16. Peneva P, Pancheva R, Nikolova S. Shedding light on respiratory problems in children with cerebral palsy. In: Medical science: recent advances and applications, vol. 2. BPI; 2025. p. 50–74.
17. Boel L, Pernet K, Toussaint M, Ides K, Leemans G, Haan J, et al. Respiratory morbidity in children with cerebral palsy: an overview. Dev Med Child Neurol. 2019;61:646–53.
18. Brandenburg JE, Fogarty MJ, Sieck GC. Why individuals with cerebral palsy are at higher risk for respiratory complications from COVID-19. J Pediatr Rehabil Med. 2020;13:317–27.
19. Garuti G, Verucchi E, Fanelli I, Giovannini M, Winck JC, Lusuardi M. Management of bronchial secretions with free aspire in children with cerebral palsy: impact on clinical outcomes and healthcare resources. Ital J Pediatr. 2016;42:7.
20. Kürtül Çakar M, Cinel G. The respiratory problems of patients with cerebral palsy requiring hospitalization: reasons and solutions. Pediatr Pulmonol. 2021;56:1626–34.
21. Blackmore AM, Gibson N, Cooper MS, Langdon K, Moshovis L, Wilson AC. Interventions for management of respiratory disease in young people with cerebral palsy: a systematic review. Child Care Health Dev. 2019;45:754–71.
22. Bax M. Diagnostic assessment of children with cerebral palsy. Lancet Neurol. 2004;3:395.
23. Knight Lozano R, Shannon H, Gilby J, Goddard S, Turner L, Marsden J. Community-based respiratory health measures in children and young people with cerebral palsy: a scoping review. Dev Med Child Neurol. 2024;66:849–62.
24. Novak I, Morgan C, Adde L, Blackman J, Boyd RN, Brunstrom-Hernandez J, et al. Early, accurate diagnosis and early intervention in cerebral palsy: advances in diagnosis and treatment. JAMA Pediatr. 2017;171:897–907.
25. Coller RJ, Singh-Verdeflor K, Eickhoff J, Chung PJ, Kloster HM, Cushing CC, et al. Preventing respiratory illness in cerebral palsy: results of a pilot randomized controlled trial. PLoS One. 2025;20:e0325970.
26. Graham D, Paget SP, Wimalasundera N. Current thinking in the health care management of children with cerebral palsy. Med J Aust. 2019;210:129–35.

27. Kolumbán E, Szabados M, Hernádfői M, Nguyen Do To U, Nagy R, Zolcsák Á, et al. Supplementary respiratory therapy improves pulmonary function in pediatric patients with cerebral palsy: a systematic review and meta-analysis. J Clin Med. 2024;13:888.
28. Gozal D. Sleep and breathing in children with cerebral palsy: it's complicated….! J Pediatr. 2025;101:101434.
29. Santoro A, Lang MBD, Moretti E, Sellari-Franceschini S, Orazini L, Cipriani P, et al. A proposed multidisciplinary approach for identifying feeding abnormalities in children with cerebral palsy. J Child Neurol. 2012;27:708–12.
30. Bear NL, Wilson A, Blackmore AM, Geelhoed E, Simpson S, Langdon K. The cost of respiratory hospitalizations in children with cerebral palsy. Dev Med Child Neurol. 2024;66:344–52.
31. Cieri ME, Brunner MMR, Condinanzi AL, Escobar J, Cuestas E. Nutritional status and dietary intake of children and adolescents with cerebral palsy. Clin Nutr ESPEN. 2023;57:391–8.
32. Fleischman A, Lerner C, Kloster H, Chung P, Klitzner T, Cushing C, et al. Adaptive intervention to prevent respiratory illness in cerebral palsy: protocol for a feasibility pilot randomized controlled trial. JMIR Res Protocols. 2024;13:e49705.
33. Carter B, Bennett CV, Jones H, Bethel J, Perra O, Wang T, Kemp A. Healthcare use by children and young adults with cerebral palsy. Dev Med Child Neurol. 2021;63:75–80.
34. Parris C, Todd H, Graham D. 227 respiratory health in cerebral palsy. BMJ; 2023.
35. Allen J, Zareen Z, Doyle S, Whitla L, Afzal Z, Stack M, et al. Multi-organ dysfunction in cerebral palsy. Front Pediatr. 2021;9:668544.
36. Vandendriessche E, Proesmans M, Ortibus E, Moens P. Complication rate after scoliosis surgery in children with cerebral palsy. Acta Orthop Belg. 2021;87:255–61.
37. Skertich NJ, Ingram M-CE, Sullivan GA, Grunvald M, Ritz E, Shah AN, Raval MV. Postoperative complications in pediatric patients with cerebral palsy. J Pediatr Surg. 2022;57:424–9.

Pain and Spasticity Management

12

Fatemeh Azizi and Nastaran Maghbouli

12.1 Case Vignette

Case Sam, a 10-year-old boy with cerebral palsy and tight legs, requiring daily care needs.

Sam uses a wheelchair and needs help with dressing and hygiene. Nights are broken by leg spasms, and diaper changes hurt. His legs feel very tight between the thighs and in the calves, and his feet tend to point down. An X-ray shows that one hip is beginning to dislocate.

What the family wants Less pain with care, better sleep, and easier mornings.

What the team does They take a stepwise approach: A small bedtime dose of a muscle relaxant; tiny amounts of botulinum toxin injected into the tight, inner-thigh and calf muscles (guided by ultrasound) to relax them for a few months; 3 weeks of gentle stretching with a series of lightweight casts; a refit of his ankle braces; and simple changes to night-time positioning. The family uses a simple 0–10 "faces" scale once a day to track pain and a brief list of home activities when the muscles are most relaxed.

What changes By 8 weeks, his pain during diapering decreases from about 7/10 to 2–3/10, and he sleeps through most nights. His hips and ankles move more comfort-

F. Azizi
Center for Orthopedic Trans-Disciplinary Applied Research, Tehran University of Medical Sciences, Tehran, Iran
e-mail: Azizi-f@alumnus.tums.ac.ir

N. Maghbouli (✉)
Department of Physical Medicine and Rehabilitation, School of Medicine, Shariati Hospital, Tehran University of Medical Sciences, Tehran, Iran
e-mail: nmaghbouli@sina.tums.ac.ir

A. Presedo et al. (eds.), *Enhancing Quality of Life in Patients with Cerebral Palsy*, https://doi.org/10.1007/978-3-032-20967-2_12

ably, and the braces no longer rub against them. At 6 months, the hip X-ray is stable. The team and family discuss future options if pain or tightness returns, including a small implanted pump that can deliver tiny doses of muscle-relaxing medicine directly to the spinal fluid.

12.2 Introduction

Injury to the developing brain can lead to a group of permanent disorders known as cerebral palsy (CP). This occurs in approximately two to three out of every 1000 live births. The most prominent characteristics are motor impairments and balance disorders, followed by pain, intellectual disabilities, inability to walk, hip displacement, speech, vision, and heterogeneous neurological disorders [1, 2]. Motor impairments may present as spasticity, dyskinesia, or ataxia, with spasticity being the most prevalent type of cerebral palsy, accounting for 80% of cases [3].

Spasticity is marked by "velocity-dependent increase in muscle tone with exaggerated tendon jerks, resulting from hyperexcitability of the stretch reflex," as one component of the upper motoneuron syndrome (UMNS) [4]. It can be classified as quadriplegic, hemiplegic, diplegic, and monoplegic. These can lead to several comorbidities, such as improper weight bearing and gait disorders, hip subluxation and dislocation, spinal deformities such as scoliosis, inability to use upper limbs for daily activities, and, most commonly, pain (75%) [5]. There is an interplay between spasticity and pain. Sustained abnormal posture, muscle spasm, joint strains, muscle weakness, and contracture can cause pain. Notably, the constant pain sensation may also lead to or exacerbate the spasticity and its management. Due to communication impairments, pain can be left undiagnosed and untreated [6].

Physical (PT) and occupational therapy (OT), oral medications such as baclofen, benzodiazepines, and tizanidine, Botulinum toxin type A (BoNT-A) injection into the contractured muscles, serial casting and orthotics, and dorsal rhizotomy are common treatment plans for spasticity and pain management [7].

Given the complex and interconnected nature of spasticity and pain, effective management necessitates a comprehensive and integrated strategy. Therefore, a coordinated multidisciplinary approach becomes paramount. In this chapter, we will synthesize the current understanding of spasticity and pain and present a comprehensive range of multidisciplinary management strategies.

12.3 Understanding Spasticity in CP

12.3.1 Pathophysiology of Spasticity

12.3.1.1 Neural Basis: Upper Motor Neuron Lesion, Disinhibition, Hyperexcitability of Stretch Reflexes

There is a widely used definition for spasticity proposed by Lance in 1980: "*motor disorder characterized by a velocity-dependent increase in the tonic stretch reflex (muscle tone) with exaggerated tendon jerks, resulting from hyperexcitability of the stretch reflex, as one component of the upper motor neurone syndrome.*" In other words, spasticity prevents the muscle from properly stretching or lengthening, especially in faster muscle movements [8]. In 2005, Pandyan et al. proposed an updated definition, arguing that the manifestations of spasticity extend beyond solely the hyperexcitability of the stretch reflex and can be observed in both active and passive conditions. Their updated version, "*disordered sensori-motor control, resulting from an upper motor neuron lesion, presenting as intermittent or sustained involuntary activation of muscles,*" offers a broader, more clinically encompassing perspective of hypertonia in the upper motor neuron syndrome [9]. However, Lance's definition remains a foundational reference, particularly for its precision in describing the physiological reflex component of spasticity.

Spasticity in CP arises from a lesion in the developing brain that disrupts the complex interplay of descending pathways. Specifically, this involves a loss of balance between critical descending inhibitory control, primarily mediated by the dorsal reticulospinal tract, and excitatory pathways to the spinal cord, such as the facilitatory medial reticulospinal and vestibulospinal tracts. This leads to an overactive spinal reflex arc, manifesting as the characteristic signs of spasticity. Furthermore, the specific clinical pattern and manifestation of spasticity often depend on the precise location and extent of the lesion. The specific pattern of spasticity (e.g., antigravity posture or paraplegia in extension vs. flexion) depends on which specific inhibitory or facilitatory pathways are most affected at different spinal cord levels. This helps explain the heterogeneity of spasticity in CP. Loss of inhibitory influences (especially from the dorsal reticulospinal tract) can lead to the "release" of flexor reflexes, resulting in prominent flexor spasms and phenomena like the clasp-knife reflex. Notably, there is also a flaccid weakness period before the initiation of the spasticity. This initial flaccidity underscores the dynamic and evolving nature of motor impairments following early brain injury, preceding the development of spasticity as chronic neural reorganization progresses [10].

12.3.1.2 Contribution of Peripheral Factors: Muscle Length Changes, Contractures

While spasticity originates from a lesion in the central nervous system, its chronic presence often leads to significant secondary changes within the muscles and connective tissues, ultimately resulting in muscle contracture. Muscle contracture is a common phenomenon observed in CP patients. This leads to a reduced range of motion (ROM) in the joint, stiffness in the affected muscles, and loss of flexibility. The long-term effects of BoNT-A injection, which primarily targets muscle tone and spasticity, often reveal few or insignificant improvements in established joint range of motion. This clinical observation suggests that while spasticity contributes to their formation, established contractures involve complex, independent structural changes within the muscle and surrounding soft tissues, necessitating targeted interventions beyond reducing spasticity alone [11]. A cohort of 359 CP children aged 2–14 years showed a decrease of nine degrees in hip abduction, 17° in hip external rotation, 25° in popliteal angle, 6° in knee extension, and 10° in dorsiflexion (which was primarily developed under 5 years of age, and remained the same after that period) over time [12].

Skeletal muscle consists of long bundles called fibers, which are comprised of myofibers with myofibril strands. Contractile units along the length of the fibers, called sarcomeres, comprise two protein filaments named actin and myosin. The sarcomeres provide the myofibers' length and cross-sectional area, producing the muscle force together. Children with typical development (TD) have both cross-sectional and longitudinal myofiber growth [13]. In CP patients, the sarcomeres are overlengthened and decreased in number (40% lower); the cross-sectional area and muscle volume are reduced, and muscle-tendon units (MTUs) are relatively shorter, with longer tendons and shorter muscle sections [14, 15]. It is also known that there is a highly significant positive correlation between the length of the sarcomeres and the intensity of contracture [16].

Muscle development and regeneration require specific stem cells known as satellite cells. CP patients have fewer of these cells than TD children, especially in spastic forms, indicating a reduced capacity for muscle regeneration [17, 18].

Collectively, these structural and cellular alterations in the muscle contribute significantly to the increased passive stiffness, reduced extensibility, and diminished functional capacity observed in individuals with spastic CP, even in the absence of active neural overactivity.

12.3.2 Clinical Manifestations and Assessment of Spasticity

12.3.2.1 Clinical Presentation: Varying Degrees, Specific Muscle Groups, Impact on Gait, Posture, and Function

The Gross Motor Function Classification System (GMFCS) is a frequently used scale for CP classification, categorizing individuals based on their self-initiated movement and daily functional abilities [19]. Level I patients are independently ambulatory with minor balance impairments, while level V patients lack neck control and require consistent assistance for daily living. A large-scale study of 3312 CP patients found that nearly 60% can walk independently (GMFCS Levels I and II), 11% use aids and instruments for walking (Level III), and 29% rely on wheelchairs for mobility (Levels IV and V) [14, 20].

Clinically, spasticity manifests as increased muscle tone, exaggerated deep tendon reflexes, clonus, and impaired selective motor control (the inability to isolate movement at a single joint). Spastic cerebral palsy, which accounts for approximately 85% of cases, presents with varying degrees of severity and distribution across the body [21]. Bilateral spastic CP, the most common subtype (45–70% of cases, particularly in preterm patients), primarily affects the lower limbs, often manifesting as paraplegia or asymmetric bilateral patterns. Common lower limb presentations include toe walking and equinus gait due to calf muscle spasticity and dorsiflexion restrictions, as well as crouch gait characterized by persistent knee and hip flexion with excessive ankle dorsiflexion. These abnormal gait patterns significantly increase the energy expenditure during walking, reduce walking speed and efficiency, and compromise balance, increasing the risk of falls. This Spasticity also profoundly influences posture, leading to sustained abnormal positioning such as hip adduction and internal rotation, knee flexion, ankle equinus, and trunk stiffness. These fixed postures can impede maintaining sitting balance, executing transfers, and achieving optimal standing alignment, often contributing to secondary orthopedic complications, such as hip dislocations and spinal deformities like scoliosis [22, 23]. Unilateral spastic CP (hemiparesis) presents with increased reflexes and various deformities primarily on one side of the body. In this type, the upper limb is more frequently affected than the lower limb. Upper limb involvement typically includes elbow flexion, wrist flexion, forearm pronation, and a fisted hand posture, severely limiting fine motor skills, reach, grasp, and overall manipulation. Consequently, tasks requiring bimanual coordination or precise hand movements become challenging [24, 25]. The gastrocnemius, hamstrings, quadriceps, hip adductors, knee, and ankle muscles are the most commonly affected lower limb muscles, while flexors and shoulder muscles are predominantly affected in the upper limb [21]. Beyond motor impairments, individuals with spastic CP may also experience various comorbidities, such as epilepsy, intellectual disorders, and linguistic and communicational problems, which can further impact their functional abilities and quality of life [26]. Finally, spastic CP can be categorized according to the neuromuscular type of impairment, which provides a more granular understanding of the underlying challenges: (1) muscle weakness, (2) short muscle tendon units (contractures), (3) muscle spasticity, and (4) impaired selective motor control (SMC) [21].

12.3.2.2 Assessment Tools

Tools are listed and explained in Table 12.1.

12.3.2.3 Impact of Spasticity on Function and Quality of Life

Spasticity significantly affects motor function, which causes a chain reaction of physical problems. It often results in characteristic gait deviations such as toe-walking (equinus gait), scissoring gait (adductor spasticity), and crouch gait (hamstring and hip flexor spasticity). These abnormal patterns lead to increased energy expenditure, reduced walking speed and efficiency, impaired balance, and a higher risk of falls [36]. Spasticity profoundly influences the ability to maintain and adjust postures. It can lead to sustained abnormal positioning of limbs and trunk, affecting sitting, balance, challenging transfers from one position to another, and hindering optimal standing alignment. Chronic abnormal postures also contribute to the development of fixed orthopedic deformities (contracture, scoliosis, pelvic obliquity, windswept hip, and hip dislocation) [37].

In the upper limbs, spasticity commonly manifests as elbow flexion, wrist flexion, forearm pronation, and fisted hand postures. These impairments affect reach, grasp, and manipulation skills, significantly limiting the ability to perform precise, coordinated movements required for Activities of Daily Living (ADL) like writing, dressing, eating, brushing, moving objects, hygiene, and other necessary daily tasks [38].

Table 12.1 Spasticity assessment tools

Assessment tool	What it measures?	Brief description	Strengths/advantages	Limitations/challenges	Clinical relevance/ purpose
Modified Ashworth Scale (MAS) [27]	Resistance to passive movement (muscle tone)	Passively move the joint through full ROM, score on a 0–5 scale	Simple, quick, widely recognized	Subjective, poor reliability for subtle changes, doesn't distinguish neural from mechanical stiffness [28]	Quick clinical assessment, general monitoring
Tardieu Scale (or Modified Tardieu Scale—MTS) [29]	Velocity-dependent resistance, catch angle (R1-R2)	Move joint at different velocities (slow, fast) to determine angles	Differentiates dynamic spasticity from fixed contracture; more objective than MAS [30]	More complex, requires training, still some subjectivity	Guiding interventions (e.g., BoNT-A injections), surgical planning
Electrophysiological Measures (e.g., H-reflex, F-wave, EMG) [31]	Neural excitability, reflex pathways, muscle activation patterns	Electrical stimulation and recording of muscle activity	Objective, quantitative, sensitive to neural changes, can differentiate reflex mechanisms	Requires specialized equipment and expertise; can be uncomfortable; primarily research tools	Research, understanding underlying mechanisms, specific diagnostic questions
Pendulum test (Wartenberg test) [32]	Stimulating the muscle stretch reflex	Passive swinging of the lower leg	Simple, quick, reproducible	Subjective, depending on muscle relaxation and sitting position.	Quick clinical assessment and spasticity degree recognition
Australian Spasticity Assessment Scale (ASAS)	Velocity-dependent increased rapid response	Rapid passive movements at different velocities to determine spasticity, score on 0–4 scale	Simple, easy, quick, reproducible	Results might be affected if the procedure is done after other spasticity assessments.	Quick clinical assessment, general monitoring
Acoustic radiation force impulse elastography (ARFI) [33]	Spatial differences in tissue spasticity and elasticity	Images made by ultrasound scanning and shear wave velocity (SWV)	Safe, reliable, objective, quantitative, non-invasive	Requires specialized equipment and expertise	Research, understanding underlying mechanisms, specific diagnostic questions

Assessment tool	What it measures?	Brief description	Strengths/advantages	Limitations/challenges	Clinical relevance/ purpose
Real-time sonoelastography (RTS) [34]	Real-time elasticity assessment	Assessing strain ratio using an ultrasound device	Simple, practical, non-invasive	Imprecise outcomes, limited interoperator reproducibility	Research, understanding underlying mechanisms
Functional Scales (e.g., GMFM—Gross Motor Function Measure) [35]	Gross motor function and capabilities	Observational assessment of motor tasks (sitting, standing, walking, etc.)	Standardized, validated, reliable, directly assesses functional abilities, sensitive to change over time, and patient-centered	Time-consuming; requires trained administrators; does not directly measure spasticity itself	Tracking progress in rehabilitation, evaluating intervention effectiveness, research, and team communication

Apart from the burden of the physical abnormalities and the associated limitations, children with spastic CP may consequently develop several mental issues, such as depression, anxiety, and self-injurious behaviors, which need extensive supervision and care [39].

12.4 Understanding Pain in Cerebral Palsy

12.4.1 Prevalence and Characteristics of Pain in CP

Pain is a highly prevalent and often debilitating co-occurring condition in individuals with CP, significantly impacting their daily lives and overall well-being. Its occurrence is widespread across the lifespan, from childhood into adulthood. Its prevalence ranges from 14% to 76%, considering the possibility of undiagnosed cases due to the low age and communication disorders they might have. The pain is higher in older ages, females, and GMFM class V. Most frequently reported pain sites are the lower limbs, head, back, abdomen, and upper limbs [40]. Primary causes of pain are known to be driven by hip dislocation or subluxation, dystonia, MSK deformities (foot and hand deformities, scoliosis, and lumbar lordosis), constipation, focal muscle spasm, muscle weakness, fatigue or overuse, spasticity, abnormal gait, contracture, post-orthopedic surgical pain, and gastroesophageal reflux [41].

12.4.2 Assessment of Pain in CP

12.4.2.1 Challenges of Pain Assessment

Pain in CP is complex, with several factors influencing the location and intensity of the pain experienced. The communication and intellectual problems also make diagnosing and assessing the pain more complicated. Effective pain assessment is essential because pain adversely impacts quality of life and restricts participation in daily activities [41].

12.4.2.2 Primary Approaches to Pain Assessment

Parents and caregivers are the primary observers of pain, noticing the child's daily behavior and changes, especially for nonverbal children or those with intellectual disabilities who may struggle with self-reporting. Caregivers' interpretation of pain in nonverbal children may include poor feeding, facial expressions, irritability, crying upon movement (such as diaper changing), and nighttime awakenings [41].

When children and youth are able to self-report, it is considered the gold standard for pain measurement. The physician may also recognize pain behavior during the primary clinical assessment and prescribe analgesics as a first-line treatment [42].

12.4.2.3 Assessment Tools

Pain assessment scales can be categorized into Patient-Reported Outcome Measures (PROMs, or self-report tools) and Observer-Reported Outcome Measures (ObsROMs) (or proxy-report). Table 12.2 describes the most commonly used scales, briefly mentioning their purpose, strengths, limitations, and clinical relevance [43–45].

12.4.2.4 Importance of History Taking and Physical Examination

Detailed history is essential, especially from caregivers who can identify subtle changes in behavior or routine. Such histories often provide the first and best clues to pain, particularly in individuals who struggle to communicate verbally. This includes perinatal, birth, intensive care unit records, developmental milestones, surgical records, medications, rehabilitation sessions' information, and current functional abilities [46].

Children with cerebral palsy are at risk of worsening musculoskeletal problems, so physical exams need to be done at different periods of time, depending on the patient's specific conditions. For movement abilities, a five-level classification system is typically used, which is covered in Sect. 3.2.1. This primarily addresses the dynamic assessment, while other tests should also be used to evaluate static responses, such as muscle tone, joint range of motion, and contracture. These tests help evaluate the condition's severity, inform treatment planning, and determine if surgery or interventions will be needed in the future. They also help track progress and detect any worsening of the condition [47].

Table 12.2 Pain assessment tools

Assessment tool	What it measures?	Brief description	Strengths/advantages	Limitations/challenges	Clinical relevance/ purpose
Faces Pain Scale-Revised (FPS-R)	Self-reported pain intensity	Child points to the face that best describes their pain (0–10 scale, faces range from happy to crying)	Visually intuitive, good for children 4–12 years, minimal cognitive demand	Relies on self-report, may not be suitable for non-verbal or severely cognitively impaired	Common for self-report in verbal children
FLACC Scale (Face, Legs, Activity, Cry, Consolability)	Observational pain assessment	The clinician observes and scores 5 behavioral categories (0–2 for each, totaling 0–10)	Suitable for non-verbal or cognitively impaired children (infants to adolescents); widely used	Subjective interpretation can be influenced by non-pain factors (e.g., hunger, fatigue)	Post-operative pain, acute pain, in children with communication difficulties
Wong-Baker FACES Pain Rating Scale	Self-reported pain intensity	Similar to FPS-R, uses a series of faces with expressions	Popular, intuitive for children, adaptable for various ages	Similar limitations to FPS-R for non-verbal/ cognitively impaired; cultural variations in facial expression interpretation	General pain assessment in children (often 3 years and up)
Visual Analogue Scale (VAS)	Self-reported pain intensity	The patient marks a point on a 10 cm line representing the severity of their pain	Sensitive to small changes, good for research	Requires fine motor skills; harder for young children or those with motor/ cognitive impairments	Older children, adolescents, adults, often in research settings
Pediatric Pain Profile (PPP)	Observational pain assessment	A 20-item behavioral rating scale. Parents rate the behavior at the child's best, and at the pain	Valid for use with people who have significant cognitive and communication limitations who are unable to self-report their pain experience. High test-retest reliability	Very low quality of evidence for cross-cultural validity	Children with severe CP and other neurological conditions, unable to communicate

Assessment tool	What it measures?	Brief description	Strengths/advantages	Limitations/challenges	Clinical relevance/ purpose
Non-Communicating Child's Pain Checklist-Revised (NCCPC-R)	Observational pain assessment	The parent observes the child, during a time period of pain and without pain	Rated as high for internal consistency and has content validity	Less feasible for clinical use due to its length and the complexity of the scoring system	Children with severe CP and other neurological conditions, unable to communicate
11-Point Numeric Rating Scale (NRS-11)	Self-reported pain intensity	Rating the past 24 h pain intensity from 0 to 10	Easy, quick, sufficient structural validity	It was rated as "insufficient" for hypotheses testing for construct validity. The quality of evidence for its properties is very low	It may be an option for routine pain intensity assessment in a subgroup of individuals with CP, but requires further psychometric testing
21-Point Numeric Rating Scale (NRS-21)	Self-reported pain intensity	A list of 21 numbers (0–100 in multiples of 5) representing the average pain intensity in the past 24 h	Easy, quick, and rated as sufficient for structural validity and hypothesis testing for construct validity	Low quality of evidence for its measurement properties	It may be an option for routine pain intensity assessment in a subgroup of individuals with CP, but requires further psychometric testing
5-Point Verbal Rating Scale (VRS-5)	Self-reported pain intensity	Five pain intensity levels: "none," "mild," "moderate," "severe," and "very severe." indicating the average pain over the past 24 h	Easy, quick, rated as sufficient for structural validity	Rated as "insufficient" for hypothesis testing for construct validity. The quality of evidence for its measurement properties is low	It may be an option for routine pain intensity assessment in a subgroup of individuals with CP, but requires further psychometric testing

(continued)

Table 12.2 (continued)

Assessment tool	What it measures?	Brief description	Strengths/advantages	Limitations/challenges	Clinical relevance/ purpose
16-Point Verbal Rating Scale (VRS-16)	Self-reported pain intensity	Sixteen descriptors represent different levels of pain intensity in the past 24 h	Easy, quick, and rated as sufficient for structural validity and hypotheses testing for construct validity	The quality of evidence for its measurement properties is low	It may be an option for routine pain intensity assessment in a subgroup of individuals with CP, but requires further psychometric testing
Adapted Chronic Pain Grade (adapted CPG)	Pain interference with daily activities, social activities, and work	A 3-item questionnaire scored from 0 (“no interference”) to 10 (“unable to carry out activities”)	It addresses pain-associated disability	Rated as “insufficient” for internal consistency and hypothesis testing. The quality of evidence for its measurement properties is low	It aims to capture the impact of pain on daily life for individuals with CP
10-item Interference Scale adapted from the Brief Pain Inventory (adapted BPI)	Interference of pain with activities over the past week (e.g., general activity, mood, mobility, sleep, self-care, social)	Includes 10 items scored from 0 (“does not interfere”) to 10 (“completely interferes”)	Addresses pain-associated disability. Rated as sufficient for internal consistency and hypothesis testing with high feasibility	The quality of evidence for its measurement properties is low. No validation of the changes from the original BPI was conducted. Its validity for people with CP has not been tested	It aims to evaluate pain interference with a broader scope of activities for individuals with CP. It has good feasibility for routine clinical use

Assessment tool	What it measures?	Brief description	Strengths/advantages	Limitations/challenges	Clinical relevance/ purpose
Questionnaire on Pain caused by Spasticity (QPS)—Self-report module	Spasticity-related pain at rest, during daily activities, active mobilization, and self-defined physically difficult activity	Contains 12 items with a 6-point response scale (0 "no hurt" to 10 "hurts worst"). It is designed for children/adolescents (2–17 years) experiencing limb spasticity-related pain	One of the few instruments with specific modules for different administrations (self-report, interview-administered, observer-report). Obtained a "sufficient" rating for content validity and reliability. It has moderate quality evidence for reliability and internal consistency (for interview and observer modules)	Internal consistency was rated "insufficient" for the self-report module. Hypothesis testing was rated "insufficient". Structural validity was rated "indeterminate". The overall quality of evidence ranges from very low to moderate	It is designed to specifically assess spasticity-related pain in children and adolescents with CP
Pain Assessment Instrument for Cerebral Palsy (PAICP)	Pain in patients with CP and hip problems	Includes 21 items/ drawings, with sections for preliminary introduction, daily situations (not painful, usually painful), and situations specifically painful for those with hip problems. It utilizes a 1–7 faces pain scale	Hypothesis testing was rated as "sufficient"	Internal consistency was rated "indeterminate," and reliability was rated "insufficient". The overall quality of evidence is very low	It is a tool specifically designed for assessing pain in patients with CP who have hip problems

(continued)

Table 12.2 (continued)

Assessment tool	What it measures?	Brief description	Strengths/advantages	Limitations/challenges	Clinical relevance/purpose
Bath Adolescent Pain Questionnaire (BAPQ)—Self-report	Impact of pain on: emotional wellbeing, physical abilities, participation, quality of life	A questionnaire designed for adolescents with chronic pain	Categorized as a pain interference tool with strong measurement properties and high feasibility	Some of the items require minor modifications for use with non-ambulant young patients. Content validity has "low" quality evidence. It has not been specifically validated for CP population	It assesses the comprehensive impact of chronic pain on adolescents, including functional aspects
Brief Pain Inventory (BPI)/Modified Brief Pain Inventory (m-BPI)—Self-report	Pain location, pain intensity, changeable factors, impact on emotional wellbeing, physical abilities, participation, quality of life, sleep	It is a comprehensive pain assessment tool	Good feasibility for routine clinical use. Categorized as a pain interference tool. It has "high" quality evidence for construct validity	Its validity for people with CP has not been tested. Some versions may need support for augmentative and alternative communication (AAC)	It provides a broad assessment of pain and its interference in daily life
Child Activity Limitations Interview (CALI-21)—Self-report	Impact of pain on physical abilities and participation	This is a 21-item questionnaire	It is categorized as a pain interference tool with strong measurement properties and high feasibility	Some of its items are not appropriate for people unable to ambulate	It assesses activity limitations experienced by children and adolescents due to chronic pain

Assessment tool	What it measures?	Brief description	Strengths/advantages	Limitations/challenges	Clinical relevance/ purpose
Cerebral Palsy Quality of Life Questionnaire—child version (CP QoL-child)—Self-report	Pain intensity, impact on emotional well-being	It is a condition-specific measure of quality of life for children with CP	It has content validity for CP	Considered less feasible for clinical use due to its length and complexity of scoring. Contains items requiring cognitive and functional skills that may not be present in some cases. It has "low" quality evidence for structural validity, internal consistency, reliability, and construct validity	It can be useful for research purposes, such as assessing surgical outcomes
Cerebral Palsy Quality of Life Questionnaire—teen version (CP QoL-teen)—self-report	Pain intensity, impact on emotional well-being, participation, quality of life	It is a quality-of-life questionnaire for adolescents with CP	It has content validity for CP	Same as for CP Qol-child	It can be useful for research purposes, such as assessing surgical outcomes

(continued)

Table 12.2 (continued)

Assessment tool	What it measures?	Brief description	Strengths/advantages	Limitations/challenges	Clinical relevance/ purpose
Fear of Pain Questionnaire (FOPQ)—Child Self-report	Impact on emotional well-being, physical abilities, and participation. It assesses pain-related fear	This questionnaire assesses fear of pain	Categorized as a pain coping tool with the strongest measurement properties and highest feasibility among coping tools. It has "moderate" quality evidence for content and structural validity, internal consistency, and construct validity	Needs modifications to improve ease of understanding and for use in complex communicational disorders. It has not been specifically validated in CP	It helps identify fear-avoidant behavior related to pain
Functional Disability Inventory (FDI)	Impact on physical abilities, participation, and sleep	It assesses difficulty with regular activities due to sickness or not feeling well	It showed greatest mapping with ICF (International Classification of Functioning, Disability and Health) core sets among measures. It is considered feasible. It was identified as addressing the impact of chronic pain on day-to-day functional abilities	Its content validity has "low" quality evidence. Some items may not be appropriate for people unable to ambulate	It helps assess the impact of pain on daily functional abilities, which is crucial for comprehensive pain management
Graded Chronic Pain Scale (GCPS)/ Revised (GCPS-R)	Pain frequency, pain intensity, impact on physical abilities, participation, and quality of life	It is used to measure and classify chronic pain grade	It is considered feasible. It has "high" quality evidence for reliability and construct validity	It has "moderate" quality evidence for content validity and structural validity. It has not been specifically validated in CP	It is used to classify chronic pain by intensity and disability

Assessment tool	What it measures?	Brief description	Strengths/advantages	Limitations/challenges	Clinical relevance/ purpose
Pain Anxiety Symptom Scale (PASS-20)	Impact on emotional well-being, physical abilities. It measures pain anxiety symptoms	This scale assesses symptoms of pain anxiety	It has "high" quality evidence for structural validity, internal consistency, and construct validity	It has poor feasibility for complex communication needs (unable to use with AAC). Its content validity has "very low" quality evidence. It has not been specifically validated in CP	It helps in assessing the level of anxiety experienced in relation to pain
Pain Burden Inventory—Youth (PBI-Y)—Self-report	Pain frequency, impact on emotional well-being, participation, physical abilities, and sleep	It is a self-reported tool that assesses the burden of pain	It is considered feasible. It has "moderate" quality evidence for content validity	It has "very low" quality evidence for internal consistency and construct validity. It has not been specifically validated in CP	It quantifies the overall burden of chronic pain experienced by young people
Pain Catastrophizing Scale (PCS)—Self-report	Impact on emotional well-being. It measures catastrophizing thoughts about pain	This scale assesses how an individual's thoughts exaggerate the threat or negative aspects of pain	It is considered feasible. It has "moderate" quality evidence for internal consistency and construct validity	It has "very low" quality evidence for content validity. It has not been specifically validated in CP	It helps understand the cognitive-affective responses to pain that can influence pain experience

(continued)

Table 12.2 (continued)

Assessment tool	What it measures?	Brief description	Strengths/advantages	Limitations/challenges	Clinical relevance/ purpose
Pain Coping Questionnaire (PCQ)—Self-report/Short Form	Impact on emotional well-being, physical abilities. It assesses coping strategies for pain	This questionnaire explores various ways individuals deal with their pain	It is categorized as a pain-coping tool with the strongest measurement properties and the highest feasibility among coping tools	It needs modifications to improve ease of understanding and for use with young people who have complex communication needs. It has "low" quality evidence for content validity, structural validity, reliability, construct validity, and responsiveness. It has not been specifically validated in CP	It helps understand how individuals manage their pain and identifies areas where coping skills might be improved
Pain Interference Index (PII)	How pain interferes with everyday life (e.g., school, activities, friends, mood, mobility, sleep)	It contains six statements about pain interference, with responses indicating the degree of interference on a numerical scale (0 = "not at all" to 6 = "very much")	It is a validated questionnaire translated into Swedish. It gives valuable information. It showed higher interference in children with pain, particularly for sleep, school work, and being with friends. It emphasizes assessing interference beyond just intensity and location	Some of its items are not appropriate for people unable to ambulate. It has "low" quality evidence for reliability, responsiveness, and construct validity	It explores the impact of pain on functional aspects of daily life, which is crucial for comprehensive pain management

Assessment tool	What it measures?	Brief description	Strengths/advantages	Limitations/challenges	Clinical relevance/ purpose
Pediatric Pain Screening Tool (PPST)	Pain location, pain frequency, impact on emotional well-being, physical abilities, participation, quality of life, and sleep	It is designed for the rapid identification of risk in youth with pain complaints	It has good feasibility for routine clinical use. It has "high" quality evidence for structural validity, internal consistency, reliability, construct validity, and responsiveness	Its validity for people with CP has not been tested. Some items are not appropriate for people unable to ambulate. It needs support for AAC	It serves as a quick screening tool for pain and its multidimensional impact
Pediatric Quality of Life- Cerebral Palsy Module (Peds QL-CP module)—Self-report	Pain location, pain intensity, and impact on sleep	It is a module designed to measure the quality of life in pediatric cerebral palsy	It has content validity for CP. It has "high" quality evidence for reliability and construct validity	It has "very low" quality evidence for structural validity and internal consistency. Some items are not appropriate for people unable to ambulate. It needs support for AAC	It assesses pain within the broader context of quality of life for children with CP
Pediatric Outcomes Data Collection Inventory (PODCI)—Self-report	Pain intensity, impact on participation, and physical abilities	This tool is part of a broader measure of health status and function	It showed the greatest mapping with ICF core sets among reviewed measures. It was identified as addressing the impact of chronic pain on day-to-day functional abilities	It is unclear if it supports AAC, and it may be difficult to use with AAC. It has "low" quality evidence for content validity, structural validity, internal consistency, construct validity, cross-cultural validity, and responsiveness	It is useful for comprehensively capturing functional information related to experiencing chronic pain

(continued)

Table 12.2 (continued)

Assessment tool	What it measures?	Brief description	Strengths/advantages	Limitations/challenges	Clinical relevance/ purpose
PROMIS Pediatric Pain Interference (PROMIS-PIS) item bank/short form (8a)—Self-report	Impact on emotional well-being, physical abilities, participation, quality of life, and sleep	This item bank is designed to measure pain interference	It has high-quality evidence for content validity (though primarily in non-CP populations). It has "high" quality evidence for reliability. It is categorized as a pain interference tool with strong measurement properties and high feasibility	Some items are not appropriate for people unable to ambulate. It needs support for AAC. It has "moderate" quality evidence for structural validity and internal consistency. It has "low" quality evidence for responsiveness	It aims to assess the impact of pain on daily life activities and general well-being
Psychological Inflexibility in Pain scale	Impact on participation, physical abilities. It measures psychological inflexibility related to pain	This scale assesses an individual's psychological flexibility in the context of pain	It has "high" quality evidence for structural validity and internal consistency	It has poor feasibility for complex communication needs (unable to use with AAC). It has "very low" quality evidence for content validity. It has not been specifically validated in CP	It assesses psychological factors that can influence the experience and management of pain
Pain Vigilance and Awareness Questionnaire (PVAQ)—Self-report	Impact on emotional well-being and changeable factors (what helps/doesn't help with pain). It measures vigilance and awareness of pain	This questionnaire measures the degree to which an individual focuses attention on pain	It is considered feasible. It has "moderate" quality evidence for structural validity, internal consistency, and construct validity	It has "very low" quality evidence for content validity. It has not been specifically validated in CP	It helps understand how much attention is paid to pain sensations, which can influence pain perception and coping

12.5 Management of Spasticity

12.5.1 General Principles

The overarching philosophy for managing spasticity in cerebral palsy is to approach it from a patient-centered and goal-oriented perspective. Management is not about simply reducing a score on a spasticity scale; it's about improving an individual's function, comfort, and overall quality of life. This requires a flexible and integrated strategy guided by three core principles: goal setting, an individualized approach, and ongoing reassessment [48].

12.5.1.1 Goal Setting

Setting goals before treatment planning is crucial, as it helps establish a clear purpose for the intervention and enables tracking of the patient's condition over time. This can be set into three principles:

1. Functional goals: These are aimed at improving a person's ability to perform daily activities, considering real-world tasks [48]. For example, a goal might be to improve a child's ability to walk a short distance with better balance, grasp an object more easily for schoolwork, or enable a teenager to dress themselves independently.
2. Comfort Goals: These focus on reducing pain, preventing complications, and enhancing well-being. A key goal might be to reduce painful spasms, alleviate discomfort caused by abnormal posturing, or improve sleep comfort [49].
3. Caregiver Goals: Acknowledge that spasticity management often significantly impacts caregivers. A goal might be to make it easier to transfer a patient, perform hygiene, or dress them. [50].

12.5.1.2 Individualized Approach

Every person with CP is unique. Their spasticity will vary in severity, location, and its impact on their life. The treatment plan should be tailored based on the individual's age and developmental stage, their gross motor function classification system (GMFCS) level, the specific muscle groups affected, and the presence of comorbidities such as pain, contractures, or other movement disorders. By using this approach, we can tailor a treatment plan that's most effective for each individual, taking into account their unique priorities [49].

12.5.1.3 Ongoing Reassessment

Spasticity and its consequences can change over time due to growth, aging, and the effects of interventions. Reassessment is crucial for monitoring the effectiveness of interventions, adjusting the treatment plan (which may require changes in medications, rehabilitation plans, or considering a new approach), and setting new goals after reaching a milestone. This may include radiographic hip and spine examinations as needed, reevaluation of GMFCS, muscle tone, passive ROM, positioning, pain, spasticity, and the efficacy of the patient's assistive devices [51, 52].

12.5.2 Non-pharmacological Interventions

Interventions like physical therapy, occupational therapy, and assistive devices are explored in greater detail in the Chap. 6. However, we'll cover each topic briefly here to help better understand spasticity and pain management.

12.5.2.1 Physical Therapy

Stretching

Stretching is a fundamental component of physical therapy for managing spasticity in cerebral palsy (CP). It aims to lengthen tight muscles and connective tissues, thereby reducing muscle tone, relieving joint strain, and improving range of motion. Regular stretching can help stabilize muscle tone, maintain or increase mobility, and reduce pain, potentially delaying the need for surgical interventions. Different types of stretching are employed, including passive stretching, where a therapist or caregiver moves the limb, and active stretching, performed by the individual if motor control allows [53].

However, the effectiveness of stretching alone in improving function in CP is somewhat limited. Studies suggest that muscle and tendon adaptations in spastic muscles are complex, and prolonged or combined interventions, such as resistive training, electrical stimulation, and orthotic use, may enhance outcomes. For example, stretching combined with strength training or antagonist muscle stimulation can improve muscle fascicle length and joint range more effectively than stretching alone. Orthoses and serial casting are often used to provide prolonged passive stretch to complement regular stretching exercises [53, 54].

Strengthening

Strengthening exercises play a vital role in the physical therapy management of spasticity in cerebral palsy (CP). Contrary to older beliefs that muscle strengthening might exacerbate spasticity, contemporary research supports that appropriately designed strengthening programs can improve muscle strength, functional ability, posture, and balance without increasing spasticity. Strengthening helps counteract muscle weakness frequently present in CP, especially in muscles opposing the spastic muscle groups, thus enhancing overall motor control and functional mobility. Exercises include resistance training with weights or bands, aquatic therapy, cycling, treadmill training, and targeted functional tasks such as sit-to-stand movements. This approach aims to enhance muscle endurance, improve joint stability, and optimize gross motor function, thereby contributing to improved performance in daily activities such as walking, dressing, and transfers. Physical therapists commonly integrate strengthening with stretching and neuromuscular re-education to provide comprehensive care tailored to individual needs [55, 56].

Positioning and Gait Training

Proper positioning techniques, applied continuously throughout the day and night, help reduce muscle tone, prevent contractures, improve joint alignment, and enhance comfort. Prolonged prone positioning, semi-reclined postures, and the use of standing frames have been shown to improve gross motor function and reduce spasticity in children with quadriplegic CP by promoting muscle stretching and better postural control [57]. Orthotic devices, such as ankle-foot orthoses (AFOs), support proper positioning of the feet and ankles, helping to improve walking efficiency and mobility [58]. Gait training focuses on developing functional walking patterns using assistive devices, strengthening the muscles involved in gait, and optimizing alignment to improve mobility and reduce compensatory movements. This training aims to improve independence, reduce pain, and enhance quality of life. Therapists often integrate positioning, stretching, strengthening, and gait training into comprehensive rehabilitation programs tailored to the patient's specific needs and functional level. Educating caregivers on maintaining therapeutic positioning at home is crucial for achieving sustained benefits [59].

Modalities

Physical therapy modalities such as heat, cold, and electrotherapy are commonly used to manage spasticity in cerebral palsy (CP), offering complementary approaches to reduce muscle tone, improve joint mobility, and alleviate pain. Cold therapy, including local cryotherapy and whole-body cryostimulation (WBC), has been shown to reduce spasticity by decreasing nerve conduction velocity and muscle spindle sensitivity, leading to temporary muscle relaxation and decreased hyperactive stretch reflexes. Studies report significant reductions in spasticity scores, improved gait parameters, and enhanced motor function following cold therapy sessions in CP patients. The effects of cold therapy are generally short-lived but can be potentiated when combined with stretching or exercise [60].

Heat therapy promotes blood flow, reduces muscle stiffness, and enhances tissue elasticity, which can improve joint range of motion and comfort. Paradoxically, both heat and cold therapies can reduce spasticity through different physiological mechanisms [61]. Electrotherapy modalities, such as neuromuscular electrical stimulation (NMES), are used to activate antagonist muscles, thereby inhibiting spastic muscles through reciprocal inhibition and improving voluntary motor control. Therapeutic ultrasound and transcutaneous electrical nerve stimulation (TENS) have also shown promise in reducing muscle tone and pain associated with spasticity [62].

12.5.2.2 Occupational Therapy

Occupational Therapy (OT) focuses on an individual's ability to participate in meaningful daily life tasks. OT addresses the motor, cognitive, sensory, and psychosocial components of function. This may include self-care activities like eating, transferring, grooming, bathing, and sleeping. Being able to perform ADL tasks independently will encourage the patient to practice, follow the treatment plans, and finally promote neuroplasticity and improve functional abilities [63].

Activities of Daily Living (ADL) Adaptation

Spasticity, with its associated muscle stiffness, limited range of motion, and impaired fine motor control, directly interferes with a person's ability to perform activities of daily living (ADLs). Occupational therapists use a two-pronged approach:

1. Adapting the individual (skill development):

   - Fine motor control: Manipulating small objects, such as picking up and sorting beads, small blocks, or pegs, helps improve the precision and control of individual fingers. OTs integrate therapy into a child's natural environment using toys and games. Examples include building with LEGOs, playing with puzzles, using clay to strengthen hand muscles, and threading beads onto a string. These activities are engaging and promote motor learning in a fun context.
   - Practicing functional tasks: The most effective therapy is often task-oriented and directly related to a person's daily life. This can include practicing fastening buttons, tying shoelaces, zipping jackets, holding and using a pencil for writing or drawing, or practicing with adaptive utensils for feeding. The therapist may use assistive devices or modify the task to ensure success as skills are developed.

Orthotics, Splints, and Casting

Orthotics, splints, and casts are essential components of the multidisciplinary management of spastic cerebral palsy, aimed at improving joint alignment, preventing contractures, reducing spasticity, and enhancing functional mobility.

Orthoses are considered a conservative treatment for spastic equinus deformity. Ankle-foot-orthoses (AFOs) are recommended for young ambulatory or partially ambulatory children with CP and dynamic equinus deformity, as they are useful for improving ankle dorsiflexion at initial contact and gross motor function [64, 65]. In children under 2 years old with spastic diplegia, a prospective, randomized, controlled trial found that AFOs increased the passive ankle dorsiflexion angle within treatment groups (spastic diplegia of GMFCS levels I and II). However, there was no significant difference in passive ankle dorsiflexion between daytime-only AFO wear and day–night AFO wear. Daytime AFO use reduced opposing muscle co-activation during ankle dorsiflexion, whereas wearing the brace day and night was linked to weaker dorsiflexion [66].

Casting contributes to gait improvement and ankle dorsiflexion at knee extension. Casting works by immobilizing and lengthening the muscle position, which can reduce spasticity and enhance gait function and ankle movement. Evidence shows that neither casting alone nor casting added to BoNT-A produces greater gains in gait or passive ankle dorsiflexion than BoNT-A alone. Serial casting remains a reasonable option for more pronounced spasticity (e.g., MAS grade 3) and is often combined with BoNT-A and targeted physiotherapy [64, 65].

The mechanisms of splints for spastic muscles are primarily designed to stretch the affected muscle, restore the joint to an ideal posture, and facilitate the growth of its sarcomeres, as described in Sect. 2.1.2. They are mainly used for the upper limbs and come in two types. One type is designed for stretching spastic muscles and preventing the contracture process, referred to as "non-functional hand splints". The other assists patients in their daily activities and is called "functional hand splints". The efficacy of these types of devices is limited in the literature, with most studies favouring the combination therapies of splints (BoNT-A and OT) over other therapies alone [67, 68].

12.5.3 Pharmacological Interventions

12.5.3.1 Oral Medications

Systemic agents, such as oral medications, are utilized when a generalized antispasticity effect is desired to treat widespread muscle stiffness affecting large areas or the entire body. In contrast, localized or segmental agents, including botulinum toxin injections or chemical denervation with phenol, are reserved for spasticity affecting a specific muscle group or a single extremity. This section will focus on the four most common oral pharmacological agents used for generalized spasticity: Baclofen, Tizanidine, Diazepam, and Dantrolene [69]. Information about their mechanism of action, indications, adverse effects, and primary clinical niche is described in Table 12.3.

Comparative Analysis and Clinical Synthesis

The fundamental difference in how these oral medications work directly explains their distinct safety profiles. Baclofen, Tizanidine, and Diazepam are all centrally acting agents that target the spinal cord or brain to inhibit excitatory neurotransmitter activity. Since these drugs exert a broad inhibitory effect on the CNS, a system responsible for alertness, coordination, and consciousness, it is a logical and direct consequence that their primary side effects are CNS-related. These common adverse effects include drowsiness, dizziness, and ataxia, and in the case of benzo diazepines, the potential for dependence and respiratory depression (Table 12.4) [70, 79].

In contrast, Dantrolene's mechanism of action is unique because it acts peripherally, directly on the skeletal muscle fiber itself. This allows it to circumvent the CNS entirely, meaning it does not cause the same CNS-related side effects as the other three drugs. However, this peripheral action introduces a new set of risks, which are a direct consequence of its therapeutic mechanism. By directly reducing muscle contraction, Dantrolene can cause dose-dependent muscle weakness and, due to its metabolic pathway, carries the non-negligible risk of hepatotoxicity [73]. This clear cause-and-effect relationship between a drug's mechanism of action and its side effect profile provides a valuable framework for understanding and comparing these medications (Table 12.5).

12.5.3.2 Botulinum Toxin Injection

The primary objective of BoNT-A therapy is to achieve a targeted reduction in muscle tone, thereby improving joint function and mobility, reducing pain, and potentially delaying the need for surgical interventions. It is crucial to understand that

Table 12.3 Most commonly used medications for spasticity

Medication	Mechanism of action	Indications	Adverse effects/ Risks	Primary clinical niche
Baclofen [70]	Gamma-aminobutyric acid beta receptor (GABA-B) agonist In presynaptic neurons, it inhibits the excitatory neurotransmitters responsible for contraction (glutamate and aspartate), and at the postsynaptic area, it brings hyperpolarization and neurotransmitter inhibition. This dual mechanism effectively inhibits the transmission of both mono- and polysynaptic reflexes at the spinal cord, providing a broad, generalized muscle-relaxing effect	Initially designed for epilepsy. Currently used for spasticity in neurological disorders	Weakness, drowsiness, dizziness, confusion, headache, nausea, vomiting Risk of withdrawal symptoms if not tapered correctly (altered mental status, seizure, hallucination, worsening of spasticity)	First-line option for generalized spasticity.
Tizanidine [71]	Alpha-2 adrenergic receptor agonist Presynaptic inhibition of motor neurons (similar to baclofen).	Spasticity in brain and spinal cord injury, and multiple sclerosis Chronic low back and neck pain	Dry mouth, drowsiness, muscle weakness, hypotension, and bradycardia Withdrawal syndrome is associated with anxiety, hypertonicity, hypertension, and reflex tachycardia	Alternative option for patients not tolerating or responding to first-line agents

(continued)

Table 12.3 (continued)

Medication	Mechanism of action	Indications	Adverse effects/ Risks	Primary clinical niche
Diazepam [72]	Enhances the action of the inhibitory neurotransmitter gamma aminobutyric acid (GABA). Specifically, it binds to the alpha and gamma subunits of the GABAA receptor, which causes a conformational change that increases the frequency of the chloride channel opening. The resulting influx of chloride ions into the neuron leads to hyperpolarization, which in turn results in broad CNS depression and muscle relaxation	A sedative to treat anxiety, panic attacks, alcohol withdrawal, seizures, and skeletal muscle spasms.	Hypotension, confusion, ataxia, drowsiness, headache, and vertigo.	Short-term or nocturnal use to facilitate physical therapy and improve sleep
Dantrolene [73]	Its action is localized within the muscle cell, where it binds to the ryanodine receptor 1 (RYR1) located in the sarcoplasmic reticulum. The ryanodine receptor is a calcium channel responsible for mediating the release of intracellular calcium, which is an essential step for initiating muscle contraction, which is inhibited by this mechanism.	Malignant hyperthermia crisis Spasticity in multiple sclerosis, brain and spinal cord injury, and CP	Dizziness, muscle weakness, fatigue, diarrhea, hepatotoxicity	Specialized agent for refractory cases of spasticity

BoNT is not a standalone treatment but rather an adjunctive component within a broader, comprehensive management plan [80].

Neuromuscular Chemo-Denervation

The mechanism of action for botulinum toxin is highly specific and localized. As a potent neurotoxin, BoNT-A acts at the neuromuscular junction (NMJ), the synapse where a motor neuron communicates with a muscle fiber. Its effect is to produce a dose-dependent, partially reversible "chemo-denervation" of the injected muscle. This process involves the toxin blocking the presynaptic release of acetylcholine (ACh), a neurotransmitter essential for triggering muscle contraction. By inhibiting

Table 12.4 Doses and titrations of antispasmodics

Medication	Age/weight range	Initial dose	Titration schedule	Maximum daily dose
Baclofen [74]	4 months-7 years	2.5 mg daily	Titrate every third day based on response	10–15 mg daily (4 month-7 years), 20–60 mg daily (>12 years)
Tizanidine [75]	Adult use (off-label for children)	2 mg every 6–8 h as needed	Increase by 2–4 mg every few days	36 mg
Diazepam [76]	1 month-1 year	250 mcg/kg	Start with a once-daily evening dose, increase to twice daily if needed	10 mg/day as an adjunctive therapy
	1–5 years	2.5 mg	Start with a once-daily evening dose, increase to twice daily if needed	10 mg/day as an adjunctive therapy
	5–12 years	5 mg	Start with a once-daily evening dose, increase to twice daily if needed	10 mg/day as an adjunctive therapy
	12–18 years	10 mg	Start with a once-daily evening dose, increase to twice daily if needed	10 mg/day as an adjunctive therapy
Dantrolene [77, 78]	<5 years	1 mg/kg/day divided twice daily	Maintenance dose: 12 mg/kg/day	Not to exceed 400 mg/24 h
	≥5 years	0.5 mg/kg once daily for 7 days	Gradually increase every 7 days	Not to exceed 100 mg four times daily

the release of ACh, BoNT effectively prevents the nerve signal from reaching the muscle. This interruption of neural transmission results in temporary muscle paralysis, which, in turn, reduces the exaggerated muscle tone and spasticity characteristic of cerebral palsy [81].

Clinical Application and Protocols

Patient selection is a critical step in maximizing the effectiveness of the treatment. BoNT is indicated for children with focal or segmental spasticity affecting a limited number of muscle groups in the upper and lower extremities [82]. It is not a suitable intervention for widespread, generalized spasticity. The most common indication in pediatric practice is the injection of the gastrocnemius (calf muscles) to correct a spastic equinus gait, often referred to as "toe-walking". Other frequently targeted

Table 12.5 Risk-benefit profiles and clinical niche

Medication	Risk-benefit
Baclofen	It is considered a first-line option for generalized spasticity due to its established efficacy and a side effect profile that is generally manageable with careful titration. The main clinical challenge is navigating its CNS depressant effects and the necessity for a slow, safe withdrawal to prevent a rebound in symptoms.
Tizanidine	Serves as an effective alternative for patients who may not respond to or tolerate Baclofen. Its use, however, is often limited by a higher incidence of adverse effects, including dry mouth and hypotension, and the requirement for regular liver function monitoring to mitigate the risk of hepatotoxicity.
Diazepam	It is particularly useful for short-term, targeted relief, especially when administered as a single bedtime dose. This strategy mitigates the primary side effect of daytime sedation, transforming the drug into a tool that can facilitate physical therapy and daily activities. However, its potential for dependence and misuse significantly limits its utility for long-term management.
Dantrolene	It is a specialized agent that is typically reserved for refractory cases of spasticity when other oral options have failed. While its unique peripheral mechanism offers a valuable therapeutic pathway, its use is carefully weighed against the non-negligible risk of severe liver damage.

muscles include the hamstrings, adductors, and key upper limb muscles such as the biceps brachii [83].

Selecting the correct target muscles requires a high degree of clinical expertise. Not all spastic muscles require injection; rather, a focused approach on the specific muscle groups causing the most significant functional impairment is essential. This precision is vital to avoid potential adverse compensatory movements. For instance, while a gastrocnemius injection can improve ankle and knee movements, it has been shown to acutely worsen hip joint motion as the child adapts to the reduced push-off ability [83]. A comprehensive biomechanical and gait analysis prior to injection is therefore essential to anticipate and manage such compensatory effects.

Dosing and Injection Techniques

The dose of botulinum toxin is meticulously tailored to each individual patient, considering factors such as body weight, the size and number of targeted muscles, the severity of the spasticity, and the patient's response to previous treatments. The potency units of different BoNT-A formulations are not interchangeable, which is a crucial aspect of safe administration. To provide clarity on this point, Tables 12.6 and 12.7 summarize comparative dosing guidelines from clinical practice.

The injections are administered intramuscularly using a small-diameter needle, such as a 27-gauge, with the dose divided across four or five sites within a large muscle to ensure adequate toxin spread. Accurate needle placement is paramount for effective "chemo-denervation." To achieve this, clinicians often utilize guidance technologies such as needle electromyography (EMG), nerve stimulation, or ultrasound. To enhance patient comfort, particularly in children, topical anesthetics like

Table 12.6 Pediatric BoNT-A sites and doses

Muscle	Recommended dose (units/kg)	Number of sites
Upper limb		
Biceps brachii	1.5–3.0	4
Brachialis	1.0–2.0	2
Brachioradialis	0.5–1.0	2
Flexor carpi radialis	1.0–2.0	2
Flexor carpi ulnaris	1.0–2.0	2
Flexor digitorum profundus	0.5–1.0	2
Flexor digitorum superficialis	0.5–1.0	2
Lower limb		
Gastrocnemius medial head	1.0–2.0	2
Gastrocnemius lateral head	1.0–2.0	2
Soleus	1.0–2.0	2
Tibialis posterior	1.0–2.0	2

Table 12.7 Adult BoNT-A sites and doses

Muscle	Recommended dose (units/kg)	Number of sites
Upper limb		
Biceps brachii	60–200	2–4
Brachioradialis	45–75	1–2
Brachialis	30–50	1–2
Pronator teres	15–25	1
Pronator quadratus	10–50	1
Flexor carpi radialis	12.5–50	1
Flexor carpi ulnaris	12.5–50	1
Flexor digitorum profundus	30–50	1
Flexor digitorum superficialis	30–50	1
Lumbricals/interossei	5–10	1
Adductor pollicis	20	1
Flexor pollicis longus	20	1
Flexor pollicis brevis/opponens pollicis	5–25	1
Lower limb		
Gastrocnemius medial head	75	3
Gastrocnemius lateral head	75	3
Soleus	75	3
Tibialis posterior	75	3
Flexor hallucis longus	50	2
Flexor digitorum longus	50	2

EMLA cream and special coolant sprays are frequently used to minimize pain at the injection site [81, 84].

The therapeutic effects of botulinum toxin are not immediate. The onset of clinical benefit, including reduced spasticity and improved joint mobility, typically begins within a few days to a week following the injection. The period of maximal and clinically useful relaxation generally lasts between 3 and 6 months. Repeat injections are a routine part of long-term management and are typically administered no sooner than 12 weeks after the previous session, or when the return of muscle tone begins to interfere with a patient's function [85, 86].

Long-Term Efficacy

The long-term efficacy of repeated BoNT injections is a crucial consideration for clinical practice. While some studies suggest a general improvement in overall gait patterns following a second injection that can last for up to a year, there are concerns that the duration of the therapeutic response may diminish after multiple injections, possibly due to increasing dynamic components of the spasticity that develop with age, with most patients benefiting from 2 to 3 injections [81, 85].

Adverse Effects

When administered at appropriate doses by experienced clinicians, botulinum toxin injections are generally safe and well-tolerated. The most common side effects are localized and mild in nature. These include temporary muscle weakness at the injection site, minor pain, bruising, or small dots of blood where the needle entered the skin. The muscle weakness is a recognized consequence of the treatment's mechanism of action and typically resolves within 1–2 weeks [85, 87].

Muscle Atrophy

A significant and often under-discussed long-term concern associated with repeated botulinum toxin injections is the potential for muscle atrophy. The temporary paralysis induced by BoNT leads to a period of muscle disuse, which can cause muscle atrophy as a direct consequence. Research has shown that muscle atrophy can persist for at least 12 months, a duration that substantially outlasts the 3- to 6-month period of therapeutic muscle relaxation. This atrophy is characterized by a loss of contractile elements, followed by their replacement with fat and connective tissue [88]. This observation has prompted questions regarding the long-term musculoskeletal health of children receiving repeated injections. The central dilemma is the use of an agent that causes weakness to manage a condition already characterized by weakness. While botulinum toxin remains a standard of care, the evidence of prolonged muscle atrophy necessitates a reevaluation of current clinical protocols, urging a more thoughtful approach to injection frequency and enhanced long-term monitoring of the effects on the injected muscles [89].

12.5.3.3 Intrathecal Baclofen

Baclofen is a gamma-aminobutyric acid (GABA) agonist that acts at the spinal cord level to reduce muscle tone. However, the efficacy of oral baclofen is often limited by its low lipid solubility and poor ability to cross the blood-brain barrier (BBB). To achieve a therapeutic effect on spasticity, a significantly larger dose is required, which often leads to systemic side effects such as sedation, drowsiness, confusion, and weakness. Intrathecal baclofen (ITB) therapy involves the surgical implantation of a pump that delivers a liquid form of baclofen directly into the cerebrospinal fluid (CSF). This bypasses the BBB, allowing for a much smaller and more precise dose to achieve a profound effect with fewer systemic side effects. This targeted delivery provides continuous, consistent control of spasticity and serves as a reversible alternative to irreversible surgical interventions such as selective posterior rhizotomy [90]. The therapy is indicated for individuals with severe, generalized spasticity that has not responded adequately to other conservative treatments, including maximal recommended oral doses of medications or botulinum toxin injections. Beyond refractory spasticity, candidacy is also considered for patients who experience intolerable side effects from oral medications [91].

Mechanism of Action

The efficacy of ITB therapy is rooted in its precise mechanism of action at the spinal cord level. Baclofen, or 4-amino-3-(4-chlorophenyl) butanoic acid, is a structural analog of GABA, the primary inhibitory neurotransmitter in the central nervous system. As a GABA-B receptor agonist, it binds to receptors located in the dorsal horn of the spinal cord. This receptor binding triggers a cascade of second messengers that ultimately leads to the hyperpolarization of the presynaptic membrane. The hyperpolarization impedes the release of excitatory neurotransmitters that are responsible for the hyperexcitability of the stretch reflex, which is the underlying cause of spasticity. By directly interrupting this spinal reflex arc, ITB therapy effectively reduces peripheral motor tone, producing a potent antispastic effect exactly where it is needed [70, 92].

Procedure of the Pump Implantation

A test dose of baclofen (e.g., 50 μg for adults) is administered via a lumbar puncture or a temporary catheter into the intrathecal space. The patient is then monitored for a period of at least 6–8 h. The effects of the test dose typically begin within 30 min to 1 h, peak at around 4 h, and last for 4–8 h. A positive response is defined as a significant reduction in spasticity and an improvement in the patient's range of motion. If the initial test dose does not produce a response, a larger dose may be administered on a different day to confirm the patient is not a candidate for the therapy.

The surgical implantation of an intrathecal baclofen (ITB) pump is a procedure that places a small, programmable pump under the skin of the abdomen. This pump is connected to a catheter that is tunneled to the intrathecal space around the spinal cord, allowing for the direct delivery of baclofen. This method is highly effective for managing severe spasticity by targeting the spinal receptors. Post-surgery, patients are monitored in the hospital for a few days to carefully adjust the baclofen dose. The initial period of recovery is crucial for physical therapists to begin working with the patient to leverage the reduction in muscle tone and initiate rehabilitation for improved mobility and function.

Complications

Intrathecal baclofen (ITB) therapy, despite its benefits, is associated with potential complications that a physical therapist should be aware of. These risks fall into three main categories. First, there are general surgical risks like infection, bleeding, and spinal fluid leaks. Second, hardware-related issues, such as catheter kinks or displacement, can impede drug delivery. Third, and most critically, are the drug-related emergencies of overdose and withdrawal. An overdose, often due to a pump malfunction or programming error, can cause severe muscle weakness and respiratory depression. Conversely, a sudden and unintentional withdrawal, for example, from a pump failure or missed refill, can be fatal. It leads to a hypermetabolic state characterized by fever, rebound spasticity, and potential organ failure.

The long-term effect of ITB therapy on scoliosis is a controversial area with mixed research findings. Some studies suggest that the therapy accelerates the progression of spinal curvature. The theory is that the beneficial reduction of spasticity in the trunk and paraspinal muscles may lead to muscle hypotonia, which can compromise spinal stability and contribute to deformity.

Conversely, other research indicates that ITB therapy does not significantly alter the natural progression of scoliosis in patients with CP. This discrepancy likely stems from the complexity of the condition itself, as well as differences in patient selection and the use of other management techniques. Given this, it is understood that scoliosis is a multifactorial issue, and ITB therapy is not its sole cause. Additionally, ITB therapy has been shown to improve hip-related issues, such as subluxation and pelvic obliquity, which may have a positive indirect effect on spinal alignment. A comprehensive management plan, including the use of an inner seat system, is crucial for mitigating the risk of scoliosis progression in patients undergoing ITB therapy.

12.5.3.4 Surgical Intervention

Orthopedic Surgery

Orthopedic surgery plays a crucial role in a comprehensive, multidisciplinary management strategy for spastic cerebral palsy. It is not a standalone solution, but a vital step in correcting fixed deformities, improving function and mobility, reducing chronic pain, and ultimately enhancing the patient's quality of life. When spasticity becomes resistant to non-surgical interventions, such as physical therapy, orthotics, or botulinum toxin injections, surgical interventions are considered. This is often a long-term, staged approach, with procedures timed to align with the child's growth and development. The ultimate goal is to enable a child to sit more comfortably, walk with greater efficiency, and perform daily activities with less discomfort [93]. This topic is comprehensively discussed in the Chap. 5. Still, we will discuss two of the most commonly used approaches, and more relevant to our topic, sections "Selective Dorsal Rhizotomy (SDR)" and "Selective Peripheral Neurotomy (SPN)."

Selective Dorsal Rhizotomy (SDR)

The neurophysiological basis of SDR is the permanent disruption of the abnormal spinal reflex arc that underlies spasticity. The procedure involves a laminectomy, in which a small section of bone is removed from the lower back vertebrae to expose the spinal cord and the nerve roots. A key step in modern SDR is the use of intraoperative neuromonitoring and electrical stimulation to identify and separate the sensory nerves (dorsal roots) from the motor nerves (ventral roots). The surgeon then selectively tests and severs a specific percentage, typically 25–30%, of the sensory nerve rootlets that are sending abnormal signals from the muscles back to the spinal cord, while carefully preserving the motor nerves and those controlling bladder and bowel function [94].

This method of identifying and cutting only the specific nerve fibers responsible for spasticity is what makes the procedure "selective." By cutting these afferent (incoming) nerve fibers, SDR effectively "detunes" the hyperactive spinal reflex arc, leading to a permanent reduction in spasticity below the level of the surgery. Following the procedure, the patient may initially feel a sense of weakness [95]. This key point in the patient's journey involves removing spasticity's 'bracing' effect, enabling new movement patterns. Intensive postoperative physical therapy is essential for SDR's success. The surgery isn't a cure for brain damage but a way to restructure the spinal nervous system for better rehabilitation and motor learning.

Patient Selection Criteria and Indications

SDR is best suited for children with spastic cerebral palsy who have the cognitive and physical ability to engage in intensive post-operative physical therapy. It is not recommended for children with non-CP diagnoses, mixed or dystonic movement patterns, or significant underlying weakness. While primarily used to improve ambulation, a "palliative SDR" approach exists for non-ambulatory children. In these cases, the goal shifts from improving walking to enhancing quality of life by reducing discomfort and making caregiving easier. The decision to proceed is a careful one, prioritizing the patient's specific goals [96, 97].

Clinical Efficacy and Outcomes: A Review of the Evidence

SDR is an effective procedure for managing spasticity in children, particularly in the lower limbs. A robust body of evidence, including meta-analyses, confirms a significant and immediate reduction in muscle tone, as measured by tools such as the Modified Ashworth Scale. Beyond spasticity relief, when SDR is followed by intensive physical therapy, it leads to improvements in gross motor function, balance, and walking capacity. Gait analysis studies have shown positive changes, such as increased ankle dorsiflexion and improved knee angles. The procedure also helps reduce pain associated with spasticity, which directly enhances a patient's quality of life [98].

The long-term efficacy of SDR is still a topic of discussion. While some long-term studies report sustained reductions in muscle tone, others find the evidence for lasting functional improvements over a decade to be inconclusive. This suggests that SDR is best viewed not as a one-time solution, but as the beginning of a lifelong management strategy that often requires "add-on" treatments like botulinum toxin injections. The ultimate success of SDR relies on the patient's and healthcare system's commitment to a demanding, long-term rehabilitation plan [99].

Postoperative Complications and Long-Term Risks

SDR is a safe procedure with low rates of major complications. In the short term, patients may experience problems with their pulmonary, bladder, or gastrointestinal systems, including constipation. Rare complications like deep wound infections or spinal fluid leaks can occur. Post-op sensory changes, such as numbness or hypersensitivity, affect about half of patients; most are temporary, but some are permanent. The primary long-term risk is spinal deformity, including lumbar lordosis and scoliosis, which is particularly prevalent during adolescence. It's key to differentiate between surgical complications and unmasked muscle weakness, as surgery clarifies baseline motor function by reducing spasticity. Any perceived function loss often results from inadequate post-op rehab to address muscle weakness [93].

Selective Peripheral Neurotomy (SPN)

Selective peripheral neurotomy (SPN) is a surgical procedure that addresses spasticity by targeting peripheral nerves, not the central spinal cord. The procedure involves cutting or partially sectioning a specific motor nerve branch that innervates a spastic muscle. This approach is fundamentally different from SDR because it directly targets the efferent (outgoing) motor pathway, rather than the afferent (incoming) sensory pathway. The goal is to eliminate the abnormal efferent information to the spastic muscle, which reduces the reflex arc and helps to restore the balance between agonist and antagonist muscles around a specific joint [100].

Patient Selection Criteria and Indications for Focal Management

SPN is mainly indicated for focal or multifocal spasticity, differentiating it from SDR's role in generalized spasticity. It's considered when a specific muscle or group causes functional issues, pain, or deformity, especially after failed localized treatments like botulinum toxin injections, which can be costly or require repeated sessions. Usually performed on patients with a Modified Ashworth Scale score of 3 or higher, SPN is often used in adults with post-stroke spasticity but is increasingly applied to pediatric CP cases with focal needs [93, 100].

Efficacy in Reducing Focal Spasticity and Improving Function

SPN has shown considerable promise in managing focal spasticity. A review of the literature suggests an 80–85% success rate in reducing localized spasticity. Systematic reviews indicate that SPN is effective for reducing spasticity in the lower limbs without negatively impacting walking speed. This is a crucial finding, as the direct targeting of motor nerves could theoretically lead to a loss of function.

Table 12.8 Key differences between Selective Dorsal Rhizotomy (SDR) and Selective Peripheral Neurotomy (SPN)

Feature	Selective Dorsal Rhizotomy (SDR)	Selective Peripheral Neurotomy (SPN)
Surgical target	Spinal nerve rootlets (dorsal roots)	Peripheral motor nerve branches
Indications	Generalized/diffuse spasticity	Focal/multifocal spasticity
Primary goal	Improved mobility and gait	Improved posture and function in a specific limb
Underlying mechanism	Permanent interruption of the spinal reflex arc	Permanent reduction of muscle tone via denervation
Patient profile	Spastic diplegia (GMFCS I–III)	Spasticity in a specific muscle/limb
Reversibility	Irreversible	Irreversible (though compensation occurs)
Role in care pathway	Definitive neurosurgical intervention for widespread spasticity	Alternative to repeated chemodenervation

Reported outcomes of SPN include improvements in muscle tone, passive range of motion in the ankle, pain, and walking speed. These functional improvements align with the core goal of the procedure: restoring a more balanced and effective movement pattern in a specific limb or joint [101].

Complications and Safety Profile

The effectiveness and safety of Selective Peripheral Neurotomy (SPN) depend on careful patient selection and a commitment to intensive postoperative rehabilitation. Short-term risks include incision infection and temporary muscle weakness due to targeting motor nerve fibers. Sensory changes can occur if sensory fascicles are involved. A major long-term challenge is the potential recurrence of spasticity, often due to nerve regrowth. Modern techniques involve resecting longer nerve segments to reduce this risk, improving long-term safety and efficacy (Table 12.8) [101].

12.6 Management of Pain

12.6.1 General Principles

A core principle of pain management is the identification and treatment of the underlying cause of pain. In cerebral palsy, this is a complex task because pain is rarely a simple, singular issue. It is instead multifactorial, stemming from both the primary consequences of the brain lesion and a wide range of secondary complications. Clinicians must adopt a rigorous, systematic diagnostic approach and resist the reflex of attributing all pain to the most apparent causes, such as spasticity or muscle contractures. A thorough "head-to-toe" examination is essential to rule out other, potentially severe, or life-threatening conditions. Table 12.9 provides a structured overview of the diverse sources of pain in cerebral palsy, reinforcing the need for a broad differential diagnosis [102].

Table 12.9 Common sources of pain in cerebral palsy

Category	Etiology	Associated conditions and details
Musculoskeletal	Spasticity and dystonia	Increased muscle tone, contractures, spasms; can be secondary to pain
	Orthopedic deformities	Hip subluxation/dislocation (most common cause of pain in children), scoliosis, joint malalignment
	Joint and bone issues	Degenerative joint disease, pathological fractures, osteoporosis
Neurological	Dystonia	Painful, involuntary muscle contractions (second most common cause of pain after hip dislocation), often triggered by movement or stress
	Neuropathic pain	Resulting from nerve damage
	Other neurological issues	Headaches, increased intracranial pressure (e.g., in children with VP shunts), and seizures
Gastrointestinal	Functional disorders	Constipation (74%), gastroesophageal reflux (50%), abdominal pain (32%)
	Anatomic issues	Intestinal volvulus (a life-threatening but rare cause of bowel obstruction) and delayed gastric emptying
Iatrogenic and other	Procedural pain	Pain from physical therapy (especially stretching), surgery, or injections
	Equipment-related	Pain from braces, splints, casts, or other devices
	Psychological	Anxiety, depression, sleep deprivation, and emotional difficulties
	Infections	Dental infections, urinary tract infections, skin, bone, or joint infections, and otitis media

Accurate and consistent pain assessment is the bedrock of effective pain management. However, in the cerebral palsy population, especially for nonverbal individuals, this task is one of the most significant clinical challenges. A principled approach to assessment must therefore be multi-dimensional, integrating validated tools, a deep understanding of behavioral cues, and the crucial input of parents and caregivers. A comprehensive list of pain assessment tools is presented in Sect. 12.4.2.3, Table 12.2.

12.6.1.1 Embracing the Biopsychosocial Model

The biopsychosocial model is the most widely accepted and effective framework for understanding and managing chronic pain. This model posits that pain is a dynamic experience resulting from a reciprocal interaction among biological, psychological, and social factors unique to each individual. A purely biological approach that focuses only on tissue damage or muscular dysfunction is inadequate for addressing the full scope of a patient's pain [103].

The three domains of the model are as follows:

- *Biological*: This domain encompasses the physiological and neurological components of pain. In CP, this includes spasticity, muscle contractures, joint issues, osteoporosis, gastrointestinal problems, and infections [104].

- *Psychological*: This domain considers the individual's cognitive and emotional state. Factors such as anxiety, depression, fear, and pain catastrophizing can significantly amplify the pain experience. Psychological approaches can also focus on improving interoceptive sensitivity—the ability to perceive and interpret internal bodily sensations—to enhance the individual's awareness and regulation of their internal states [105].
- *Social*: This domain includes environmental and relational factors that influence the pain experience. These include family culture, caregiver support, school attendance, access to healthcare, and peer relationships [104, 105].

A key aspect of this model is understanding how components influence each other cyclically. For instance, a child's pain (biological) can cause social withdrawal, anxiety, and frustration (psychological). Conversely, psychological factors like low mood or pain catastrophizing often relate more to functional disability than pain intensity. Family distress can lead to overprotective behavior (social), reinforcing a child's pain-avoidance and worsening deconditioning and distress. This vicious cycle justifies a multimodal, interdisciplinary approach, as one intervention cannot break it. The schematic below illustrates this dynamic [106].

12.6.1.2 The Multidisciplinary and Interdisciplinary Team Approach

The complex, multifactorial nature of pain in CP cannot be adequately addressed by a single clinician. It necessitates a coordinated, team-based approach to care. The most effective model is an interdisciplinary team, which is distinct from a traditional multidisciplinary one. In a multidisciplinary team, each specialist provides their own recommendation and shares their findings in parallel. In an interdisciplinary team, the professionals are "interdependent" and work collaboratively toward a unified resolution [105].

A comprehensive pain management team for CP may include a pediatrician, neurologist, psychologist, orthopedic surgeon, physical therapist, occupational therapist, and speech therapist. Collaboration among these professionals is essential. A systematic review on interdisciplinary pain programs for children with chronic pain showed these programs improve pain, disability, anxiety, depression, and school attendance. This evidence indicates that a collaborative, integrated effort leads to functional restoration. A physical therapist may focus on gait and flexibility while a psychologist addresses fear of movement, all coordinated with a pain specialist to manage nociception. The collective effort results in lasting improvements greater than individual contributions [107].

12.6.2 Non-pharmacological Interventions

12.6.2.1 The Foundational Role of Physical Therapy

The goals of physical therapy interventions are not simply to alleviate existing pain but also to prevent the onset and progression of secondary impairments, maximize physical functioning, and restore, maintain, and promote overall fitness and quality of life. By addressing the biomechanical and physiological origins of pain, physical therapy enables individuals to overcome physical limitations, increase independence, and engage more fully in a healthy and active lifestyle.

Mechanisms and Benefits of Therapeutic Exercise

Exercise interventions like stretching, strengthening, and endurance training improve muscle strength, flexibility, balance, posture, sensory integration, and cardiorespiratory fitness to address discomfort. They prevent secondary impairments by stopping muscles from shortening and losing movement, thus avoiding painful contractures and joint deformities [108].

The evidence base for therapeutic exercise in CP is robust, yet certain areas present apparent contradictions that require a nuanced interpretation. For example, a meta-analysis involving children with CP found no significant difference in a global measure of gross motor function (GMF) following exercise interventions [109]. In stark contrast, another meta-analysis concluded that physical exercise could significantly improve GMF in children with CP [110]. This discrepancy is not a sign of intervention failure but rather a reflection of the methodological heterogeneity across the studies. A closer examination of the first meta-analysis reveals that, although GMF did not change globally, there were significant improvements in underlying components, such as gait speed and muscle strength. These improvements are clinically meaningful as they directly reduce the biomechanical strain that causes pain. The second study, which found a positive effect on GMF, likely included a different patient cohort or a different mix of intervention types, leading to a different outcome. The existence of these contrasting findings underscores the need for standardized reporting of patient characteristics, intervention protocols, and outcome measures in future research.

Evidence-Based Dosing of Exercise (the FITT Principle)

To maximize therapeutic benefit and ensure safety, exercise interventions for individuals with CP should be prescribed using the FITT (frequency, intensity, time, type) principle. A review of randomized controlled trials (RCTs) provides specific guidance on these parameters.

- *Frequency*: Recommendations from RCTs suggest a training frequency of two to four sessions per week. For individuals who are highly deconditioned, it is often more practical and advisable to begin with one to two sessions per week and gradually increase the frequency as they adapt. Intensive training, defined as at least two sessions per week, is generally considered more beneficial than less frequent, distributed therapy [111].
- *Intensity*: Exercise intensity should align with guidelines from the American College of Sports Medicine (ACSM), which are often measured relative to an individual's maximal effort. Specific metrics include a target of 60–80% of maximum heart rate (HRmax), 40–80% of heart rate reserve (HRR), or 50–65% of peak oxygen consumption [111].

- *Time*: Sessions should be at least 20 min in duration, though some studies have reported positive effects with sessions lasting up to 60 min or more [111].
- *Type*: The types of exercises prescribed should be regular, purposeful, continuous, and rhythmic, and should engage major muscle groups. Effective activities identified in studies include running, cycling, swimming, propelling a wheelchair, and strength training [111].

Transcutaneous Electrical Nerve Stimulation (TENS) and Functional Electrical Stimulation (FES)

Transcutaneous Electrical Nerve Stimulation (TENS) and Functional Electrical Stimulation (FES) are non-invasive modalities that utilize low-level electrical currents applied to the skin to achieve therapeutic effects. The analgesic mechanism of TENS is believed to involve the activation of inhibitory pain pathways in the central nervous system, which reduces central excitability and consequently pain perception [112]. FES, on the other hand, is specifically designed to restore function by inducing muscle contractions during a specific task or activity [113]. The evidence supports the use of these modalities, with a systematic review of seven trials showing that TENS significantly improved gross motor function, gait velocity, hand function, and health-related quality of life. The review also noted that TENS was safe, with any adverse events being rare, mild, and self-resolving [112].

Hydrotherapy (Aquatic Therapy)

Hydrotherapy, also known as aquatic therapy, is a therapeutic intervention that utilizes the unique properties of water to facilitate movement and alleviate pain. The buoyancy of water reduces the compressive forces on joints, alleviating stress and allowing for easier, more fluid movement. The warmth of the water helps to soothe muscle tension and reduce spasms, while hydrostatic pressure can improve blood circulation and reduce swelling. Evidence from meta-analyses has shown that hydrotherapy significantly improves gross motor functions in children and adolescents with CP, with the most notable benefits observed in programs that last for more than 10 weeks. It also shows a positive trend in improving fine motor functions and is reported to reduce discomfort during exercises, which can improve patient motivation and participation. Hydrotherapy offers a safe and supportive environment for patients to build strength and flexibility, eliminating the risk of injury associated with land-based exercises [114].

Role of Positioning and Assistive Devices

Therapeutic positioning is a crucial yet often overlooked aspect of physical therapy, vital for managing pain and preventing secondary issues in individuals with CP. It aims to maintain skeletal alignment, prevent or accommodate deformities, and provide a stable support base for functional activities. Proper positioning is crucial for achieving pain relief, particularly from poor posture, misaligned joints, and pressure points. Using tools like standing frames can promote healthy hip development, prevent dislocation, and boost bone density, reducing future pain. It also lessens stiffness, tone, and uncontrolled movements, enhancing comfort [115].

12.6.2.2 Occupational Therapy (OT)

Occupational therapy (OT) occupies a unique and critical position in the non-pharmacological management of pain for individuals with cerebral palsy (CP). While other disciplines may focus on isolated aspects of physical function, the core tenet of OT is to promote health and well-being through an individual's engagement in meaningful daily activities, or "occupations." This patient-centered approach is particularly vital in the context of CP, where pain frequently originates not only from primary neurological impairments but also from the secondary biomechanical consequences of limited movement and function. For instance, pain can arise from muscle stiffness, joint misalignment, and poor posture, all of which are exacerbated when individuals struggle to perform daily tasks such as eating, dressing, or moving around [7].

Task-Oriented and Intensive Bimanual Training

Central to occupational therapy is the use of hands-on, task-oriented interventions that are driven by the principles of motor learning and neuroplasticity. These intensive training methods aim to improve functional abilities and reduce pain by enhancing motor control and coordination. Two prominent examples are Hand-Arm Bimanual Intensive Therapy (HABIT) and Constraint-Induced Movement Therapy (CIMT).

HABIT is a highly intensive approach that focuses on the coordinated use of both arms in functional and playful activities, with a goal of improving bimanual coordination and independence. This approach is often provided at high intensity, for instance, 6 h/day over 10–15 days, reflecting a deliberate effort to leverage the brain's capacity for change through repetition. The evidence for intensive bimanual training is strong, indicating its effectiveness in enhancing functional independence and coordination. CIMT, in contrast, involves constraining the less-affected or stronger limb to encourage and strengthen the use of the more-affected limb. By forcing the use of the weaker arm, the individual builds new neural pathways and skills, which can lead to long-term improvements in function [116].

Sensory Integration and Sensory Processing Interventions

Pain perception in CP can be significantly influenced by a child's ability to process sensory information. Sensory Integration Therapy (SIT) is a play-based, clinical approach that helps children organize and respond appropriately to sensory stimuli, such as touch, sight, and proprioception. Proprioception, the body's sense of its position and movement in space, is particularly important. Deficits in this area can lead to poor body awareness, muscle tone, and motor control, which can directly contribute to discomfort and pain. Occupational therapists use SIT to provide structured sensory input, helping children regulate their responses. Activities may include using swings and balance beams to stimulate the vestibular system, working with textured materials like rice or soft sand to desensitize tactile receptors, or engaging in tasks that provide deep pressure and joint compression to enhance proprioception. While SIT is considered to offer many therapeutic prospects and has shown positive results in some comparative studies for improving balance and gross motor function, the overall evidence base remains limited [117].

Psychological Interventions

Cognitive Behavioral Therapy (CBT)

Cognitive behavioral therapy has emerged as a first-line psychosocial treatment for a wide spectrum of chronic pain syndromes, including those affecting special populations like children. It is a structured, goal-oriented, and multi-component treatment that addresses the interconnectedness of thoughts, feelings, and actions. The primary objective of CBT for chronic pain is not simply to eliminate the pain but to improve the individual's quality of life and daily functioning by modifying maladaptive cognitions and dysfunctional behavioral patterns. Its efficacy is well-supported by evidence from numerous randomized controlled trials and systematic reviews for a variety of conditions, including low back pain, headaches, and fibromyalgia [118].

Somatic Interventions

Progressive muscle relaxation (PMR) involves systematically tensing and relaxing muscle groups to increase awareness and release tension, thereby promoting relaxation. Neurobiological studies support its effects; an fMRI study showed that while simple muscle tensing activates broad brain areas, PMR specifically decreases activity in regions such as the superior frontal gyrus (SFG), inferior frontal gyrus (IFG), and posterior cingulate cortex (PCC). This reduction helps exclude distractions and fosters focus, validating PMR's role in relaxation and pain management [119].

Virtual reality (VR) represents the next generation of distraction-based therapy. Its immersive and engaging nature allows it to deeply absorb a patient's attention, making them able to ignore aversive stimuli more effectively than traditional methods. Beyond simple distraction, VR provides a safe, interactive, and motivating environment for therapy, and is being actively explored for neurorehabilitation and physical therapy in children with CP. As a pain management tool, its ability to create a "corrective psychological and physiological environment" makes it a promising area for further research, particularly in the context of pain exposure therapy [120].

Biofeedback is an evidence-based behavioral intervention that teaches patients to consciously control and self-regulate involuntary physiological processes. Using electronic sensors, biofeedback provides real-time data about bodily functions, such as heart rate, muscle tension, or skin temperature, via visual or auditory displays. Patients learn to make subtle changes in their thoughts and behavior to achieve responses such as muscle relaxation or a lowered heart rate. Seeing and understanding physiological data helps patients actively participate in their own care, especially for conditions like CP, where they often feel a lack of control. Biofeedback offers a tangible, real-time view of progress [121].

Complementary and Alternative Medicine (CAM)

CAM encompasses practices and products that fall outside conventional medicine. 'Integrative medicine' uses CAM therapies backed by strong evidence alongside standard treatments. Many with chronic disabilities, including CP, use CAM, often driven by personal health philosophies rather than dissatisfaction with conventional care. This approach emphasizes supplementing, not replacing, traditional treatments, forming a core part of multidisciplinary care.

Acupuncture

Acupuncture, a key part of traditional Chinese medicine with a long history, helps alleviate symptoms of cerebral palsy, like pain and motor issues. It works by inserting fine needles into specific points to restore the flow of energy and enhance overall health. Today, it's often used as a complementary therapy. Literature indicates that the effectiveness of acupuncture varies depending on the specific technique employed. For example, electroacupuncture (EA) is more effective than traditional acupuncture in reducing muscle tone in children with spastic CP, and scalp acupuncture beats conventional rehab in treating pediatric CP. This differentiation highlights that acupuncture is not a singular therapy, but rather a group of specialized techniques, and practitioners must consider the specific therapeutic method when targeting clinical outcomes [122].

Massage Therapy

Massage therapy is one of the most widely used complementary and alternative therapies for children with CP. Surveys indicate that its use is particularly common, with some reports suggesting that as many as 80% of families with a child with CP have utilized massage at some point, and parents of children with special needs are almost twice as likely to use it compared to the general population [123]. This high rate of use reflects a strong belief in its benefits among parents and caregivers. Beyond pain relief, parents and caregivers report that massage therapy can improve calmness, enhance social and communication skills, regulate bowel habits, and improve sleep patterns. The evidence for massage therapy's effectiveness in managing spasticity and pain is promising but mixed. A systematic review that included 11 studies with 297 children with CP found that massage significantly decreased muscle tone in children with the spastic type of the condition. The therapy has been reported to decrease hypertonicity, alleviate chronic pain, and improve range of motion, providing a valuable component of a comprehensive treatment plan [124].

Music Therapy

Music therapy is an evidence-based system of clinical interventions, particularly a subfield known as neurologic music therapy (NMT). It operates on the principle of auditory-motor coupling, using music as a versatile stimulus to activate and reorganize neural networks. The therapeutic benefit is rooted in the brain's innate capacity for neuroplasticity, where consistent and structured musical engagement can facilitate improvements in motor control, gait, and emotional well-being by strengthening connections between the sensory and motor cortices. This process provides a powerful rehabilitative cue that helps to retrain and improve dysfunctional neural pathways [125, 126].

12.6.2.3 Pharmacological Pain Management

Non-opioid Analgesics: Acetaminophen and NSAIDs

These agents are considered the first line of defense for mild-to-moderate nociceptive pain in children and adults with CP. They are often used to manage pain from musculoskeletal issues, inflammation, and general discomfort [127].

Acetaminophen: Frequently the initial treatment for mild to moderate pain, acetaminophen's mechanism of action is thought to involve the activation of descending serotonergic pathways and the inhibition of prostaglandin synthesis in the central nervous system. It is widely used and available in oral, rectal, and intravenous formulations. While generally safe, hepatotoxicity is a rare but serious risk, particularly with prolonged use or supratherapeutic doses, necessitating a limitation on intake [128].

Nonsteroidal Anti-inflammatory Drugs (NSAIDs): NSAIDs, such as ibuprofen, are effective first-line agents, especially for pain with an inflammatory component. Their mechanism involves the inhibition of cyclooxygenase (COX) enzymes, which are responsible for producing pro-inflammatory prostaglandins. This dual analgesic and anti-inflammatory action makes them particularly useful for pain associated with musculoskeletal issues. Some evidence suggests ibuprofen may be more effective than acetaminophen for certain types of acute pain. While adverse events are uncommon in pediatric patients, NSAIDs are associated with gastrointestinal issues, bleeding, and a risk of kidney failure [128].

Opioid Analgesics

Opioids are powerful analgesics reserved for the management of severe, acute pain, such as that experienced in postoperative pain, with morphine, fentanyl, and oxycodone being common options. They block pain signals in the brain and spinal cord. However, in the CP population, opioids pose high risks. Recent studies show adults with CP are more likely to be prescribed opioids for longer and in higher doses. This is concerning because opioids often aren't effective for the complex, non-nociceptive pain many with CP experience. One study found nearly 80% of adults with mixed pain phenotypes received non-perioperative opioids, indicating dependence on a high-risk drug class for less responsive pain [129].

The risk–benefit ratio for opioids in this population is unfavorable, especially long-term. Patients with CP are vulnerable and more prone to severe opioid side effects like respiratory depression, sedation, constipation, and dependence. Long-term use is also linked to cognitive issues, memory problems, and a higher risk of substance use disorder. Persistent pain in CP drives a clinical demand for relief that, without effective alternatives, can lead to inappropriate, prolonged opioid use. Clinicians should seek specialist advice and try less risky analgesics first [129].

Medications for Neuropathic Pain

Gabapentin and pregabalin are cornerstone treatments for neuropathic pain. They are considered a first-line therapy for this pain phenotype in adults, with growing evidence for their use in pediatric populations, particularly in the CP community.

Gabapentinoids do not bind to GABA receptors, as their names might suggest. Instead, they bind to the alpha-2-delta subunit of voltage-gated calcium channels in the central nervous system, particularly in the dorsal horn of the spinal cord. This binding reduces the influx of calcium, thereby inhibiting the release of excitatory neurotransmitters such as glutamate and Substance P. This mechanism makes them highly effective for targeting the central neuropathic pain component often present in CP [130, 131]. Gabapentinoids have a side effect profile that includes CNS effects like dizziness, drowsiness, fatigue, and ataxia, which are worse with opioids, raising the risk of respiratory depression. Slow tapering helps prevent withdrawal symptoms like anxiety, sleep issues, and seizures [132].

Oral Muscle Relaxants and Antispasmodics

This topic is thoroughly covered in Sect. 4.3.

Antidepressants

Antidepressants are a valuable class of adjuvant analgesics, particularly in the management of chronic pain. While their primary indication is for mood disorders, they have a separate mechanism as coanalgesics, modulating pain signals in the central nervous system. Tricyclic antidepressants (TCAs) and serotonin-norepinephrine reuptake inhibitors (SNRIs) are often used for this purpose. The high prevalence of depression and anxiety in individuals with chronic illness makes antidepressants a dual-purpose therapy that can address both psychological and physiological components of pain. Although there is a lack of high-quality studies on their use for pain in children, clinical experience suggests a favorable risk-benefit profile when used at low doses [133].

Topical Analgesics

For localized pain or procedural pain (e.g., prior to injections), topical agents can be a useful adjunctive therapy. These agents, available as creams, patches, or ointments, contain active ingredients such as lidocaine, a local anesthetic that blocks pain signals, or capsaicin and menthol, which act as counterirritants to distract the brain from the sensation of pain [134].

12.6.2.4 Interventional Pain Procedures

Nerve Blocks: Diagnostic and Therapeutic Applications

Temporary peripheral blocks with local anesthetics serve as a reversible "test" to simulate the effects of permanent motor blocks. They temporarily interrupt nerve signals to assess potential functional response, gait impact, and the benefit of reducing spasticity. This safe, controlled test helps determine permanent procedures, such as neurolytic blocks or surgery, thereby minimizing risks [135].

In their therapeutic role, neurolytic blocks, which involve the injection of agents like phenol or alcohol, provide more prolonged relief than local anesthetics. These blocks are easy to perform, effective, and relatively inexpensive, making them a viable option for long-term spasticity management. Common peripheral sites targeted for these procedures include the pectoral nerve loop, as well as the median, obturator, and tibial nerves, depending on the location of the most debilitating or painful spasticity [135].

Targeted Muscular, Spinal, and Neurosurgical Interventions
The use of BoNT-A, intrathecal baclofen, and selective dorsal rhizotomy is thoroughly discussed in Sects. 4.3.2, 4.3.3, and 4.3.4.6.

12.7 The Interplay of Spasticity and Pain Management

12.7.1 Distinguishing Pain from Spasticity

While spasticity is a core feature of CP and a well-recognized cause of pain, the relationship between the two is intricate and not always a simple cause-and-effect chain. The hypertonia and involuntary muscle movements associated with spasticity can be directly painful, but they also initiate a cascade of secondary complications that become long-term sources of chronic pain. Therefore, an effective management strategy must acknowledge and address the dynamic, bidirectional nature of this relationship, where spasticity leads to pain, and pain, in turn, can exacerbate spasticity [136, 137].

12.7.2 Contradictions in the Literature

A thorough review of the literature reveals a nuanced and at times contradictory picture regarding the direct correlation between spasticity reduction and pain relief. While some studies, particularly those involving BoNT-A, have found a significant reduction in pain following spasticity treatment, a study found that there is no significant direct relationship between the reduction of spasticity and pain relief in children with CP following BoNT-A treatment [136, 138]. In other studies in adults, spasticity measures, such as the Modified Ashworth Scale, do not consistently correlate with pain levels; however, self-reported spasm frequency does show a moderate association with pain severity. Additionally, there is evidence that no significant differences exist in pain measures across GMFCS levels, suggesting that pain affects individuals differently, regardless of their functional ability [139, 140].

These contradictory findings suggest that while spasticity management is a powerful tool for pain reduction, especially in preventing long-term deformities, a successful strategy must also consider other sources of pain and the direct analgesic effects of treatments.

12.8 Parent and Caregiver Support

Parents and caregivers play a crucial role in managing spasticity and pain. Good outcomes depend on clear goal-setting, informed choices about tone treatments, reliable pain monitoring at home, and timely escalation when red flags appear. Major guidelines (NICE) and specialty pathways (AACPDM) emphasize shared decision-making, family-friendly education, and structured follow-up for children and young people with CP [141].

12.8.1 Help Families Tell "Tone" from "Pain"

Caregivers often see day-to-day changes first. Teach simple distinctions:

Spasticity/tone feels like "tightness" that varies with speed, position, or emotion; dystonia looks like twisting or abnormal postures that "come and go." Both can cause discomfort and limit function, but not all increases in tone equal pain. AACPDM's pathways (including dystonia) encourage plain-language education and team review when function or comfort changes [142, 143].

12.8.2 Use Caregiver-Friendly Pain Tools

For children who cannot self-report, teach parents one observational tool and use it consistently:

- r-FLACC (lets families add child-specific behaviors).
- NCCPC-R/NCCPC-PV (validated for severe cognitive impairment).
- Pediatric Pain Profile (PPP) (20-item behavior checklist used by parents).

12.8.3 Prepare Families for Each Spasticity Pathway

Table 12.10 provides families with a general understanding of each treatment type, what they can do at home, what they can expect, and the red flags that may require urgent action.

Table 12.10 Caregiver support guide

Treatment	What families do at home	What to expect	Red flags/call now
Oral medications (baclofen, diazepam, etc.)	Give on schedule; track function + side effects; never stop abruptly.	Calmer muscles; watch for sleepiness/ constipation.	Excess sedation, breathing concerns, abrupt stoppage.
BoNT-A injections	Stretch/position as advised; goal-based practice daily (e.g., dressing, standing); orthosis use if prescribed.	Peak effect 2–6 weeks; fades by ~3–6 months.	Worsening weakness, new pain/swelling; no functional gains → tell team.
Serial casting	Skin checks each day; keep dry; elevate if sore; return for scheduled changes.	Gradual ROM gain; walking may feel different.	Skin breakdown, wet/loose cast, fever, severe pain.
AFOs/orthoses	Break-in schedule; sock under brace; report redness >30 min after removal.	Better heel-strike/ stride; energy savings.	Pressure sores, pain → review fit/design.
ITB pump	Keep refill dates; know emergency plan; carry info card.	Reduced painful spasms; easier care.	Withdrawal: high fever, agitation, severe spasticity. Overdose: somnolence, hypotonia, breathing issues. Urgent care.
SDR	Support intensive PT blocks; daily home exercises; track endurance and balance.	Less spasticity; gradual strength/ skill gains.	New weakness/falls without a plan; uncontrolled pain; missed rehab.

12.9 Guide for Multidisciplinary Team

Effective spasticity and pain care rests on a coordinated team plan that families can understand and run at home. Current guidance stresses: (1) shared decisions and family-centered goals, (2) clear differentiation of spasticity vs dystonia vs pain, (3) standardized assessment (tone and pain), (4) evidence-based tone pathways (oral agents, BoNT-A, casting/orthoses, ITB, SDR) with required therapy dose, and (5) proactive surveillance for preventable pain (hips, skin/device issues), with rapid escalation for red flags [141, 143].

12.9.1 Speak the Same "Tone and Pain" Language

Use plain terms with families: spasticity (velocity-dependent stiffness), dystonia (twisting postures/fluctuating tone), and pain (often multifactorial). Follow AACPDM's dystonia care pathway to guide pharmacologic/neurosurgical options when dystonia causes interference [143]. Treat pain as a parallel target, not just a symptom of tone. Use one caregiver-friendly observational tool (e.g., r-FLACC, NCCPC, PPP) for children who cannot self-report; apply it consistently to see trends and judge response [144].

12.9.2 Standardize Assessment and Outcomes

Tone: Modified Ashworth/Tardieu for documentation; function: GMFM/goal attainment; comfort/ease-of-care outcomes after BoNT-A or ITB [83].

Pain: daily caregiver ratings with the chosen tool; note triggers (positioning, orthoses fit, constipation, dental/skin issues) [142].

12.9.3 Choose Tone Interventions

- Oral medications (e.g., baclofen, diazepam): balance function vs sedation; plan slow titration and weaning [141].
- BoNT-A: set functional goals (hygiene, orthosis tolerance, dressing); pair with task-specific therapy during the 2–6-week "window." Evidence supports gains in comfort and ease of care, particularly in non-ambulatory children, when combined with therapy [83].
- Serial casting/orthoses: casting improves ROM; AFOs improve ankle kinematics/stride length (benefits vs skin/comfort trade-offs) [145].
- Intrathecal baclofen (ITB): agree on refill schedule and emergency plan; teach overdose vs withdrawal signs (withdrawal can be life-threatening) [70].
- Selective dorsal rhizotomy (SDR): consider in carefully selected ambulant children; ensure families understand irreversibility and the mandatory post-op rehab dose [146].

12.10 Conclusion

Effective management of pain and spasticity in cerebral palsy represents a complex, lifelong endeavor that requires a nuanced and multimodal approach, progressing from foundational rehabilitative therapies and pharmacological interventions to more advanced surgical and technological solutions. While these individual treatments—ranging from oral medications and targeted botulinum toxin injections to the continuous delivery of intrathecal baclofen and the selective neurosurgical procedure of dorsal rhizotomy—are essential, the core of successful care lies not merely in the selection of a specific modality but in its implementation within a truly collaborative, family-centered model. This framework marks a profound paradigm shift from traditional, hierarchical service delivery to an integrated, transdisciplinary approach, where a dedicated team of specialists, including physical medicine and rehabilitation experts, surgeons, and therapists, works in shared partnership with the patient and their family, who are empowered as the central decision-makers. This holistic structure is vital for addressing the inherent paradox of cerebral palsy: that a static brain injury often leads to progressive, secondary conditions, such as chronic pain and contractures, that profoundly impact functional independence and quality of life in adulthood. Though current interventions may have limitations, such as temporary effectiveness or variable patient responses, the future of the field is characterized by a two-pronged research effort: one that is refining symptomatic management with cutting-edge technologies like non-invasive brain stimulation and exoskeletons, and another that is proactively charting a course toward prevention and even a potential cure through advances in genetic research, regenerative medicine, and therapeutic hypothermia. Ultimately, the journey of managing pain and spasticity is a continuous, integrated, and deeply personal one, with a collective commitment from a sophisticated healthcare team, empowered families, and a dynamic research community that is not just making life more manageable but is fundamentally reshaping the lifelong experience of cerebral palsy.

References

1. Novak I, Hines M, Goldsmith S, Barclay R. Clinical prognostic messages from a systematic review on cerebral palsy. Pediatrics. 2012;130:e1285–e312.
2. Vitrikas K, Dalton H, Breish D. Cerebral palsy: an overview. Am Fam Physician. 2020;101:213–20.
3. Centers for Disease Control and Prevention. Cerebral palsy. Updated March 17, 2025. Available from: https://www.cdc.gov/cerebral-palsy/about/index.html.
4. Rivelis Y, Zafar N, Morice K. Spasticity. Treasure Island: StatPearls [Internet]; 2018.
5. Wahyuni LK. Multisystem compensations and consequences in spastic quadriplegic cerebral palsy children. Front Neurol. 2023;13:1076316.
6. Ostojic K, Paget SP, Morrow AM. Management of pain in children and adolescents with cerebral palsy: a systematic review. Dev Med Child Neurol. 2019;61:315–21.
7. Peck J, Urits I, Kassem H, Lee C, Robinson W, Cornett EM, et al. Interventional approaches to pain and spasticity related to cerebral palsy. Psychopharmacol Bull. 2020;50:108–20.
8. Barnes MP. An overview of the clinical management of spasticity. In: Barnes MP, Johnson GR, editors. Upper motor neurone syndrome and spasticity: clinical management and neurophysiology. 2nd ed. Cambridge: Cambridge University Press; 2008. p. 1–8.
9. Pandyan A, Gregoric M, Barnes M, Wood D, Wijck FV, Burridge J, et al. Spasticity: clinical perceptions, neurological realities and meaningful measurement. Disabil Rehabil. 2005;27:2–6.
10. Brown P. Pathophysiology of spasticity. J Neurol Neurosurg Psychiatry. 1994;57:773–7.
11. Tedroff K, Granath F, Forssberg H, Haglund-Akerlind Y. Long-term effects of botulinum toxin A in children with cerebral palsy. Dev Med Child Neurol. 2009;51:120–7.
12. Nordmark E, Hägglund G, Lauge-Pedersen H, Wagner P, Westbom L. Development of lower limb range of motion from early childhood to adolescence in cerebral palsy: a population-based study. BMC Med. 2009;7:1–11.
13. Hill J, Olson E. Muscle 2-volume set: fundamental biology and mechanisms of disease. London; Waltham: Academic Press; 2012.
14. Handsfield GG, Williams S, Khuu S, Lichtwark G, Stott NS. Muscle architecture, growth, and biological remodelling in cerebral palsy: a narrative review. BMC Musculoskelet Disord. 2022;23:233.

15. Mathewson MA, Ward SR, Chambers HG, Lieber RL. High resolution muscle measurements provide insights into equinus contractures in patients with cerebral palsy. J Orthop Res. 2015;33:33–9.
16. Pontén E, Gantelius S, Lieber RL. Intraoperative muscle measurements reveal a relationship between contracture formation and muscle remodeling. Muscle Nerve. 2007;36:47–54.
17. Robinson KG, Crowgey EL, Lee SK, Akins RE. Transcriptional analysis of muscle tissue and isolated satellite cells in spastic cerebral palsy. Dev Med Child Neurol. 2021;63:1213–20.
18. Loomis T, Kulkarni VA, Villalba M, Davids JR, Leach JK, Smith LR. Muscle satellite cells and fibro-adipogenic progenitors from muscle contractures of children with cerebral palsy have impaired regenerative capacity. Dev Med Child Neurol. 2025;67:77–86.
19. Palisano R, Rosenbaum P, Walter S, Russell D, Wood E, Galuppi B. Development and reliability of a system to classify gross motor function in children with cerebral palsy. Dev Med Child Neurol. 1997;39:214–23.
20. Reid SM, Carlin JB, Reddihough DS. Using the gross motor function classification system to describe patterns of motor severity in cerebral palsy. Dev Med Child Neurol. 2011;53:1007–12.
21. Clewes K, Hammond C, Dong Y, Meyer M, Lowe E, Rose J. Neuromuscular impairments of cerebral palsy: contributions to gait abnormalities and implications for treatment. Front Hum Neurosci. 2024;18:1445793.
22. Yeargin-Allsopp M, Van Naarden BK, Doernberg NS, Benedict RE, Kirby RS, Durkin MS. Prevalence of cerebral palsy in 8-year-old children in three areas of the United States in 2002: a multisite collaboration. Pediatrics. 2008;121:547–54.
23. Peixoto MV, Duque AM, Carvalho SD, Gonçalves TP, Novais APDS, Nunes MAP, editors. Epidemiological characteristics of cerebral palsy in children and adolescents in a Brazilian northeast capital. 2021.
24. Kulak W, Sobaniec W. Comparisons of right and left hemiparetic cerebral palsy. Pediatr Neurol. 2004;31:101–8.
25. Bodur M, Özmen AH, Okan MS. Clinical phenotypes and etiological risk factors in children with cerebral palsy: a retrospective study. Inn J Pediatr. 2024;34:e143328.
26. Amoghimath R, Gowda V, Benakappa A. Comorbidities and their relationship to subtype of cerebral palsy in a tertiary care hospital in South India. Indian J Cereb Palsy. 2016;2:204408.
27. Bohannon RW, Smith MB. Interrater reliability of a modified Ashworth scale of muscle spasticity. Phys Ther. 1987;67:206–7.
28. Ansari NN, Naghdi S, Moammeri H, Jalaie S. Ashworth scales are unreliable for the assessment of muscle spasticity. Physiother Theory Pract. 2006;22:119–25.
29. Haugh A, Pandyan A, Johnson G. A systematic review of the Tardieu scale for the measurement of spasticity. Disabil Rehabil. 2006;28:899–907.
30. Patrick E, Ada L. The Tardieu Scale differentiates contracture from spasticity whereas the Ashworth Scale is confounded by it. Clin Rehabil. 2006;20:173–82.
31. Nourizadeh M, Shadgan B, Abbasidezfouli S, Juricic M, Mulpuri K. Methods of muscle spasticity assessment in children with cerebral palsy: a scoping review. J Orthop Surg Res. 2024;19:401.
32. Szopa A, Domagal–Skaszopa M, Kidoń Z, Syczewska M. Quadriceps femoris spasticity in children with cerebral palsy: measurement with the pendulum test and relationship with gait abnormalities. J Neuroeng Rehabil. 2014;11:1–10.
33. Bilgici MC, Bekci T, Ulus Y, Ozyurek H, Aydin OF, Tomak L, Selcuk MB. Quantitative assessment of muscular stiffness in children with cerebral palsy using acoustic radiation force impulse (ARFI) ultrasound elastography. J Med Ultrason. 2018;45:295–300.
34. Öztürk M, Sayinbatur B. Real-time ultrasound elastography of the Achilles tendon in patients with cerebral palsy: is there a correlation between strain ratio and biomechanical indicators? J Med Ultrason. 2018;45:143–8.

35. Palisano RJ, Avery L, Gorter JW, Galuppi B, McCoy SW. Stability of the gross motor function classification system, manual ability classification system, and communication function classification system. Dev Med Child Neurol. 2018;60:1026–32.
36. Armand S, Decoulon G, Bonnefoy-Mazure A. Gait analysis in children with cerebral palsy. EFORT Open Rev. 2016;1:448–60.
37. Sato H. Postural deformity in children with cerebral palsy: why it occurs and how is it managed. Physical therapy research. 2020;23:8–14.
38. Basit A, Querishi MS, Arif MI. Need assessment of an interventional package for development of fine motor skills of children with cerebral palsy. Palarch's J Archaeol Egypt/Egyptol. 2021;18:1483–99.
39. McMorris C, Lake J, Lunsky Y, Dobranowski K, Fehlings D, Bayley M, et al. Adults with cerebral palsy: physical and mental health issues and health service use patterns. Int Rev Res Dev Disabil. 2015;48:115–49.
40. Mckinnon CT, Meehan EM, Harvey AR, Antolovich GC, Morgan PE. Prevalence and characteristics of pain in children and young adults with cerebral palsy: a systematic review. Dev Med Child Neurol. 2019;61:305–14.
41. Penner M, Xie WY, Binepal N, Switzer L, Fehlings D. Characteristics of pain in children and youth with cerebral palsy. Pediatrics. 2013;132:e407–e13.
42. Tedroff K, Gyllensvärd M, Löwing K. Prevalence, identification, and interference of pain in young children with cerebral palsy: a population-based study. Disabil Rehabil. 2021;43:1292–8.
43. Caravau H, Rosa AF, Rocha NP, Silva AG. Pain assessment in cerebral palsy: a systematic review of measurement properties and evaluation using the COSMIN checklist. Disabil Rehabil. 2022;44:909–19.
44. Smith NL, Gibson N, Bear N, Thornton AL, Imms C, Smith MG, Harvey AR. Measurement properties and feasibility of chronic pain assessment tools for use with children and young people with cerebral palsy. Disabil Rehabil. 2025;47:840–54.
45. Schiariti V, Oberlander TF. Evaluating pain in cerebral palsy: comparing assessment tools using the international classification of functioning, disability and health. Disabil Rehabil. 2019;41:2622–9.
46. Jersak T, Noritz G. Evaluation of pain in adults with childhood-onset disabilities and communication difficulties. Front Neurol. 2021;12:722971.
47. Sarathy K, Doshi C, Aroojis A. Clinical examination of children with cerebral palsy. Indian J Orthop. 2019;53:35–44.
48. Rajiv S, Alison C. Real-life outcomes in spasticity management: features affecting goal achievement. BMJ Neurol Open. 2020;2:e000015.
49. Brandão MB, Oliveira RH, Mancini MC. Functional priorities reported by parents of children with cerebral palsy: contribution to the pediatric rehabilitation process. Braz J Phys Ther. 2014;18:563–71.
50. Mavis Mallory M, Joseph Ngmenesegre S, Yaa Nyarko A, Margaret WK. Family caregivers' experience of care with a child with cerebral palsy: the lived experiences and challenges of caregivers in a resource-limited setting in northern Ghana. BMJ Paediatr Open. 2023;7:e001807.
51. Bøttcher L, Stadskleiv K, Berntsen T, Christensen K, Korsfelt Å, Kihlgren M, Ödman P. Systematic cognitive monitoring of children with cerebral palsy—the development of an assessment and follow-up protocol. Scand J Disabil Res. 2016;18:304–15.
52. Rasmussen HM, Nordbye-Nielsen K, Møller-Madsen B, Johansen M, Ellitsgaard N, Pedersen CR, et al. The Danish cerebral palsy follow-up program. Clin Epidemiol. 2016;8:457–60.
53. Mehraban Jahromi M, Vlček P, Grünerová LM. Stretching exercises in managing spasticity: effectiveness, risks, and adjunct therapies. Eur J Transl Myol. 2024;34:12455.
54. Kalkman BM, Bar-On L, O'Brien TD, Maganaris CN. Stretching interventions in children with cerebral palsy: why are they ineffective in improving muscle function and how can we better their outcome? Front Physiol. 2020;11:131.

55. Merino-Andrés J, García de Mateos-López A, Damiano DL, Sánchez-Sierra A. Effect of muscle strength training in children and adolescents with spastic cerebral palsy: a systematic review and meta-analysis. Clin Rehabil. 2022;36:4–14.
56. Dodd KJ, Taylor NF, Damiano DL. A systematic review of the effectiveness of strength-training programs for people with cerebral palsy. Arch Phys Med Rehabil. 2002;83:1157–64.
57. Rauf W, Sarmad S, Khan I, Jawad M. Effect of position on gross motor function and spasticity in spastic cerebral palsy children. J Pak Med Assoc. 2021;71:801–5.
58. Ricardo D, Raposo MR, Cruz EB, Oliveira R, Carnide F, Veloso AP, João F. Effects of ankle foot orthoses on the gait patterns in children with spastic bilateral cerebral palsy: a scoping review. Children. 2021;8:903.
59. Booth AT, Buizer AI, Meyns P, Oude Lansink IL, Steenbrink F, van der Krogt MM. The efficacy of functional gait training in children and young adults with cerebral palsy: a systematic review and meta-analysis. Dev Med Child Neurol. 2018;60:866–83.
60. Elanchezhian C, Swarnakumari P. Efficacy of cold therapy and passive stretching to improve gait in spastic diplegic cerebral palsy children. J Pediatr Perspect. 2019;7:10109–18.
61. Shamsoddini A, Amirsalari S, Hollisaz MT, Rahimnia A, Khatibi-Aghda A. Management of spasticity in children with cerebral palsy. Iran J Pediatr. 2014;24:345–51.
62. Greve KR, Joseph CF, Berry BE, Schadl K, Rose J. Neuromuscular electrical stimulation to augment lower limb exercise and mobility in individuals with spastic cerebral palsy: a scoping review. Front Physiol. 2022;13:951899.
63. Peters C, Chang A, Morales A, Barnes K, Allegretti A. An integrative review of assessments used in occupational therapy interventions for children with cerebral palsy. Cadernos Brasileiros de Terapia Ocupacional. 2019;27:168–85.
64. Ayala L, Winter S, Byrne R, Fehlings D, Gehred A, Letzkus L, et al. Assessments and interventions for spasticity in infants with or at high risk for cerebral palsy: a systematic review. Pediatr Neurol. 2021;118:72–90.
65. Klaewkasikum K, Patathong T, Woratanarat P, Woratanarat T, Thadanipon K, Rattanasiri S, Thakkinstian A. Efficacy of conservative treatment for spastic cerebral palsy children with equinus gait: a systematic review and meta-analysis. J Orthop Surg Res. 2022;17:411.
66. Zhao X, Xiao N, Li H, Du S. Day vs. day-night use of ankle-foot orthoses in young children with spastic diplegia: a randomized controlled study. Am J Phys Med Rehabil. 2013;92:905–11.
67. Jackman M, Novak I, Lannin N. Effectiveness of hand splints in children with cerebral palsy: a systematic review with meta-analysis. Dev Med Child Neurol. 2014;56:138–47.
68. Lidman GRM, Nachemson AK, Peny-Dahlstrand MB, Himmelmann KME. Long-term effects of repeated botulinum neurotoxin A, bimanual training, and splinting in young children with cerebral palsy. Dev Med Child Neurol. 2020;62:252–8.
69. Peck J, Urits I, Crane J, McNally A, Noor N, Patel M, et al. Oral muscle relaxants for the treatment of chronic pain associated with cerebral palsy. Psychopharmacol Bull. 2020;50:142–62.
70. Ghanavatian S, Derian A. Baclofen. Treasure Island: StatPearls [Internet]; 2024.
71. Malanga G, Reiter RD, Garay E. Update on tizanidine for muscle spasticity and emerging indications. Expert Opin Pharmacother. 2008;9:2209–15.
72. Bounds CG, Patel P. Benzodiazepines. Treasure Island: StatPearls [Internet]; 2024.
73. Krause T, Gerbershagen M, Fiege M, Weisshorn R, Wappler F. Dantrolene–a review of its pharmacology, therapeutic use and new developments. Anaesthesia. 2004;59:364–73.
74. Ertzgaard P, Campo C, Calabrese A. Efficacy and safety of oral baclofen in the management of spasticity: a rationale for intrathecal baclofen. J Rehabil Med. 2017;49:193–203.
75. Dai AI, Aksoy SN, Demiryürek AT. Comparison of efficacy and side effects of oral baclofen versus tizanidine therapy with adjuvant botulinum toxin type A in children with cerebral palsy and spastic equinus foot deformity. J Child Neurol. 2016;31:184–9.
76. Mathew A, Mathew MC, Thomas M, Antonisamy B. The efficacy of diazepam in enhancing motor function in children with spastic cerebral palsy. J Trop Pediatr. 2005;51:109–13.
77. Pinder RM, Brogden RN, Speight TM, Avery GS. Dantrolene sodium. Drugs. 1977;13:3–23.
78. Ratto D, Joyner RW. Dantrolene. Treasure Island: StatPearls [Internet]; 2018.

79. Mathew A, Mathew M. Bedtime diazepam enhances well-being in children with spastic cerebral palsy. Pediatr Rehabil. 2005;8:63–6.
80. Kaya Keles CS, Ates F. Botulinum toxin intervention in cerebral palsy-induced spasticity management: projected and contradictory effects on skeletal muscles. Toxins (Basel). 2022;14:772.
81. Unlu E, Cevikol A, Bal B, Gonen E, Celik O, Kose G. Multilevel botulinum toxin type A as a treatment for spasticity in children with cerebral palsy: a retrospective study. Clinics. 2010;65:613–9.
82. Strobl W, Theologis T, Brunner R, Kocer S, Viehweger E, Pascual-Pascual I, Placzek R. Best clinical practice in botulinum toxin treatment for children with cerebral palsy. Toxins. 2015;7:1629–48.
83. Multani I, Manji J, Hastings-Ison T, Khot A, Graham K. Botulinum toxin in the management of children with cerebral palsy. Paediatr Drugs. 2019;21:261–81.
84. Farag SM, Mohammed MO, El-Sobky TA, El Kadery NA, El Zohiery AK. Botulinum toxin A injection in treatment of upper limb spasticity in children with cerebral palsy: a systematic review of randomized controlled trials. JBJS Reviews. 2020;8:e0119.
85. Fattal-Valevski A, Domenievitz D, Giladi N, Wientroub S, Hayek S. Long-term effect of repeated injections of botulinum toxin in children with cerebral palsy: a prospective study. J Child Orthop. 2008;2:29–35.
86. Sozbilen MC, Evren SK. Long-term efficacy and safety of repeated botulinum toxin a applications based on function and anesthesia type in children with cerebral palsy. J Orthop. 2022;29:22–7.
87. Joshi TN, Joshi S. Adverse effects of botulinum neurotoxin A in spasticity management. Int J Nutr Pharmacol Neurol Dis. 2011;1:126–33.
88. Kaya Keles CS, Ates F. Botulinum toxin intervention in cerebral palsy-induced spasticity management: projected and contradictory effects on skeletal muscles. Toxins. 2022;14:772.
89. Valentine J, Stannage K, Fabian V, Ellis K, Reid S, Pitcher C, Elliott C. Muscle histopathology in children with spastic cerebral palsy receiving botulinum toxin type A. Muscle Nerve. 2016;53:407–14.
90. Hasnat MJ, Rice JE. Intrathecal baclofen for treating spasticity in children with cerebral palsy. Cochrane Database Syst Rev. 2015;2015:Cd004552.
91. Cho SR. Intrathecal Baclofen therapy: pros and cons. Ann Rehabil Med. 2023;47:1–3.
92. Brennan PM, Whittle IR. Intrathecal baclofen therapy for neurological disorders: a sound knowledge base but many challenges remain. Br J Neurosurg. 2008;22:508–19.
93. Banawal LK, Chandrol V, Ratre S, Yadav YR, Bajaj J. Surgical approach for spasticity: a systematic review. Indian J Neurosurg. 2025;14:S7–S19.
94. Grunt S, Fieggen AG, Vermeulen RJ, Becher JG, Langerak NG. Selection criteria for selective dorsal rhizotomy in children with spastic cerebral palsy: a systematic review of the literature. Dev Med Child Neurol. 2014;56:302–12.
95. DuDley RW, PaRolin M, GaGnon B, Saluja R, Yap R, Montpetit K, et al. Long-term functional benefits of selective dorsal rhizotomy for spastic cerebral palsy. J Neurosurg Pediatr. 2013;12:142–50.
96. Nicolini-Panisson RD, Tedesco AP, Folle MR, Donadio MVF. Selective dorsal rhizotomy in cerebral palsy: selection criteria and postoperative physical therapy protocols. Rev Paul Pediatr. 2018;36:9.
97. Wang KK, Munger ME, Chen BP, Novacheck TF. Selective dorsal rhizotomy in ambulant children with cerebral palsy. J Child Orthop. 2018;12:413–27.
98. Otero-Luis I, Martinez-Rodrigo A, Cavero-Redondo I, Moreno-Herráiz N, Araya-Quintanilla F, Lever-Megina CG, Saz-Lara A. Efficacy of selective dorsal rhizotomy in the treatment of spasticity in children with cerebral palsy: a systematic review and meta-analysis. J Neurosurg Pediatr. 2025;35:571–80.
99. Tedroff K, Hägglund G, Miller F. Long-term effects of selective dorsal rhizotomy in children with cerebral palsy: a systematic review. Dev Med Child Neurol. 2020;62:554–62.

100. Ploegmakers DJM, Van Duijnhoven HJR, Duraku LS, Kurt E, Geurts ACH, De Jong T. Efficacy of selective neurotomy for focal lower limb spasticity: a systematic review. J Rehabil Med. 2024;56:jrm39947.
101. Fan J, Milosevic R, Wang S. Selective peripheral neurotomy (SPN) as a treatment strategy for spasticity. Brain Sci Adv. 2020;6:30–41.
102. Rinde ER, Anderzén-Carlsson A, Jahnsen RB, Andersen RD. Children with cerebral palsy and their parents have different experiences of pain management: a qualitative study. Children. 2024;11:1055.
103. Meints SM, Edwards RR. Evaluating psychosocial contributions to chronic pain outcomes. Prog Neuro-Psychopharmacol Biol Psychiatry. 2018;87:168–82.
104. Williams E, Coghill J. Understanding and managing pain in children with cerebral palsy. Paediatr Child Health. 2023;33:17–22.
105. Bruce BK, Weiss KE, Ale CM, Harrison TE, Fischer PR. Development of an interdisciplinary pediatric pain rehabilitation program: the first 1000 consecutive patients. Mayo Clin Proc Innov Qual Outcomes. 2017;1:141–9.
106. Collins AB. Chronic pediatric pain management: a review of multidisciplinary care and emerging topics. Curr Phys Med Rehabil Rep. 2019;7:30–9.
107. Liossi C, Johnstone L, Lilley S, Caes L, Williams G, Schoth DE. Effectiveness of interdisciplinary interventions in paediatric chronic pain management: a systematic review and subset meta-analysis. Br J Anaesth. 2019;123:e359–e71.
108. Gonzalez NA, Sanivarapu RR, Osman U, Latha Kumar A, Sadagopan A, Mahmoud A, et al. Physical therapy interventions in children with cerebral palsy: a systematic review. Cureus. 2023;15:e43846.
109. Liang X, Zhujiang T, Guojun Y, Jianguo C, Jinggang W, Qing L, Turong C. Effectiveness of exercise interventions for children with cerebral palsy: a systematic review and meta-analysis of randomized controlled trials. J Rehabil Med. 2020;53:2733.
110. Yang G, Su H, Yang M, Chang J. The effect of physical exercise on gross motor function in children with cerebral palsy: a meta-analysis. Int J Hum Mov Sports Sci. 2022;10:581–91.
111. Verschuren O, Peterson MD, Balemans AC, Hurvitz EA. Exercise and physical activity recommendations for people with cerebral palsy. Dev Med Child Neurol. 2016;58:798–808.
112. Vance CGT, Dailey DL, Chimenti RL, Van Gorp BJ, Crofford LJ, Sluka KA. Using TENS for pain control: update on the state of the evidence. Medicina. 2022;58:1332.
113. Garzon LC, Switzer L, Musselman KE, Fehlings D. The use of functional electrical stimulation to improve upper limb function in children with hemiplegic cerebral palsy: a feasibility study. J Rehabil Assist Technol Eng. 2018;5:2055668318768402.
114. Tao Y, Cao Z, Shin MC, Chen M, Han S. The effects of hydrotherapy on athletic ability in children with cerebral palsy: a systematic review and meta-analysis. PLoS One. 2025;20:e0325517.
115. Shekari Z, Sadeghian Afarani R, Fatorehchy S, Bakhshi E, Shahshahani S, Mousavi E. Relationship between postural asymmetry, balance, and pain in children with spastic cerebral palsy. Pediatr Neurol. 2024;155:84–90.
116. Ouyang R-G, Yang C-N, Qu Y-L, Koduri MP, Chien C-W. Effectiveness of hand-arm bimanual intensive training on upper extremity function in children with cerebral palsy: a systematic review. Eur J Paediatr Neurol. 2020;25:17–28.
117. Warutkar VB, Kovela RK, Warutkar V. Review of sensory integration therapy for children with cerebral palsy. Cureus. 2022;14:e30714.
118. Ehde DM, Dillworth TM, Turner JA. Cognitive-behavioral therapy for individuals with chronic pain: efficacy, innovations, and directions for research. Am Psychol. 2014;69:153.
119. Kobayashi S, Koitabashi K. Effects of progressive muscle relaxation on cerebral activity: an fMRI investigation. Complement Ther Med. 2016;26:33–9.
120. Won AS, Bailey J, Bailenson J, Tataru C, Yoon IA, Golianu B. Immersive virtual reality for pediatric pain. Children. 2017;4:52.
121. MacIntosh A, Lam E, Vigneron V, Vignais N, Biddiss E. Biofeedback interventions for individuals with cerebral palsy: a systematic review. Disabil Rehabil. 2019;41:2369–91.

122. Hu J, Wang X, Liu X, Xia T, Liu Q, Zhang X, Hu Y. Effectiveness and safety of acupuncture for children with cerebral palsy: an overview of systematic reviews. Eur J Integr Med. 2022;56:102199.
123. Glew GM, Fan MY, Hagland S, Bjornson K, Beider S, McLaughlin JF. Survey of the use of massage for children with cerebral palsy. Int J Ther Massage Bodywork. 2010;3:10–5.
124. Topcu ZG, Tomaç H. The effectiveness of massage for children with cerebral palsy: a systematic review. Adv Mind Body Med. 2020;34:4–13.
125. Yang S, Suh JH, Kwon S, Chang MC. The effect of neurologic music therapy in patients with cerebral palsy: a systematic narrative review. Front Neurol. 2022;13:852277.
126. Vinolo-Gil MJ, Casado-Fernandez E, Perez-Cabezas V, Gonzalez-Medina G, Martin-Vega FJ, Martin-Valero R. Effects of the combination of music therapy and physiotherapy in the improvement of motor function in cerebral palsy: a challenge for research. Children. 2021;8:868.
127. Sansone L, Gentile C, Grasso EA, Di Ludovico A, La Bella S, Chiarelli F, Breda L. Pain evaluation and treatment in children: a practical approach. Children. 2023;10:1212.
128. Beecham E, Candy B, Howard R, McCulloch R, Laddie J, Rees H, et al. Pharmacological interventions for pain in children and adolescents with life-limiting conditions. Cochrane Database Syst Rev. 2015;2015:Cd010750.
129. Peterson MD, O'Leary M, Ashbaugh K, Haapala H, Schmidt M, Kamdar N, Hurvitz EA. Medication and therapy profiles for pain and symptom management among adults with cerebral palsy. Mayo Clin Proc Innov Qual Outcomes. 2025;9:100597.
130. Hauer JM, Solodiuk JC. Gabapentin for management of recurrent pain in 22 nonverbal children with severe neurological impairment: a retrospective analysis. J Palliat Med. 2015;18:453–6.
131. Sills GJ. The mechanisms of action of gabapentin and pregabalin. Curr Opin Pharmacol. 2006;6:108–13.
132. Nwankwo A, Koyyalagunta D, Huh B, D'Souza RS, Javed S. A comprehensive review of the typical and atypical side effects of gabapentin. Pain Pract. 2024;24:1051–8.
133. Baltenberger EP, Buterbaugh WM, Martin BS, Thomas CJ. Review of antidepressants in the treatment of neuropathic pain. Mental Health Clinician. 2015;5:123–33.
134. Faccioli S, Ehsani A, Kaleci S, Tonini G, Tagliani I, Vetrano M, Sassi S. Procedural pain management in patients with cerebral palsy undergoing botulinum toxin injection: a systematic review and meta-analysis. Toxins. 2025;17:317.
135. Novikov VA, Umnov VV, Zharkov DS, Barlova OV, Mustafaeva AR, Vissarionov SV. Prognostic efficiency of diagnostic blockade as a method of modeling the result of selective neurotomy of the motor branches of the median nerve in patients with cerebral palsy. Pediatr Traumatol Orthop Reconstr Surg. 2024;12:173–83.
136. Wong C. The relationship between pain and spasticity and tell-tale signs of pain in children with cerebral palsy. Toxins. 2023;15:152.
137. Peck J, Urits I, Kassem H, Lee C, Robinson W, Cornett EM, et al. Interventional approaches to pain and spasticity related to cerebral palsy. Psychopharmacol Bull. 2020;50:108.
138. Kurenkov A, Bursagova B, Artemenko A. Assessment of spasticity-related pain in cerebral palsy and the efficacy of its treatment with incobotulinumtoxin A (literature review). Neurol Neuropsychiatry Psychosomatics. 2024;16:94–101.
139. Smith JM, Field TS. Pain in adults with cerebral palsy: measuring the contribution of spasticity. Dev Med Child Neurol. 2020;62:271.
140. Flanigan M, Gaebler-Spira D, Kocherginsky M, Garrett A, Marciniak C. Spasticity and pain in adults with cerebral palsy. Dev Med Child Neurol. 2020;62:379–85.
141. guideline N. Cerebral palsy in under 25s: assessment and management 25 January 2017. Available from: https://www.nice.org.uk/guidance/ng62/chapter/Recommendations#pain-discomfort-and-distress.
142. Hauer J, Houtrow AJ, HOSPICE SO, PALLIATIVE MEDICINE COCWD. Pain assessment and treatment in children with significant impairment of the central nervous system. Pediatrics. 2017;139:e20171002.

143. Fehlings D, Agnew B, Gimeno H, Harvey A, Himmelmann K, Lin J-P, et al. Pharmacological and neurosurgical management of cerebral palsy and dystonia: clinical practice guideline update. Dev Med Child Neurol. 2024;66:1133–47.
144. Chan AY, Ge M, Harrop E, Johnson M, Oulton K, Skene SS, et al. Pain assessment tools in paediatric palliative care: a systematic review of psychometric properties and recommendations for clinical practice. Palliat Med. 2022;36:30–43.
145. McGrath TM, Palmer ST. Integrated hip surveillance pathways for pain, function and quality of life in children with cerebral palsy: a systematic literature review. Eur J Paediatr Neurol. 2024;53:166–73.
146. guidance Ip. Selective dorsal rhizotomy for spasticity in cerebral palsy 15 December 2010 [IPG373]. Available from: https://www.nice.org.uk/guidance/ipg373.

Psychological and Emotional Well-Being of Individuals with Cerebral Palsy

13

Kaveh Same and Mahtab Motamed

13.1 Introduction

Yasmin is a 14-year-old girl with a diagnosis of spastic diplegic cerebral palsy, classified as GMFCS Level III. She uses a walker daily and has mild dysarthria but is cognitively intact and attends a mainstream school with special educational support. Yasmin's grades have been average; however, her teachers have been voicing concern as they have recently noticed growing problems in her concentration and declining participation in class activities.

During a routine follow-up, Yasmin's mother also expressed concern about changes in her daughter's behavior. She had become increasingly withdrawn, often avoiding social gatherings and exhibiting intense worry about her appearance and others' opinions of her. She frequently compares herself to classmates and becomes visibly distressed when unable to participate in physical activities like others. She recently began expressing reluctance to go to school, saying that she was afraid of getting bullied. When asked further, it was revealed that a group of classmates had mocked her gait and walker.

Initial assessments by a pediatric psychologist suggested clinically significant symptoms of social anxiety and emerging signs of depressive mood. Yasmin reported feeling "different" and "not enough," describing herself as "a burden" to others

K. Same
Michael Ogon Laboratory for Orthopaedic Research, Orthopaedic Hospital Speising, Vienna, Austria

Doctoral Programme MedUni Vienna, Medical University of Vienna, Vienna, Austria
e-mail: kaveh.same@oss.at

M. Motamed (✉)
Psychiatry Department, School of Medicine, Tehran University of Medical Sciences, Tehran, Iran
e-mail: mmotamed@tums.ac.ir

A. Presedo et al. (eds.), *Enhancing Quality of Life in Patients with Cerebral Palsy*, https://doi.org/10.1007/978-3-032-20967-2_13

around her. She also reported recurring thoughts of wishing she were "normal," and occasional feelings of hopelessness. Pain and fatigue from her muscle tone issues were found to exacerbate her emotional distress, particularly in the afternoons. She also demonstrated symptoms of inattentiveness, but due to her physical disabilities, hyperactivity was not readily observable, making ADHD screening more nuanced.

A comprehensive care plan was developed by a multidisciplinary team that involved:

- *Individual cognitive-behavioral therapy (CBT)* focused on managing anxiety, body image concerns, and developing coping strategies for peer interactions.
- *School-based interventions*, including anti-bullying support and mobility-inclusive physical education modifications.
- *Family counseling sessions* to support emotional validation and reduce parental stress.
- *Occupational therapy* to enhance participation in leisure activities and boost self-efficacy.

Three months later, Yasmin showed improved mood and school performance and had re-engagement with a small group of peers in a shared art class, which became a source of pride and enjoyment for her. The psychologist noted gradual improvements in self-esteem and reduced school-related anxiety. She continues regular CBT and participates in a school peer support group for students with disabilities.

13.1.1 Overview

Faced with a myriad of lifelong complications that require near-constant medical attention and management, patients with cerebral palsy (CP) are usually forced to adjust their life plans and activities accordingly and cope with the implications and effects of their condition on their choices. With the disease ever present, this chronic battle begins at the same time as the very first steps of their psychological development, influencing their mental maturation and character formation since birth.

In their "Isle of Wight" study, Rutter and others have demonstrated that the presence of psychiatric disorders will be higher in children with neurological disease [1]. Such a profound impact of a condition on one's mental development and health warrants the need for equally detailed and extensive research; however, such attempts are hindered by the significantly varied nature of the disease and its accompanying symptoms. As Liptak points out, "variability is a hallmark of CP," and based on the severity of the symptoms and presence or absence of mental capacity deficits, the degree by which CP will affect the psychological and physical well-being of the individual can vary [2]. The current chapter will try to serve as an overview of the challenges that individuals with CP and those around them face in dealing with mental health issues throughout their lives.

13.1.2 Mental State

To gain a proper perspective into the mental state of individuals with CP, the best starting point would be to ask them what they think about themselves and their identity, challenges, and aspirations. In a qualitative study conducted to help understand and assess the "lived experiences" of those affected with CP [3], while introducing themselves, the participants usually began by stating their daily activities and societal roles rather than their exact medical diagnosis or condition, an observation that the authors interpreted as an effort by the subjects not to be defined by their illness and as a sign of their striving to achieve "normality" through social participation. The individuals also did not talk about CP-related goals when asked about their ambitions and dreams. That being said, it is crucial to point out that "Participation is not necessarily inclusion" [4], and truly, many individuals in the study reported high levels of depression and anxiety at least partly due to CP-related difficulties that prevented them from pursuing their goals. Furthermore, participants shared how the lack of a definitive diagnosis regarding their mental health issues could keep them from being able to benefit from the available supporting services, leading to the development of unhealthy coping mechanisms such as drug abuse in some cases.

Apart from its profound influence on the individual's ability to participate in daily physical activities, CP also impacts the patient's body image and how they see themselves. This becomes especially important as these children go through adolescence. Some studies have demonstrated that overall, adolescents with CP tend to have a more negative body image compared with their non-CP counterparts [5]. While others have found differing results in this regard [6], the existence of such evidence suggests the need for careful consideration of this phenomenon in CP patients' therapy and rehabilitation sessions and its implications on the individual's overall self-confidence.

Comparing life values and definitions of happiness, success, and health between adults with CP and non-CP controls, researchers reported CP individuals to share the same overall definitions of all three domains: success was defined as the ability to reach one's goals while being happy and having a purpose in life, happiness as being able to spend time with loved ones and to take part in one's favorite recreational activities, and finally health as having a good mind-body balance and being healthy in both dimensions. Still, differences were observed, especially regarding how one could obtain such goals and their lived experiences. Individuals with CP more strongly emphasized the importance of tenacity and persistence in achieving success, while they acknowledged having experienced negative feelings during their life and in social encounters, many of which they believed to have been influenced by their condition. Furthermore, many stated that they felt like they needed to achieve "more" compared with others to be considered equally successful [7].

Lastly, regarding their hopes and aspirations, in a qualitative narrative study, adolescents with CP were asked about their favorite out-of-school activities, important people in their lives, their short-term goals, and their long-term hopes, dreams, and aspirations, using several interview and qualitative data collection techniques [8]. The researchers classified the responses into three main themes:

1. Keeping close relationships with family and friends in the future: Participants may have somewhat differed from typical adolescents in this regard, as they expressed strong desires to maintain a close relationship with their family and acknowledged their family's important role in their physical and emotional well-being. They also expressed their desire to maintain close contact with their friends and additionally stated the wish to have a pet in the future.
2. Choosing their own future life: Consistent with previous research [9], the responses clearly indicated that individuals wanted to be able to choose their own path in life. While some had clear ideas of what job they wanted to have, all participants emphasized the importance of continuing their education and its role in their future.
3. Future Hobbies and interests: All participants reported a wish to have hobbies and leisure activities in the future. Their responses clearly showed their desire for "independently" choosing their favorite pastime activities, while they also took into consideration their physical capabilities.

Overall, studies indicate that while individuals with CP strive for the same goals and aspirations as everyone else, their disability has a considerable impact on their life experiences, their view of themselves, and their choices and future dreams.

13.1.3 Challenges

A lifelong disability with a significant impact on the individual's self-view and life experiences, living with CP can have serious negative consequences on mental health, especially as individuals go through major mental-development phases of life, such as adolescence. To that end, it is crucial to gain a better understanding of the specific mental-health challenges that might affect those with CP. Assessing the risks of different mental disorders in children with CP, individuals were found to show a higher risk for anxiety, behavior, and conduct problems, and the presence of multiple morbidities. However, the researchers found the risk of depression and attention-deficit/hyperactivity disorder (ADHD) to be the same as in the control group. Interestingly, social factors were shown to play a significant role in the observed elevated risk: after adjustment for "difficulty with friendships," the odds for anxiety, behavior and conduct problems, and multimorbidity were no longer increased compared with the controls while adjustment for "bully victimization" showed a decrease in the odds of behavior and conduct problems, and multimorbidity [4]. Other studies have also reported a higher prevalence of mental disorders in the CP population. However, the exact nature of the observed disorders varies in different studies, with some having reported very high rates of ADHD and autism [10, 11].

Due to the presence of CP during all major mental development phases of the child, its impact on the individual's psyche and therefore the exact nature of the potential mental disorders arising as a result of it will differ during the person's different life stages, therefore, the next section will review the most important mental health challenges affecting individuals with CP during each period of their life.

13.2 Period-Specific Mental Health Disorders

13.2.1 Childhood and Adolescence

Cerebral palsy is increasingly understood as a condition associated with significant neurodevelopmental and psychiatric comorbidities. Factors such as chronic pain, sleep disturbances, limited mobility, and societal stigma serve as additional risk factors for developing mental health conditions. Emerging evidence also suggests common genetic and neurobiological pathways between CP and certain neurodevelopmental disorders, warranting the need for further investigation into the prevalence and clinical presentation of such comorbidities.

13.2.1.1 Neurodevelopmental Disorders

The National Institute for Health and Care Excellence (NICE) in the UK now explicitly recommends the assessment of autism spectrum disorder (ASD) and attention-deficit/hyperactivity disorder (ADHD) in children and adolescents with CP.

Autism Spectrum Disorder (ASD)

The prevalence of ASD in children with CP has been reported across a wide range, from 2% to around 30%. Such a wide range reflects significant heterogeneity in diagnostic criteria, study populations, and methodologies. The risk appears to be particularly high in children with co-occurring intellectual disability, prematurity, and visual impairments. Conversely, CP has been identified in approximately 2–4% of autistic individuals [12]. These figures emphasize a bidirectional relationship that warrants routine screening for ASD symptoms in clinical settings, especially when intellectual and sensory impairments are present.

Early and accurate diagnosis of ASD in individuals with CP is essential, as timely intervention can enhance quality of life, support adaptive functioning, and improve the individual's compliance with therapy and educational or rehabilitation programs. That being said, diagnosing Autism in individuals with CP poses considerable difficulties for clinicians. Many symptoms of ASD, such as restricted interests, repetitive behaviors, or difficulties with social communication, may be overlooked or misinterpreted as typical for CP. Furthermore, such symptoms may wrongly be solely attributed to motor or cognitive impairments. This diagnostic overshadowing can delay proper identification and intervention. A detailed assessment, particularly a detailed developmental history, is crucial. Clinicians must carefully evaluate not only speech and language development but also social communication skills, social cognition, emotional capabilities, and the presence of repetitive or ritualistic behaviors and limited interests. These domains are central to an accurate diagnosis of ASD and should not be overlooked, even in the context of motor or intellectual impairments associated with CP.

Management of co-occurring ASD and CP requires a multidisciplinary approach, involving collaboration between neurologists, psychiatrists, developmental pediatricians, therapists, and educators. Interventions such as behavioral therapies, occupational therapy, and structured social skills training can be especially beneficial. Pharmacological treatments, including the use of atypical antipsychotics for aggression or severe behavioral challenges, should be considered with caution. While these medications may help manage behavioral symptoms, their possible side effects, especially those affecting the patient's movement and physical abilities, must be carefully weighed, as they may exacerbate mobility issues in patients with CP.

Attention-Deficit/Hyperactivity Disorder (ADHD)

ADHD is another frequently co-occurring neurodevelopmental disorder in CP. Prevalence estimates vary widely, from 19% to 35%, depending on the study design and assessment tools used. A meta-analysis estimated the pooled prevalence at approximately 7.2%. The higher rates observed in clinical samples suggest underrecognition in broader community settings and the need for systematic evaluation of attentional and behavioral symptoms in this population [12].

Diagnosing ADHD in individuals with CP can be particularly complex and often underrecognized. One of the main challenges lies in the altered or limited expression of core ADHD symptoms—especially hyperactivity—due to motor impairments. Children with CP may not display overt physical restlessness or excessive movement, which can lead clinicians and caregivers to overlook the possibility of ADHD. As a result, inattentive symptoms, which may manifest more subtly, are frequently missed or misattributed to cognitive delays or fatigue. To address this diagnostic challenge, a thorough clinical evaluation is essential, including a detailed history focusing on attention span, task persistence, impulse control, and academic performance. Input from parents, teachers, and other caregivers can provide valuable insights into behaviors across different settings.

Timely identification and treatment of ADHD in children with CP is crucial, as it can significantly improve self-esteem, academic achievement, social functioning, and overall quality of life. Early intervention may also help prevent the development of secondary mental health issues such as anxiety, depression, or oppositional behavior.

Management typically involves a combination of pharmacotherapy and psychotherapy. Stimulant medications or non-stimulant alternatives can be effective in improving attention and reducing impulsivity, though careful monitoring for side effects—particularly in the context of existing neurological or medical conditions—is necessary. Behavioral interventions, parent training programs, cognitive-behavioral strategies, and educational support can further enhance outcomes by addressing both the core symptoms and the broader functional impacts of ADHD.

13.2.1.2 Behavioral Symptoms

As mentioned above, children with CP often present with a complex interplay of physical, cognitive, and emotional challenges. In clinical practice, it is not uncommon to encounter children with CP who appear emotionally distressed but are unable to effectively communicate their feelings due to intellectual disabilities or impairments in speech and language. In such cases, behavior often becomes their primary mode of expression. Emotional states such as pain, frustration, boredom, and the impact of social stigma are frequently externalized through behavioral symptoms, making it essential for clinicians to interpret these cues carefully. Studies using standardized assessment tools have demonstrated elevated levels of behavioral problems compared to typically developing (TD) peers.

According to findings from the Child Behavior Checklist (CBCL), total problem scores in children with CP fell within the clinically abnormal range in 24–31% of cases. Nearly half (46%) had at least one clinically concerning subscale score. Affective and anxiety-related problems were among the most prevalent (23–24%), followed by oppositional defiant problems (10%). The overall pooled prevalence based on CBCL scores was 28% (95% CI: 0.22–0.36), with moderate heterogeneity [13]. Similarly, results from the Strengths and Difficulties Questionnaire (SDQ) revealed significant emotional and behavioral concerns. Total difficulties were reported in 19–67% of cases, with emotional symptoms ranging from 17% to 30%. Peer relationship problems were particularly prevalent, reaching rates as high as 87% in some studies. The pooled estimate for clinically significant SDQ scores was 35% (95% CI: 0.20–0.59), though substantial heterogeneity ($I^2 = 96.4\%$) highlights variability across studies [13].

13.2.1.3 Depression and Anxiety

Large-scale epidemiological data confirm a heightened burden of internalizing disorders in children and adolescents with CP. In a study involving 3544 individuals with CP and 71,080 typically developing peers, anxiety was diagnosed in 23% of those with CP, compared to 9% in the TD group. Depression, though less common, was observed in 3% of children with CP, versus 5% in TD peers [14]. Notably, the likelihood of developing these conditions increased with the severity of motor impairment. Individuals classified within Gross Motor Function Classification System (GMFCS) levels III–V had significantly higher odds of receiving a mental health diagnosis than those at levels I–II (OR = 1.23; 95% CI: 1.09–1.40; $p = 0.001$). These findings underscore the importance of considering the functional impact of motor impairments when evaluating emotional well-being.

13.2.1.4 Other Psychiatric Disorders

The same large-scale study also documented the prevalence of several other psychiatric disorders in the CP population:

- *Obsessive-Compulsive Disorder (OCD)*: Diagnosed in 7% of individuals with CP, compared to only 1% in the TD group.

- *Conduct or Impulse Control Disorders*: Present in 14% of those with CP, versus 5% in TD peers.
- *Trauma- and Stressor-Related Disorders*: Found in 10% of individuals with CP, slightly higher than the 8% in TD controls.
- *Suicidal Ideation*: Reported in 2% of children with CP and 5% of TD children.

Importantly, gender differences were also observed. Males with CP were more likely than females to be diagnosed with conduct or impulse control disorders (OR = 1.41; 95% CI: 1.16–1.73) and ADHD (OR = 1.41; 95% CI: 1.15–1.73) [14].

13.2.1.5 Psychosocial Stressors and Bullying

In addition to clinical diagnoses, psychosocial stressors such as bullying contribute significantly to mental health problems in children with CP. Studies consistently report that children with CP are more likely to experience peer victimization, which in turn increases the risk for depression, anxiety, and social withdrawal. Stigma and social exclusion further exacerbate these challenges, limiting opportunities for social integration and emotional development [4].

13.2.2 Adulthood

While a considerable body of research focuses on children with CP, findings from pediatric populations cannot be directly generalized to adults. Adult-specific studies remain limited, and many fail to distinguish between individuals with CP who also have intellectual disabilities and those who do not. The relationship between mental health problems and factors such as medical comorbidities, physical limitations, social determinants, and psychological influences is complex and often bidirectional.

13.2.2.1 Prevalence of Mental Health Disorders in Adults with CP

Evidence indicates that adults with CP experience significantly higher rates of mental health disorders compared to the general population. These include mood disorders (especially depression), anxiety disorders, psychotic disorders, personality disorders, behavioral problems, and self-injurious behavior. Substance use disorders appear to be an exception, with some studies showing a lower prevalence in the CP population.

In their cross-sectional analysis on the prevalence of mental health disorders using data from a large U.S. insurance claims database, Whitney et al. analyzed records from 8.7 million adults, identifying 7348 individuals with CP—of whom 5052 had CP alone and 2296 had CP with comorbid neurodevelopmental disorders, such as intellectual disabilities, autism spectrum disorders, or epilepsy. Adults with CP were found to have a higher prevalence of mental health disorders compared to those without CP across nearly all diagnostic categories. Mood affective disorders were present in 28.6% of women and 19.5% of men with CP, compared to 14.3% and 8.1% respectively in the general population. Anxiety disorders affected 28.6%

of women and 19.5% of men with CP, in contrast to 18.0% and 11.1% among those without CP. Schizophrenia and other psychotic disorders were also more common, affecting 3.2% of women and 2.8% of men with CP, compared to just 0.6% and 0.7% in adults without CP. Overall, adults with both CP and neurodevelopmental disorders exhibited similar or higher rates of mental health disorders compared to those with CP alone, except substance-related disorders, which were lower in men with comorbid neurodevelopmental disorders [4].

A clinical study of 501 adults with CP in the United States reported that 39% met diagnostic criteria for an anxiety disorder and 31% met criteria for major depressive disorder. In another study examining psychiatric service utilization over 2 years, 33.7% of adults with CP received a psychiatric diagnosis, compared to 24.7% of controls. Adults with CP were over twice as likely to be diagnosed with psychotic disorders, personality disorders, and bipolar disorder. Conversely, they were less likely to be diagnosed with substance use disorders (prevalence ratio: 0.76) [15].

Another large population-based study, which included 1705 adults with CP and 5115 matched controls, found an increased adjusted hazard ratio (HR) for depression: 1.28 (95% CI: 1.09–1.51), and an increased HR for anxiety: 1.40 (95% CI: 1.21–1.63). Furthermore, when stratified by the presence of intellectual disability, adults with CP without ID had significantly higher risks of developing depression (HR: 1.44; 95% CI: 1.20–1.72) and anxiety (HR: 1.55; 95% CI: 1.28–1.87). Adults with CP and comorbid ID did not show the same elevated risk for these conditions, possibly due to underdiagnosis or diagnostic overshadowing. However, there are inconsistencies in the literature, with some studies reporting increased risk of most psychiatric conditions in the presence of an intellectual disability [16]. These findings underscore the importance of differentiating mental health outcomes based on cognitive functioning, as mental health needs may manifest differently in those with and without intellectual disabilities.

Despite the increasing number of individuals with cerebral palsy (CP) surviving into adulthood, the topic of sexuality in this population remains under-discussed and frequently overlooked in both clinical care and public discourse. Findings from recent studies reveal that while a significant portion of adults with CP are sexually active or have sexual experience, only a small fraction have ever received sexuality education tailored to their needs as individuals with disabilities. Common physical challenges such as muscle spasms, discomfort, and difficulties with positioning can interfere with sexual intimacy, yet these issues are rarely addressed proactively by healthcare providers. Many individuals, particularly those with more severe functional limitations, report reduced opportunities for romantic or sexual relationships, which may negatively impact their quality of life. Importantly, participants who had sexual experiences often noted positive effects on self-esteem, highlighting the importance of intimacy and sexual expression as integral aspects of well-being.

Psychosexual functioning in adults with CP also varies significantly depending on gender, marital status, and ambulatory ability. Unmarried men with CP are particularly vulnerable, showing significantly lower scores in sexual knowledge, drive, experience, satisfaction, and overall sexual functioning compared to their able-bodied peers. In contrast, unmarried women with CP reported fewer differences, except in body image concerns. Married individuals with CP, regardless of gender, often face heightened psychological distress and reduced sexual satisfaction—particularly among women. Non-ambulatory individuals are also at greater risk of psychosexual dysfunction, with markedly lower levels of sexual information, experience, and satisfaction. Despite these findings, sexual health is rarely included in routine clinical assessments for individuals with CP. Clinicians must be encouraged to initiate sensitive, inclusive conversations about sexuality, body image, and emotional intimacy, and to provide tailored support and referrals. Integrating sexual health into comprehensive care not only promotes autonomy and dignity but also addresses a core human need that remains underserved in adults with CP [17, 18].

13.2.2.2 Gaps in Knowledge

Despite growing recognition of the mental health burden in adults with CP, major gaps remain:

- Most studies are cross-sectional, limiting understanding of causal relationships
- Longitudinal research is needed to evaluate how mental health trajectories evolve over time
- The pattern of mental health service utilization in adults with CP remains poorly understood
- There is a lack of evidence-based interventions tailored to the specific needs of this population

Given these gaps, clinical guidelines should emphasize routine screening for mental health symptoms in adults with CP, with particular attention to functional status and comorbid intellectual disability.

13.2.3 Late Adulthood

Recent projections by the Government of Canada suggest that by 2031, the population of adults aged 65 and older living with CP is expected to triple [19]. Despite this demographic shift, healthcare systems remain largely unprepared, often lacking integrated services and professionals trained in the lifelong and evolving needs of individuals with CP. Too frequently, CP is mistakenly regarded solely as a pediatric condition, leaving many aging adults underserved.

As people with CP transition into later adulthood, they face early-onset challenges in critical life domains such as employment, health, mobility, and independent living. These changes can lead to premature isolation, limited access to meaningful social roles, and a heightened risk of mental health conditions, particularly depression and anxiety [20].

A key concern is loneliness, which is notably more prevalent among adults with CP—especially those over 40—compared to non-disabled peers aged 60 or older. Research using the UCLA Loneliness Scale confirms that both verbal communicators and individuals relying on augmentative and alternative communication (AAC) report high levels of loneliness. Importantly, this loneliness appears to be unrelated to the method of communication but is significantly influenced by loss of function, social exclusion, and limited community engagement [21].

13.2.3.1 Functional Decline and Emotional Health

As adults with CP age, the progressive deterioration in motor function, coupled with chronic pain and fatigue, frequently contributes to reduced participation in daily and social activities. This loss of engagement can exacerbate feelings of purposelessness and distress, creating a cycle that further undermines mental well-being. Additionally, the severity of fatigue was associated with depressive symptoms [22].

13.2.3.2 Clinical Tips for Healthcare Providers Working with Elderly Individuals with CP

- *Adopt a lifespan perspective*: Recognize that CP is a lifelong condition with evolving physical, psychological, and social implications. Avoid framing it as solely a pediatric disorder.
- *Screen proactively for mental health issues*: Take psychiatric history and utilize validated tools such as the PHQ-9 for depression or GAD-7 for anxiety.
- *Refer to specialists familiar with disability*: When mental health concerns arise, prioritize referrals to clinicians who have experience working with individuals with neurodevelopmental disorders and physical disabilities.
- *Address early losses holistically*: Support older adults in identifying areas of decline—such as mobility, employment, or independence—and work collaboratively to find adaptive solutions.
- *Promote access and participation*: Encourage involvement in community activities, vocational training, or volunteer work. Facilitate connections to services that can improve access to transportation, assistive devices, or social engagement.
- *Monitor for chronic pain and fatigue*: These are often underreported but have a significant impact on mental health. A multidisciplinary approach involving physiotherapy, occupational therapy, and pain management can be beneficial.
- *Foster continuity of care*: Collaborate with primary care providers, rehabilitation specialists, and mental health professionals to build a coordinated, person-centered care plan.
- *Validate identity and contribution*: Employment or purposeful daily activity can provide structure, identity, and social contact. Explore avenues for preserving or reestablishing these elements in the patient's life.

13.3 Quality of Life and Emotional Well-Being

13.3.1 Quality of Life

As a physical disability with profound impact on mental health and physical function, CP can affect the individual's quality of life (QoL) in a multitude of ways. Following the same logic as before, one of the best starting points would be to look at what children and adolescents with CP think about their own subjective quality of life status and its contributing factors.

In a qualitative study on adolescents with CP, subjective QoL was found to be influenced by an interplay of intrinsic and extrinsic factors. Among the intrinsic factors were the individual's perception and view of themselves and their abilities to overcome challenges, as well as their level of physical capabilities and CP severity. Interestingly, it was observed that those with more severe forms of the disease compared themselves with those with even greater levels of disability, usually describing their situation as "better" than others they knew. The opposite was observed in patients with less debilitating forms of CP, as they compared themselves with those without the disease and stated their "disadvantages". As for extrinsic factors, a wide range of elements were identified to influence their perceived QoL, chief among them being their family and friends. As expected of their age, friends played a major role both in providing approval and support, as well as providing opportunities for shared experiences and activities. The interaction between the intrinsic and extrinsic factors was proved to be very important, as it included both how others viewed them and their own ability to take part in activities of their choosing. The latter was found to be one of the most important factors contributing to their overall subjective QoL. Ultimately, when asked to rate their overall QoL, all rated it to be eight or above on a scale of 1–10 [23].

Taking a more classic approach, a survey was conducted to compare a questionnaire-based QoL score for young adults with CP with that of typically developed controls. Results indicated that those with CP experienced lower QoL scores in physical, psychological, and role function [24]. Interestingly, further analysis revealed no association between level of motor function and mobility, and the psychological domain of the QoL, pointing to more complex interactions between the elements influencing the perceived psychological QoL. On the other hand, in a study comparing adults with CP with the general population, similar QoL scores were found in both groups [25] with no notable differences, an outcome which the researchers concluded indicated the high adaptive capabilities of individuals with CP in coping with their unique situation and its demands.

13.3.2 Assessment

Several assessment tools and questionnaires exist for the assessment of QoL in children, with some especially designed for use in individuals with CP. Three of the more widely used examples will be discussed here briefly.

- Child Health Questionnaire (CHQ): One of the oldest and most widely used questionnaires for the assessment of health-related QoL in children, CHQ was developed for the evaluation of physical and psychological well-being of 5–18-year-old children. Available both as self-administered and parent-administered versions, the questionnaire also has a shortened form. Most items require taking into account the past 4 weeks, along with a single-item scale requiring consideration of changes in health in the last year [26].

- KIDSCREEN: Another widely used questionnaire designed for the assessment of health-related QoL, the classic version has 52 items in ten dimensions. The questionnaire is extensively validated, especially in European countries [27].
- CP QoL-Child and CP QoL-Teen: Designed specifically for individuals with CP, both versions of the questionnaire are available in self-report or caregiver-administered versions. During the initial development, they were validated using both CHQ and KIDSCREEN for comparison. Each questionnaire measures QoL in seven dimensions; however, the exact title and scope of dimensions differ between QoL-Child and CP QoL-Teen and are as follows [28]:
  - CP QoL-Child:
    - Social well-being and acceptance
    - Feelings about functioning
    - Participation and physical health
    - Emotional well-being and self-esteem
    - Access to services
    - Pain and impact of disability
    - Family health
  - CP QoL-Teen:
    - General well-being and participation
    - Feelings about functioning
    - Communication and physical health
    - School wellbeing
    - Access to services
    - Social wellbeing
    - Family health

13.3.3 Contributing Factors

Using CHQ, motor function and other function limitations were shown to be among the most prominent predictors of the physical aspect of the QoL in school-age children with CP. However, they did not appear to have a similar effect on the psychosocial aspect. In contrast, behavioral difficulties and dysfunctional social skills were found to be associated with the psychological aspect of QoL [29]. Other studies have also investigated the effect of physical activity and function on QoL. Regarding the relationship between physical functioning and QoL as assessed by the QoL-Child questionnaire, function has been found to be associated with all questionnaire-defined domains of the QoL except that of "Access to service," albeit with varying degrees. Moreover, using "self-reported" responses, a significant relation between function and "Emotional well-being" was not observed [30]. Still, others have reported children with CP to have overall similar QoL scores compared with the general population using the KIDSCREEN questionnaire. Furthermore, motor function has been found to be associated only with the "school environment" dimension of the questionnaire, while the type of received education (special vs. regular) was the one variable associated with the physical well-being domain of the QoL. Finally, age was the only variable found to be associated with psychological well-being [31].

Looking at other possible determinants, studies have demonstrated the association between participation in leisure activities, diversity of activities, and their enjoyment, and different dimensions of QoL in children with CP, including the psychological aspect of QoL [32]. Investigating the effect of recurrent musculoskeletal pain on mental health and health-related QoL, results indicated a relation between the two, with higher pain levels associated with more mental health problems and lower health-related QoL [33]. Interestingly, such a correlation was only observed in self-reported data and was not present in the proxy-reported (i.e., by parents or guardians of the child) results, a finding that emphasizes the importance of child-reported data collection for the clinician and decision makers to make a truly informed decision.

13.4 Parents and Caregivers

Understanding the effects of caring for an individual with CP on their immediate caregivers is vital for ensuring that proper levels of care can be provided to the child, especially considering the chronic nature of the disease and the proven importance of family support and care in the well-being of the patient. In a cross-sectional study of 158 mothers of children with CP, researchers reported that mothers spent an average of 6.0 h per day during weekdays caring for their child's needs. Their results further indicated a clear association between the mothers' psychological problems and both their actual spent time, and their perceived "time pressure" [34]. Others have demonstrated that mothers of children with CP had significantly lower QoL than those of typically developing children. Several personality traits were also found to be associated with the mother's mental health and QoL; extraversion was correlated with better mental health, while neuroticism and psychoticism were negatively correlated with mental health and QoL [35]. In their study on 161 caregivers in Ireland, Byrne et al. reported that poorer health was observed in the parents of children with CP compared with the general population, and women had worse health than men [36]. Guillamón also reported similar results, finding parents of children with CP to show an overall low QoL and mental health [37]. Lastly, a systematic review including fourteen studies concluded depression and anxiety to be significantly more prevalent in the parents of children with CP, and the amount of time spent on the child by the caregiver was found to be associated with the chance of mental illness [38].

Interestingly, uncertainties seem to exist regarding the effects of a child's disease severity and levels of motor activity on caregivers' QoL and mental health. Naletilić et al. found motor function levels to have no influence on the mother's QoL [35]. Similarly, others also reported no difference in health based on the child's level of "dependence" [36]. On the other hand, in a comparison of the impacts of walking and non-walking children with CP on the mental health of their primary caregivers, researchers have reported significant differences in the parents' anxiety levels and their sense of restriction in daily living between the two groups [39]. Similar findings were also reported in a review, in which the authors stated that at least in some of the included articles, the severity of the child's disorder was reported to be a risk factor for the parents' chance of mental illness [38].

Regardless of the specific findings, the present results clearly show the potential negative impacts of caring for a child with CP on the mental health and QoL of their primary caregivers. Such a fact, along with the proven positive consequences of effective family support on the emotional and mental well-being of the child, emphasizes the need for functional and accessible supportive services for the primary caregivers of children with CP, to alleviate the strains of caring for the child, and not only improving the parents' mental health and QoL, but also allowing the child to benefit from it.

13.5 Conclusion and Future

Children and adults with CP face a high prevalence of mental health challenges across the lifespan, ranging from internalizing disorders such as anxiety and depression to neurodevelopmental conditions like ADHD and autism spectrum disorder. These mental health issues are often underrecognized and undertreated due to diagnostic overshadowing, communication barriers, and insufficient clinical training in integrated care. The variability in symptom presentation and functional abilities necessitates a personalized, multidisciplinary approach that addresses both psychological and physical health. Despite striving for similar aspirations, social roles, and quality of life as their typically developing peers, individuals with CP encounter significant obstacles—such as stigma, exclusion, and unmet emotional needs—that impact their well-being. Their caregivers, too, face heightened psychological distress and reduced quality of life, further highlighting the need for systemic interventions that consider the family as a unit of care.

Future efforts must prioritize longitudinal research to better understand the evolution of mental health symptoms over time and to identify predictive risk and resilience factors in CP. Development and implementation of tailored, evidence-based interventions—including early screening protocols, inclusive mental health education, adaptive psychotherapies, and community-based support systems—are critical. Healthcare systems should integrate mental health evaluation into routine care across all stages of life and ensure access to trained professionals who can recognize and manage psychiatric comorbidities in this population. Importantly, research must also focus on understudied domains such as aging with CP, sexuality, and service utilization to foster a truly lifespan-oriented model of care. Empowering individuals with CP through accessible mental health services and meaningful participation in society will significantly enhance their autonomy, dignity, and overall quality of life.

References

1. Rutter M. A neuropsychiatric study in childhood. In: Clinics in developmental medicine nos 35/36. London: Spastics International Medical Publications (Mac Keith Press); 1970.
2. Liptak GS, Accardo PJ. Health and social outcomes of children with cerebral palsy. J Pediatr. 2004;145(2 Suppl):S36–41.
3. Hanes JE, Hlyva O, Rosenbaum P, Freeman M, Nguyen T, Palisano RJ, et al. Beyond stereotypes of cerebral palsy: exploring the lived experiences of young Canadians. Child Care Health Dev. 2019;45(5):613–22.
4. Whitney DG, Peterson MD, Warschausky SA. Mental health disorders, participation, and bullying in children with cerebral palsy. Dev Med Child Neurol. 2019;61(8):937–42.
5. Hammar GR, Ozolins A, Idvall E, Rudebeck CE. Body image in adolescents with cerebral palsy. J Child Health Care. 2009;13(1):19–29.
6. King GA, Shultz IZ, Steel K, Gilpin M, Cathers T. Self-evaluation and self-concept of adolescents with physical disabilities. Am J Occup Ther. 1993;47(2):132–40.
7. Gannotti ME, Blanchard Y, Blumberg L, LaRocco D. Shared meanings of success, happiness, and health among adults with cerebral palsy and physiotherapists: implications for practice and research. Disabil Rehabil. 2019;41(11):1321–30.
8. Cussen A, Howie L, Imms C. Looking to the future: adolescents with cerebral palsy talk about their aspirations–a narrative study. Disabil Rehabil. 2012;34(24):2103–10.
9. Yeung PH, Passmore AE, Packer TL. Active citizens or passive recipients: how Australian young adults with cerebral palsy define citizenship. J Intellect Dev Disabil. 2008;33(1):65–75.
10. Gillberg C. Mental health problems in cerebral palsy: comprehensive management for children and their families. Dev Med Child Neurol. 2020;62(2):154.
11. Påhlman M, Gillberg C, Himmelmann K. Autism and attention-deficit/hyperactivity disorder in children with cerebral palsy: high prevalence rates in a population-based study. Dev Med Child Neurol. 2021;63(3):320–7.
12. Craig F, Savino R, Trabacca A. A systematic review of comorbidity between cerebral palsy, autism spectrum disorders and attention deficit hyperactivity disorder. Eur J Paediatr Neurol. 2019;23(1):31–42. https://doi.org/10.1016/j.ejpn.2018.10.005.
13. Downs J, Blackmore AM, Epstein A, Skoss R, Langdon K, Jacoby P, et al. The prevalence of mental health disorders and symptoms in children and adolescents with cerebral palsy: a systematic review and meta-analysis. Dev Med Child Neurol. 2018;60(1):30–8.
14. Bhatnagar S, Mitelpunkt A, Rizzo JJ, Zhang N, Guzman T, Schuetter R, et al. Mental health diagnoses risk among children and young adults with cerebral palsy, chronic conditions, or typical development. JAMA Netw Open. 2024;7(7):e2422202-e.
15. McMorris CA, Lake J, Dobranowski K, McGarry C, Lin E, Wilton D, et al. Psychiatric disorders in adults with cerebral palsy. Res Dev Disabil. 2021;111:103859.
16. Smith KJ, Peterson MD, O'Connell NE, Victor C, Liverani S, Anokye N, et al. Risk of depression and anxiety in adults with cerebral palsy. JAMA Neurol. 2019;76(3):294–300.
17. Newell A, Liang N, Moskowitz J, Lee N, Pan XN, Kim H. Exploring the sexual experiences and challenges of individuals with cerebral palsy. J Pediatr Rehabil Med. 2024;17(1):35–45.
18. Cho S-R, Park ES, Park CI, Na S-I. Characteristics of psychosexual functioning in adults with cerebral palsy. Clin Rehabil. 2004;18(4):423–9.
19. Amankwah N, Oskoui M, Garner R, Bancej C, Manuel DG, Wall R, et al. Original quantitative research-cerebral palsy in Canada, 2011–2031: results of a microsimulation modelling study of epidemiological and cost impacts. Health Promot Chronic Dis Prev Can. 2020;40(2):25.

20. Svien LR, Berg P, Stephenson C. Issues in aging with cerebral palsy. Top Geriatr Rehabil. 2008;24(1):26–40.
21. Balandin S, Berg N, Waller A. Assessing the loneliness of older people with cerebral palsy. Disabil Rehabil. 2006;28(8):469–79.
22. Van Der Slot WM, Nieuwenhuijsen C, Van Den Berg-Emons RJ, Bergen MP, Hilberink SR, Stam HJ, et al. Chronic pain, fatigue, and depressive symptoms in adults with spastic bilateral cerebral palsy. Dev Med Child Neurol. 2012;54(9):836–42.
23. Shikako-Thomas K, Lach L, Majnemer A, Nimigon J, Cameron K, Shevell M. Quality of life from the perspective of adolescents with cerebral palsy: "I just think I'ma normal kid, I just happen to have a disability". Qual Life Res. 2009;18(7):825–32.
24. Jiang B, Walstab J, Reid SM, Davis E, Reddihough D. Quality of life in young adults with cerebral palsy. Disabil Health J. 2016;9(4):673–81.
25. Schmidt S, Markwart H, Rapp M, Guyard A, Arnaud C, Fauconnier J, et al. Quality of life and mental health in emerging adults with cerebral palsy compared to the general population. Health Qual Life Outcomes. 2022;20(1):61.
26. Landgraf JM. Child health questionnaire (CHQ). In: Encyclopedia of quality of life and well-being research. Springer; 2024. p. 772–7.
27. Ravens-Sieberer U, Gosch A, Rajmil L, Erhart M, Bruil J, Power M, et al. The KIDSCREEN-52 quality of life measure for children and adolescents: psychometric results from a cross-cultural survey in 13 European countries. Value Health. 2008;11(4):645–58.
28. Davis E, Mackinnon A, Davern M, Boyd R, Bohanna I, Waters E, et al. Description and psychometric properties of the CP QOL-teen: a quality of life questionnaire for adolescents with cerebral palsy. Res Dev Disabil. 2013;34(1):344–52.
29. Majnemer A, Shevell M, Rosenbaum P, Law M, Poulin C. Determinants of life quality in school-age children with cerebral palsy. J Pediatr. 2007;151(5):470–5. 5.e1–3.
30. Shelly A, Davis E, Waters E, Mackinnon A, Reddihough D, Boyd R, et al. The relationship between quality of life and functioning for children with cerebral palsy. Dev Med Child Neurol. 2008;50(3):199–203.
31. Kato M, Arai H, Komatsu K, Tateyama K, Nishikawa T. The lower the physical function, the higher the quality of life in Japanese adolescents with cerebral palsy. Phys Occup Ther Pediatr. 2023;43(6):713–24.
32. Badia M, Longo E, Orgaz MB, Gómez-Vela M. The influence of participation in leisure activities on quality of life in Spanish children and adolescents with cerebral palsy. Res Dev Disabil. 2013;34(9):2864–71.
33. Ramstad K, Loge JH, Jahnsen R, Diseth TH. Self-reported mental health in youth with cerebral palsy and associations to recurrent musculoskeletal pain. Disabil Rehabil. 2015;37(2):144–50.
34. Sawyer MG, Bittman M, La Greca AM, Crettenden AD, Borojevic N, Raghavendra P, et al. Time demands of caring for children with cerebral palsy: what are the implications for maternal mental health? Dev Med Child Neurol. 2011;53(4):338–43.
35. Naletilić M, Tomić V, Ostojić L, Damjanović VM, Grabovac M. Personality traits and quality of life of mothers who have children with cerebral palsy. Psychiatr Danub. 2017;29(Suppl 4):793–803.
36. Byrne MB, Hurley DA, Daly L, Cunningham CG. Health status of caregivers of children with cerebral palsy. Child Care Health Dev. 2010;36(5):696–702.
37. Guillamón N, Nieto R, Pousada M, Redolar D, Muñoz E, Hernández E, et al. Quality of life and mental health among parents of children with cerebral palsy: the influence of self-efficacy and coping strategies. J Clin Nurs. 2013;22(11–12):1579–90.
38. Barreto TM, Bento MN, Barreto TM, Jagersbacher JG, Jones NS, Lucena R, et al. Prevalence of depression, anxiety, and substance-related disorders in parents of children with cerebral palsy: a systematic review. Dev Med Child Neurol. 2020;62(2):163–8.
39. Svedberg LE, Englund E, Malker H, Stener-Victorin E. Comparison of impact on mood, health, and daily living experiences of primary caregivers of walking and non-walking children with cerebral palsy and provided community services support. Eur J Paediatr Neurol. 2010;14(3):239–46.

Educational Support and Inclusive Education

14

Sarina Zare and Nastaran Maghbouli

14.1 Case Study

Consider an 8-year-old boy with congenital neuropathy. Despite significant motor challenges—being wheelchair-bound due to severe spinal scoliosis, with both distal and proximal disabilities that prevent him from holding a pencil—he demonstrates exceptional cognitive abilities. His intelligence is above average, and he communicates fluently in both his native language, Persian, and in English.

Yet, despite these remarkable strengths, he has been placed in an exceptional school where the majority of students have cognitive impairments. This decision was made not because of his intellectual capacity, but because normal schools lack the facilities and inclusive strategies to accommodate a child with his physical needs. As a result, his potential for academic and personal growth is underutilized, highlighting the urgent need for more inclusive and supportive educational systems.

14.2 Introduction

Cerebral palsy (CP) is a lifelong motor disorder that affects children's movement, communication, cognition, and behavior, presenting unique challenges in educational settings [1–3]. Access to education on an equal basis is a fundamental human right, yet students with CP often face barriers that limit participation, academic achievement, and social inclusion [4–6]. Educational support and inclusive

S. Zare
School of Medicine, Tehran University of Medical Sciences, Tehran, Iran

N. Maghbouli (✉)
Department of Physical Medicine and Rehabilitation, School of Medicine, Shariati Hospital, Tehran University of Medical Sciences, Tehran, Iran
e-mail: nmaghbouli@sina.tums.ac.ir

A. Presedo et al. (eds.), *Enhancing Quality of Life in Patients with Cerebral Palsy*, https://doi.org/10.1007/978-3-032-20967-2_14

education aim to address these challenges by providing equitable learning opportunities within mainstream classrooms while tailoring strategies to individual needs.

Inclusive education emphasizes the integration of children with disabilities into regular schools, fostering social cohesion, reducing stigma, and promoting personal and academic development [4–6]. Complementary educational support strategies, such as individualized education plans (IEPs), assistive technologies, and parent and school collaboration, help children with CP engage meaningfully in learning and extracurricular activities.

This chapter explores the educational barriers faced by children with CP, the strategies and systems that facilitate learning, the critical role of families and multidisciplinary teams, and the challenges and future directions for inclusive education. By examining these elements, the chapter highlights how targeted support and inclusive practices can enhance the quality of life and long-term outcomes for students with cerebral palsy.

14.3 What Is Inclusive Education?

Access to education on an equal basis is a fundamental human right, and schools are expected to accommodate all students, with and without disability, and provide inclusive education. Inclusive education is an approach that seeks to provide equitable learning opportunities for all students, including those with disabilities, within mainstream educational settings [4]. Historically, education for children with disabilities was often provided in segregated institutions, limiting their social participation and access to the same curriculum as their peers. Over recent decades, educational policies and international agreements have increasingly emphasized the right of all children to learn together, leading to the development and implementation of inclusive education frameworks worldwide [5, 6]. The importance of inclusive education lies in its potential to foster social cohesion, reduce stigma, and improve academic and personal outcomes by ensuring that children with disabilities are active participants in the learning community. According to the 2022 American Academy of Pediatrics (AAP) and American Academy for Cerebral Palsy and Developmental Medicine (AACPDM) Cerebral Palsy guidelines, a multidisciplinary network of providers should be involved to address the medical, developmental, socio-emotional, academic, and future needs of children with CP [7].

14.4 Educational Barriers Faced by CP Patients

Cerebral palsy (CP) is the most common motor disorder in childhood and causes motor dysfunction that results in lifelong impairments [1, 2]. Children with CP may also experience differences in sensation, perception, cognition, communication, and behavior. Communication difficulties are highly prevalent, with approximately 80% having delayed or disordered speech production [3] and 55% demonstrating reduced functional communication skills [8]. These limitations affect daily activities, peer interaction, and participation in school tasks.

Learning difficulties are also common. Many children with CP develop learning disabilities before the start of formal schooling [9, 10], with specific challenges in areas such as mathematics and reading [11, 12]. These academic difficulties, combined with the functional limitations of CP, can contribute to a sense of alienation from school and low levels of student engagement—factors strongly associated with poor academic performance and higher school dropout rates [13]. Environmental and social factors further compound these challenges. Students with CP may face obstacles in navigating school buildings, experience reduced social inclusion, and encounter difficulties in preparing for and taking examinations or completing homework [13].

The long-term educational achievements of individuals with CP vary widely. Reported rates of university degree completion range from 2% [14] to 5% [15] and 24% [16]. Employment outcomes also differ, with rates reported at 36% [14], 45% [17], 68% [18], and 79% [19]. These disparities highlight the significant impact of educational barriers on life opportunities.

A shortage of school-based support systems and broader societal support can limit independence, access to higher education, and employment opportunities [20]. The demands of meeting the needs of a child with CP can also place considerable stress on families, affecting their social, emotional, and financial resources [21].

14.5 Educational Support Systems and Strategies

All children with cerebral palsy have the potential to learn, and it's essential to promote their participation not only in education but also in after-school and community activities [7]. Recognizing and addressing their diverse needs through tailored educational support systems ensures that learning environments are accessible, engaging, and inclusive. Such strategies aim to remove barriers to participation, foster academic achievement, and enhance social integration, ultimately contributing to improved quality of life for children with CP.

1. *Parents' Strategies*

Parents play a key role in supporting the educational participation of children with CP. The majority of parents adopt either an Autonomy Allowance (AA) or Acceptance and Support (AS) parental style. Most parents reported using supportive practices to promote autonomous behaviors related to their children's school routines, including helping them manage school responsibilities such as being punctual to class and completing homework [13].

Family support is a crucial facilitator for children with CP, along with encouragement from friends and broader society. Adequate family time dedicated to healthcare and educational support contributes positively to children's engagement in activities. However, overprotection or insufficient time devoted to these supports can limit children's participation and autonomy in school and community activities [22].

2. *Individualized Education Programs (IEPs)*

An Individualized Education Program (IEP) is a document developed for a learner with special needs that specifies the strategies, services, and measures used to monitor achievement. The IEP identifies the specific needs of the learner, which may range from minimal support for some students to detailed plans involving educational modifications, adaptive technologies, or healthcare interventions for others [23]. By addressing these needs, IEPs help ensure that the quality of education meets the diverse requirements of learners. They enable students to progress at their own pace and accommodate major differences in what is learned, how much is learned, and the standards used to evaluate performance [24].

In the United States, IEPs have enhanced teaching for students with cerebral palsy by applying universal design principles, reducing the need for later adaptations. These programs consider environmental requirements, such as providing quiet spaces and allowing freedom of movement, and include testing accommodations to ensure fair assessment. Additional supports may include scheduled breaks and instruction in interpersonal and self-help skills, further promoting participation and success in educational settings [25].

You can see some examples of IEPs for disabled students on Children's Hemiplegia and Stroke Association website at https://chasa.org/individualized-education-program-examples/.

3. *Assistive technologies*

Innovations in technology have greatly expanded the possibilities for supporting the education of children with special needs, including those with CP [26]. Assistive technologies encompass a range of tools and devices designed to help students overcome barriers to learning, communication, and participation in educational activities. These technologies can include robots, smartphone applications, computer-based equipment, and speech-generating devices, all aimed at enhancing cognitive skills, academic performance, and independence [27, 28].

Robots have been increasingly used for educational purposes in children with CP, helping to improve cognitive skills [29] and promote hands-on learning activities, such as mathematics exercises [30]. The Lego robots and CRS A465 robotic systems have been shown to enhance children's learning and cognitive skills in educative activities. The Lego robots were used to help children demonstrate cognitive skills beyond standardized tests, improve abilities over time, and actively participate in school activities. They applied robots to show understanding of subjects like math and social studies and could even operate them with speech-generating devices, though performance declined with complex tasks. The IROMEC robot is another versatile system used with CP patients. It has the potential to support children in movement functions, learning knowledge, communication and interactions

[31]. However, these robots are relatively few and require technical adaptations and programming to be usable by children, parents, therapists, and educators. Interdisciplinary teams using a user-centered design approach are essential for developing new, low-cost robots for this population [32].

Mobile applications also offer innovative assistive solutions. The SmartAbility Android application supports the education of students with CP by identifying the most accessible ways for them to interact with learning materials and participate in class. By using smartphone sensors to detect a student's physical abilities—such as head movements, blinking, speech clarity, or limb motion—SmartAbility can recommend personalized assistive technologies, including eye-gaze communication systems, voice-controlled software, switch-access devices, or adapted keyboards. These tools can then be integrated into the learning environment, allowing students to type, communicate, navigate educational software, and access online resources more independently [33].

High-tech assistive technologies, including computer-based equipment and speech-generating devices, help bridge the gap between students' needs and their abilities. CP students can use these technologies to overcome communication barriers [27, 28]. When a need for assistive technology is identified, health professionals are responsible for assessment, training, implementation, and evaluation of outcomes. Collaboration among all stakeholders—including students, parents, teachers, and therapists—is essential for successful implementation [34]. There is also a clear need for guidelines and training opportunities to help stakeholders' access and effectively use these technologies [35].

Assistive devices are tools designed to enhance the physical functioning of individuals with disabilities or to reduce environmental barriers, thereby increasing their independence and opportunities for participation [36]. These devices range from low-tech tools such as pencil grips to high-tech ones like power wheelchairs [37, 38].

4. *School and social support*

Children with cerebral palsy (CP) rely primarily on support from family members, while friends serve as an important external source of social support. Attending school or group training programs can further facilitate participation, as friends may encourage children to engage in activities [22]. However, some caregivers reported receiving little or no support from rehabilitation professionals [39, 40].

The inclusive and welcoming environment of the school is highly valued by both children with CP and their families. Physical accessibility is a key factor, and accommodations such as wheelchair access and ramps are necessary to ensure full participation in school activities. In addition, sufficient staff should be available, and school personnel should be trained to meet the educational, social, and physical needs of students with CP effectively. An inclusive school culture is characterized by a central understanding that children with CP can learn. To foster this culture, it is also important to educate other students to promote a welcoming environment for peers with disabilities. Such a culture promotes active care for these students and proactive planning to accommodate their individual needs [41].

5. *Involving families in educational planning*

A key factor in facilitating the academic success of children with cerebral palsy (CP) is effective collaboration between families, schools, and external organizations. Parents can engage with the school even before enrollment, helping to ensure that their child's needs are understood and addressed from the start. Early involvement also increases parental confidence and fosters a stronger partnership with educators [41].

Parental involvement is crucial because parents know their child's abilities, preferences, and challenges better than anyone else. They can provide valuable input on individualized learning goals, suggest necessary accommodations or assistive technologies, and participate in developing the student's Individualized Education Plan (IEP). Families can also help monitor progress, reinforce learning strategies at home, and communicate regularly with teachers and therapists. Involving parents in educational planning not only supports academic achievement but also promotes social and emotional development, empowering children with CP to participate fully in school and community life.

14.6 Role of Multidisciplinary Collaboration

Effective education and support for children with CP require collaboration among a multidisciplinary team, including parents, teachers, therapists, healthcare professionals, and school staff [7, 41]. Such collaboration ensures that the child's educational, social, and physical needs are addressed in a coordinated and comprehensive manner. Parents provide insight into their child's abilities and challenges, while teachers and school staff implement classroom strategies, accommodations, and inclusive practices. Therapists and healthcare providers contribute expertise on physical, cognitive, and communication interventions, and assistive technologies are integrated based on professional assessments [34, 35]. This team-based approach fosters a consistent support system, promotes active participation in learning, and enhances overall academic and social outcomes for children with CP.

14.7 Case Studies of Inclusive Education

An illustrative example of inclusive educational support for children with cerebral palsy is the implementation of Conductive Education (CE)-based programs [42] in Victoria, Australia. Introduced over the past decade, these programs were designed to offer a structured, group-based educational approach for children aged 12–36 months, emphasizing independence and social participation. Unlike traditional neurodevelopmental therapies, CE is not a medical treatment but an educational system led by a "conductor"—a professional who integrates the roles of teacher and therapist. The CE model incorporates rhythmic songs, verbal instructions, and specialized equipment such as plinths and ladder-back chairs to facilitate motor and cognitive development. In a rigorous study conducted by Reddihough et al., 66 children with CP were assessed over a 6-month period, with 34 randomly assigned to either CE-based or traditional programs and 32 self-selecting their preferred intervention. Both groups received comparable therapy hours to ensure parity in intensity.

The results revealed that children in CE-based programs made developmental gains similar to those in traditional therapy, with improvements noted across gross motor function, expressive language, and caregiver-reported coping. Notably, CE participants showed higher scores in expressive language and play, while traditional program participants demonstrated slightly greater gains in cognitive measures and physical function. Caregivers of children in CE programs also reported reduced stress and improved coping, suggesting a positive psychosocial impact. Despite these promising outcomes, the study faced several challenges, including difficulties in randomizing participants due to family preferences, cultural adaptations of the Hungarian CE model, and the need for substantial funding and professional collaboration. Nevertheless, the CE-based approach exemplifies how inclusive education can be tailored to meet the developmental and social needs of young children with CP, offering families an empowering alternative to conventional therapy.

14.8 Challenges and Future Directions

Despite the availability of educational support systems and inclusive strategies, children with cerebral palsy (CP) continue to face multiple challenges in accessing quality education. Barriers include limited school-based support, insufficiently trained staff, physical accessibility issues, and gaps in the use of assistive technologies [20, 30, 35, 41]. Overprotection by families or inadequate engagement in school and community activities can also limit participation and autonomy [22]. In addition, assistive technologies are often expensive and not easily accessible for all families, creating inequalities in educational opportunities. To be effective, these tools require personalization to each child's needs, which demands close collaboration among a multidisciplinary team including occupational therapists, speech therapists, psychiatrists, physicians, and the child's parents. Furthermore, clear responsibility must be defined at the institutional and governmental levels to ensure sustainable support, provision, and monitoring of these services. Future efforts should focus on strengthening multidisciplinary collaboration, expanding the availability and affordability of assistive technologies, providing targeted training for teachers and school staff, and developing clear guidelines for parents and professionals on implementing individualized support plans [34, 35]. Promoting inclusive school cultures and ensuring ongoing evaluation of educational interventions will be critical for improving academic outcomes and overall quality of life for children with CP.

14.9 Conclusion

The education of children with cerebral palsy is shaped by both opportunities and challenges. While inclusive education and tailored support strategies provide a pathway toward equity, barriers such as insufficient resources, lack of trained staff, and limited access to assistive technologies continue to hinder progress. The case of the 8-year-old boy presented at the beginning of this chapter illustrates the consequences of inadequate inclusive systems: a child with remarkable cognitive and linguistic abilities is placed in a segregated school, not because of intellectual limitations, but due to a lack of accommodations in mainstream education. Such cases underscore the urgent need for systemic change.

Moving forward, inclusive education must be seen not merely as a legal or policy requirement, but as an ethical commitment to recognizing the potential of every child. Strengthening multidisciplinary collaboration, personalizing educational supports, and fostering inclusive school cultures are essential steps. By ensuring accessibility, affordability, and accountability in educational systems, we can empower children with cerebral palsy to reach their full potential and contribute meaningfully to their communities.

References

1. Lennon N, Church C, Miller F. Patient-reported mobility function and engagement in young adults with cerebral palsy: a cross-sectional sample. J Child Orthop. 2018;12(2):197–203.
2. Novak I, Mcintyre S, Morgan C, Campbell L, Dark L, Morton N, et al. A systematic review of interventions for children with cerebral palsy: state of the evidence. Dev Med Child Neurol. 2013;55(10):885–910.
3. Mei C, Reilly S, Reddihough D, Mensah F, Morgan A. Motor speech impairment, activity, and participation in children with cerebral palsy. Int J Speech Lang Pathol. 2014;16(4):427–35.
4. UNESCO P. Policy guidelines on inclusion in education. Paris (Fr). 2009.
5. Graves P, Tracy J. Personal viewpoint education for children with disabilities: the rationale for inclusion. J Paediatr Child Health. 1998;34(3):220–5.
6. Jenkins JR, Jewell M, Leicester N, Jenkins L, Troutner NM. Development of a school building model for educating students with handicaps and at-risk students in general education classrooms. J Learn Disabil. 1991;24(5):311–20.
7. Jawed A, Mowry M. Strengthening equitable access to care and support for children with cerebral palsy and their caregivers. Children. 2023;10(6):994.
8. Kristoffersson E, Dahlgren Sandberg A, Holck P. Communication ability and communication methods in children with cerebral palsy. Dev Med Child Neurol. 2020;62(8):933–8.
9. Michel E, Roethlisberger M, Neuenschwander R, Roebers CM. Development of cognitive skills in children with motor coordination impairments at 12-month follow-up. Child Neuropsychol. 2011;17(2):151–72.
10. Jenks KM, van Lieshout EC, de Moor J. The relationship between medical impairments and arithmetic development in children with cerebral palsy. J Child Neurol. 2009;24(5):528–35.
11. Frampton I, Yude C, Goodman R. The prevalence and correlates of specific learning difficulties in a representative sample of children with hemiplegia. Br J Educ Psychol. 1998;68(1):39–51.
12. Bottcher L, Flachs EM, Uldall P. Attentional and executive impairments in children with spastic cerebral palsy. Dev Med Child Neurol. 2010;52(2):e42–e7.

13. Pereira A, Moreira T, Lopes S, Nunes AR, Magalhães P, Fuentes S, et al. "My child has cerebral palsy": parental involvement and children's school engagement. Front Psychol. 2016;7:1765.
14. Van der Dussen L, Nieuwstraten W, Roebroeck M, Stam H. Functional level of young adults with cerebral palsy. Clin Rehabil. 2001;15(1):84–91.
15. Maestro-Gonzalez A, Bilbao-Leon MC, Zuazua-Rico D, Fernandez-Carreira JM, Baldonedo-Cernuda RF, Mosteiro-Diaz MP. Quality of life as assessed by adults with cerebral palsy. PLoS One. 2018;13(2):e0191960.
16. Hergenröder H, Blank R. Subjective well-being and satisfaction with life in adults with spastic cerebral palsy: a pilot study of a randomized sample. Dev Med Child Neurol. 2009;51(5):389–96.
17. Benner JL, Hilberink SR, Veenis T, van der Slot WM, Roebroeck ME. Course of employment in adults with cerebral palsy over a 14-year period. Dev Med Child Neurol. 2017;59(7):762–8.
18. van der Slot W, Nieuwenhuijsen C, van den Berg-Emons RJ, Wensink-Boonstra AE, Stam HJ, Roebroeck M, Netherlands TRGSW. Participation and health-related quality of life in adults with spastic bilateral cerebral palsy and the role of self-efficacy. J Rehabil Med. 2010;42(6):528–35.
19. Jacobson DN, Lowing K, Hjelmarsson E, Tedroff K. Exploring social participation in young adults with cerebral palsy. J Rehabil Med. 2019;51(3):167–74.
20. Shrader MW, Church C, Lennon N, Shields T, Salazar-Torres JJ, Howard JJ, Miller F. Well-being of ambulatory adults with cerebral palsy: education, employment, and physical function of a cohort who received specialized pediatric care. Front Neurol. 2021;12:732906.
21. Sipal R, Schuengel C, Voorman J, Van Eck M, Becher J. Course of behaviour problems of children with cerebral palsy: the role of parental stress and support. Child Care Health Dev. 2010;36(1):74–84.
22. Earde PT, Praipruk A, Rodpradit P, Seanjumla P. Facilitators and barriers to performing activities and participation in children with cerebral palsy: caregivers' perspective. Pediatr Phys Ther. 2018,30(1).27–32.
23. Cowin R. Postsecondary education in British Columbia: public policy and structural development, 1960–2015. UBC Press; 2018.
24. Agumba SOR. Implementation of individualized education programme for effective teaching of learners with cerebral palsy in two special primary schools, Kisumu County, Kenya. Unpublished Master' s Thesis, Kenyatta University; 2017.
25. Eason AI, Whitbread K. IEP and inclusion tips for parents and teachers. (No Title). 2006.
26. Cook A, Encarnação P, Adams K. Robots: assistive technologies for play, learning and cognitive development. Technol Disabil. 2010;22(3):127–45.
27. Copley J, Ziviani J. Barriers to the use of assistive technology for children with multiple disabilities. Occup Ther Int. 2004;11(4):229–43.
28. Henderson S, Skelton H, Rosenbaum P. Assistive devices for children with functional impairments: impact on child and caregiver function. Dev Med Child Neurol. 2008;50(2):89–98.
29. Encarnação P, Alvarez L, Rios A, Maya C, Adams K, Cook A. Using virtual robot-mediated play activities to assess cognitive skills. Disabil Rehabil Assist Technol. 2014;9(3):231–41.
30. Cook A, Adams K. Access to hands-on mathematics measurement activities using robots controlled via speech generating devices: three case studies. Disabil Rehabil Assist Technol. 2014;9(4):286–98.
31. Van Den Heuvel RJ, Lexis MA, Janssens RM, Marti P, De Witte LP. Robots supporting play for children with physical disabilities: exploring the potential of IROMEC. Technol Disabil. 2017;29(3):109–20.
32. Miguel Cruz A, Rios Rincon AM, Rodriguez Dueñas WR, Quiroga Torres DA, Bohórquez-Heredia AF. What does the literature say about using robots on children with disabilities? Disabil Rehabil Assist Technol. 2017;12(5):429–40.
33. Whittington P, Dogan H, Phalp K, Jiang N. Detecting physical abilities through smartphone sensors: an assistive technology application. Disabil Rehabil Assist Technol. 2022;17(8):974–85.
34. Jones J, Stewart H. A description of how three occupational therapists train children in using the scanning access technique. Aust Occup Ther J. 2004;51(3):155–65.

35. Karlsson P, Johnston C, Barker K. Influences on students' assistive technology use at school: the views of classroom teachers, allied health professionals, students with cerebral palsy and their parents. Disabil Rehabil Assist Technol. 2018;13(8):763–71.
36. Scherer MJ. Living in the state of stuck: how assistive technology impacts the lives of people with disabilities. Third edition. 2005; 122–123.
37. Østensjø S, Carlberg EB, Vøllestad NK. The use and impact of assistive devices and other environmental modifications on everyday activities and care in young children with cerebral palsy. Disabil Rehabil. 2005;27(14):849–61.
38. Butler P, Farmer S, Stewart C, Jones P, Forward M. The effect of fixed ankle foot orthoses in children with cerebral palsy. Disabil Rehabil Assist Technol. 2007;2(1):51–8.
39. Davis E, Shelly A, Waters E, Boyd R, Cook K, Davern M. The impact of caring for a child with cerebral palsy: quality of life for mothers and fathers. Child Care Health Dev. 2010;36(1):63–73.
40. Pfeifer LI, Silva DBR, Lopes P, Matsukura T, Santos JLF, Pinto MPP. Social support provided to caregivers of children with cerebral palsy. Child Care Health Dev. 2014;40(3):363–9.
41. Bourke-Taylor HM, Cotter C, Lalor A, Johnson L. School success and participation for students with cerebral palsy: a qualitative study exploring multiple perspectives. Disabil Rehabil. 2018;40(18):2163–71.
42. Reddihough DS, King J, Coleman G, Catanese T. Efficacy of programmes based on conductive education for young children with cerebral palsy. Dev Med Child Neurol. 1998;40(11):763–70.

Transitioning to Adulthood 15

Tina Alinia and Saeed Pourhassan

Case Presentation

A 19-year-old man with spastic diplegic cerebral palsy (GMFCS III) walks short distances with forearm crutches and uses a wheelchair for community mobility. He has been followed in a pediatric rehabilitation center by a multidisciplinary team including neurology, physiatry, therapy services, and social work.

His comorbidities include well-controlled epilepsy on anticonvulsant therapy and chronic hip and back pain, which has worsened over the past 2 years. He completed high school and is interested in graphic design but worries that daily fatigue will limit college or employment opportunities.

Socially, he has few friends but feels isolated as most peers are at university. He wishes for independence and hopes to live alone, but he and his parents feel unprepared. His parents have always managed his medical care, and with the upcoming transition to adult providers, the family views the process with uncertainty.

T. Alinia
School of Medicine, Tehran University of Medical Sciences, Tehran, Iran

S. Pourhassan (✉)
Internal Medicine Department, School of Medicine, Shariati Hospital, Tehran University of Medical Sciences, Tehran, Iran

A. Presedo et al. (eds.), *Enhancing Quality of Life in Patients with Cerebral Palsy*, https://doi.org/10.1007/978-3-032-20967-2_15

15.1 Introduction

Cerebral palsy has been considered a pediatric condition throughout history. The advances in the neonatal and pediatric fields have led to an increase in the survival rate of children with CP. Currently, many of the individuals with CP survive into adulthood, and with proper care, the life expectancy in the milder forms of the condition could be similar to that of the normal population [1]. This in turn leads to issues regarding the quality and readiness of the medical services and support systems for this population. Transitioning from the coordinated and multi-disciplinary healthcare system for the pediatric population to the unprepared and insufficient system for young adults can be described as falling off a cliff [2].

Transition should not be viewed as merely a transfer of records or the treating physician, but as a planned and purposeful process requiring coordination between pediatric and adult services [3]. Studies have shown that the current reality falls short of this ideal [4]. Unsuccessful transition is associated with negative outcomes, health deterioration, increased hospitalization and emergency care requirements, poor adherence to treatments, poor follow-up and development of preventable secondary health conditions [5]. Receiving age-appropriate care as the medical and personal needs of young adults with chronic lifelong diseases, improves their quality of life. The emotional and mental burden of adulthood as well as the responsibilities and expectations of adults in society, often without prior experience or preparation, further complicates this transition. Feeling "thrust into adulthood" suddenly, with many services being revoked or altered after high school education, issues with finding and managing appropriate education and employment services as well as activities of daily life independently have been reported by young adults with CP as some of the issues with this transition [6].

The difficulties seen during transition are not simply a natural result of growing older with a disability; they mostly come from the way our medical systems are divided and organized. The success of pediatrics in improving survival has revealed a major weakness in how care continues after childhood. The adult medical system is mostly built to treat acute illnesses or chronic diseases that begin in adulthood, and it usually does not have the training, resources, or team-based approach needed for complex conditions that start in childhood, such as neurodevelopmental disorders. This chapter suggests that instead of relying on a pediatric-focused model, care should be continuous throughout life. In this approach, transition is an important phase that makes sure health, function, and quality of life are supported across the person's whole lifespan.

15.2 The Changing Health Landscape of Adults with Cerebral Palsy

For a successful transition, the adult healthcare system must include doctors who understand the unique health course of people with cerebral palsy. It is a mistake to think of CP in adulthood as something fixed and unchanging. Although the brain injury itself is not progressive, its musculoskeletal and physiological effects change over time and can cause many secondary health problems [7, 8].

15.2.1 Differentiating the Injury from Its Effects

Adults with CP often develop problems due to years of living with changes in movement and body mechanics. Moving and mobility tasks require much more effort for them since individuals with CP are unable to use their muscles to their maximal strength [9]. This ongoing strain speeds up the aging process and can cause chronic pain, fatigue, and further muscle weakness [10]. These issues are not signs that the brain injury is getting worse, but rather predictable results of living with CP and its impairments over time. Because of this, adult healthcare providers should not dismiss new or worsening symptoms as "just part of CP" and need to carefully look for other treatable conditions that may be present.

15.2.2 Common Health Problems in Adults with CP

Regular screening and early management of newly developed health problems are very important. Adults with CP are at higher risk of developing chronic diseases, and these conditions often appear earlier than in the general population [11]. Individuals with cerebral palsy are also at a greater risk of developing combinations of multiple morbidities and chronic conditions [12].

Musculoskeletal Decline: The bones and joints are under constant abnormal forces and often not used properly. Over time, this causes joint contractures, worsening scoliosis, and early osteoarthritis, especially in hips and knees. Osteoporosis is also very common, which makes fragile fractures more likely. This comes from lack of mobility, poor nutrition, and sometimes long-term use of medicines like anticonvulsants [13, 14].

Neurological Problems: Although the original brain injury in CP does not progress, new neurological problems can appear in adulthood. Stroke is about twice as common as in the general population, even after adjusting for other risk factors [15]. Myelopathy, particularly Cervical spondylotic myelopathy and lumbar myelopathy, is another concern, because abnormal posture and movements lead to early spine degeneration. Symptoms like hand numbness, worsening gait, or bowel and bladder changes should be assessed quickly with spinal imaging. Screening for cervical myelopathy has been suggested to start from the third decade of life in order to provide appropriate treatment and better prognosis [16–18] Cognitive changes also need attention. Adults with CP with comorbidities like epilepsy or intellectual disability have been reported to have a higher risk of developing dementia. Alzheimer's disease and related dementia, especially early-onset types, have been reported to have higher incidence in adults with CP [19, 20].

Cardiometabolic Disease: Many adults with CP live with low physical activity and have higher body fat with less muscle mass; the progressive decrease in function can help understand the reason behind this [21]. This raises the chance of conditions such as high blood pressure, impaired glucose handling, dyslipidemia, heart failure, and ischemic heart disease, which can happen at a younger age compared to the general population [22]. The increased risk for cardiovascular and metabolic diseases in adults with CP, as well as the younger age at disease presentation observed in this population, suggests early screening for risk factors of such conditions. Continuous monitoring of factors such as obesity, blood pressure, and cholesterol should be performed, and patients should be educated regarding dietary habits, smoking, and mobility [23].

Pain and Fatigue: Chronic pain and fatigue are very common, disabling, and undertreated in this population. Pain affects most adults with CP, with reports as high as 70% [24]. Chronic fatigue is also very common and affects the vast majority of adults with CP and significantly disrupts their quality of life [11]. Doctors must separate "primary fatigue" (from nervous system inefficiency) from "secondary fatigue" caused by pain, poor sleep, depression, deconditioning, or side effects of medications. Treatment should combine different approaches: energy-saving methods ("pacing"), exercise to improve efficiency, better sleep hygiene, and management of possible underlying issues like pain or mood problems [25].

Mental Health: Mental health problems are a major comorbidity in this population and are often overlooked. In adults with CP, many symptoms are wrongly explained as part of their disability. Studies show a higher rate of depression, anxiety, and schizophrenia compared to the general population. The risk is even greater in people with intellectual disability or autism [26, 27]. These are not just reactions to disability but real and treatable medical conditions that reduce quality of life and function. Regular screening for mental health is very important. Screening tools should be adapted to the communication and cognitive needs of adults with CP. This may include the use of simplified language, visual support, or augmentative and alternative communication systems.

Table 15.1 provides a summary of key health concerns in adults with CP.

Table 15.1 Common adult health concerns in cerebral palsy: a clinical guide for proactive screening and management

Health domain	Specific condition	Key points & red flags	Initial management/ referral considerations
Neurological	Myelopathy	New or progressive weakness (especially in a previously stable patient), new sensory changes (numbness, tingling), gait deterioration, or new bowel/bladder dysfunction.	Urgent spinal imaging (MRI). Referring to Neurology/ Neurosurgery.
	Stroke	Acute onset of focal neurological deficits. Risk is about twice that of the general population, even after adjusting for traditional risk factors [1].	Follow standard acute stroke protocol. Aggressive secondary prevention and management of vascular risk factors.
	Dementia/Cognitive Decline	New, functionally significant memory loss or decline in executive function. Higher risk with comorbid epilepsy/ intellectual disability [1].	Formal neuropsychological testing to establish a baseline and monitor changes. Differentiate from depression or medication effects.
Musculoskeletal	Osteoarthritis	Chronic joint pain (hip, knee, spine), stiffness, and functional decline. Often occurs decades earlier.	Radiographic imaging. Refer to Orthopedics, and Physical Therapy for pain management, bracing, and surgical evaluation.
	Osteoporosis	Increased risk of fragility fractures.	Consider baseline DEXA scan, especially in non-ambulatory individuals or those on long-term anticonvulsants. Ensure adequate vitamin D/calcium intake.

(continued)

Table 15.1 (continued)

Health domain	Specific condition	Key points & red flags	Initial management/ referral considerations
Mental health	Depression & Anxiety	High prevalence [2] overlaps with and exacerbates pain and fatigue. Avoid diagnostic overshadowing.	Routine screening with validated and adapted tools. Refer to Psychology/ Psychiatry. Integrate mental health support into the core care plan.
Cardiometabolic	Hypertension, diabetes, heart disease	Increased prevalence and earlier onset. Often linked to physical inactivity and altered body composition [3].	Routine screening as per general population guidelines, but with heightened awareness starting in young adulthood. Emphasize lifestyle modification and refer to cardiology/ endocrinology as needed.
General	Chronic pain	Prevalence of 65–70% [4]. Can be musculoskeletal or neuropathic. Strongly impacts function and quality of life.	Multimodal approach: physiatry, physical therapy, pain psychology, non-opioid pharmacotherapy. Address underlying causes.
	Chronic fatigue	Overwhelming exhaustion disproportionate to activity. Differentiate primary vs. secondary causes (sleep, pain, mood, deconditioning) [5].	Promote energy conservation strategies and physical conditioning. Optimize sleep hygiene. Screen for and treat depression and pain. Refer to occupational and physical therapy.

Refs. [11, 21, 24, 25, 26]

15.3 A Framework for Successful Transition: From Theory to Practice

The transition between pediatric and adult healthcare is difficult, but not impossible. Over the years, research and clinical experience have led to many good models and guidelines for transition. The main problem is not about knowing what to do, but rather about putting it into practice. System and financial barriers often stop this from happening. Studies have suggested that while many clinics report having a structured transition program, they might lack many key components, and very few programs can manage to successfully transfer all patients to adult care [28, 29]. This shows a clear gap between research and practice and highlights the need for clinicians not only to use best practices in their own work but also to push for system-wide changes that make transition possible.

15.3.1 Foundational Principles and Models

Transition is not just a single step, but an ongoing and complex process. Several evidence-based models provide useful guidance for this process:

- *The Six Core Elements of Health Care Transition (HCT)*: Published by Got Transition and supported by multiple American medical societies, this toolkit gives a practical, quality-focused approach. The six elements are: (1) establishing a clear transition policy, (2) tracking and monitoring patients as they approach transition age, (3) assessing their readiness for transition, (4) making a comprehensive transition plan, (5) managing the actual transfer of care with a "warm handoff," and (6) ensuring transition completion and integration into adult-centered care [30]. The effectiveness of this toolkit has been assessed by multiple studies and significant improvements in the transition process have been observed [31].
- *NICE Guidelines (UK)*: The National Institute for Health and Care Excellence guidelines stress having clear and documented care pathways. They recommend the involvement of the young patient's general practitioner, pediatric and adult clinicians with interest in CP, and a coordinator or "named worker" to guide the process. They also highlight that functional problems—like difficulties in mobility, communication, or swallowing—can change over time, and this must be included in planning [3].
- *CanChild's "Best Journey to Adult Life"*: This model was developed with strong input from patients and families. It sees transition as a journey with three phases: preparation, the actual move, and arrival in adult care. It is based on six themes: the need for collaborative policies, stronger capacity for communities and individuals, the role of a "Navigator," access to clear information, the importance of education, and continuous research [32].

Even though these models use different terms, they all agree on key principles: transition must be planned, patient-centered, flexible, thorough, and well-coordinated. The first important step is for patients, families, and both pediatric and adult teams to understand that the two systems have very different cultures and ways of working [33] (Table 15.2).

Table 15.2 Contrasting care models: pediatric vs. adult healthcare [1]

Feature	Pediatric care	Adult care
Philosophy of care	Family-centered, developmental focus. Emphasis on reaching potential.	Patient-centered, disease/problem focus. Emphasis on managing conditions.
Team structure	Care is coordinated by a multidisciplinary team (MDT) with joint visits.	Care is fragmented and referral based. Patients are responsible for coordinating multiple specialists.
Decision-making	Doctors and parents usually make decisions together.	The patient makes their own decisions and is expected to advocate for themselves.
Family role	Parents are main caregivers, primary advocates, and legal decision-makers.	Family acts as support, but only with the consent of the adult patient.
Communication	Clinics regularly update and communicate with families.	The patient is responsible for reaching out to providers.
Setting	Care is often centralized in children's hospitals or specialized centers.	Care is spread across multiple community clinics, hospitals, and private offices.
Visit style	Appointments are longer, with focus on development, prevention, and family education.	Appointments are shorter and often focused on a specific problem or complaint.
Provider expertise	Providers have deep knowledge of developmental disabilities and their comorbidities.	Provider expertise is often disease-specific (e.g., cardiology, pulmonology), with limited training in childhood-onset disabilities.

Ref. [33]

15.3.2 The Multidisciplinary Transition Team: Roles and Collaboration

Transition cannot be managed by one clinician alone. It requires a collaborative effort between pediatric and adult care providers.

- *Pediatric Team*: This team usually includes a pediatrician, pediatric neurologist, and/or physiatrist, physical/occupational/speech therapists, and a social worker, and is responsible for the initiation of transitioning process. Their main tasks are to start discussing transition early (around ages 12–14), help the teenager learn about their health and how to manage it by themselves, and prepare a clear medical summary. This summary should include history, current providers, medications, equipment, and the care plan.
- *Adult Team*: The receiving team must include clinicians willing and able to care for this population. The team should include a primary care doctor, an adult neurologist and/or physiatrist, therapists, and mental health specialists. Their role is to join the planning process before transfer, accept the patient into their care, and provide ongoing care with an understanding of the specific needs of adults with CP.

- *Transition Coordinator/Navigator*: This role is very important for a successful transition. Often a nurse specialist or social worker, the coordinator is the main contact for the family. They organize communication between pediatric and adult teams, help arrange appointments, connect the family with community resources (like job training or housing services), and make sure the transfer is smooth, so the patient does not get lost in the system [3, 34].

15.3.3 The Transition Timeline: Step by Step

Moving from pediatric to adult care should not happen suddenly at the age of 18. It is better to see it as a gradual and step-by-step process, where the young person slowly learns new skills and gains knowledge.

- *Phase 1: Preparation (Ages 12–14)*: At this stage, the pediatric team starts talking with the adolescent and family about the future and the idea of moving to adult care. The focus is on building foundational self-care skills. The adolescent should learn the names and uses of their medications, understand their diagnosis in basic terms, and start speaking for themselves during part of the medical visit.
- *Phase 2: Planning (Ages 15–17)*: A formal, written transition plan is created, often with a checklist such as the Six Core Elements. Possible adult providers are identified and contacted. The conversations also include education after high school, work options, independent living, and legal or financial issues. If possible, meetings with the future adult care team should be arranged, which usually helps with better outcomes.
- *Phase 3: Transfer (Ages 18–22+)*: At this point, the main medical responsibility is transferred to the adult care team. The exact timing should depend on the young person's readiness, not on age alone. A full and updated medical summary is given to the adult team. For a defined period, usually the first 6–12 months, the pediatric team should stay available to consult and support the adult providers and make the process smoother.
- *Phase 4: Integration (Post-Transfer)*: The adult team makes sure that the young adult is fully included in their system. This means having a main primary care physician (PCP) who coordinates care, arranging regular follow-up visits, and continuing to support the young adult in their health and life goals [28, 35].

15.4 Domains of Adult Life: A Practical and Holistic View

If transition is focused only on medical needs, it is not complete and can even be called a failed transition. The main goal is to help the young person succeed in all areas of adult life. Research on transition in cerebral palsy (CP) shows that a planned and holistic process is necessary for the best long-term medical and psychosocial results [29]. In contrast, a poor transition process can lead to problems such as unstable housing, unemployment, and difficulties in making relationships.

Health, social, and economic issues are closely connected. For example, pain and fatigue, which are very common in adults with CP, can limit education and job opportunities. This can then cause financial problems and limited housing choices. Social isolation may follow, and this is strongly linked with depression and anxiety, which are more common in adults with CP than in the general population [27]. Depression and anxiety, in turn, increase the perception of pain and fatigue, creating a cycle that is difficult to break. Because of this, the clinician's role must go beyond medical treatment and also include attention and support in social, educational, and economic areas.

15.4.1 Building Autonomy and Self-Determination

The most important principle of transition is moving from care directed by parents or doctors toward care where the young person is the main decision-maker.

Developing Self-Advocacy

During adolescence, doctors should gradually change their focus from parents to the patient. Young people need to be encouraged to express their concerns, ask questions, make their own appointments, and manage their medications [36]. Resources such as GotTransition® can help both families and adolescents with this process [37]. If these skills are not developed before the legal age of adulthood, a "competency gap" may appear, and families may feel forced to use very restrictive legal measures.

Legal Decision-Making

At age 18, parents usually lose the legal right to make decisions for their child. This change requires preparation and planning.

- *Guardianship (Conservatorship)*: In this process, the court takes away the person's right to make decisions and gives this authority to a guardian. This is sometimes necessary for people with very severe cognitive problems who cannot participate in decisions. However, it is often used too quickly and should only be the last option, because it takes away basic personal rights [38].
- *Supported Decision-Making (SDM)*: This is the better alternative for most people with disabilities, including CP. In SDM, the individual keeps all their legal rights and decision power. They choose trusted supporters (for example, family or friends) to help them understand information, consider options, and communicate their choices. SDM supports autonomy and independence and is a strong tool for empowerment. Clinicians should know about SDM and guide families to use it whenever possible [38, 39] (Table 15.3).

Table 15.3 Guardianship vs. Supported Decision-Making (SDM) [1, 2]

Feature	Guardianship	Supported Decision-Making (SDM)
Decision-maker	The court-appointed guardian	The individual with a disability
Legal rights	Rights are removed from the individual and transferred to the guardian	The individual retains all legal rights and authority
Philosophy	Focus is on protection by replacing the person's judgement	Focus is on empowerment and self-determination, with support in decision-making
When appropriate	Individuals with profound cognitive impairments who cannot participate in the decision-making process	Most individuals with disabilities can participate in decision-making with support

Refs. [38, 39]

15.4.2 Education and Vocation

Work is an important part of adult identity, social life, and financial independence.

The Employment Gap

Although most adults with CP consider employment a top priority, they face many barriers and usually have much lower employment rates than the general population. Studies suggest the rate of employment in adults with cerebral palsy to be about 39%, compared to about 82% of their peers within the general population, which is very low [40]. The most important predictors of employment are higher education and cognitive ability, but physical limitations and social prejudice also play a major role [41].

Vocational Support

Government-supported vocational rehabilitation (VR) programs can help many people with CP, but they are not used enough. For those who participate, almost half find successful employment, which shows there is a gap between what these programs can do and what is actually achieved. Research highlights some key services that lead to success, such as on-the-job training, job placement assistance, job coaching, and the use of assistive technology [42, 43]. Physicians and transition teams should know about their local VR programs and make timely referrals. This referral is not just paperwork—it can be a life-changing intervention.

15.4.3 Independent Living and Community Participation

Planning for housing and daily living is an important part of transition. Many young adults with CP continue to live with their parents, not by choice but because of limited affordable housing and lack of community support. Access to personal assistance is the most important factor for independent living. Studies have demonstrated higher rates of independent living and participation in society in settings with higher access to personal assistance availability [44, 45]. Transition planning should therefore include housing options, such as living alone with personal care assistants, supported apartments, or group homes. It is also important to prevent isolation by encouraging participation in community activities, recreational programs, and peer support groups.

15.4.4 Sexuality and Intimate Relationships

Sexuality is an important part of human life and well-being, but it is often ignored in the care of people with disabilities. This can leave young adults with CP feeling invisible and unprepared.

Desire and Experience
Studies show that adults with CP have the same needs for love, intimacy, and sexuality as their peers. However, they are less likely to be in a relationship or to have sexual experiences [46]. The reason is not lack of desire, but many barriers.

Barriers
Barriers include physical problems such as pain, spasticity, fatigue, and difficulties with positioning. Emotional and social barriers include low self-esteem, social anxiety, fear of rejection, and fewer chances for dating. Educational barriers are also very common: many young adults with CP have never had sexuality discussed in rehabilitation and even less have received sex education adapted to their disability [46, 47].

The Clinician's Role
Clinicians should take an active role in creating a safe and confidential space to discuss sexuality and relationships. Talking about these issues in a respectful and routine way helps normalize them and allows young adults to ask questions. Frameworks such as the CDC's "5 P's" (Partners, Practices, Protection from STIs, Past history of STIs, Pregnancy) can guide these conversations. Clinicians must be non-judgmental, speak directly to the patient, keep confidentiality, and when needed, refer to other professionals such as counselors or therapists who can address specific physical or emotional concerns [48, 49].

15.4.5 Financial Planning and Benefits

Financial stability is essential for independence. Many adults with CP rely, at least partly, on government benefits like SSI (Supplemental Security Income) and aid for medical conditions. These programs are critical for covering basic needs like food, housing, and healthcare; however, they have very strict limits on income and assets. For example, individuals usually must have less than a certain amount in countable assets to stay eligible for SSI. This rule system can create a "poverty trap" because people may fear saving money or receiving help lest they lose their essential benefits [50].

Special Needs Trusts (SNTs)

A Special Needs Trust, also called a Supplemental Needs Trust, is a key tool to help individuals keep their eligibility for benefits. It is a legal trust where assets can be held for a person with CP without the assets counting against benefit limits [51].

How SNTs Work

A trustee manages the funds in the SNT, and the money is used for "supplemental needs", things that improve quality of life but are not covered by government programs, such as education, hobbies, travel, dental care, transportation, or assistive devices. There are different types of SNTs:

- *First-party SNTs*: Funded by the individual's own money (e.g., settlement funds).
- *Third-party SNTs*: Funded by others like parents or grandparents.

All types share the same purpose: to add support without replacing government benefits [51].

Clinicians should advise families to consult an attorney who specializes in special-needs planning as part of transition or estate planning. This advice is more than simple financial counsel—it is a vital clinical intervention that addresses a major barrier to independence and well-being.

15.5 Conclusion: The Clinician's Role in Supporting Full-Life Care

Transition from pediatric to adult care is a crucial moment for individuals with cerebral palsy. It can either lead to a healthy, fulfilling adult life or lead to decline in well-being. The current system remains fragmented and fails many people. Even so, every clinician can make a difference by approaching care with knowledge and a holistic perspective.

Key Clinical Responsibilities

- *Start early*: Begin transition discussions and planning by ages 12–14.
- *Use a structured process*: Use a formal transition policy and checklist (e.g., based on the Six Core Elements) to address all domains.
- *Recognize CP beyond childhood*: CP does not stop at reaching adulthood. Actively screen for and manage evolving adult health issues like pain, fatigue, neurological, and cardiometabolic conditions.
- *Prioritize mental health*: Make mental health checks routine, avoid diagnostic overshadowing, and ensure access to psychological services.
- *Promote autonomy*: Discuss legal decision-making before adulthood and help families understand Supported Decision-Making as a rights-respecting option instead of guardianship.

- *Think holistically*: Ask about education, work, social life, relationships, and money. Use a multidisciplinary team to refer patients to social workers, job services, psychologists, and legal or financial experts when needed.
- *Create a medical home*: The goal of transition is for the young adult to join an adult-care system with a dedicated primary care provider who coordinates their ongoing care.

Improving transition care requires more than one clinician's effort; it demands support on a more general level. Clinicians, who see the consequences of system failure firsthand, have a unique role to:

- Integrate adult neurodevelopmental care into medical education.
- Support new funding models that allow time-consuming care coordination.
- Encourage the development of comprehensive, multidisciplinary lifespan-care centers.

By combining both clinical and advocacy roles, we can help reduce the "transition cliff" and ensure that every person with cerebral palsy can navigate adulthood and live a long, healthy, and meaningful life.

Patient Discussion

This case highlights the common challenges faced during the transition from pediatric to adult care in cerebral palsy. Many young adults describe the process as stepping off a "cliff," reflecting the sudden loss of coordinated pediatric support. A successful transition requires a planned approach that addresses not only medical issues but also psychosocial, educational, and vocational needs.

His worsening musculoskeletal pain and fatigue are expected secondary effects of CP rather than signs of a static disorder. An adult care team, including a primary physician and an adult neurologist or physiatrist, should monitor and manage these issues, especially risks like early osteoarthritis and osteoporosis. His feelings of isolation and anxiety also underline the importance of routine mental health screening, as depression and anxiety are common but often missed in this population.

Promoting independence means teaching him to manage appointments, medications, and decision-making for his own care. Vocational rehabilitation services can provide job coaching and assistive technologies that make careers such as graphic design more suitable despite fatigue. Planning for independent living should also include accessible housing and possible personal assistance to support participation in the community.

Using a structured framework, such as the Six Core Elements, the pediatric and adult teams can coordinate a smooth transfer, ensure continuity of care and supporting his path toward a healthier, more independent adult life.

15.6 A Practical Guide for Parents and Caregivers

Supporting your child with cerebral palsy as they move into adulthood can feel difficult, but starting early and planning step by step will make the process smoother. This guide offers practical advice to help you and your child through this important stage.

1. *Start Early and Build Skills*
   The transition should begin long before age 18. It is best to start conversations with your child and their doctors around ages 12–14. The focus in these years is to increase independence.
   - *Health literacy*: Teach your child to know the names of their condition, medicines, and allergies. Encourage them to speak during part of each clinic visit.
   - *Self-management*: Slowly involve them in tasks like refilling prescriptions or booking appointments. These small steps build confidence for later.
2. *Build the Adult Care Team*
   Adult healthcare is less coordinated than pediatric care, and patients must take more responsibility.
   - *Find the right doctors*: With help from your pediatric team, look for a primary care doctor who can be the new "medical home" and specialists such as an adult neurologist or physiatrist who work with childhood-onset disabilities.
   - *Ask for a smooth transfer*: A smooth transfer happens when the pediatric and adult teams communicate directly. A nurse or social worker can help coordinate. Make sure a full medical summary is sent to the new providers.
3. *Plan Beyond Medical Needs*
   Good health is only one part of adult life. The transition plan should also cover education, work, living, and finances.
   - *Education and work*: If your child wants to work, connect with your local vocational rehabilitation (VR) services. These programs offer training, job coaching, and technology support.
   - *Independent living*: Discuss housing early. Options include accessible apartments, supported living, or personal care services.
   - *Financial planning*: Benefits such as SSI can help but have strict limits on income and savings. A lawyer who knows special needs planning can explain tools like a Special Needs Trust (SNT), which protects savings while keeping benefits.
4. *Support Autonomy*
   At age 18, your child is legally an adult, and parents no longer make decisions for them. Planning for this change is important.
   - *Guardianship as last resort*: Full guardianship takes away legal rights and should only be used for severe cognitive disability.
   - *Supported decision-making (SDM)*: In most cases, SDM is better. Your child keeps all rights but chooses trusted people to help understand information and make choices. This respects their independence while providing support.

5. *Care for the Whole Person*

   Your child has the same needs for friendship, love, and purpose as anyone else.

   - *Mental health*: Adults with CP have a higher risk of depression and anxiety. Encourage open conversations and include mental health in regular care.
   - *Relationships and sexuality*: Sexual health is part of normal adult life but often ignored in disability care. Create a safe space for questions and ask doctors to discuss these topics privately and respectfully.

15.7 Guide for Multidisciplinary Teams

Multidisciplinary teamwork is the cornerstone of successful transition and lifelong care for individuals with cerebral palsy (CP). No single clinician can address the complex medical, functional, and psychosocial needs of this population. Instead, care should be coordinated through an integrated team that combines medical, therapeutic, and social expertise, with the patient and family at the center.

Team Composition and Roles

- *Primary Care Physician* serves as the medical home, ensuring continuity and coordination of care across specialties.
- *Neurologists and Physiatrics* address neurological symptoms, musculoskeletal complications, spasticity management, and long-term rehabilitation needs.
- *Therapists (physical, occupational, and speech language)* guide functional independence, communication strategies, and adaptive equipment use.
- *Mental Health Specialists* screen for and treat depression, anxiety, and other psychiatric comorbidities, which are often overlooked.
- *Social Workers and Transition Coordinators* connect patients with community resources, vocational programs, housing options, and financial planning tools.
- *Specialist Consultants* (orthopedics, cardiology, gastroenterology, gynecology/urology) should be engaged as health issues evolve.

Principles of Collaboration

The team must adopt a *shared-care model* where communication is open, records are unified, and decisions are patient-centered. Regular multidisciplinary meetings and case conferences improve alignment of goals. Transition planning should begin early, with both pediatric and adult teams overlapping during the transfer period. Importantly, the young adult should be included as an active participant, promoting autonomy and supported decision-making rather than passive dependence.

Broader Goals

Beyond medical treatment, the team should address domains such as education, employment, sexuality, and financial stability, recognizing that these directly influence health outcomes. In resource-limited settings, prioritizing coordination, early planning, and use of available community supports can help reduce the "transition cliff" and ensure continuity of care.

References

1. Blair E, Langdon K, McIntyre S, Lawrence D, Watson L. Survival and mortality in cerebral palsy: observations to the sixth decade from a data linkage study of a total population register and National Death Index. BMC Neurol. 2019;19(1):111.
2. Turner S, Nash C, Goodwin J, Smith J, Fairhurst C, Cadwgan J. Transition and life-long care for adults with cerebral palsy: a patient group 'too hard to impact!'are we still sending young people 'off a cliff'? J Eval Clin Pract. 2025;31(1):e70011.
3. UK NGA. Cerebral palsy in under 25s: assessment and management. London: National Institute for Health and Care Excellence (NICE); 2017.
4. While A, Forbes A, Ullman R, Lewis S, Mathes L, Griffiths P. Good practices that address continuity during transition from child to adult care: synthesis of the evidence. Child Care Health Dev. 2004;30(5):439–52.
5. Ryan JM, Fortune J, Walsh A, Norris M, Kerr C, Hensey O, et al. Transition from child to adult health services for young people with cerebral palsy in Ireland: a mixed-methods study protocol. BMJ Open. 2020;10(12):e041425.
6. Bagatell N, Chan D, Rauch KK, Thorpe D. "Thrust into adulthood": transition experiences of young adults with cerebral palsy. Disabil Health J. 2017;10(1):80–6.
7. Bromham N, Dworzynski K, Eunson P, Fairhurst C. Cerebral palsy in adults: summary of NICE guidance. BMJ. 2019;364:l806.
8. Ryan JM, Albairami F, Hamilton T, Cope N, Amirmudin NA, Manikandan M, et al. Prevalence and incidence of chronic conditions among adults with cerebral palsy: a systematic review and meta-analysis. Dev Med Child Neurol. 2023;65(9):1174–89.
9. Stackhouse SK, Binder-Macleod SA, Lee SC. Voluntary muscle activation, contractile properties, and fatigability in children with and without cerebral palsy. Muscle Nerve. 2005;31(5):594–601.
10. Shortland A. Muscle deficits in cerebral palsy and early loss of mobility: can we learn something from our elders? Dev Med Child Neurol. 2009;51:59–63.
11. Smith SE, Gannotti M, Hurvitz EA, Jensen FE, Krach LE, Kruer MC, et al. Adults with cerebral palsy require ongoing neurologic care: a systematic review. Ann Neurol. 2021;89(5):860–71.
12. Cremer N, Hurvitz EA, Peterson MD. Multimorbidity in middle-aged adults with cerebral palsy. Am J Med. 2017;130(6):744. e9–e15.
13. Gajdosik CG, Cicirello N. Secondary conditions of the musculoskeletal system in adolescents and adults with cerebral palsy. Phys Occup Ther Pediatr. 2002;21(4):49–68.
14. Whitney DG, Hurvitz EA, Devlin MJ, Caird MS, French ZP, Ellenberg EC, et al. Age trajectories of musculoskeletal morbidities in adults with cerebral palsy. Bone. 2018;114:285–91.
15. Wu CW, Huang SW, Lin JW, Liou TH, Chou LC, Lin HW. Risk of stroke among patients with cerebral palsy: a population-based cohort study. Dev Med Child Neurol. 2017;59(1):52–6.
16. Harada T, Ebara S, Anwar MM, Okawa A, Kajiura I, Hiroshima K, et al. The cervical spine in athetoid cerebral palsy: a radiological study of 180 patients. J Bone Joint Surg Br Vol. 1996;78(4):613–9.
17. Sakai T, Yamada H, Nakamura T, Nanamori K, Kawasaki Y, Hanaoka N, et al. Lumbar spinal disorders in patients with athetoid cerebral palsy: a clinical and biomechanical study. Spine. 2006;31(3):E66–70.

18. Guettard E, Ricard D, Roze E, Elbaz A, Anheim M, Thobois S, et al. Risk factors for spinal cord lesions in dystonic cerebral palsy and generalised dystonia. J Neurol Neurosurg Psychiatry. 2012;83(2):159–63.
19. Mahmoudi E, Lin P, Kamdar N, Gonzales G, Norcott A, Peterson MD. Risk of early-and late-onset Alzheimer disease and related dementia in adults with cerebral palsy. Dev Med Child Neurol. 2022;64(3):372–8.
20. Smith KJ, Peterson MD, Victor C, Ryan JM. Risk of dementia in adults with cerebral palsy: a matched cohort study using general practice data. BMJ Open. 2021;11(1):e042652.
21. Whitney DG, Hurvitz EA, Ryan JM, Devlin MJ, Caird MS, French ZP, et al. Noncommunicable disease and multimorbidity in young adults with cerebral palsy. Clin Epidemiol. 2018;10:511–9.
22. Whitney DG. 5-year risk of "adult-onset" chronic diseases during childhood and adolescent transitioning for individuals with cerebral palsy. Prev Med Rep. 2022;29:101933.
23. Heyn PC, Tagawa A, Pan Z, Thomas S, Carollo JJ. Prevalence of metabolic syndrome and cardiovascular disease risk factors in adults with cerebral palsy. Dev Med Child Neurol. 2019;61(4):477–83.
24. van der Slot WM, Benner JL, Brunton L, Engel JM, Gallien P, Hilberink SR, et al. Pain in adults with cerebral palsy: a systematic review and meta-analysis of individual participant data. Ann Phys Rehabil Med. 2021;64(3):101359.
25. Brunton LK, McPhee PG, Gorter JW. Self-reported factors contributing to fatigue and its management in adolescents and adults with cerebral palsy. Disabil Rehabil. 2021;43(7):929–35.
26. Whitney DG, Warschausky SA, Ng S, Hurvitz EA, Kamdar NS, Peterson MD. Prevalence of mental health disorders among adults with cerebral palsy: a cross-sectional analysis. Ann Intern Med. 2019;171(5):328–33.
27. Smith KJ, Peterson MD, O'Connell NE, Victor C, Liverani S, Anokye N, et al. Risk of depression and anxiety in adults with cerebral palsy. JAMA Neurol. 2019;76(3):294–300.
28. Mitchell DL, Shlobin NA, Winterhalter E, Lam SK, Raskin JS. Gaps in transitional care to adulthood for patients with cerebral palsy: a systematic review. Childs Nerv Syst. 2023;39(11):3083–101.
29. Bolger A, Vargus-Adams J, McMahon M. Transition of care in adolescents with cerebral palsy: a survey of current practices. PM R. 2017;9(3):258–64.
30. Transition® G. Six Core Elements of Health Care Transition™ 3.0: The National Alliance to Advance Adolescent Health; 2020. Available from: https://www.gottransition.org/six-core-elements/.
31. Jones MR, Hooper TJ, Cuomo C, Crouch G, Hickam T, Lestishock L, et al. Evaluation of a health care transition improvement process in seven large health care systems. J Pediatr Nurs. 2019;47:44–50.
32. S SDFMLMHHB-GJFMYNG. "The Best Journey to Adult Life" for youth with disabilities: an evidence-based model and Best Practice Guidelines for the transition to adulthood for youth with disabilities. Hamilton: McMaster University, Can Child Centre for Childhood Disability Research; 2009. Available from: https://canchild.ca/research-in-practice/transitions/best-practice-guidelines/?utm_source=chatgpt.com.
33. Hurvitz EA, Whitney DG, Waldron-Perrine B, Ryan D, Haapala HJ, Schmidt M, et al. Navigating the pathway to care in adults with cerebral palsy. Front Neurol. 2021;12:734139.
34. Pringsheim T, Batla A, Shalash A, Sahu JK, Cosentino C, Ebrahimi-Fakhari D, et al. Transitional care for young people with movement disorders: consensus-based recommendations from the MDS task force on pediatrics. Mov Disord Clin Pract. 2023;10(5):748–55.
35. Freeman M, Stewart D, Cunningham CE, Gorter JW. Information needs of young people with cerebral palsy and their families during the transition to adulthood: a scoping review. J Transit Med. 2019;1(1):20180003.
36. Burke R, Spoerri M, Price A, Cardosi A-M, Flanagan P. Survey of primary care pediatricians on the transition and transfer of adolescents to adult health care. Clin Pediatr. 2008;47(4):347–54.
37. White PH, Cooley WC. Supporting the health care transition from adolescence to adulthood in the medical home. Pediatrics. 2018;142(5):e20182587.

38. Salzman L. Guardianship for persons with mental illness-a legal and appropriate alternative. Louis UJ Health L & Pol'y. 2010;4:279.
39. Blanck P, Martinis JG. "The right to make choices": the national resource center for supported decision-making. Inc. 2015;3(1):24–33.
40. Benner JL, Hilberink SR, Veenis T, van der Slot WM, Roebroeck ME. Course of employment in adults with cerebral palsy over a 14-year period. Dev Med Child Neurol. 2017;59(7):762–8.
41. Donkervoort M, Roebroeck M, Wiegerink D, Van der Heijden-Maessen H, Stam H, Netherlands TRGSW. Determinants of functioning of adolescents and young adults with cerebral palsy. Disabil Rehabil. 2007;29(6):453–63.
42. Huang IC, Holzbauer JJ, Lee EJ, Chronister J, Chan F, O'neil J. Vocational rehabilitation services and employment outcomes for adults with cerebral palsy in the U nited S tates. Dev Med Child Neurol. 2013;55(11):1000–8.
43. Ma Z, Dhir P, Perrier L, Bayley M, Munce S. The impact of vocational interventions on vocational outcomes, quality of life, and community integration in adults with childhood onset disabilities: a systematic review. J Occup Rehabil. 2020;30(1):1–21.
44. von Granitz H, Sonnander K, Reine I, Winblad U. Do personal assistance activities promote participation in society for persons with disabilities in Sweden? A five-year longitudinal study. Disabil Rehabil. 2022;44(15):3973–81.
45. Pettersson K, Rodby-Bousquet E. Living conditions and social outcomes in adults with cerebral palsy. Front Neurol. 2021;12:749389.
46. Wiegerink D, Roebroeck M, Bender J, Stam H, Cohen-Kettenis P, Netherlands TRGSW. Sexuality of young adults with cerebral palsy: experienced limitations and needs. Sex Disabil. 2011;29(2):119–28.
47. Wiegerink DJ, Roebroeck ME, Donkervoort M, Stam HJ, Cohen-Kettenis PT. Social and sexual relationships of adolescents and young adults with cerebral palsy: a review. Clin Rehabil. 2006;20(12):1023–31.
48. Breuner CC, Mattson G, Adelman WP, Alderman EM, Garofalo R, Marcell AV, Powers ME, Upadhya KK, Yogman MW, Bauer NS, Gambon TB. Sexuality education for children and adolescents. Pediatrics. 2016;138(2):e20161348.
49. Marcell AV, Burstein GR, Committee on Adolescence, Braverman P, Adelman W, Alderman E, et al. Sexual and reproductive health care services in the pediatric setting. Pediatrics. 2017;140(5):e20172858.
50. Stapleton DC, O'Day BL, Livermore GA, Imparato AJ. Dismantling the poverty trap: disability policy for the twenty-first century. Milbank Q. 2006;84(4):701–32.
51. Lacey RP, Nadler HD. Special needs trusts. Fam Law Q. 2012;46(2):247–67.

Traditional and Complementary Medicine in Cerebral Palsy

16

Mohammad Sadegh Adel-Mehraban, Azadeh Zarei, Niusha Esmaealzadeh, and Roodabeh Bahramsoltani

16.1 Introduction

Cerebral palsy (CP) is a complex neurodevelopmental disorder dramatically affecting motor function, coordination, and overall quality of life. Conventional medicine employs different therapeutic modalities for the management of condition, including physiotherapy, occupational therapy, and pharmacological interventions; though the limitation of these therapies, as well as the complex nature of the disease, attracts the attention of scientists to traditional, complementary, and alternative medicine as an adjuvant to the conventional treatment strategies. Recent studies have begun to illuminate the potential of such integrative strategies in enhancing motor function and promoting holistic wellness in children with CP [1].

Traditional and integrative medicine (TIM) is defined as a category of treatment modalities, including acupuncture, herbal medicine, massage therapies, and mind-body interventions, rooted in ancient healing systems of different countries all over the world. These interventions offer a holistic approach, i.e., considering all

M. S. Adel-Mehraban · A. Zarei
Department of Traditional Persian Medicine, School of Persian Medicine, Tehran University of Medical Sciences, Tehran, Iran
e-mail: sadeghadel@gmail.com; azarei@tums.ac.ir

N. Esmaealzadeh
Department of Traditional Pharmacy, School of Persian Medicine, Tehran University of Medical Sciences, Tehran, Iran
e-mail: n-esmaealzadeh@tums.ac.ir

R. Bahramsoltani (✉)
Department of Traditional Pharmacy, School of Persian Medicine, Tehran University of Medical Sciences, Tehran, Iran

PhytoPharmacology Interest Group (PPIG), Universal Scientific Education and Research Network (USERN), Tehran, Iran
e-mail: rbahramsoltani@sina.tums.ac.ir

A. Presedo et al. (eds.), *Enhancing Quality of Life in Patients with Cerebral Palsy*, https://doi.org/10.1007/978-3-032-20967-2_16

physical and mental aspects of the whole body instead of focusing on the specific organ showing the disease symptom. Additionally, the personalized approach of TIM designs specific treatments based on the condition of each patient rather than a general prescription for all patients suffering from a specific disease [2].

Although current number of studies assessing TIM approaches in CP patients is not that high, available data suggest promising effects of some of these treatment methods such as massage and acupuncture. Traditional Chinese medicine (TCM) has been widely adopted in several parts of the world, and emerging evidence from cohort studies in Taiwan indicates that TCM, when combined with conventional rehabilitation, may improve functional outcomes in children with CP [1]. Also, Ayurveda, which originates from India and has an emphasis on herbal remedies and lifestyle modifications, has been suggested by systematic reviews and meta-analyses to improve spasticity and motor control among pediatric patients with CP [2].

Recent clinical protocols have started to evaluate integrative medicine rehabilitation programs, which combine conventional therapies with traditional modalities such as acupuncture and herbal treatments, further confirming the promising role of TIM in CP patients [3].

Considering the growing interest in clinical application of TIM approaches in patients with CP, this chapter reviews the scientific foundations, preclinical studies, and clinical evidence of different TIM modalities in the management of these patients.

16.2 Role of Acupuncture in CP

Traditional Chinese medicine (TCM) is a holistic medical system consisting of prevention, diagnosis, and treatment of disease, which dates back about 3000 years [4] spreading beyond regions, mostly in Northeast Asia [5]. The central principle of TCM is the concept of Yin and Yang, which describes two opposite substances mutually complementary inside the human body. Based on this theory, TCM explains the interaction of the main organs (Zang), the assistant organs (Fu), the extraordinary organs, vital energy of qi, and meridians [6]. On this foundation, TCM offers syndrome differentiation followed by suggested TCM medical intervention methods, including acupuncture, herbal remedies, moxibustion, etc., to recover the balance of various body functions [4].

Acupuncture, literally meaning needle penetration, is the practice of placing small needles into particular acupoints, which are the areas to let qi flow into meridians, according to TCM [6]. Under this theory, health stems originate in the alignment of qi, as the vital energy of the body, which provides optimal function of organs and body homeostasis, and the role of acupuncture is to remove any blockage, deficiency, or excess that disrupts the function of qi [7]. The TCM physician accesses the qi through meridians, specific channels through which qi flows [8]. Over the past 40 years, acupuncture has emerged as a medical modality all around the world and evolved as one of the most utilized therapeutic methods of complementary and alternative systems in the United States, so that in 1 year, millions of people preferred acupuncture to manage different diseases [9]. Expanding the relationship between Eastern and Western acupuncture accelerated the progression, evolution, and acceptance of acupuncture. Since the Consensus Development Conference on Acupuncture in 1997 introduced acupuncture as an extensively utilized method by physicians, dentists, and acupuncturists, as well as the National Institute of Health (NIH) survey in 2007 that estimated millions of adults and children use acupuncture, world organizations have recommended acupuncture as a treatment method [10].

The desire of the patient to pursue treatment using acupuncture is the prime factor in determining whether or not to recommend acupuncture. Although acupuncture or even its placebo (sham acupuncture) makes positive effects for the patients [9], like other therapeutic methods, the effectiveness of acupuncture is associated with the physician or healthcare giver who provides the treatment [4]. From the viewpoint of medical ethics, the primary tenet of medicine is not to harm; nonetheless, acupuncture has very few restrictions. Acupuncture can be used even in high-risk conditions such as pregnancy and pediatrics. Using anticoagulants is not a restriction either [7]. Most acupuncturists avoid acupuncture if there is an active infection or a lesion of cutaneous malignancy due to the threat of the expansion of the infectious area or spread of the malignant cells [11]. Studies showed only two particular contraindications warrant special attention: using acupuncture for patients with an automatic implantable cardioverter-defibrillator (AICD) is not restricted, but they should avoid electrical stimulation, which is a form of performing acupuncture. Furthermore, patients who suffer from or are predisposed to specific psychological diseases such as psychosis or delusions should avoid acupuncture [11]. Contrary to prohibitions and restrictions, acupuncture has been applied for various purposes such as acute and chronic pain and peripartum and chemotherapy-induced nausea [7]. Moreover, pediatric patients increasingly use acupuncture for a variety of diseases such as asthma, post-operative symptoms, nausea and vomiting, pain, cancer complications, and CP [12–14]. According to a United States survey, more than 30% of pediatric pain centers proposed acupuncture in their health care services [15]. Fortunately, acupuncture is well-tolerated by children with a low rate of adverse event incidence [16].

16.2.1 Different Acupuncture Methods

Acupuncture needles are mainly stainless steel, sterile, flexible needles with the long ranging from 0.1 to 10 cm. Shorter needles are needed to penetrate thinner tissues. Usually, the abdomen and back use thick and long needles, and the head and neck and extremities use thin and short needles. Generally, each session involves inserting 5–20 needles at selected acupuncture points that remain for 10–20 min. The patients rest in a supine position, relax, and have a gentle sensation upon insertion of needles with a quick, minimized pain [7, 10].

Since the inception of acupuncture to the present, from its discovery to recent Western acceptance, scientists have progressively integrated the traditional science of acupuncture and the growing evidence to establish new techniques and devices to improve the treatment modalities [9]. Hence, different acupuncture types have been advanced out of the integrative medicine—besides manual pressure or manual acupuncture—including electricity acupuncture (electroacupuncture), laser acupuncture, fire acupuncture, acupoint injection, and acupuncture microsystems. The application of different modalities is in the same way, thought to intervene in the flow of qi in simple needle penetration [6].

Manual acupuncture A guide tube made of plastic might be useful for the placement of very thin needles. The acupuncturist inserts the needle with a quick move at the selected acupoint. Usually, patients feel a sensation of tugging, numbness, or gentle radiculopathy with a radiation within the skin, called de-qi in TCM-while inserting the needle, which is a sign for proper intervention. Needles will remain at the identified point for 10–20 min and might be twisted as a manipulation according to the practitioner's opinion [17].

Electroacupuncture (EA) Electrical stimulation of a certain acupoint consists of passage of an electric current via two needles by an electrical pulse generator that adjusts the stimulus. EA is similar to manual acupuncture in the point selection method; however, EA stimulates a larger area (acu-zone) rather than an acupoint [18].

Laser acupuncture Scientists began to experiment the laser acupuncture in the 1950s, utilizing focused light instead of a needle. Due to the proven safety and efficacy of laser acupuncture, as well as manual acupuncture, it is viable in many medical settings, especially practical pediatric patients who often refuse needles [19].

Acupressure Pressing acupoints by the use of a protruding plastic button or even with a finger can stimulate specific points to increase the qi flow and get similar therapeutic results as manual acupuncture [20].

Fire acupuncture In this therapeutic method, a thick or thin needle will be burned red on a gentle flame and quickly puncture identified points and parts on the body. The fire needle adjusts the immunity of the body and regulates the blood circulation to counter diseases. Fire needle is safe and easy to operate with no side effects and recent clinical studies showed its positive effects in pain management [21].

Acupoint injection This method is derived from the intramuscular injection, a technique that stimulates an acupoint by injecting a liquid agent, mostly herbal extract, to prevent or treat diseases. These liquid agents include different Chinese herbal extracts, Western medicine treatments, vitamins, bee venom, or even normal saline solution. Injecting these agents in certain acupoints causes a synergistic effect on stimulating the acupoint. This modality shows more sustained effects than manual acupuncture and specific systematic effects compared to simple intramuscular injection [22].

Acupuncture microsystems While traditional systemic acupuncture organizes acupoints into linear sequences (meridians), each with specific functions, microsystem acupuncture employs specific patterns of local points on parts of the body—such as the auricle, scalp, or tongue—that reflect the corresponding functions of systemic acupoints [23]. Microsystem points are representative of the systemic point of a corresponding organ and are detectable only when stimulated [24].

- *Scalp acupuncture*: Consists of inserting thin acupuncture needles into head acupoints. Scalp acupuncture minimizes general side effects while maintaining acupuncture effectiveness [25].
- *Tongue acupuncture*: This technique treats health problems by placing an acupuncture needle on the tongue. There is a forty-point tongue map corresponding to various organs of the body [26].
- *Auricular acupuncture*: This method consists of placing the needles in diverse areas on the ear to influence the whole body. TCM postulates that different body organs correlate with the ear; thus, manipulating the ear affects the related part of the body [27].

16.2.2 CP Syndrome Differentiation According to TCM

TCM demonstrates a significant role in the enhancement of the physical function and alleviation of comorbidities of children with CP. According to the Diagnosis and Treatment of Common Pediatric Diseases in TCM 2022 guideline [28], CP has been categorized into five distinct syndrome differentiations: (1) liver and kidney deficiency, (2) heart and spleen deficiency, (3) blood stasis and phlegm accumulation, (4) spleen deficiency with hyperactivity of the liver, and (5) spleen and kidney deficiency. Moreover, this guideline offers treatments of TCM for CP rehabilitation. Recent studies showed that TCM interventions, including oral medications or acupuncture, restore the motor functions, improve the immune function, decrease recurrent infections, enhance digestion and absorption, and alleviate drooling and constipation in pediatric patients with CP. TCM improves their intelligence, memory, speech, muscle spasm, joint range of motion, and activities of daily living (ADL) in children with CP [29].

16.2.3 Experimental Studies

Recent preclinical studies have investigated the therapeutic effects of various acupuncture modalities in animal models of CP, including manual acupuncture and EA applied to both body and scalp regions [25, 30–34] (Table 16.1). The most

Table 16.1 Experimental and clinical studies evaluating the effects of acupuncture on cerebral palsy

Subject/sample size	Age/gender	Intervention method/duration	Acupoints	Control	Outcomes	Adverse effects	References
			Animal studies				
CP rat model/56	7 d/NR	Electroacupuncture of body and scalp	Baihui (GV20) and right Zusanli (ST36), scalp motor area	No treatment, exercise	↑ Rotarod test ↔ Cylinder test, wire hanging grid test ↑ Contralateral subventricular zone, thickness of the corpus callosum, and integrated optical density	NR	[30]
CP rat model/36	7 d/NR	Electroacupuncture/4 day per week, 4 w	Baihui (GV 20) and Zusanli (ST 36)	No treatment, exercise	↑ Motor asymmetry improvement ↔ Lesion size	NR	[31]
CP rat model/50	7 d/male	Electroacupuncture/3 day per week, 3 w	Baihui (GV 20) and Zusanli (ST 36)	No treatment, exercise	↑ Rotarod test (motor function and catwalk test) ↑ Cylinder test and passive avoidance test (memory function) ↑ Corpus callosum thickness	NR	[32]

CP rat model/180	7 d/both	Scalp electroacupuncture/3 treatment course of 7 consecutive days with 2 d interval	3 methods: standard international scheme, Jiaoshi program, and Jin three-needle scheme	No treatment	↑ Motor function ↓ Brain pathologic changes ↑ Nervous system structure ↓ Neuron-specific enolase ↑ ATPase activity	NR	[33]
CP rat model/30	7 d/NR	Scalp acupuncture	Baihui (GV20), Sishencong (EX-HN1), Zhisanzhen, Niesanzhen	Sham acupuncture	↑ Suspension time ↓ Slope experiment ↓ Tactile experiment ↓ Escape latency time ↓ Hippocampal injury	NR	[25]
CP rat model/94	10 d/NR	Electroacupuncture/2 w	Scalp acupoint: motor area	Healthy model	↑ Motor function ↑ Cognition function ↑ Suspension time ↓ Brain damage	NR	[34]

(continued)

Table 16.1 (continued)

Subject/sample size	Age/gender	Intervention method/duration	Acupoints	Control	Outcomes	Adverse effects	References
			Human studies				
Randomized controlled trial on spastic CP children/50	11 m–12 y/both	Scalp, body, and auricular acupuncture/24 w	NR	No treatment	GMFCS: ↑ Function of legs or hands 68% vs. 0% ↑ Sleep quality 53% vs. 0% ↑ Mood 32% vs. 12% ↑ Speech or drooling 37% vs. 6% ↑ Bowel movements 21% vs. 0% ↑ Cognition 21% vs. 0% ↓ Ocular muscle stiffness 61% vs. 39% ↑ Happiness due to vision correction 17% vs. 22%	NR	[37]

Randomized controlled trial on CP children/33	3.52–16.8 y/both	Tongue acupuncture/40 daily sessions, each session 15 s. Cross over after 2 w wash out	Xian You, Di Men, and bilateral Xian Zuo	Sham acupuncture	↑ GMFM, ↑ PEDI (self-care, mobility, and self-care assistance sub scores)	Initial crying, fear, minor pain only in first sessions	[26]
Uncontrolled trial on CP children/140	2 m–14 y/both	Manual body acupuncture in combination with other treatments/1 m	NR	No control group	↑ Motor function, ↑ social adaptation	NR	[38]
Randomized controlled trial on spastic CP children/80	NR	Scalp acupuncture plus exercise/NR	Baihui (GV 20) and Sishencong (EX-HN 1)	Exercise only	↑ GMFM, ↑ WeeFIM, TER: 92.5% vs. 72.5%	NR	[12]
Randomized controlled trial on CP children/116	Mean: 28.5 m/both	Electroacupuncture, tuina, and rehabilitation/5 daily sessions per week for 12 w, crossover after 4 weeks wash out	Different points on scalp, trunk, and limbs	Only rehabilitation	No ↑ risk of seizure frequency	2 new onset seizure	[83]
Randomized controlled trial on CP children with acute diarrhea/60	1–24 m/both	Warming moxibustion/10–15 min twice daily, 6 d	Shenque (RN8)	Diosmectite	After 6 days: TER: 83.3% vs. 80%, ↑ MER After 3 days: ↓ diarrhea arresting time, ↑ stool exam normalization, ↓ rotavirus reversion	NR	[84]

(continued)

Table 16.1 (continued)

Subject/sample size	Age/gender	Intervention method/duration	Acupoints	Control	Outcomes	Adverse effects	References
Randomized controlled trial on spastic CP children/120	NR	Add on manual acupuncture/once daily, 3 m	4 points between Yuzhen (BL 9) and Tianzhu (BL 10)	Rehabilitation training	Marked improvement (44.83% vs. 28.81%) TEF: 91.38% vs. 84.75% ↓ Modified Ashworth scale ↑ GMFM	NR	[13]
Randomized controlled trial on spastic CP children/115	12–72 m/both	Scalp and body, manual and electroacupuncture/5 sessions per week, 12 w, cross over after 4 w interval	NR	Rehabilitation training	↑ GMFM ↑ PEDI selfcare ↑ PEDI mobility ↔ PEDI social ↑ GMFCS	NR	[43]
Randomized controlled trial on CP children/60	2–12 y/both	Scalp acupuncture/9 courses of 10 consecutive days with 2 d interval	Yu's sector Method: parietal region and sub-occipital region	Rehabilitation training	↑ Berg balance ↑ ADL	NR	[39]
Randomized controlled trial on CP children/200	1–7 y/both	Add on manual acupuncture/every 2 d, 3 courses of 10 sessions with 15 d interval	13 points of the governor vessel, Shenshu (BL 23), Taixi (KI 3), Yanglingquan (GB 34), Zusanli (ST 36), Sanyinjiao (SP 6), Shenting (GV 24), Qianding (GV 21), Baihui (GV 20), and Sishencong (Ex-HN 1)	Rehabilitation training	TER: 87% vs. 55% ↑ GMFM ↑ GDS Significant skull CT/MRI improvement	None	[48]

Randomized controlled trial on CP children/74	Mean: 32.5/both	Add on scalp acupuncture	Sishencong (EX-HN 1), scalp motor area, scalp balance area Shenshu (BL 23) Taixi (KI 3), and Zusanli (ST 36)	Rehabilitation training	↑ GMFM ↓ Modified Ashworth scales	None	[85]
Randomized controlled trial on spastic CP children/40	1–4 y/both	Add on laser acupuncture/2 sessions per week for 3 m	Yanglingquan (GB 34), Hegu (LI4), Zhouliao (LI12), Taichong (Liv3)	Physiotherapy	↓ Muscle tone ↑ Wrist ROM ↑ Ankle ROM ↑ ROM total score ↑ GMFM	NR	[19]
Randomized controlled trial on spastic CP children/55	20 m–12 y/both	Scalp, body and auricular acupuncture/weeks 1–4 three times per week, weeks 5–8 twice per week, weeks 9–12 once per week, and weeks 13–24 once every other Week: 30 sessions, 6 m every other week, and weeks 9–24, once every month: 10 sessions, 6 m	NR	Non-therapeutic play time	↑ GMFM ↑ WeeFIM mobility domain	NR	[77]

(continued)

Table 16.1 (continued)

Subject/sample size	Age/gender	Intervention method/duration	Acupoints	Control	Outcomes	Adverse effects	References
Uncontrolled trial on CP children/36	NR/both	Scalp acupuncture and auricular acupuncture/3–20 sessions	Foot motor and sensory area, motor area, speech I area, speech II area, balance area, vision area, apraxia area, and I vision area	No control group	TER: 91.7% 33.9% completely recovered, 38.9% marked improvement, 38.9% some effect, 8.3% no effect	NR	[27]
Randomized controlled trial on spastic CP children/52	15–75 m/both	Scalp acupuncture plus exercise/5 days per week, 3 m	Motor area, balance zone, foot motor sensory area, sensory area, and language area	Rehabilitation training	↑ GMFM ↑ ADL	NR	[86]

Non-randomized controlled trial on CP children/423	NR/both	Injection at acupoints/10 sessions once every 2 d	Sishencong (EX-HN 1), Baihui (GV 20), Neiguan (PC 6), Quchi (LI 11), Jianzhen (SI 9), Naoshu (SI 10), Tianzong (SI 11), Xiaohai (SI 8), Shouwuli (LI 13), Jianyu (LI 15), Jianliao (TE 14), Naohui (TE 13), Waiguan (TE 5), Tianfu (LU 3), Chize (LU 5), Hegu (LI 4), Zuwuli (LR 10), Yinbao (LR 9), Huantiao (GB 30), Xuanzhong (GB 39), Fengshi (GB 31), Xuehai (SP 10), Ququan (LR 8), Weizhong (BL 40), Zusanli (ST 36), Fenglong (ST 40), Chengshan (BL 57), Shenmai (BL 62), Taichong (LR 3), Shenshu (BL 23), Pishu (BL 20), and Weishu (BL 21)	Injection at non-acupoints: vitamin B1, vitamin B12, monosialotetrahexose ganglioside sodium, Xingnaojing	↑ GMFM ↑ FMFM	NR	[87]

(continued)

Table 16.1 (continued)

Subject/sample size	Age/gender	Intervention method/duration	Acupoints	Control	Outcomes	Adverse effects	References
Non-randomized controlled trial on spastic CP children/113	Mean: 3.65 y/both	Add on manual body and scalp acupuncture/NR	Conception vessel, governor vessel, hand-Yangming, hand-Jueyin, foot-Yangming, foot-taiyin, and scalp acupoints: motor area, balance area, sensory area, tremor-control area, foot motor-sensory area, vision area, speech area (II and III), Baihui, and Sishencong	Rehabilitation training	↑ TER ↓ PDMS ↓ Ashworth scale ↑ GMFM ↑ Barthel index ↑ GDS ↓ IL-6, TNF-α	NR	[16]
Randomized controlled trial on spastic CP children/25	Mean: 66.85 m/both	Wrist-ankle manual acupuncture/5 days a week, for 4 weeks	Professor Zhang acupoints: upper 4, upper 5, lower 1, and lower 4	Transcranial magnetic stimulation	↑ GMFM ↓ Motor evoked potential latency ↔ Motor evoked potential amplitude and duration	NR	[49]
Randomized controlled trial on spastic hemiplegic CP children/90	Mean: 9.87 y/both	Add on manual acupuncture/first 2 weeks: 5 d per week, next 2 weeks: 3 days per week, next 2 weeks: 2 days per week, next 2 weeks: 1 day per week	Baxie (EX-UE9), Hegu (LI4), Houx (SI3), Shousanli (LI10), and Quchi (LI11)	Occupational therapy plus sham acupuncture	↓ NCCPC-R ↑ Squeeze dynamometry ↑ Manual muscle test ↔ Modified Ashworth scale ↑ Box and block test	None	[88]

Non-randomized controlled trial on spastic CP children/168	Mean: 7.56 y/both	Manual acupuncture/12 w, 5 sessions per week	Scalp acupoints: motor area, foot movement sensation area, and balance area. Body acupoints: Ganshu (BL18), Pishu (BL20), Taichong (LR3), Taibai (SP3), Yanglingquan (GB34), and Sanyinjiao (SP6)	Rehabilitation training	↓ Modified Ashworth scale ↑ GMFM ↑ 6MWD ↑ WeeFIM	None	[44]
Case report on CP child/1	6 m/male	Manual acupuncture/3 courses of 10 consecutive sessions with 1 m interval	Scalp acupoints: Shenting (GV24), Benshen (GB13), Sishencong (EX-HN1), motor area, foot-motor sensory area, second speech area, and balance area Body acupoints: Jiaji (EX-B2), Juliao (GB29), Huantiao (GB30), Chengfu (BL36), and Zhibian (BL54)	None	↑ Responsiveness ↑ Motor functions ↓ Brain injury	NR	[42]

↑ increased/improved significantly, ↓ decreased significantly, ↔ no significant change, *GMFM* gross motor function measure, *GMFCS* Gross Motor Functional Classification System, *m* month, *w* week, *y* year, *d* day, *NR* not reported, *PEDI* Pediatric Evaluation of Disability Index, *TER* total effective rate, *WeeFIM* Pediatric Functional Independence Measure, *fMRI* functional magnetic resonance imaging, *MER* markedly effective rate, *ADL* activity of daily living, *FMFM* Fine Motor Function Measure, *IL-6* interleukin 6, *TNF-α* tumor necrosis factor alpha, *PDMS* Peabody Developmental Motor Scale, *GDS* Gesell's Developmental Schedule, *ATPase* adenosine triphosphatase, *NCCPC-R* non-communicating children's pain checklist-revised scale, *6MWD* 6-minute walking distance measurement, *ROM* range of motion commonly used acupoints included Baihui (GV20), Zusanli (ST36), and scalp motor area, besides Sishencong (EX-HN1), Zhisanzhen, and Niesanzhen as extra acupoints. The effects of acupuncture were compared to exercise or sham acupuncture, and outcomes were assessed using rotarod test, cylinder test, wire hanging grid test, catwalk test, passive avoidance test, and pathological studies.

A study by Kim et al. showed EA enhanced the locomotor performance of rats during rotarod test and the function of contralateral subventricular zone (SVZ) after hypoxia-ischemia, as well as behavioral recovery and neurogenesis [30]. EA improved the motor coordination and memory by modulating the myelin component and proliferation and differentiation of neuronal progenitor cells through overexpression of key proteins in neuron generation [30]. Another study by Kim et al. on rats showed significant improvements in neuronal markers and astrocyte markers, as well as motor asymmetry recovery following EA. EA reduced the cleaved caspase-3, a brain injury marker, explaining the cause of neuron apoptosis inhibition, despite no change in lesion size [31]. Similar to previous studies, Pak et al. revealed that EA of Baihui (GV 20) and Zusanli (ST 36) acupoints significantly alleviated motor and cognition dysfunctions (in cylinder, rotarod, and catwalk tests) and restored structural changes in corpus callosum and oligodendrogenesis via activating cAMP response element binding protein [32]. Myelin components in the white matter are generated by myelin-forming mature oligodendrocytes, which can be differentiated with the help of EA [31].

The brain microenvironment of neurons during brain development and the synaptic growth of the cell body are the key to nerve regeneration and functional reconstruction. Moreover, nerve cell growth factors, nerve growth-associated protein, and neurotransmitters are important components of the brain microenvironment, which are the key to nerve regeneration and functional reconstruction [35]. For instance, neuron-specific enolase (NSE) expression is positively correlated with the severity of brain tissue injury, and ATPase has important effects on nerve cell proliferation, cell differentiation, providing the energy needed to maintain ion gradients both inside and outside the nerve cells, synthetic metabolism, neurotransmitter release and uptake, transport between neuronal cell bodies and axons, cell membrane integrity, and information transfer [36]. Wang et al. performed specific methods (Jiaoshi or Jin three-needle methods) of scalp EA in CP rat models. They showed that scalp EA can significantly improve the motor function and recover nervous system pathological changes and modulate the level of ATPase and NSE [33]. Not only the stimulation of famous acupoints (e.g., GV20 and ST36) show the abovementioned effects, but also extra acupoints such as Zhisanzhen and Niesanzhen affect hippocampal injury and improve the sensory-motor functions and cognition (e.g., in increasing suspension time and decreasing slope experiment, tactile experiment, and scape latency time) [25]. Wu et al. compared the effects of EA on CP and healthy rat pups. After a single EA treatment session, an increase of 20.48% in left cerebral cortical blood flow was observed compared to post-ischemic levels. In contrast, CP group, which was left untreated, exhibited sparse and disordered cortical cell arrangement, reduced cell bodies, and evidence of nuclear fragmentation. These pathological symptoms were significantly alleviated in the EA-treated group. Consequently, rats that received EA exhibited better results in gait analysis and maze experiments [34].

16.2.4 Human Studies

In addition to preclinical studies, numerous human studies—including randomized controlled trials and case reports—have evaluated acupuncture in children with CP aged 2 months to 16 years (Table 16.1). Rather than initial crying, minor pain, or fear, especially in the first session, no serious side effects were reported. Most of the treatment protocols employed body acupuncture and several studies investigated microsystems, including tongue acupuncture, scalp acupuncture, and auricular acupuncture. Patients received a variety of acupuncture modalities such as manual acupuncture, electroacupuncture, laser acupuncture, and acupoint injection. The most commonly used acupoints in body acupuncture were included Sishencong (EX-HN 1), Baihui (GV20), Shenshu (BL23), Yanglingquan (GB34), Zusanli (ST36), Hegu (LI4), Taichong (LR3), Taixi (KI3), Sanyinjiao (SP6), Shenting (GV24), Quchi (LI11), Huantiao (GB30), and Pishu (BL20).

Duncan et al. investigated the effects of manual acupuncture on pediatric CP with spasticity. They showed that manual acupuncture of the scalp, body, and ear can significantly improve the function of hands and legs. Also, acupuncture enhanced nervous system activity such as sleep quality, mood, speech, drooling, cognition, bowel movements, and ocular muscle stiffness. They reported that patients were happy due to the correction of vision [37]. Parents of children with CP were also satisfied with outcomes such as the running and jumping of the children, enough sleep, increased vocabulary, no need for oxygen supplementation during winter, and elimination of toe walking after receiving acupuncture [37]. Acupuncture can significantly improve social adaptation, as well as motor function [38]. Study of Wang et al. showed that adding acupuncture to rehabilitation treatment results in higher "marked improvement" score and total effective rate and improved Ashworth scale and gross motor function measure (GMFM) score [13]. Scalp acupuncture significantly enhances the ADL score and Berg balance score in children with CP compared to rehabilitation treatment [39]. Neuroplasticity is the ability of the brain to adjust its structure and improve its function in response to body alterations or changes in the external environment. Neuroplasticity is one of the essential mechanisms that occur in the brain that recovers motor function after injuries [40]. Astrocytes and microglia are two cell types that are manipulated by acupuncture to regulate neuroplasticity. Acupuncture stimulates these cells to produce and release various factors with neurotrophic functions, such as brain-derived neurotrophic factor (BDNF) and nerve growth factor (NGF) [41]. Hence, as reported in a case study by Zhixiong et al., manual acupuncture can improve the motor function via alleviating the brain injury [42].

Two studies evaluated the effects of tongue acupuncture and electroacupuncture on the pediatric evaluation of disability index (PEDI) of pediatric patients with CP. While tongue acupuncture was superior to sham acupuncture in improvement of PEDI subscales (self-care, mobility, and self-care assistance) [26], electroacupuncture of the body plus scalp manual acupuncture showed significant improvements only in self-care and mobility subscales compared to rehabilitation training [43]. Furthermore, two studies assessed the effects of scalp acupuncture on the pediatric functional independence measure (WeeFIM) [12, 44]. Wang et al. showed significant effects of acupuncture compared to rehabilitation training in decreasing modified Ashworth scale, WeeFIM scale, 6-min walking distance measurement, and GMFM [44]. Adding scalp acupuncture to exercise remarkably improved the total effective rate from 72.5% to 92.5%, which means a significant improvement in motor functions [12]. They showed that acupuncture is an effective method to reduce muscle tone in spastic muscle groups, improve joint mobility, and enhance gross motor function and walking ability in children with CP [12].

Laser acupuncture can reduce the muscle tone and improve the GMFM score, total score of range of motion (ROM), and specific ROM of wrist and ankle in spastic CP [19]. Core symptoms identified for spastic CP encompassed "Motor Dysfunction", "Impaired Speech", "Delayed Development", "Limb Stiffness", "Rigidity in the limbs", "Intellectual Impairment", "Timidity and susceptibility to startle responses", "Muscle Wasting", and "Pale or Dull Complexion". The clinical manifestations of spastic CP are essentially consistent with the TCM pattern "liver exuberance and spleen weakness" [45]. Accordingly, selected acupoints used in the study of Wang et al. have been shown to regulate muscle contracture, muscle weakness, posture abnormalities, and stimulate brain electrical activity. Additionally, they increase the secretion of neurotransmitters and improve blood circulation in brain tissue, thereby improving clinical efficacy [44]. Acupuncture can promote the activation of the motor cortex and repair damage, effectively relieving muscle spasms in the limbs and improving the function of the gross motor nerve [46]. Acupuncture can promote the activation of deep spinal stabilizing muscles, increase muscle strength, and improve movement control so that children can obtain more muscle strength and exercise opportunities for limb movement control required for effective movement; thus, improving the movement function of the trunk and lower limbs of the children to a greater extent, improving their gross motor function, further improving the static and dynamic balance ability of sitting and standing, and improving their walking ability [47].

Computed tomography (CT) and magnetic resonance imaging (MRI) encephalopathic manifestations of pediatric CP include periventricular leukomalacia, leukodystrophy, or the brain's frontal and temporal lobe cortex dysplasia with periventricular leukomalacia and leukodystrophy. A study by Liu et al. showed significant amelioration of imaging findings post-acupuncture treatment, compared to rehabilitation training aligns with clinical findings, such as improvement of GMFM and Gessel developmental scale [48]. In addition, Li et al. investigated the effects of acupuncture on corticospinal tract conductivity by detecting the electrophysiological indices such as motor evoked potential latency, amplitude of motor evoked potential, and motor evoked potential duration. The corticospinal tract is the descending nerve conduction tract that controls the voluntary movement of skeletal muscles and the development of pyramidal tracts in bilateral cerebral hemispheres of children with CP is slower than that of normal children. They showed that it plays a certain role and significance in improving neurophysiological function [49]. Moreover, as inflammatory factors often lead to abnormal blood-brain barrier function and brain damage in patients with CP, recent studies showed that acupuncture can reduce the serum level of interleukin 6 (IL-6) and tumor necrosis factor (TNF)-α to enhance cerebral microcirculation to alleviate the brain damage [16].

Conclusively, acupuncture modulates the post-ischemic brain functional reconstruction, leading to enhancement of the brain's neuroplasticity. Hence, the enhanced neuroplasticity has become a goal to integrate acupuncture in the treatment plan of patients with neurological deficits, such as CP, and a new target of research to investigate the corresponding mechanisms for these actions. Neuroplasticity and the brain's capacity to compensate the neurological deficits are highest in pediatrics, and early intervention is essential to recover neurological functions in children with CP. Clinical and experimental evidence has documented the potential of acupuncture to ameliorate neurological deficits, particularly motor function impairment, spasticity, and cognitive impairment. These effects are related to the ability of acupuncture to promote spontaneous neuroplasticity after brain injury. Specifically, acupuncture can stimulate neurogenesis, activate axonal regeneration and sprouting, and improve the structure and function of synapses. These processes modify the neural network and function of the damaged brain area, producing the improvement of various skills and adaptability. These findings suggest that acupuncture can be used alongside conventional treatments for the alleviation of CP symptoms.

16.3 Role of Massage in CP

Massage therapy is highly effective in comprehensive treatments, whether as a preventive measure or as a rehabilitative practice. This method helps reduce stress, relieve pain, and increase blood circulation, all of which support the body's natural healing ability. Beyond physical benefits, massage can also improve mental health by reducing anxiety and creating a sense of calm. In conventional medicine, physiotherapy and rehabilitation often utilize massage to relax muscles, reduce edema, and improve mobility in patients with musculoskeletal issues such as back pain, sports injuries, and post-surgical recovery. Neural therapeutic approaches, like neurorehabilitation, use massage to enhance nerve function and reduce symptoms such as muscle spasms or weakness after a stroke or nerve injuries [50].

Different medical schools consider massage for addressing various health conditions, especially those involving the musculoskeletal, nervous, and brain systems. TCM employs techniques like Tui Na, which work on energy channels to restore balance and facilitate healing. Similarly, Ayurveda uses Abhyanga, an oil massage that balances doshas and promotes physical and mental well-being. Another significant advancement is the integration of massage into complementary and alternative medicine, where it is used to manage symptoms of neurological disorders and enhance nerve function, such as in Parkinson's disease, depression, and cerebral palsy [51, 52].

Massage is also one of the complementary methods for improving the quality of life in individuals with conditions like CP. Its positive effects include reducing muscle tension, improving blood circulation, increasing flexibility, and decreasing muscular pain. This can help individuals move more easily and perform body rotations better, sometimes leading to reduced spasticity and improved movement control. Additionally, massage can have a positive impact on patients' mood and psychological stress, increasing feelings of relaxation and comfort [53].

Utilizing massage as part of a comprehensive treatment plan can play an important role in enhancing the quality of life for these patients.

16.3.1 Experimental Studies

There are some preclinical investigations evaluating the effect of massage in CP (Table 16.2). In an animal study conducted on a rat model of CP, 18 rats were examined 5 days after birth. The rats were divided into two groups of nine: intervention and control. In this model, the massage steps include rubbing the spine and both sides of the spine for 1 min, pressing and kneading the spine for 5 min, and the muscles on both sides of the spine for 5 min, pressing and kneading the sensitive local acupoints in the spine for 2 min twisting for 1 min, rubbing midline from the forehead to the back of the brain for 1 min. This intervention was carried out for 6 days, with a one-day break between massage sessions. In total, the animals received therapeutic massages for 61 days. The therapeutic effect at the end of the intervention was determined as an increase in balance, motor function, growth and development, growth hormone levels, and temperature of sensitive areas of the back in the intervention group compared to the control group [50].

In another study conducted on 7-day-old young rats, 18 rats received a massage of specific areas related to TCM meridian points and pathways until the 40th day after birth. The treatment protocol in this study was as follows: First, massage of the four limb acupoints, including Quchi (LI11) and Zusanli (ST36); second, massage of the abdomen acupoints Zhongwan (RN12), Tianshu (ST25), Guanyuan (CV4), and Qihai (CV6); and finally, massage of the abdomen of the rats. The treatment results showed that massage, in addition to reducing the number of hind limb slips, can increase motor function, as well as growth and development [53].

In a study conducted on a group of 3-day-old young rats, 30 male rats were examined. In this study, the rats received a special massage on different areas of the body and corresponding to some acupuncture points. This massage included rubbing the middle of the spine, on both sides of the spine along the bladder meridian, the heads and limbs once a day from P7 to P49 and lasted for approximately 20 min each time. The results of the study showed that performing these massage movements can lead to increased motor function, learning, and memory, and on the other hand, reduce the expression of NLRP3 in the hippocampus [51].

Table 16.2 Studies evaluating the effect of massage in cerebral palsy

Subject, sample size	Age	Intervention method/duration	Control	Outcomes	Adverse effects	References
		Animal studies				
18 infant rats	5 days after birth	Rubbing the spine and both sides of the spine for 1 min. Pressing and kneading the spine for 5 min, and the muscles on both sides of the spine for 5 min pressing and kneading the sensitive local acupoints in the spine for 2 min twisting for 1 min. Rubbing midline from the forehead to the back of the brain for 1 min intervention for 6 days, then 1 day rest for 61 days		↑ Weight gain, ↑ Balance ability ↑ Motor function, ↑ Growth and development ↑ GH ↑ Temperature of sensitive parts of the back	–	[50]
18 young rats	7 days after birth	First, massage of four limb acupoints, including Quchi (LI11) and Zusanli (ST36); second, massage of the abdomen acupoints Zhongwan (RN12), Tianshu (ST25), Guanyuan (CV4), and Qihai (CV6); and finally, massage of the abdomen of the rats until 40th day	–	↑ Motor function ↑ Growth and development ↓ The number of hind limb slips	–	[53]
30 male rat pups	3 days after birth	Rubbing the middle of the spine, on both sides of the spine along the bladder meridian, the heads and limbs once a day from P7 to P49 and lasted for approximately 20 min each time	–	↑ Body weight ↑ Motor performance ↑ Learning and memory ↓ Expression of NLRP3 in the hippocampi	–	[51]

(continued)

Table 16.2 (continued)

Subject, sample size	Age	Intervention method/duration	Control	Outcomes	Adverse effects	References
11 male rats	Neonatal	Tuina treatment p4–p31	–	↑ Weight loss ↓ Weakness of limb strength ↓ Disorders of neurological reflexes ↑ Learning ↑ Memory functions ↑ 5 hmC and Tet2 levels in the cerebral temporal cortex	–	[52]
		Human studies				
40 children with CP	1–7 years	Single-blind clinical trial Swedish massage for 30 min, 3 times a week for 3 months + routine occupational therapy (Rood and Bobath techniques) for 3 months Assessed before treatment and about 3 months later (1 week after the last massage therapy session)	Routine occupational therapy (Rood and Bobat techniques) for 3 months	↑ Tonicity in upper limbs and trunk	–	[54]
40 children with CP	1–7 years	Single-blind clinical trial Swedish massage for 30 min before every OT session evaluated at the beginning of the study and 3 months later	–	No significant effects	–	[55]

113 children with CP	1–5 years	Single-blind clinical trial Acupuncture + Massage therapy governor vessel, bladder meridian and large intestine meridian as main meridians. Massage techniques, such as rolling, kneading, patting and pushing d 5 times per week, 1 time/d, 20 min/time, for three consecutive months	Bobath's exercise therapy, twice a day, 30 min/time, for three consecutive months baclofen tablets (2.5 mg/time, 4 times/d) and intravenous injection of ganglioside (20 mg/time) containing glucose injection at 0.05 g/mL or sodium chloride injection	↑ Effective rate ↓ IL-6 ↓ TNF-α	–	[16]
168 children with CP	2–7 years	Non-randomized clinical trial Acupuncture + Tuina along meridians, acupoint pressure, abnormal local muscle tuina, and abnormal posture correction Once a day, 20–30 min each time	–	↓ MAS ↑ GMFM ↑ 6MWD ↑ WeeFIM	–	[44]
115 children with CP	1 month –13 years	Single-blind clinical trial PT and conventional rehabilitation (3 months)	Conventional rehabilitation	↑ Motor function	–	[56]
70 children with CP	2–5 years	Single-blind clinical trial Once a day, 6 times a week, 3 courses (Spleen-invigorating and qi-benefiting pediatric massage) Kai-opening Tianmen (3–6 times or 3–5 min) Tui-pushing Kangong (30–50 times) EX-HN 5 (30–50 times) Rou-kneading Erhougaogu (30–50 times) GB 20 (100 times) BL 13 (until hot) Fen-parting hand yin-yang (100–300 times) from Xiaotianxin to the lateral sides of the hand for 100–300 times Flexed the child's thumb Bu-reinforcing Feijing (100–500 times) Bu-reinforcing Shenjing (100–500 times)	Conventional rehabilitation	↑ Serum IgG, IgA, IgM ↓ Recurrent respiratory tract infection ↑ Immune function	–	[57]

(continued)

Table 16.2 (continued)

Subject, sample size	Age	Intervention method/duration	Control	Outcomes	Adverse effects	References
40 children with CP	3–15 years	Single-blind clinical trial Neurodevelopmental treatment (45–60 min) + reflexology to the sole of the foot (caterpillar, birds' beak, tornado, butterfly, hooking, tearing), twice a week, 20 min, 8 weeks	Neurodevelopmental treatment (45–60 min)	↔ GMFM ↓ Constipation	–	[58]
264 children with CP	2 months –14 years	Single-blind clinical trial Acupuncture + Moment massage 2 months	Acupuncture	↑ DQ ↑ Effective rate	–	[59]

IL-6 Interleukin-6, *TNF-α* tumor necrosis factor-α, *GH* growth hormone, *MAS* Modified Ashworth Muscle Tension Scale, *GMFM-88* The Gross Motor Function Test, *6MWD* The 6-Minute Walking Distance Measurement, *WeeFIM* Children's Functional Independence Rating Scale, *P7–49* Postnatal day7–49, *NLRP3* NACHT, LRR and PYD domains-containing protein 3, *5-hmC* 5-methylcytosine, *Tet* ten-eleven translocation, *PT* Pediatric Tuina, *EX-HN 5* Rou-kneading Taiyang, *GB 20* Rou-kneading Fengchi, *BL 13* Ca-scrubbing Feishu, *MCRT* Combined microcurrent reflexotherapy, *DQ* development quotient

Another study on 11 neonatal male rats, which was accompanied only by Tuina massage at points p4–p31 in the intervention group, showed that this type of treatment can help weight loss, learning, memory functions, 5 hmC and Tet2 levels in the cerebral temporal cortex. The treatment results also showed a reduction in weakness of limb strength disorders of neurological reflexes in this intervention [52].

16.3.2 Human Studies

There are also clinical studies on the effect of massage on patients—mostly children—with CP. In a single-blind clinical trial conducted on 40 children with CP aged 1–7 years, the intervention group received Swedish massage for 30 min, 3 times a week for 3 months in addition to routine occupational therapy (Rood and Bobat techniques). Patients were assessed before treatment and about 3 months later (1 week after the last massage therapy session). The results of this study showed that receiving a massage intervention can increase tonicity in upper limbs and trunk [54]. However, a similar study with the same protocol by the same team in 2007 did not show any specific therapeutic effects [55].

In a single-blind clinical trial conducted on 115 children with CP aged 1–5 years, subjects were divided into two control and intervention groups. Both groups received initial treatments including Bobbett exercise therapy (twice a day, 30 min per session, for three consecutive months), baclofen tablets (2.5 mg per session, 4 times a day), and intravenous ganglioside injection (20 mg per session) containing glucose at a rate of 0.05 g/mL or sodium chloride injection. The intervention group also received acupuncture and special massages on the governor vessel, bladder meridian, and colon meridian as the main meridians. Massage techniques, such as rolling, kneading, tapping, and pressing, were performed 5 times a week, once a day, 20 min each time, for three consecutive months. The treatment results showed that the effective rate was increased; while the levels of IL-6 and TNF-α were decreased in the group receiving massage [16].

In a non-randomized clinical trial conducted on 168 children aged 2–7 years with CP, the intervention group received, in addition to acupuncture, Tuina massage along the meridians, pressure on acupuncture points, local Tuina massage of abnormal muscles, and correction of abnormal body posture. This therapeutic intervention was performed once a day, each time for 20–30 min. The treatment results showed a decrease in the Modified Ashworth Muscle Tension Scale and an increase in the GMFM, 6MWD, and WeeFIM factors [44].

Another study, conducted as a single-blind clinical trial on 113 children with CP, also examined the effects of Tuina massage on children. In this study, children with CP aged between 1 month and 13 years were enrolled in the study and divided into two intervention and control groups. The intervention group received pediatric Tuina for 3 months in addition to conventional rehabilitation. This massage resulted in a significant increase in motor function in the intervention group compared to the control group [56].

In another clinical trial, 70 children with CP, aged 2–5 years, were divided into two groups. The control group received only conventional rehabilitation treatments. The intervention group received specific instruction for massage once a day, six times a week for three courses. The massage program in this group was as follows: Spleen-invigorating and qi-benefiting pediatric massage, known as Kai-opening Tianmen (3–6 times or 3–5 min), Tui-pushing Kangong (30–50 times), EX-HN 5 (30–50 times), Rou-kneading Erhougaogu (30–50 times), GB 20 (100 times), BL 13 (until hot), Fen-parting hand yin-yang (100–300 times), from Xiaotianxin to the lateral sides of the hand for 100–300 times, Flexed the child's thumb:Bu-reinforcing Feijing (100–500 times), and Bu-reinforcing Shenjing (100–500 times). The results of this study showed that the intervention, in addition to reducing recurrent respiratory tract infection in children with CP, could increase serum IgG, IgA, IgM, and their immune function [57].

In another clinical trial, 40 children aged 3–15 years with CP were divided into two groups. Both groups received neurodevelopmental treatment for 45–60 min a day for 8 weeks as baseline treatment. The intervention group also received reflexology to the sole of the foot (caterpillar, birds' beak, tornado, butterfly, hooking, tearing), twice a week, 20 min each time. The study showed that despite no change in GMFM, constipation in patients in the intervention group was significantly reduced [58].

Studies show that combining massage with acupuncture can also have more promising therapeutic effects for patients with CP. In this regard, a study was conducted with a sample size of 264 children with CP who were between the ages of 2 months and 14 years. In this study, the intervention group, in addition to receiving acupuncture, received Moment massages for 2 months. This intervention increased the development quotient and effective rate of the group receiving acupuncture with massage [59].

In sum, clinical trials showcased various massage techniques that significantly improved motor functions, muscle tonicity, and overall development in children with CP when compared to control groups. Notably, interventions combined with acupuncture yielded even better results. In vivo studies using rat models demonstrated positive effects of targeted massage on balance and motor skills, suggesting potential mechanisms that may be effective in human subjects. Overall, these findings highlight the promising role of massage therapy as an integrative approach for enhancing motor abilities and overall well-being in children with CP.

16.4 Role of Herbal Medicine in CP

There is a rising tendency toward the application of herbal medicine for the prevention and treatment of diseases. This application should be rather evidence-based or evidence-informed. In case of CP, the body of evidence is thin, and the number of qualified studies is not sufficient (Table 16.3). In this part, an attempt was made to review the collected literature with the proper level of evidence. As an example, a recent study has been performed on the *Pistacia atlantica* Desf. leaf extract

Table 16.3 Herbal Medicine interventions in cerebral palsy

Subject, sample size	Age, sex	Plant, part/ phytochemical/ formulation	Model/Study design	Control	Dose, duration	Outcomes	Adverse effects	References
Wistar rats 8 pregnant rats (No. of neonatal NS)	Pregnant rats (NS, female) neonatal rats (day 0–45), mixed sex	*Pistacia atlantica* Desf. Methanolic extract (MEPaL) of the leaves	Hypoxia-induced CP	Saline	100 mg/kg & 150 mg/kg, i.p. 21 days, P.N. Outcomes measured up to day 45	↑ Motor activity Balance GSH TAC ↓ ALB NO GSSG TOC OSI	NS	[60]
Sprague-Dawley rats/10 pregnant rats, 40 neonatal	Neonates (day 15–40), equally mixed sex	Baimai ointment	Prenatal: LPS exposure Postnatal hypoxia-ischemia -induced CP	Saline (healthy rats) Placebo ointments (CP rats)	1.5 mL/day, topical, day 7–40 (33 days)	↑ Motor function Movement distance Movement velocity Rotarod retention time Histone H3.3/H4 Astrocyte activity Neurotrophic factors ↓ Peripherin/PKC delta. IL-1α TNF-α IFN-γ	NS	[61]

(continued)

Table 16.3 (continued)

Subject, sample size	Age, sex	Plant, part/ phytochemical/ formulation	Model/Study design	Control	Dose, duration	Outcomes	Adverse effects	References
Male Swiss white mice, 45	NS, male	*Costus afer* Ker Gawl., aqueous extract of stem	Ethanol-induced neurodegeneration	Distilled water (vehicle control) Ethanol (5 g/kg, memory-impaired group)	100 mg/kg, 200 mg/kg, 500 mg/kg, 28 days	↑ Spontaneous alternation in T-maze SOD ↓ Oxidative stress MDA NO_2 TNF-α IL-6	NS	[62]

Male Sprague-Dawley rats, 26	7-day-old, male	Tanshinone IIA from *Salvia miltiorrhiza* Bunge	Spastic CP (induced by carotid artery ligation)	Saline	20 mg/kg, 35 days	↑ Holding time Number of repetitions in holding tests nNOS expression VEGF expression ↓ Time spent searching Number of mistakes in radial arm water maze TNF-α IL-1β IL-6 MCP-1 COX-2 iNOS expression NF-κB p-p38MAPK ↔ Neuronal integrity in brain tissue	NS	[63]
Children with CP, 140	2 months–14 years, male (65.7%), female (34.3%)	Chinese medicine herbs, NS	Retrospective clinical case series	–	–, 6 months, 10 sessions each	↑ Motor capacity Social adaptation	NS	[38]

Abbreviations: *ALB* anxiety-like behaviors, *CP* cerebral palsy, *GSH* glutathione, *GSSG* glutathione disulfide, *i.p.* intraperitoneal injection, *LPS* lipopolysaccharide, *MDA* malondialdehyde, *NO* nitric oxide, NO_2 nitrite, *NS* not specified, *OSI* oxidative stress index, *P.N.* postnatal, *SOD* superoxide dismutase, *TAC* total antioxidant capacity, *TOC* total oxidant capacity

(MEPaL) to understand whether it can ameliorate signs of motor dysfunction in a prenatal model of hypoxia, induced by 7% O_2 for 3 h in pregnant rats. The offspring displayed obvious signs of neural damage by impairing locomotor activity, imbalance, and anxiousness. The main cause of this damage was attributed to oxidative stress due to reactive oxygen species (ROS). The administration of 100 mg/kg and 150 mg/kg of MEPaL could decrease the levels of oxidative stress biomarkers, including nitric oxide (NO), and oxidative stress index (OSI), and lead to an increase in antioxidant capacity markers, such as total antioxidant capacity (TAC), glutathione disulfide (GSSG), and GSH. Considering open-field and rotarod tests for anxiety and balance, MEPaL could significantly reduce anxiety and improve motor coordination and balance vs. negative control group. MEPaL's high content of antioxidant phytochemicals, such as α-pinene and polyphenol substances, is perceived to be the main actor in reducing ROS-activated damages, especially in the striatum and cerebellum [60]. In another study, the proteomic disturbance with induction of CP by 200 μg/kg lipopolysaccharide (LPS) and hypoxia-ischemia, was examined. Baimai ointment was topically applied on the dorsal skin of the CP rats from day 7 to 40. To evaluate the motor function, open-field and rotarod tests were performed. After the treatment trial, both the proteome status and behavioral tests were observed. In the group treated with Baimai ointment, the disturbed proteomes of the hippocampus and motor cortex were significantly restored, and the neuroinflammatory biomarkers such as TNF-α and IL-1α, as well as mitogen-activated protein kinases (MAPKs), were suppressed [61]. The role of the motor cortex and hippocampus in the development of CP is significant; therefore, in 2024, Odey et al. examined the aqueous extract *Costus afer* Ker Gawl. stems in an ethanol-induced model of neural degeneration, in which the damage was exerted in the hippocampus, cerebellum, and prefrontal cortex of mice. Ethanol damaged spatial memory by oxidative stress induced by ROS. Administration of 100, 200, and 500 mg/kg of *C. afer* extract diminished oxidative stress markers such as nitrite, malondialdehyde (MDA), TNF-α, and IL-6. It also raised the level of superoxide dismutase (SOD) back to normal. The scores in the T-maze spontaneous alternation test were also improved [62].

In a model of spastic CP, active ingredient of *Salvia miltiorrhiza* Bunge, tanshinone IIA, was tested to understand whether it can ameliorate motor and cognition impairment. Zhang et al. performed a carotid artery ligation for the induction of CP in neonatal rats. It was observed that tanshinone IIA could improve both scores of holding and water maze, and suppress inflammatory factors and pathways, namely, COX-2, iNOS, TNF-α, IL-1β, IL-6, phosphorylated (p-) nuclear factor (NF-κB), and vascular endothelial growth factor (VEGF). These results show anti-inflammatory, antioxidant, and pro-angiogenic properties of tanshinone IIA [63].

Very few clinical studies have considered herbal medicine for the management of CP in children. One of these studies was performed in 2005 by Zhou et al. In this case series, 140 children with CP who were introduced to the children's hospital of Zhejiang University, China, from 1991 to 1998, were monitored. They underwent TCM methods for the amelioration of the motor dysfunction. Later on, rehabilitation methods, along with massage, orthopedic hand manipulation, auricular seed pressure, massage, occupational therapy, language therapy, and physiotherapy, were added. During a six-month course of treatment, 139 patients showed improvement in motor function. Social adaptability, which is challenging in children with CP, was also ameliorated in 133 patients. In this case, it seems that the combination of herbal medicines, with their anti-inflammatory properties and acupuncture's neurotransmitter-stimulating effects, helped the patients. Also, occupational and language therapy could boost their everyday skills and communication [38].

Although most of the mentioned studies were in preclinical stages, herbal medicine can be offered as a complementary therapy to improve neuro-muscular activities, affecting both peripheral neurons and the central nervous system.

16.5 Other CAM Interventions in CP

Other CAM therapeutic methods have been represented in Table 16.4.

16.5.1 Ayurveda

Ayurveda, a traditional Indian medicinal system, is one of the most ancient traditional medical schools with specific philosophical and experimental foundations. Ayurveda offers a holistic approach, as a complete medical system, and personalized medicine that comprises all psychophysical, philosophico-spiritual, and ethical health. From the viewpoint of Ayurveda, each cell inheres and expresses pure intelligence, the so-called self-healing capacity [64]. Matter of anything in the universe is believed to be composed of five fundamental elements (called *Mahabhutas*), which contain the properties of space or ether (*Akasha*), wind (*Vayu*), fire (*Tejas*), water (*Jala*), and earth (*Prithivi*) [65]. These basic elements merge to arrange three *Doshas*, known as *Vata*, *Pitta*, and *Kapha*, which are the psychophysiological basis governing a variety of functions of the body. *Vata* is made of the lighter elements, mostly space and air. Fire and water form the *Pitta*, and *Kapha* is made of water and earth, which are the heavier elements. The role of *Vata* is to regulate any movement or communication in the body, e.g., the flow of blood through vessels, heart contraction, inhalation and exhalation, food passage through the gastrointestinal tract, and the transmission of neural impulses. *Pitta* manages the digestive function and metabolism of the body, including the regulation of energy, appetite, and the endocrine system. The role of *Kapha* is to maintain the structure and body integrity, including the strength and stability of the body and fluid balance. The proportion of *Vata*, *Pitta*, and *Kapha* is unique for each person, which is the basis of the psychophysiological functions of the body [66].

Some studies investigated the effects of Ayurvedic treatments on CP. A randomized clinical trial showed language, performance, gross motor, and fine motor improvements in children with CP following Ayurvedic treatment [67]. Ayurveda can significantly improve the growth and development of children, reduce the spasticity [68], and enhance the joints' range of motion [69]. A case study reported a

Table 16.4 Other complementary and alternative interventions in the treatment of cerebral palsy

Subject/sample size	Age/gender	Intervention method/duration	Control	Outcomes	Adverse effects	References
Randomized controlled trial on spastic CP children/50	11 m–12 y/ both	Craniosacral and myofascial release techniques of osteopathy	No treatment	↑ Function of legs or hands 61% vs. 0% ↑ Sleep quality 39% vs. 0% ↑ Mood 30% vs. 12% ↑ Speech or drooling 4% vs. 6% ↑ Bowel movements 26% vs. 0% ↑ Cognition 4% vs. 0% ↓ Ocular muscle stiffness 43% vs. 39% ↑ Happiness due to vision correction 38% vs. 22%	NR	[37]
Non-randomized controlled trial on spastic CP children/16	Mean: 28.2 m/4 m	Homeopathy/4 m	Placebo	No significant difference in brain and spinal reflexes and automatic reactions	NR	[81]
Randomized controlled trial on spastic CP children/24	1–5 y/NR	Homeopathy/3 m	Placebo	↔ Muscle tone	NR	[82]
Randomized controlled trial on spastic CP children/55	20 m–12 y/ both	Cranial osteopathy/weeks 1–4 once per week, weeks 5–8 once every other week, and weeks 9–24, once every month: 10 sessions, 6 m	Non-therapeutic play time	↑ Gross motor function ↑ WeeFIM mobility domain	NR	[77]

Randomized controlled trial on CP children/142	5–12 y/both	Cranial osteopathy/3 sessions within 10 w and 3 within 6 m	No treatment	↔ Gross motor function ↔ CHQ	None	[89]
Randomized controlled trial on CP children/40	2–10 y/both	Oral Ayurvedic treatment /twice per day, 2 d	Anal same Ayurvedic treatment	↑ Language ↑ Performance ↑ Gross motor function ↑ Fine motor function	NR	[67]
Case series of spastic CP children/8	3–10 y/NR	Ayurvedic treatment/3 courses of 18 days with 12 d interval	Basic Ayurvedic treatment	↑ Growth and development ↓ Spasticity	NR	[68]
Randomized controlled trial on CP children/123	2–10 y/both	Ayurvedic treatment/1 g/d, 60 d	Placebo	↑ ADL ↑ Gross motor function ↑ Fine motor function ↑ Mental function	NR	[71]
Randomized controlled trial on CP children/98	2–10 y/both	Ayurvedic treatment/2 g/d, 60 d	Placebo	↑ Mental function ↑ Gross motor function ↑ Fine motor function	NR	[90]
Case study of a spastic CP child/1	3 y/male	Ayurvedic treatment/3 courses of 22 d with 14 d interval: 90 d	None	↑ TER: 15% ↑ ROM: elbow and knee ↓ Spasticity	NR	[69]
Randomized controlled trial on spastic CP children/32	3–8 y/both	Ayurvedic treatment/3 courses of 15 days with 15 d interval: 90 d	Basic Ayurvedic treatment	↓ Ashworth scale	NR	[91]

(continued)

Table 16.4 (continued)

Subject/sample size	Age/gender	Intervention method/duration	Control	Outcomes	Adverse effects	References
Case study of a spastic CP child/1	5 y/male	Ayurvedic treatment/3 courses of 17 d with 14 d interval: 90 d	None	↑ Gross motor function ↑ Language ↑ QoL ↑ Anthropometric indices ↓ Spasticity ↓ Drooling	NR	[70]
Uncontrolled trial on CP children/14	1–12 y/both	Ayurvedic treatment/3 courses of 17 d with 15 d interval: 81 d	None	↓ Ashworth scale ↑ Gross motor function ↔ QoL	NR	[72]
Uncontrolled trial on CP children/13	5–16 y/both	Reiki protocol/8 w	None	↓ Pain while lying down ↓ Anger ↔ Sadness, stress, muscle spasticity, and hair cortisol	NR	[92]

↑ increased significantly, ↓ decreased significantly, ↔ no significant change, *WeeFIM* Pediatric Functional Independence Measure, *NR* not reported, *m* month, *w* week, *y* year, *d* day, *GMFCS* Gross Motor Functional Classification System, *CHQ* children health questionnaire, *ADL* activity of daily living, *ROM* range of motion, *QoL* quality of life, *TER* total effective rate remarkable increase in motor function, mental function, anthropometric indices, and the score of quality of life [70, 71] as well as reducing the Ashworth scale and drooling [70, 72]. Ayurvedic textbooks stated the broad utility of medicinal plants in the improvement of health and the immune system. Ayurvedic botanical prescriptions consist of natural active phytochemicals such as flavonoids, terpenes, and polyphenols. Studies on Ayurvedic approaches claim that these treatments might play a role through epigenetic mechanisms [73]; however, the exact mechanism of action of Ayurvedic treatments remained to be determined in future studies.

16.5.2 Osteopathy

Osteopathy is one of the complementary and alternative medical systems that considers the body as a cohesive functional unit and emphasizes the body's innate ability to self-heal and regulate homeostasis. Osteopathic therapies consist of manipulating bones, tissues, and joints of the body to reach the healthy state [74] based on four principal tenets: (1) the human body is an integrated unit composed of body, mind, and spirit, (2) the body itself has the ability to self-regulate, and self-healing to preserve health, (3) the body structure is closely linked to the function of organs, and (4) the root of rational and reasonable management of health problems is understanding and utilizing above-mentioned three principles [75]. Techniques of osteopathy comprise manipulating lymphatic pathways, raising the rib cage, diaphragmatic release, myofascial manipulation, ligamentous tension release, and muscle energy techniques, as well as cranial manipulation, which is a unique and substantial technique of osteopathy [74].

A systematic review showed the potential of osteopathic treatment in reducing pain and improving physical function in patients with musculoskeletal problems such as neck pain, low back pain, migraine, or irritable bowel syndrome [76]. In addition, a randomized controlled clinical trial by Duncan et al. reported that craniosacral and myofascial release techniques of osteopathy can significantly improve the function of legs and hands, sleep quality, mood, bowel movements, and cognition [37]. While Wyatt et al. reported no remarkable change in the overall health score of children with CP after receiving osteopathy, another study by Duncan et al. reported significant improvement in gross motor function and mobility domain of the pediatric functional independence measure (WeeFIM) score [77]. Parents of children with CP reported that osteopathy increased the happiness of children due to vision correction by reducing the ocular muscle stiffness [37].

16.5.3 Homeopathy

The term homeopathy, as a medical system, originates in the Greek term "homoios", which means "similar", and the word "pathos", which means "enduring from disease". Based on principles of homeopathy, an illness with a particular group of manifestations can be treated by a medication that produces a similar group of manifestations in a healthy individual, so-called "the law of similars". The doctrine of "like cures like" is the fundamental basis of homeopathic medicine, which results in the rule of management of the disease: use like to treat the like [78]. According to the homeopathic holistic point of view, the totality of disease manifestations guides the physician to select the proper medication. For instance, exposing to cutting onion results in watery eyes and runny nose that look like the manifestations of common cold. Hence, following the simile tenet, homeopathic dilution of *Allium cepa* L. is utilized in the management of common cold and hay fever [79].

Although recent studies showed clinical effects of homeopathic remedies on postoperative ileus, muscle soreness, prophylaxis of migraine, influenza, and rheumatic conditions [80], clinical trials on pediatric CP reported no significant changes (regarding muscle tone, brain reflexes, spinal reflexes, and automatic reactions) comparable with placebo [81, 82].

16.6 Conclusions and Future Perspective

As reviewed in this chapter, TIM approaches have attracted increasing attention in the multidisciplinary management of CP. Among the various modalities evaluated, acupuncture and massage therapy provide the most acceptable levels of evidence supporting their safety and efficacy as an adjuvant to the CP standard care. Acupuncture has demonstrated promising effects on spasticity, motor function, and quality of life, potentially due to regulating neuroplasticity and central nervous system regulation. Likewise, massage therapy demonstrated beneficial effects on reducing muscle stiffness, improving circulation, and relaxation.

On the other hand, the evidence for other traditional practices such as herbal medicine and osteopathy remains limited with respect to the quality and quantity of the available studies. Meanwhile, modalities like homeopathy and energy therapies (e.g., Reiki, therapeutic touch) have not demonstrated reproducible or scientifically validated effects in CP, calling for a more cautious stance on their clinical application.

The discrepancy of CP presentations, i.e., variations in motor disability, cognition, sensory impairments, and comorbidities, further makes the evaluation of TIM therapies complicated. Therefore, large-scale RCTs with a personalized approach, coupled with neuroimaging techniques, electrophysiological measurements, and validated functional scales, are necessary. Additionally, systematic reviews and meta-analyses are essential to sum up the results of different TIM modalities. Standardization of outcome measures-e.g., GMFM, PEDI, and quality-of-life indices—is also important to ensure comparability of the results across different studies. In case of herbal interventions, phytochemical profiling and standardization of the administered medicine, as well as consideration of possible herb-drug interactions between natural medicines and CP conventional medicines seems necessary. Also, in case of osteopathic treatments, biomechanical modeling and patient-centered outcome tracking would be beneficial to provide a better overview of the effectiveness.

To sum up, while acupuncture and massage therapy currently represent the most evidence-supported TIM modalities in CP care, a long path still lies a head of our understanding of other TIM practices. Nevertheless, the promising results of the currently-available preliminary research suggest future studies to be performed for further assessment of safety and efficacy of different TIM approaches in patients with CP.

16.6.1 Parents and Caregiver Support

Despite the promising results of traditional and complementary medicines in CP patients, clinical application of these methods should be approached with caution due to the limited body of supporting evidence. Among different complementary treatment approaches, acupuncture and massage are the most evident ones; however, it should be noted that due to the complicated conditions of CP patients, individual response to such treatments may vary considerably. Caregivers and parents are strongly advised to seek for the consultation of a qualified specialist in this field before initiating any of these methods. Also, such interventions must always be undertaken upon permission and supervision of the patient's physician. This is particularly critical in case of using herbal medicine and natural supplements due to the possibility of herb-drug interaction between patient's conventional drugs and these supplements. Medicinal plants may cause pharmacokinetic and/or pharmacodynamic interactions with conventional medicines. Such interactions can appear through mechanisms such as induction/inhibition of drug-metabolizing enzymes, multidrug-resistant pumps, and agonistic/antagonistic activity on receptors or channels mutual with the conventional drugs can alter drug absorption, distribution, metabolism, or excretion, which may result in decreasing therapeutic efficacy or increasing the risk of adverse effects. Therefore, simultaneous intake of these supplements should be carefully monitored by a qualified specialist to prevent any probable adverse effects.

16.6.2 Guide for Multidisciplinary Teams

Different treatments approaches have been reported from traditional and complementary medicine to manage the symptoms in CP patients. These include acupuncture, massage, herbal medicine, osteopathy, homeopathy, and energy healing. While acupuncture and massage have shown promising outcomes in clinical studies to manage muscle spasticity, speech, motor function, and gastrointestinal complications; evidence on other approaches is limited and thus, future well-designed studies are still needed. With respect to herbal medicine and natural supplements, only a few preclinical studies are available and clinical evidence is dramatically limited. It should be noted that some general natural therapies such as those reducing the anxiety may be helpful in CP patients since they can increase pain threshold and relax patients so that they have a better cooperation with the caregivers; however, due to the possibility of herb-drug interaction between these supplements and conventional medicines, caution should be undertaken when using such interventions in these patients. Further research is needed to confirm the safety and efficacy of natural supplements in simultaneous use with conventional medicine in CP patients. In case of homeopathy and energy healing methods, available evidence seems unreliable due to the limited number and low quality of the current reports; therefore, such interventions are not generally recommended until stronger evidence is provided.

References

1. Liao H-H, et al. Complementary traditional Chinese medicine use in children with cerebral palsy: a nationwide retrospective cohort study in Taiwan. BMC Complement Altern Med. 2017;17:1–12.
2. Rocha A, et al. A systematic review and meta-analysis focusing on the use of ayurvedic medicine in cerebral palsy. J Ayurveda Integr Med. 2024;15(5):101035.
3. Lee M-J, et al. Integrative medicine rehabilitation for children with cerebral palsy: a study protocol for a multicenter pragmatic randomized controlled trial. Trials. 2020;21:1–10.
4. Li L, et al. The role of Chinese medicine in health maintenance and disease prevention: application of constitution theory. Am J Chin Med. 2019;47(03):495–506.
5. Yu W, et al. Traditional Chinese medicine and constitutional medicine in China, Japan and Korea: a comparative study. Am J Chin Med. 2017;45(01):1–12.
6. Hu Q, et al. End-to-End syndrome differentiation of Yin deficiency and Yang deficiency in traditional Chinese medicine. Comput Methods Prog Biomed. 2019;174:9–15.
7. Van Hal M, Dydyk A, Green M. Acupuncture [Updated 2023 Jul 24]. In: StatPearls. Treasure Island: StatPearls Publishing; 2024.
8. Anderson BJ, et al. Interdisciplinary relationship models for complementary and integrative health: perspectives of Chinese medicine practitioners in the United States. J Altern Complement Med. 2019;25(3):288–95.
9. Smith CL, et al. The state of 21st century acupuncture in the United States. J Pain Res. 2024;17:3329–54.
10. Jishun J, Mittelman M. Acupuncture: past, present, and future. Los Angeles: SAGE Publications Sage CA; 2014. p. 6–8.
11. Kwon S, et al. Safety of acupuncture in patients taking newer oral anticoagulants: a retrospective chart review study. Evid Based Complement Alternat Med. 2018;2018(1):8042198.
12. Ji YH, et al. Therapeutic effect of scalp-acupuncture combined with exercise therapy on spastic cerebral palsy of the child. Zhongguo Zhen Jiu. 2008;28(10):723–6.
13. Wang SQ, et al. Randomized controlled clinical trials for acupuncture treatment of spastic cerebral palsy children by bilateral horizontal puncturing from Yuzhen (BL 9) to Tianzhu (BL 10). Zhen Ci Yan Jiu. 2011;36(3):215–9.
14. Wang C, et al. Trends in the utilization of acupuncture among children in Taiwan from 2002 to 2011: a nationwide population-based study. BMC Complement Altern Med. 2019;19:1–8.
15. Lin Y-C, et al. Use of complementary and alternative medicine in pediatric pain management service: a survey. Pain Med. 2005;6(6):452–8.
16. Chen K, et al. Meridian acupuncture plus massage for children with spastic cerebral palsy. Am J Transl Res. 2021;13(6):6415–22.
17. Wang TH, et al. Comparison of physical electrical conductivity and acupuncture de-qi sensation between stainless steel needling and supercritical fluid-treated needling. Biom J. 2021;44(6 Suppl 2):S267–74.
18. Hahm TS. Electroacupuncture. Korean J Anesthesiol. 2009;57(1):3–7.

19. Dabbous OA, et al. Laser acupuncture as an adjunctive therapy for spastic cerebral palsy in children. Lasers Med Sci. 2016;31(6):1061–7.
20. Lee EJ, Frazier SK. The efficacy of acupressure for symptom management: a systematic review. J Pain Symptom Manag. 2011;42(4):589–603.
21. Lu L, et al. Efficacy and safety of fire needle vs conventional acupuncture in the treatment of postherpetic neuralgia: a protocol for systematic review and meta analysis. Medicine (Baltimore). 2020;99(41):e22563.
22. Sha T, et al. An update on acupuncture point injection. QJM: Int J Med. 2016;109(10):639–41.
23. Simma I, et al. Immediate effects of microsystem acupuncture in patients with oromyofacial pain and craniomandibular disorders (CMD): a double-blind, placebo-controlled trial. Br Dent J. 2009;207(12):E26.
24. Gleditsch J. The "very point" technique: a needle based point detection method. Acupunct Med. 1995;13(1):20–1.
25. Jianyi X, et al. Scalp acupuncture Yikang therapy on Baihui (GV20), Sishencong (EX-HN1), Zhisanzhen, Niesanzhen improves neurobehavior in young rats with cerebral palsy through Notch signaling pathway. J Tradit Chin Med. 2023;43(2):337–42.
26. Sun JG, et al. Randomised control trial of tongue acupuncture versus sham acupuncture in improving functional outcome in cerebral palsy. J Neurol Neurosurg Psychiatry. 2004;75(7):1054–7.
27. Lü XL, et al. Treatment of cerebral palsy with Chinese scalp acupuncture. World J Acupunct Moxibustion. 2017;27(2):62,73–6,73.
28. Lao L, Xu L, Xu S. Traditional chinese medicine. In: Integrative pediatric oncology. Springer; 2012. p. 125–35.
29. Xuefeng W, Bingxiang M. Chinese rehabilitation guideline for cerebral palsy (2022) Chapter 5: rehabilitation treatment of traditional Chinese medicine [J]. Chin J Pract Pediatr. 2022;37(18):1365–76.
30. Kim HN, et al. Comparative analysis of the beneficial effects of treadmill training and electroacupuncture in a rat model of neonatal hypoxia-ischemia. Int J Mol Med. 2017;39(6):1393–402.
31. Kim H, et al. Combination of constraint-induced movement therapy with electroacupuncture improves functional recovery following neonatal hypoxic-ischemic brain injury in rats. Biomed Res Int. 2018;2018:8638294.
32. Pak ME, et al. Combined therapy involving electroacupuncture and treadmill exercise attenuates demyelination in the corpus callosum by stimulating oligodendrogenesis in a rat model of neonatal hypoxia-ischemia. Exp Neurol. 2018;300:222–31.
33. Wang Z, et al. Effects of three kinds of head acupuncture therapies on regulation of brain microenvironment and rehabilitation of nerve function in rats with cerebral palsy. J Tradit Chin Med. 2021;41(2):276–83.
34. Wu ZF, et al. Electroacupuncture activates the peroxisome proliferators-activated receptor pathway to improve the phenotype of cerebral palsy. CNS Neurosci Ther. 2024;30(7):e14876.
35. Savaskan NE, et al. Neurodegeneration in the brain tumor microenvironment: glutamate in the limelight. Curr Neuropharmacol. 2015;13(2):258–65.
36. Li R, et al. Single injection of a novel nerve growth factor coacervate improves structural and functional regeneration after sciatic nerve injury in adult rats. Exp Neurol. 2017;288:1–10.
37. Duncan B, et al. Parental perceptions of the therapeutic effect from osteopathic manipulation or acupuncture in children with spastic cerebral palsy. Clin Pediatr. 2004;43(4):349–53.
38. Zhou XJ, Zheng K. Treatment of 140 cerebral palsied children with a combined method based on traditional Chinese medicine (TCM) and western medicine. J Zhejiang Univ Sci B. 2005;6(1):57–60.
39. Zhang P-y, Hu F-f. Influence of cluster needling at scalp acupoints combined with rehabilitation training on balance functions of children with cerebral palsy. World J Acupunct Moxibustion. 2012;22(4):23–31.
40. Norman SL, Wolpaw JR, Reinkensmeyer DJ. Targeting neuroplasticity to improve motor recovery after stroke: an artificial neural network model. Brain Commun. 2022;4(6):fcac264.

41. Qin S, et al. The impact of acupuncture on neuroplasticity after ischemic stroke: a literature review and perspectives. Front Cell Neurosci. 2022;16:817732.
42. Zhixiong X, et al. Acupuncture on intrauterine growth restriction associated brain injury: case study including use of magnetic resonance imaging. J Tradit Chin Med. 2023;43(3):602–5.
43. Duncan B, et al. Evaluating intense rehabilitative therapies with and without acupuncture for children with cerebral palsy: a randomized controlled trial. Arch Phys Med Rehabil. 2012;93(5):808–15.
44. Wang X, et al. Acupuncture and Tuina treatment for gross motor function in children with spastic cerebral palsy: a monocentric clinical study. Neuropsychiatr Dis Treat. 2023;19:1875–86.
45. Wang X, Pang F, Du XG. Analysis of traditional Chinese medicine symptoms in children with spastic cerebral palsy: a data mining study. J Multidiscip Healthc. 2024;17:913–22.
46. Chen Z, et al. Effects of traditional Chinese medicine combined with modern rehabilitation therapies on motor function in children with cerebral palsy: a systematic review and meta-analysis. Front Neurosci. 2023;17:1097477.
47. Wright BD. Acupuncture for the treatment of neuromuscular conditions in dogs and cats, with emphasis on intervertebral disc disease. J Am Holist Vet Med Assoc. 2021;63:23–33.
48. Liu ZH, et al. Clinical observation on treatment of clearing the Governor Vessel and refreshing the mind needling in neural development and remediation of children with cerebral palsy. Chin J Integr Med. 2013;19(7):505–9.
49. Li J, et al. Evaluating the effects of 5-Hz repetitive transcranial magnetic stimulation with and without wrist-ankle acupuncture on improving spasticity and motor function in children with cerebral palsy: a randomized controlled trial. Front Neurosci. 2021;15:771064.
50. Gao T, et al. Enhancing the development and growth of infant cerebral palsy rats using selective spinal manipulations. J Vis Exp. 2024;(204):e65659.
51. Niu F, et al. Spinal Tuina improves cognitive impairment in cerebral palsy rats through inhibiting pyroptosis induced by NLRP3 and caspase-1. Evid Based Complement Alternat Med. 2021;2021:1028909.
52. Zhang Y, et al. Tuina massage improves cognitive functions of hypoxic-ischemic neonatal rats by regulating genome-wide DNA hydroxymethylation levels. Evid Based Complement Alternat Med. 2019;2019:1282085.
53. Qiao R, et al. Abdominal massage to improve motor dysfunction in rats with cerebral palsy. J Vis Exp. 2023;(198):e65625.
54. Alizad V, Sajedi F, Vameghi R. Muscle tonicity of children with spastic cerebral palsy: how effective is Swedish massage? Iran J Child Neurol. 2009;3(2):25–9.
55. Alizad V, et al. Swedish massage and abnormal reflexes of children with spastic cerebral palsy. Iran Rehabil J. 2007;5(5–6):30–3.
56. Zhao Y, et al. Enhancing motor function in children with cerebral palsy: a comparative study of pediatric tuina and conventional rehabilitation. J Bodyw Mov Ther. 2025;41:1–7.
57. Jie-shan X, et al. Clinical observation on spleen-invigorating and qi-benefiting pediatric massage for treating recurrent respiratory tract infection in children with cerebral palsy due to qi deficiency of spleen and lung. J Acupunct Tuina Sci. 2021;19(2):110–6.
58. Elbasan B, Bezgin S. The effects of reflexology on constipation and motor functions in children with cerebral palsy. Pediatr Neonatol. 2018;59(1):42–7.
59. Zhang XL. Influence of acupuncture with massage on the movement development of children with spastic cerebral palsy. Chin J Clin Rehab. 2005;9(7):116–7.
60. Nasri H, et al. The effects of MEPaL on oxidative stress and motor function in the rats affected by prenatal hypoxia. Brain Behav. 2024;14(6):e3539.
61. Wang T, et al. Proteomic changes in the hippocampus and motor cortex in a rat model of cerebral palsy: effects of topical treatment. Biomed Pharmacother. 2021;133:110844.
62. Odey AI, et al. Stem extract from Costus afer (Bush cane) prevents ethanol-induced neuronal degeneration in mice via an antioxidant-inflammatory pathway. Phytomed Plus. 2024;4(4):100653.

63. Zhang WL, et al. Neuroprotective effect of tanshinone IIA weakens spastic cerebral palsy through inflammation, p38MAPK and VEGF in neonatal rats. Mol Med Rep. 2018;17(1):2012–8.
64. Chauhan A, et al. Ayurvedic research and methodology: present status and future strategies. Ayu. 2015;36(4):364–9.
65. Sharma H. Ayurveda: science of life, genetics, and epigenetics. Ayu. 2016;37(2):87–91.
66. Valiathan M. The legacy of Caraka. Orient Blackswan; 2003.
67. Shailaja U, Rao Prasanna N, Arun Raj GR. Clinical study on the efficacy of samvardhana ghrita orally and by matrabasti in motor disabilities of cerebral palsy in children. Int J Res Ayurveda Pharm. 2013;4(3):373–7.
68. Bhinde SM, et al. Management of spastic cerebral palsy through multiple Ayurveda treatment modalities. Ayu. 2014;35(4):462–6.
69. Bhinde SM. A case study on the Ayurvedic management of cerebral palsy. Anc Sci Life. 2015;34(3):167–70.
70. Niraj SK, Varsha S. A case study on the ayurvedic managment of spastic cerebral palsy due to birth asphyxia. J Nat Remedies. 2019;19(3):153–61.
71. Shailaja U, et al. Exploratory study on the ayurvedic therapeutic management of cerebral palsy in children at a tertiary care hospital of Karnataka, India. J Tradit Complement Med. 2014;4(1):49–55.
72. Upasana S, Mahapatra Arun K, Rajagopala S. The effect of Murcchita Tila Taila based Panchakarma procedure and Balapanchamrita yoga In the management of cerebral palsy in children: a single arm prospective clinical trial. Ayushdhara. 2021;7(6):3004–8.
73. Sharma H, Clark CS. Ayurvedic healing: contemporary Maharishi Ayurveda medicine and science. 2nd ed. Singing Dragon; 2011.
74. Chila AG, Carreiro JE, A.O. Association. Foundations of osteopathic medicine. Lippincott Williams & Wilkins; 2011.
75. Roberts A, et al. Osteopathic manipulative medicine: a brief review of the hands-on treatment approaches and their therapeutic uses. Medicines (Basel). 2022;9(5):33.
76. Zipp CR, et al. An overview of systematic reviews on the efficacy and safety of osteopathic techniques. J Bodyw Mov Ther. 2025;42:1186–97.
77. Duncan B, et al. Effectiveness of osteopathy in the cranial field and myofascial release versus acupuncture as complementary treatment for children with spastic cerebral palsy: a pilot study. J Am Osteopath Assoc. 2008;108(10):559–70.
78. Fisher P. What is homeopathy? An Introduction. FBE. 2012;4(5):1669–82.
79. Taragi S. Common cold, fever and its homeopathic management in pediatric age group. Int J Adv Eng Manage (IJAEM). 2024;6:377–83.
80. Ernst E. A systematic review of systematic reviews of homeopathy. Br J Clin Pharmacol. 2002;54(6):577–82.
81. Sajedi F, et al. The effect of adding homeopathic treatment to rehabilitation on abnormal reflexes of children with spastic cerebral palsy. Iran Rehabil J. 2007;5(5–6):34–9.
82. Sajedi F, et al. The effect of adding homeopathic treatment to rehabilitation on muscle tone of children with spastic cerebral palsy. Complement Ther Clin Pract. 2008;14(1):33–7.
83. Wu Y, et al. Randomized controlled trial of traditional Chinese medicine (acupuncture and Tuina) in cerebral palsy: part 1 – any increase in seizure in integrated acupuncture and rehabilitation group versus rehabilitation group? J Altern Complement Med. 2008;14(8):1005–9.
84. Zhang HY, Lu SF, Xiao N. Effect of warming moxibustion on Shenque acupoint for the treatment of acute diarrhea in children with infantile cerebral palsy. Chin J Integr Med. 2009;15(6):454–7.
85. Wang J, Sun KX, Wu XB. Effect of individualized needling on gross motor function in cerebral palsy infants. J Acupunct Tuina Sci. 2013;11(1):13–8.
86. Gao J, et al. Rehabilitation with a combination of scalp acupuncture and exercise therapy in spastic cerebral palsy. Complement Ther Clin Pract. 2019;35:296–300.
87. Sun Y, Chen H, Wu C. Effect of the medication injection site on treatment efficacy in pediatric cerebral palsy: conventional sites vs acupoints. J Tradit Chin Med. 2019;39(5):716–21.

88. Zhao FY, et al. Occupational therapy with or without combined acupuncture on upper limb pain and hand functions in children with spastic hemiplegic cerebral palsy: a three-arm randomized, placebo-controlled trial. World J Acupunct Moxibustion. 2022;32(1):1–8.
89. Wyatt K, et al. Cranial osteopathy for children with cerebral palsy: a randomised controlled trial. Arch Dis Child. 2011;96(6):505–12.
90. Shailaja U, et al. Clinical study on the efficacy of Rajayapana Basti and Baladi Yoga in motor disabilities of cerebral palsy in children. Ayu. 2014;35(3):294–9.
91. Arun Raj G, et al. Effectiveness of Ayurveda treatment modalities in the management of spasticity in children with cerebral palsy at a tertiary care teaching hospital of Southern India. Int J Res Ayurveda Pharm. 2018;9(2):96–100.
92. Love L, et al. A study of Reiki therapy on unpleasant symptoms in children with cerebral palsy. Complement Ther Clin Pract. 2022;46:101529.

Cerebral Palsy Emergent Situations

17

Ali Labaf, Mohammad Eftekhari, and Saeed Aqavil-Jahromi

17.1 Case Presentation

A 4-year-old boy with cerebral palsy was brought to your emergency department by his mother. She reported that he had been bedridden due to severe spasticity and scoliosis, and had a tracheostomy and a percutaneous endoscopic gastrostomy (PEG) feeding tube for the past 2 years. He had not had a bowel movement for 6 days, had been vomiting after each feeding for 5 days, and had fever, grunting, and altered consciousness and no eye contact for the past 2 days. On examination, in response to painful stimuli, the child did not open his eyes, moaned, and did not move his limbs. Vital signs were: BP 65/40 mmHg, PR 140 bpm, RR 19 breaths/min, T 38.5 °C, SpO_2 88%. The tracheostomy stoma was clean, but purulent secretions were present within the tube. Lung auscultation revealed coarse crackles at the base of the right lung. Abdominal examination demonstrated distension, tympanic percussion, generalized tenderness, and no evidence of a distended bladder. The PEG tube bag contained fecal material. The limbs were mottled and cold, but not edematous. No pressure ulcers were found.

A. Labaf (✉)
Emergency Medicine, Hakim Children's Hospital, Tehran University of Medical Science, School of Medicine, Tehran, Iran
e-mail: alabaf@tums.ac.ir

M. Eftekhari · S. Aqavil-Jahromi
Emergency Medicine, Tehran University of Medical Science, School of Medicine, Tehran, Iran
e-mail: smeftekhari@tums.ac.ir; saqavil@sina.tums.ac.ir

A. Presedo et al. (eds.), *Enhancing Quality of Life in Patients with Cerebral Palsy*, https://doi.org/10.1007/978-3-032-20967-2_17

17.2 Introduction

Cerebral palsy (CP) has a prevalence of 2 to 4 per 1000 live births [1, 2] and accounts for approximately 0.4% of pediatric emergency department (ED) visits, the majority of whom require hospitalization [3]. This condition is a non-progressive, permanent motor disorder resulting from brain injury sustained during the fetal or early infancy period [1]. Depending on its severity, CP encompasses a wide spectrum of motor symptoms and is often associated with neurologic, respiratory, gastrointestinal, urinary, and musculoskeletal comorbidities. The diagnosis is typically clinical, based on serial history and examinations, and supported by ancillary tests to rule out other treatable or "CP-mimicking" conditions, usually within the first years of life [4].

▶ Patients with a previous diagnosis who have achieved reliable communication generally have milder motor and associated disorders, and their diagnostic and therapeutic processes do not significantly differ from the general population. However, patients without a prior diagnosis presenting for the first time to the ED (e.g., fever or seizures) pose considerable diagnostic and management challenges for clinicians. On the other hand, symptoms such as constipation or spasticity in children with chronic diseases like CP may be mistakenly attributed to the underlying condition without thorough evaluation, when in fact they could indicate serious issues such as bowel obstruction or seizures. The greater the severity of motor impairment, the higher the likelihood and severity of cognitive and other comorbidities, which in turn increases the risk for emergent situations [5].This chapter will first address the challenges in vital sign measurement and resuscitation, and then focus on diagnostic and management challenges of common emergencies leading to ED presentations, particularly those with higher Gross Motor Function Classification System (GMFCS) levels.

17.3 Challenges in Vital Sign Measurement

There are reports of dysautonomia in patients with CP compared to a control group with normal motor development. They exhibited higher systolic and diastolic blood pressure, heart rate, and respiratory rate, as well as lower blood oxygen saturation and oral body temperature [6].

▶ Using appropriately sized equipment, especially the blood pressure cuff, is essential. The width of the cuff should be at least 40% of the arm length, and the bladder length should cover 80% of the arm's circumference. A too-narrow cuff will overestimate blood pressure, while one too-wide will underestimate it [7]. Given the prevalence of mouth breathing in many of these patients, oral thermometers are likely to yield falsely low temperature readings; therefore, the tympanic thermometer is probably the best tool for measuring peripheral temperature in this population [8, 9].

17.4 Challenges in Resuscitation

Before reviewing the clinical manifestations of CP patients, it is essential—regardless of the underlying diagnosis—to address the challenges that may arise while managing the critical steps of airway, breathing, and circulation ("ABC"). Due to the common comorbidities associated with cerebral palsy, such as spasticity and contractures, as well as a history of prior hospitalizations and medical interventions (including prolonged intubation, tracheostomy, or multiple venipunctures), it is essential to be prepared for potential difficulties during seemingly routine procedures. This includes basic airway management and establishing intravenous access. Without prior mental preparation, clinicians may face catastrophic scenarios such as "cannot intubate, cannot ventilate" after administration of intubation medications without having an alternative plan ready. Therefore, several practical recommendations regarding ABC management are warranted:

17.4.1 Airway

- Familiarize yourself in advance with the concepts, algorithms, and techniques for managing anatomically and/or physiologically difficult airways so that you can promptly choose and implement appropriate preparations when required [10–13]. When intubation is expected to be difficult, consider using advanced techniques like video laryngoscopy or fiber optics, extra-glottic devices, and surgical approaches.

17.4.2 Breathing

- Due to oropharyngeal anomalies and swallowing dysfunction [14], a proper mask fit may not be achievable, resulting in ineffective positive pressure ventilation and a higher risk of aspiration. Spasticity and scoliosis may result in restrictive lung disease, requiring careful selection of ventilator settings tailored to the patient's condition. To improve mask ventilation, consider inserting an oropharyngeal airway, positioning the lower edge of the mask inside the lower lip (i.e., over the mucosa), or packing the cheeks with gauze [15].

▶ After successful intubation, the tidal volume for ventilator settings should be determined based on ideal body weight rather than total body weight. Once you select either volume-controlled or pressure-controlled ventilation, settings must be rechecked and tailored according to the underlying disease, current respiratory and hemodynamic status, blood gas analysis, and ventilator measurements [16].

17.4.3 Circulation

▶ In the setting of hemodynamic instability, allow a limited time (e.g., 5 min) for obtaining peripheral venous access and consider using advanced techniques from the beginning. Favor anatomic sites with higher success rates, such as the basilic vein on the dorsal aspect of the forearm, the saphenous vein on the distal and anterior surface of the tibia, and the external jugular vein. The application of topical nitroglycerin can facilitate local venodilation and ease venous access. Ultrasound guidance may also be utilized to access veins that are difficult to locate, such as the basilic vein on the medial aspect of the arm. If peripheral access remains unsuccessful, promptly proceed to intraosseous or central venous access.

17.5 Patients Without a Prior Diagnosis

> Any presentation requiring a thorough neurological assessment, such as fever with or without seizure in an infant, is challenging. Important examinations, such as primitive reflexes, may be absent or exaggerated due to the underlying disease [17].

Given the non-progressive nature of CP, obtaining a detailed history of previous function and developmental milestones is essential for evaluating these children. Six clinical features recommended by international experts [18] for assessment of possible CP include:

- Hand preference develops before 12 months of age,
- Sustained clenching or fisted posture of the hands after 4 months of age,
- Stiffness or tightness in the legs between 6 and 12 months of age,
- Persistence of head lag beyond 4 months of age,
- Inability to sit without support by 9 months of age,
- Consistent asymmetry of posture and movements after 4 months of age.

Changes in clinical signs compared to baseline are also highly significant. For example, new-onset dysphagia in a child who previously could swallow, or spasticity in a limb that was not previously spastic, suggests a new process. Finally, it is important to recognize that some treatable disorders, such as creatine deficiencies, can mimic CP [19]. Therefore, in children with atypical features or suspected complicated diagnoses, consultation with experts in the field is essential.

17.6 Common Presentations

The most common comorbidities among children with CP presenting to the EDs are, respectively, epilepsy, the presence of a feeding tube, and an intrathecal baclofen pump. The most frequent reasons for their emergency visits are respiratory problems, injury or poisoning, neurological issues, and digestive complaints, respectively. These comorbidities, ED visit frequency, ambulance arrival, triage acuity, and hospitalization rates, including intensive care unit (ICU) admission, increase with higher GMFCS levels [3, 20].

17.6.1 Respiratory Problems

► Respiratory problems are the most common reason for ED visits among patients with CP. The most significant risk factor associated with these complications is dysphagia, followed by higher GMFCS levels [21, 22]. The most frequent diagnoses leading to hospitalization in these patients are pneumonia due to chronic aspiration, followed by bronchiolitis and tracheostomy-related complications, respectively [23]. These patients typically present with a combination of symptoms, including fever, grunting, cough, oxygen desaturation, increased secretions, and sputum production [22, 23]. During hospitalization, the majority of these patients require oxygen supplementation, and approximately half will need invasive ventilatory support. In addition to potentially carrying pathogenic bacteria such as Pseudomonas and Klebsiella, CP patients also have a high risk of co-infection with respiratory viruses. Many of them also suffer from structural lung parenchymal abnormalities, such as atelectasis or bronchiectasis. As a result, it can be inferred that these patients often require ICU admission, ventilatory support, and treatment with multiple antibiotics [23].

17.6.1.1 Tracheostomy Care

CP patients may require permanent tracheostomy for various reasons, such as progressive weakness of the pharyngeal musculature with increasing age [24, 25]. These patients frequently present to the ED, and their visits may be unrelated to their tracheostomy [26]. Providing education and establishing better communication with their families, as well as certain preventive surgical interventions [27], can enhance their quality of life and also reduce the workload on healthcare [26]. Given the high likelihood of encountering such patients in the ED [23], a brief discussion of the approach to tracheostomy complications is warranted.

▶ In CP patients with a tracheostomy who present with respiratory distress, differential diagnoses include both causes unrelated to the tracheostomy (e.g., pneumonia, pulmonary embolism, and pneumothorax), as well as tracheostomy complications itself. Tracheostomy is most often performed electively in the operating room, but it can also be placed emergently using the percutaneous dilational tracheostomy technique. Although complications are more common with the latter, obtaining a history regarding the method and indication for tracheostomy is essential. The most critical question is the timing of tracheostomy placement. This is because the incidence, likelihood, and categories of tracheostomy complications differ depending on the time since placement. Tracheostomy complications are generally divided into early and late categories. Early complications, defined as those occurring within 3 weeks after placement, are primarily surgical (e.g., pneumomediastinum) and typically occur during hospitalization; they are thus less frequently encountered in the ED. Late complications are defined as occurring more than 3 weeks after placement and include obstruction, dislodgement, equipment failure, infection, anatomic disruption, and hemorrhage [25].

For a better understanding of potential complications, a brief description of tracheostomy components and routine care is provided below. The most common type of tracheostomy encountered consists of three parts: 1. The outer cannula, which includes a cuff and flanges; the tube size is indicated on this part, 2. The inner cannula, which typically sits inside the outer cannula. An important point is that bag-mask ventilation can only be performed by attaching the bag to the top of this part, not the outer cannula and 3. The obturator, which is used only during insertion or replacement of the tracheostomy tube and fits inside the outer cannula.

▶ The care of a tracheostomy aims to achieve three primary goals: 1. Prevention of secretion buildup in the tube through regular cleaning and air humidification, 2. Prevention of infection and stoma injury, and 3. Prevention of tracheal mucosa injury by the cuff while ensuring adequate ventilation by proper pressure adjustment. In summary, the external part of the outer cannula (and, if present, the dressing) should be cleaned once daily. The inner cannula should be removed and soaked in half-strength hydrogen peroxide solution for 15 min. Air humidification is provided by a heat-moisture exchanger for ambulatory patients needing low-flow oxygen, and by regular saline nebulization for those requiring long-term ventilation. The cuff is inflated in cases that need positive pressure ventilation or are at risk of aspiration, and its pressure should be maintained below 25 mmHg [28].

▶ Suctioning may be required to improve oxygenation or ventilation, or for sampling airway secretions. Although there are no absolute contraindications to suctioning, it is essential to note that the procedure can increase intracranial pressure, damage the airway epithelium, and cause dysrhythmias. Therefore, complete cardiopulmonary monitoring should be prepared before suctioning. The patient should be sedated or paralyzed if necessary. Before suctioning, humidified air should be provided to thin secretions, and preoxygenation should be performed. All preparations for closed or open and aseptic suctioning must be ensured. The appropriate suction catheter size should be half of the tracheostomy tube's diameter. Suction depth should be set just slightly beyond the end of the tracheostomy tube. The negative pressure should be less than 80 mmHg in infants and less than 150 mmHg in adults. The procedure should not last longer than 15 s. It should also be noted that instilling saline into the airway has not been proven to improve suctioning effectiveness [29, 30].

- Tracheostomy tube replacement may be necessary for reasons such as damage to a part of the tube (e.g., the cuff), failure to resolve tube obstruction with suctioning or cleaning, the need to change the tube size, routine scheduled tube replacement (recommended within a maximum of 3 months), or replacing an uncuffed tracheostomy with a cuffed one. After about 1 week, the tract and stoma typically become canalized, but before this, removing the outer cannula can prevent re-establishing the lumen and increase the risk of creating a false passage. In these situations, it is essential to prepare an appropriately sized tracheostomy tube and at least one smaller size in case the initial size is not suitable. Additionally, monitoring equipment, alternative airway devices (such as for difficult oral tracheal intubation), and suction equipment should be readily available. A tracheal hook may be needed to hold the stoma open, and you might also require a bougie, a red rubber catheter, or a fiberoptic scope to perform the Seldinger technique [31]. In most cases, however, the tract is well established. After preoxygenation, the tracheostomy tube can be removed by disconnecting tube attachments and deflating the cuff. The new tube, coated with a water-based lubricant, can be gently inserted with the patient in a semi-sitting position and extended neck. The obturator is then replaced with the inner cannula, and, if necessary, the cuff is inflated and the tube is connected to a ventilator.

- Hemorrhage from a tracheostomy site can be a complication of the tracheostomy itself or may originate from the lungs. Tracheostomy bleeding commonly results from irritation of the granulation tissue around the stoma, tracheitis, or may originate from the pharynx or gastrointestinal tract if a fistula is present. About 10% of bleeding from a tracheostomy occurs because of fistulation to nearby blood vessels. The innominate artery is the vessel most commonly involved, which can lead to nearly 100% mortality [32]. Every episode of bleeding from a tracheostomy, even if small in volume and self-limited, must be evaluated for serious causes such as vascular fistulas. Due to the risk of life-threatening diagnoses, prompt notification of the surgical team is crucial. If the bleeding is not superficial and visible, and a vascular fistula is suspected, increasing cuff inflation to tamponade the most common fistula site can help to control and temporarily stop the bleeding. Superficial hemorrhage can be managed using hemostatic agents, injection of lidocaine with epinephrine (1:100,000), local pressure, chemical or electric cauterization, or suturing. It is essential to avoid forcibly removing any blood clots.

► The risk of anterior fistulization is not the only concern; posterior tracheal fistulas can also develop between the trachea and esophagus. It can occur due to mucosal injury caused by tube insertion, excessive cuff pressure, or pressure from a nasogastric or orogastric tube. These factors may ultimately lead to the formation of a tracheoesophageal fistula [33]. This diagnosis should be considered in patients who develop respiratory symptoms during feeding or have a history of recurrent pneumonia. It should be confirmed with imaging such as bronchoscopy, barium esophagography, or mediastinal CT scan. Management, in addition to surgery, includes placement of a nasogastric or orogastric tube, cessation of oral feeding, positioning the cuff distal to the fistula, and administration of broad-spectrum antibiotics.

17.6.2 Neurologic Problems

17.6.3 Assessment of the Level and Content of Consciousness

In patients without motor, visual, or cognitive impairment, scoring systems such as the Glasgow Coma Scale (GCS) and the Full Outline of Unresponsiveness (FOUR) score are commonly used [34]. However, there is currently no separate scoring system specifically for CP patients. These patients may have visual or speech impairments, dysphagia, and may be unable to react to stimuli due to their motor dysfunction. Thus, currently, clinical assessment can rely on changes compared to the patient's baseline condition, including eye opening or closing, even the slightest change in facial expression, or minimal withdrawal from pain, as well as signs such as tachycardia or tachypnea in response to pain. Furthermore, in critically ill patients, the use of the Bispectral Index (BIS) can also be helpful [35].

► If a CP patient truly has a superimposed acute disorder of consciousness (e.g., after a new injury), neurobehavioral tools like Coma Recovery Scale–Revised (CRS-R), Coma/Near-Coma Scale (CNCS), Level of Cognitive Functioning Assessment Scale (LOCFAS), and Post-Acute Level of Consciousness Scale might have limited use, but always need careful contextualization. However, these scales are neither validated nor widely appropriate for routine level or content of consciousness assessment in children with CP [36].

17.6.3.1 Seizure

Between 15% to 70% of patients with CP, depending on the severity and type of their condition, have epilepsy. The most common type is partial epilepsy, particularly in patients with hemiplegia, who often experience the self-limited focal epilepsy variant. Therefore, it is essential to closely monitor any unusual movements or changes in muscle tone compared to the patient's baseline condition to avoid missing partial seizures. Generalized tonic-colonic seizures are more frequently observed in patients with spastic tetraplegia and diplegia [14, 37].

► Epilepsy was defined as ≥2 afebrile seizures occurring beyond the neonatal period. A history of neurological problems and epilepsy is an important risk factor for status epilepticus. This condition refers to a seizure event with or without convulsive movements lasting more than 5 min, or recurrent seizures occurring before the end of the postictal phase of the previous seizure. The management of epilepsy and status epilepticus is similar to that in patients without CP. Therefore, while investigating underlying causes such as hypoglycemia, electrolyte disturbances, central nervous system infections, etc., benzodiazepines should be administered as initial treatment. If seizure did not cease after administering appropriate anticonvulsant drugs, a continuous infusion of antiepileptic medications should be considered. Meanwhile, careful attention to securing the airway is necessary. Simultaneously, consultation with a neurologist is recommended in critical patients [38, 39].

17.6.3.2 Spasticity

► Various treatments are available for spasticity in CP patients, including physiotherapy and occupational therapy, as well as botulinum toxin injections for focal spasms. When treating spasticity, and after ruling out other potential diagnoses like seizures, appropriate medication can be started based on the patient's weight and previous use of these drugs. The following medications may be considered in order of priority: baclofen, benzodiazepines such as diazepam and clonazepam, dantrolene, and tizanidine [40, 41].

17.6.4 Gastrointestinal Problems

17.6.4.1 Constipation

Constipation in patients with intellectual disability is defined as hard stool passage or fewer than three bowel movements per week. This issue is observed in approximately 75% of CP patients and is among the top five causes of hospitalization in young adults with CP [42, 43].

- Abdominal examination in CP patients has low diagnostic accuracy in detecting signs of peritoneal irritation. Thus, there is a risk of delayed diagnosis of surgical conditions in this population. The most common surgical emergency is intestinal volvulus, which tends to occur in locations other than the sigmoid colon and cecum more frequently in these patients compared to the general population. Therefore, a high index of clinical suspicion, combined with the appropriate use of paraclinical investigations (e.g., imaging), is essential for evaluating bowel obstruction.
- The treatment of functional constipation in this population currently follows standard protocols used for the general population, as no specific treatment guidelines have yet been developed or validated specifically for patients with intellectual disabilities [42, 44].

17.6.4.2 Feeding Tube

Dysphagia and pulmonary aspiration are observed in about 90% and 40% of patients with CP, respectively [43]. Approximately 6% of pediatric tertiary ED visits are attributed to feeding tube issues, including malfunctions or dislodgements. Almost 90% of these visits are due to tube dislodgement, and about 90% of these cases are managed and discharged by emergency clinicians [45].

- The two main types of feeding tubes are gastrostomy tubes (G-tubes) and gastrojejunal tubes (GJ-tubes). Each type has various tube designs and tip shapes for secure placement. Unfortunately, most emergency patients do not carry documentation indicating the specific type of their tube. If there is a surgical scar at the site of the stoma, it is more likely to be a GJ-tube, which should not be removed in the ED. In the absence of a surgical scar, it is likely a G-tube, which terminates in the stomach or jejunum. The stoma and its tract to the skin typically take about 1–3 weeks to form adhesions and become mature [46, 47].
- If the tube has been dislodged and the tract is confirmed to be mature, it should be promptly replaced with a lubricated Foley catheter to prevent stoma closure, which can occur within hours. To ensure that the Foley is placed in the stomach and not in the peritoneum, air can be insufflated using a syringe, and auscultation performed over the stomach. The Foley should then be secured approximately 1 cm from the skin using tape or a bolster to prevent migration. If there is uncertainty about whether the original tube terminated in the stomach or jejunum, the Foley catheter balloon should not be inflated, because inflation within the jejunum may lead to bowel obstruction. During removal, the inner crossbar of the original tube may detach; in adults, it is often passed rectally, whereas in pediatric patients, endoscopic retrieval may be necessary [48].

- Patients may also present to the ED due to tube clogging. Gentle irrigation can be attempted, but is often ineffective. Additional tools such as a declogger, a Fogarty catheter, or tube replacement may be required. Patients may also present with vomiting and high residuals of feeding solution (normal gastric residual volume is less than 100 cc). This may be due to distal migration causing obstruction or non-tube-related causes such as volvulus. These complications, as well as leakage of feeding material into the peritoneal cavity and resulting peritonitis, generally require consultation with gastroenterology and/or surgery specialists [46].

17.6.5 Urinary Retention

- CP patients commonly have lower urinary tract dysfunction, which has been associated with urinary retention. Most of them present to the hospital with another reason (e.g., pulmonary problems), have a reversible cause of retention such as post-anesthesia, constipation, urinary tract infection, and escalating medication. These cases can be managed with caretaker education of clean intermittent catheterization every 6 h or as needed, and a urologic follow-up [49]. Other aspects of urinary retention, like indications for requesting paraclinics, are the same as those for other patients.

17.7 Analgesia and Sedation

- Patients with cerebral palsy (CP) often experience both chronic pain, like that from hip displacement and muscle spasms, and acute pain in various parts of the body, such as the head and abdomen. They also frequently undergo multiple medical procedures and hospital visits. Pain intensity in these patients has been assessed using tools such as the Visual Analog Scale (VAS) and the Wong-Baker FACES Scale, and others. However, individuals with higher GMFCS levels often have limited verbal and motor ability to express pain. This likely explains why, in a systematic review on pain management in children with CP, which included 57 studies, only 23 reported the use of a pain assessment scale [50]. As a result, it is recommended to administer analgesics during any potentially painful medical condition (e.g., bowel obstruction, cellulitis, etc.) even in the absence of obvious signs of pain.
- These patients with pain also face significant stress and anxiety during procedures. However, anxiety scales have not been systematically studied or validated in this population. Like all patients, they need appropriate procedural sedation and analgesia. It is crucial to consider their unique anatomical differences and potential hepatic or renal dysfunction when choosing sedation and analgesic agents [51].

17.8 Conclusion

Patients with CP present to ED for a wide range of conditions, most frequently respiratory problems, injury or poisoning, neurological issues, and digestive complaints. A higher GMFCS level is associated with increased clinical complexity and greater challenges in acute management. Comparing the patient's current status with their baseline condition remains the most reliable method for detecting new pathological events.

This chapter reviewed key diagnostic and therapeutic considerations for CP patients in the emergency setting, including:

- Challenges in airway, respiratory, and circulatory management;
- Situations in which the diagnosis of CP should be suspected in previously undiagnosed individuals and the importance of considering mimicking disorders;
- Differences in managing respiratory, gastrointestinal, urinary, and pain-related problems; and.
- Specific aspects of tracheostomy and feeding tube care.

Awareness of these condition-specific challenges, combined with a systematic approach, can facilitate timely diagnosis, optimize decision-making, and improve outcomes for patients with CP in ED.

17.9 Parent and Caregiver Guide for Children with Cerebral Palsy (CP)

17.9.1 When you Should Suspect CP

Seek an evaluation if your baby shows any of these signs: Stiff or tight legs between 6–12 months, favoring one hand before 12 months, persistent head lag after 4 months, cannot sit without support by 9 months, and uneven or "asymmetric" movements.

17.9.2 General Tips

Always keep a copy of your child's medical history, their medication list, and an emergency care plan with you. It is advisable to also keep these documents on your mobile phone.

Learn what's normal for your child—such as their usual movement, alertness, and feeding—so you can spot changes quickly.

Use the right-sized blood pressure cuff for your child.

An ear (tympanic) thermometer is most accurate for fever checks in children with CP.

Keep your child upright after meals to lower the risk of aspiration.

Keep a regular bowel routine, with fluids, fiber, and prescribed stool softeners or laxatives if allowed.

Watch for bloating, vomiting, and abdominal distention or pain—these could mean a gastrointestinal obstruction.

Children with CP may not always show pain clearly—look for signs like irritability and facial grimacing.

Learn to spot subtle seizures, such as brief stiffening, lip smacking, or eye flickers.

Keep prescribed seizure rescue medicine at home and learn how to use it.

Warning signs for a respiratory problem: grunting, noisy breathing, blue lips, or extra secretions.

Constipation, infections, or some medicines can cause urinary problems.

If your child had problems with urination, you would consult with your doctor.

If advised, learn clean intermittent catheterization.

17.9.3 During Emergency Department Visits

Bring all medical records for your doctor.

Children with CP have additional health problems or body positions that can make emergency procedures more challenging. Stay calm and let the doctors know if there were difficulties in the past.

Intravenous lines may be tricky to place; nurses and doctors might use the leg, neck, or even bone instead.

Assume pain is present after injuries, procedures, or infections, even if your child can't say so.

17.9.4 Tracheostomy Tube

If recommended, learn basic suctioning or safe positioning techniques.

Clean the outer part of the tube daily; clean the inner cannula as instructed.

Use humidified air or a nebulizer as advised by their doctor.

Consult with your doctor about replacing tube every 3 months or sooner.

Redness, pus, or blood around the site can be signs of infection.

Any bleeding from the tracheostomy is an emergency—get help immediately.

Coughing with feeding or frequent pneumonia may signal a fistula—ask your doctor.

17.9.5 Feeding Tube

Keep medical records of the tube placement, including type and time.

If the feeding tube comes out, get to the ED as soon as possible to prevent closure of the stoma.

Watch for redness, swelling, or leakage at the site.

Don't force a blocked tube—get medical help.

Vomiting or belly swelling could mean the tube is in the wrong place or blocked—this is urgent.

References

1. Rosenbaum P, Paneth N, Leviton A, Goldstein M, Bax M, Damiano D, et al. A report: the definition and classification of cerebral palsy April 2006. Dev Med Child Neurol Suppl. 2007;109(suppl 109):8–14.
2. Oskoui M, Coutinho F, Dykeman J, Jetté N, Pringsheim T. An update on the prevalence of cerebral palsy: a systematic review and meta-analysis. Dev Med Child Neurol. 2013;55(6):509–19.
3. Meehan E, Williams K, Reid SM, Freed GL, Babl FE, Sewell JR, et al. Comparing emergency department presentations among children with cerebral palsy with general childhood presentations: a data linkage study. Dev Med Child Neurol. 2017;59(11):1188–95.
4. Patel DR, Neelakantan M, Pandher K, Merrick J. Cerebral palsy in children: a clinical overview. Transl Pediatr. 2020;9(Suppl 1):S125–s35.
5. Murphy N. Emergency department visits for children with cerebral palsy: what triggers the call for help? Dev Med Child Neurol. 2017;59(11):1110.
6. Ibrahim AI, Muaidi QI, Alghamde AA. Abnormalities of vital signs in children with cerebral palsy: relationship to physical disabilities. J Dev Phys Disabil. 2018;30(1):55–67.
7. Bur A, Herkner H, Vlcek M, Woisetschläger C, Derhaschnig U, Delle Karth G, et al. Factors influencing the accuracy of oscillometric blood pressure measurement in critically ill patients. Crit Care Med. 2003;31(3):793–9.
8. Park S-H, Lee HS, Kwack MJ, Cho YS, Kang C-B. Systematic review and meta-analysis of the diagnostic accuracy of an infrared tympanic thermometer for use with adults. Int J Nurs. 2014;1(2):115–34.
9. Giuliano KK, Giuliano AJ, Scott SS, MacLachlan E, Pysznik E, Elliot S, et al. Temperature measurement in critically ill adults: a comparison of tympanic and oral methods. Am J Crit Care. 2000;9(4):254–61.
10. Fiadjoe JE, Nishisaki A, Jagannathan N, Hunyady AI, Greenberg RS, Reynolds PI, et al. Airway management complications in children with difficult tracheal intubation from the Pediatric Difficult Intubation (PeDI) registry: a prospective cohort analysis. Lancet Respir Med. 2016;4(1):37–48.
11. Torun AÇ, Sarı ME, Köksal E, İbiş S. Comparing the intubation effectiveness of two different laryngoscopes in patients with cerebral palsy. Cumhur Dent J. 2018;21(2):123–9.
12. Capone CA, Emerson B, Sweberg T, Polikoff L, Turner DA, Adu-Darko M, et al. Intubation practice and outcomes among pediatric emergency departments: a report from National Emergency Airway Registry for children (NEAR4KIDS). Acad Emerg Med. 2022;29(4):406–14.
13. Kornas RL, Owyang CG, Sakles JC, Foley LJ, Mosier JM. Evaluation and management of the physiologically difficult airway: consensus recommendations from Society for Airway Management. Anesth Analg. 2021;132(2):395–405.
14. Pruitt DW, Tsai T. Common medical comorbidities associated with cerebral palsy. Phys Med Rehabil Clin. 2009;20(3):453–67.
15. Racine SX, Solis A, Hamou NA, Letoumelin P, Hepner DL, Beloucif S, et al. Face mask ventilation in edentulous patients: a comparison of mandibular groove and lower lip placement. Anesthesiology. 2010;112(5):1190–3.
16. Hite RD. Mechanical ventilation in restrictive lung disease. In: A practical guide to mechanical ventilation; 2011. p. 173–94.
17. Zafeiriou DI, Tsikoulas IG, Kremenopoulos GM. Prospective follow-up of primitive reflex profiles in high-risk infants: clues to an early diagnosis of cerebral palsy. Pediatr Neurol. 1995;13(2):148–52.

18. Boychuck Z, Andersen J, Bussières A, Fehlings D, Kirton A, Li P, et al. International expert recommendations of clinical features to prompt referral for diagnostic assessment of cerebral palsy. Dev Med Child Neurol. 2020;62(1):89–96.
19. Leach EL, Shevell M, Bowden K, Stockler-Ipsiroglu S, van Karnebeek CDM. Treatable inborn errors of metabolism presenting as cerebral palsy mimics: systematic literature review. Orphanet J Rare Dis. 2014;9(1):197.
20. Paget S, Ostojic K, Goldsmith S, Nassar N, McIntyre S. Determinants of hospital-based health service utilization in cerebral palsy: a systematic review. Arch Phys Med Rehabil. 2022;103(8):1628–37.
21. Blackmore AM, Bear N, Blair E, Langdon K, Moshovis L, Steer K, et al. Predicting respiratory hospital admissions in young people with cerebral palsy. Arch Dis Child. 2018;103(12):1119–24.
22. Marpole R, Blackmore AM, Gibson N, Cooper MS, Langdon K, Wilson AC. Evaluation and management of respiratory illness in children with cerebral palsy. Front Pediatr. 2020;8:333.
23. Kürtül Çakar M, Cinel G. The respiratory problems of patients with cerebral palsy requiring hospitalization: reasons and solutions. Pediatr Pulmonol. 2021;56(6):1626–34.
24. Kontorinis G, Thevasagayam MS, Bateman ND. Airway obstruction in children with cerebral palsy: need for tracheostomy? Int J Pediatr Otorhinolaryngol. 2013;77(10):1647–50.
25. Gustave J, Shenoy A. Medical management of tracheostomy in the child with cerebral palsy. In: Miller F, Bachrach S, Lennon N, O'Neil ME, editors. Cerebral palsy. Cham: Springer; 2020. p. 937–48.
26. Meier JD, Valentine KJ, Hagedorn C, Hartling C, Gershan W, Muntz HR, et al. Emergency department use among children with tracheostomies: avoidable visits. J Pediatr Rehabil Med. 2015;8(2):105–11.
27. Schmidt R, Tsang C, Barth P. Surgical management of tracheostomies and tracheal diversion in children with cerebral palsy. In: Miller F, Bachrach S, Lennon N, O'Neil ME, editors. Cerebral palsy. Cham: Springer; 2020. p. 829–39.
28. Minsley M, Wrenn S. Long-term care of the tracheostomy patient from an outpatient nursing perspective. Orl-head Neck Nurs. 1996;14(4):18–22.
29. Vanner R, Bick E. Tracheal pressures during open suctioning. Anaesthesia. 2008;63(3):313–5.
30. Tenaillon A, Boiteau R, Perrin-Gachadoat D, Burdin M. Humidification and aspiration of the respiratory tract in patients with mechanical ventilation. Rev Prat. 1990;40(25):2315–9.
31. Young JS, Brady WJ, Kesser B, Mullins D. A novel method for replacement of the dislodged tracheostomy tube: the nasogastric tube "guidewire" technique. J Emerg Med. 1996;14(2):205–8.
32. Scalise P, Prunk SR, Healy D, Votto J. The incidence of tracheoarterial fistula in patients with chronic tracheostomy tubes: a retrospective study of 544 patients in a long-term care facility. Chest. 2005;128(6):3906–9.
33. Reed MF, Mathisen DJ. Tracheoesophageal fistula. Chest Surg Clin. 2003;13(2):271–89.
34. Brun FK, Fagertun VH, Larsen MH, Solberg MT. Comparison of Glasgow Coma Scale and Full Outline of UnResponsiveness score to assess the level of consciousness in patients admitted to intensive care units and emergency departments: a quantitative systematic review. Aust Crit Care. 2025;38(1):101057.
35. Kim YS, Won YJ, Jeong H, Lim BG, Kong MH, Lee IO. A comparison of Bispectral index and entropy during Sevoflurane anesthesia induction in children with and without Diplegic Cerebral palsy. Entropy. 2019;21(5):498.
36. Molteni E, Canas LS, Briand M-M, Estraneo A, Font CC, Formisano R, et al. Scoping review on the diagnosis, prognosis, and treatment of pediatric disorders of consciousness. Neurology. 2023;101(6):e581–e93.
37. Cooper MS, Mackay MT, Dagia C, Fahey MC, Howell KB, Reddihough D, et al. Epilepsy syndromes in cerebral palsy: varied, evolving and mostly self-limited. Brain. 2022;146(2):587–99.
38. Coppler PJ, Elmer J. Status epilepticus: a neurologic emergency. Crit Care Clin. 2023;39(1):87–102.
39. Kurz JE, Goldstein J. Status epilepticus in the pediatric emergency department. Clin Pediatr Emerg Med. 2015;16(1):37–47.

40. Reilly M, Liuzzo K, Blackmer AB. Pharmacological management of spasticity in children with cerebral palsy. J Pediatr Health Care. 2020;34(5):495–509.
41. Lumsden DE, Crowe B, Basu A, Amin S, Devlin A, DeAlwis Y, et al. Pharmacological management of abnormal tone and movement in cerebral palsy. Arch Dis Child. 2019;104(8):775–80.
42. Vande Velde S, Van Renterghem K, Van Winckel M, De Bruyne R, Van Biervliet S. Constipation and fecal incontinence in children with cerebral palsy: overview of literature and flowchart for a stepwise approach. Acta Gastro-Enterol Belg. 2018;81(3):415–8.
43. Del Giudice E, Staiano A, Capano G, Romano A, Florimonte L, Miele E, et al. Gastrointestinal manifestations in children with cerebral palsy. Brain Dev. 1999;21(5):307–11.
44. Aboelmaaty SA, Gomaa IA, Pachon MEP, Rumer KK. Surgical abdominal emergencies among patients with cerebral palsy: a case report and review article. World J Colorectal Surg. 2024;13(2):54–7.
45. Wong A-L, Meehan E, Babl FE, Reid SM, Catto-Smith A, Williams K, et al. Paediatric emergency department presentations due to feeding tube complications in children with cerebral palsy. J Paediatr Child Health. 2019;55(10):1230–6.
46. Bruckstein AH. Managing the percutaneous endoscopic gastrostomy tube. Postgrad Med. 1987;82(3):143–6.
47. Torosian MH. Feeding by tube enterostomy. Surg Gynecol Obstet. 1980;150:918–27.
48. Korula J, Harma C. A simple and inexpensive method of removal or replacement of gastrostomy tubes. JAMA. 1991;265(11):1426–8.
49. Cornwell LB, Ewing E, Algra J, Chiang GJ. Acute urinary retention in pediatric cerebral palsy: is there an optimal management strategy? J Pediatr Urol. 2021;17(4):527.e1–7.
50. Vinkel MN, Rackauskaite G, Finnerup NB. Classification of pain in children with cerebral palsy. Dev Med Child Neurol. 2022;64(4):447–52.
51. Rabach I, Peri F, Minute M, Aru E, Lucafò M, Di Mascio A, et al. Sedation and analgesia in children with cerebral palsy: a narrative review. World J Pediatr. 2019;15(5):432–40.

Ethical Considerations in Cerebral Palsy 18

Maryam Modabber, Alireza Parsapour, and Ehsan Shamsi Gooshki

18.1 Introduction

Neurology, particularly in the context of caring for individuals with cerebral palsy (CP), is increasingly confronted with a wide range of complex ethical challenges. With a prevalence of approximately 1 in 500 live births and an estimated 17 million people affected worldwide, CP is the most common cause of physical disability in children [1, 2]. The *World Health Organization (WHO)*, in collaboration with the *Global Burden of Disease Study (GBD)* estimated that approximately 1.2% of children under 5 years of age (≈12 per 1000) are living with CP, with more than 90% of the cases occurring in low- and middle-income countries (LMICs), compared to a prevalence of about 0.6% (5.8 per 1000) in high-income settings [3, 4]. These geographic and economic disparities reflect inequities in social determinants of health, risk factors as well as in access to preventive and rehabilitative care [5].

CP encompasses a broad clinical spectrum, ranging from relatively mild motor impairments to complex, multi-dimensional limitations in mobility, speech, cognition, and development [6]. The condition could impose not only a heavy physical health burden but also profound and long-lasting psychological, social, and financial strains on affected individuals, families, and communities. Economic analyses reveal that direct medical expenses account for only part of this burden; indirect and non-medical costs, such as caregiving, transportation, home adaptation, and assistive devices, represent a significant share [7]. A global systematic review on the

M. Modabber · A. Parsapour
Medical Ethics and History of Medicine Research Center, Tehran University of Medical Sciences, Tehran, Iran

E. Shamsi Gooshki
Monash Bioethics Center, Monash University, Melbourne, VIC, Australia
e-mail: Ehsan.shamsigooshki@monash.edu

A. Presedo et al. (eds.), *Enhancing Quality of Life in Patients with Cerebral Palsy*, https://doi.org/10.1007/978-3-032-20967-2_18

economic burden of cerebral palsy found that healthcare costs for children with CP were 10–26 times greater than those for typically developing children, and expenses increased proportionally with the severity of gross motor impairment [8]. For instance, a study in Spain found that the mean annual societal cost per child with cerebral palsy was €102,135, with caregiver productivity losses accounting for 59.37% (€60,638), special education costs 8.75% (€8932), out-of-pocket expenses 6.89% (€7041), and medical care costs 3.72% (€3801) [9]. Consequently, the economic burden of CP and the complexity of its clinical needs frequently place decision-making at the intersection of ethics and resource allocation.

Since CP begins at birth and persists throughout a person's entire lifespan, it is considered a chronic condition. Its long-term nature affects and involves a wide range of stakeholders, including patients, families including other siblings, social support systems, healthcare facilities, and healthcare professionals. Individuals with CP face lifelong challenges influenced by the disabilities as the result of the neurological deficit, the wide range of physical and mental manifestations of the disease dependent on the characteristics of neurological damage, ongoing therapeutic and rehabilitation needs and shifting demands across the life course, from childhood to adulthood and old age and complex socio-economic and cultural factors that influences them. The ethical challenges around CP are shaped in this complex and multilateral environment where moral rights and responsibilities of different players contribute to creating a wide range of different ethical challenges in both clinical research and healthcare from theoretical and applied points of views. These complexities are mostly rooted in social and ethical debates around disability, vulnerability, the quality of life of CP patients and their caregivers, broader equity-based concerns and sensitive end-of-life decisions in some CP Cases, such as whether or not to initiate CPR, in a context of imbalanced power dynamics among main role players. Therefore, the challenges could include examples such as limitations in expressing autonomy, ambiguities in informed consent in borderline cases, marginalization, neglect or abuse of CP patients. Other factors such as progressive development of medical technologies such as brain-computer interface boosted by introduction of artificial intelligence (AI), declining level of public trust toward healthcare system reinforced by misinformation and disinformation widely populated by social media makes these challenges more difficult to be addressed. Specifically, the advent of novel technologies (e.g., experimental Stem Cell interventions) and related clinical research raises new questions about the ethical methodology of trials and the protection of vulnerable participants [10]. Recent scholarship has explicitly examined these evolving ethical implications within changing scientific and social landscapes. On the other hand, chronic nature of this medical condition makes the long-lasting patient–professional relationship vulnerable. The increasing number of legal lawsuits against physicians, high prevalence of defensive [11] and unnecessary medical practices out of fear of legal litigations and vulnerability of families to various therapeutic claims by traditional healers, complementary medicine practices and even new technology developers makes the situation more complicated.

The complex interaction of clinical, social, and economic factors in CP, combined with its lifelong impact and global disparities in care, gives rise to a range of ethical challenges that require careful and thoughtful consideration. Addressing these challenges calls for nuanced decision-making by patients, families, and healthcare providers alike. When ethical dilemmas cannot be easily resolved, seeking formal clinical ethics consultation or support from clinical ethics support services such as trained clinical ethicists, clinical ethics response groups and clinical ethics committees or even seeking can help clarify options and reduce the moral distress experienced by all parties involved. In settings without an established ethics committee, seeking informal advice by consulting experienced healthcare professionals can offer valuable guidance. For centers that care for a large number of children with CP, developing specialized clinical ethics services may be especially beneficial to address recurring and complex ethical issues. The following sections will discuss these dilemmas in greater depth, exploring how they arise in different contexts and their implications for stakeholders in both clinical practice and research.

18.2 Ethical Considerations in the Clinical Care of Cerebral Palsy

18.2.1 Active Participation in Treatment Decisions

Informed consent (IC) is a cornerstone of care for individuals with CP, underpinned by the principle of respect for autonomy and plays an important role in shaping patient–physician relationship. Despite the ethical necessity and significance IC enjoys a global acceptance from an ethical perspective and is supported by some influential international documents such as those introduced by the *World Medical Association (WMA)* and local laws, its practice is widely influenced by contextual factors such as those related to the role of families specifically in relation to patients with limited physical or mental abilities [12]. The capacity to provide valid IC requires the ability to comprehend and retain information, engage in reciprocal questioning, evaluate relevant details, and justify a decision. Importantly, the process of IC should not be reduced to an administrative formality; rather, it represents an opportunity to build a strong bridge of collaboration between the individual, families and the care team. When a patient has decisional capacity, family involvement may be valuable given their role as caregivers, but such involvement must remain aligned with the patient's best interests and autonomy. Excluding competent patients with cerebral palsy from decision-making—whether by overemphasizing the role of families or by invoking cultural diversity as justification—is ethically unacceptable. This concern is particularly relevant in countries with more family-centered cultures and in situations involving vulnerable groups, such as women in certain cultural contexts, where the patient's voice may be at greater risk of being marginalized.

However, some individuals with CP may face cognitive or communicative challenges that complicate decision-making. Participation in this process is not only a legal and ethical right but also a commitment emphasized in international instruments such as the *Convention on the Rights of Persons with Disabilities (CRPD)* [13]. According to this framework, all persons with disabilities—including those requiring "greater intellectual support"—have the right to express themselves freely, make choices, and play an active role in decisions affecting their lives. While cognitive impairments may hinder full understanding of complexities or consequences, this does not warrant the complete withdrawal of participation in ones' medical decisions; rather, it calls for *supported decision-making* [14, 15]. Such an approach necessitates careful assessment of decision-making capacity, using standardized tools such as the *MacArthur Competence Assessment Tool for Clinical Research (MacCAT-CR)* when necessary including for borderline cases [16], or structured clinical interviews [17]. Supplementary strategies, including presenting information in simplified language [17, 18], *employing augmentative and alternative communication (AAC)* systems [19], and consulting other professionals while prioritizing the individual's expressed preferences, can facilitate this process.

In cases of moderate-to-severe cognitive impairment, *surrogate consent* is provided by parents or legal guardians. Nevertheless, ethical principles emphasize the importance of seeking the patient's *assent*, even when expressed nonverbally—through emotional cues or gestures [20]. Failure to uphold these principles can result in *healthcare-related trauma*, eroding trust in medical systems and leading to treatment non-compliance and even withdrawal [21]. To address these challenges, multi-step consent protocols, visual tools such as infographics or educational videos [22], and multidisciplinary consultation sessions with psychiatrists, psychologists and social workers are recommended. These approaches, particularly when adapted to the unique needs of children and adolescents, help prevent marginalization and safeguard dignity [23].

A common misconception among both the public and healthcare professionals is the assumption that all individuals with CP experience cognitive impairment. This bias stems from limited awareness of the heterogeneous nature of CP, where some individuals present solely with motor impairments while retaining intact cognitive and emotional capacities. Evidence shows that approximately 45% of children with CP have an intellectual disability (IQ < 70), whereas the remainder range from typical cognition to mild or moderate impairments [24]. Negative preconceptions—often operating as *stigma*—can originate from society, families, or healthcare providers. Beliefs that individuals with CP are incapable of independent decision-making or require lifelong support foster discrimination, social exclusion, and diminished self-esteem. Qualitative studies among adults with CP reveal frequent experiences of belittlement and underestimation of their capacities, limiting participation in professional and social domains [25]. Beyond stigma and discrimination, *ableism* [26] perpetuates marginalization by disregarding potential capabilities and denying opportunities for independent decision-making.

To counter these barriers, it is essential to acknowledge the full *spectrum of CP*, which encompasses spastic, dyskinetic, ataxic, and mixed subtypes—each with distinct motor and cognitive profiles. Individualized cognitive assessments, using standardized tests such as WISC or WAIS [27], particularly motor-free or motor-adapted versions, are crucial to avoid unwarranted generalizations. Educational programs for healthcare professionals and the public on effective communication with individuals with CP can reduce stigma [25], supported by campaigns that highlight abilities rather than limitations.

Furthermore, each individual with CP should be recognized as a human being with intrinsic worth and unique capacities—not merely as a "patient" or "disabled person." This perspective is reinforced through inclusive policies and social support systems. Article 3 of the CRPD specifically underscores respect for the dignity of individuals with CP, advocating their active involvement in decision-making, equitable access to healthcare and education, and efforts to reduce stigma. Collectively, these measures enhance quality of life and mental well-being [28].

Sometimes disagreements arise between parents and physicians when parental decisions are not aligned with the patient's best interests as understood through objective medical knowledge. Parents are generally recognized as the primary surrogate decision-makers for their children, and their subjective understanding of what serves the child's best interest is usually respected. However, the scope of parental discretion in medical decision-making is not absolute [29]. When healthcare providers judge that a parental decision exposes a child with cerebral palsy to an unjustified risk of harm, various strategies may be employed to address the challenge. Often, seemingly unacceptable decisions—such as refusing beneficial interventions—stem from a lack of accurate understanding about the nature, necessity, or risks of a procedure. For example, in some clinical settings parents may be reluctant to consent to a lumbar puncture due to misinformation or disinformation. In such cases, disputes can often be resolved through deeper communication and empathetic dialogue. In more serious situations, however, further steps such as seeking a court order may be necessary.

18.2.2 Palliative and Rehabilitative Care

As previously discussed, CP is a heterogeneous condition in which the degree of disability ranges from minimal to severe. Palliative care for individuals with CP encompasses a set of interventions aimed at alleviating symptoms and enhancing the quality of life for both the patient and their family. Its primary goal is to manage distressing symptoms and ensure comfort, even when curative treatments are no longer feasible [30]. Palliative care thus addresses the physical, psychosocial, and spiritual dimensions of life for individuals with life-limiting conditions [31].

With the increasing life expectancy of individuals with CP, the need for palliative care in adulthood has become more pronounced. Adults with CP frequently encounter secondary health complications, including chronic pain, degenerative arthritis and osteoporosis. These conditions significantly impact quality of life, underscoring the importance of comprehensive strategies for symptom relief and pain management [32]. Contrary to the common misconception, palliative care is not restricted to the terminal stage of illness. Early identification of palliative needs from the time of diagnosis is critical [33]. An integrated approach strengthens both the individual's quality of life and the family's support system [34].

Several tools have been developed to better identify palliative care needs, such as the *Edmonton Symptom Assessment Scale (ESAS)* and the *Paediatric Palliative Screening Scale (PaPaS)* [30].

Effective palliative care for individuals with CP must be personalized, adaptable to disease progression, and built upon a multidisciplinary framework involving physicians, nurses, psychologists, occupational therapists, and physiotherapists [34, 35]. A comprehensive treatment plan may include physiotherapy, speech therapy, and pharmacological interventions for spasticity, as well as non-pharmacological strategies such as neurotherapy, biofeedback, and orthopedic support [34, 36, 37]. Central to this approach is ensuring patient well-being, improving quality of life, and supporting family members. Family involvement in palliative and rehabilitative planning is therefore of critical importance [38].

Despite its value, palliative care for individuals with CP faces significant challenges. A key barrier is the shortage of professionals with sufficient knowledge and commitment to serving this population. Pediatricians are often more familiar with treating children, while adult healthcare providers may lack expertise in CP, reducing their confidence in delivering appropriate care [39]. Additionally, the transition from a generally comprehensive pediatric services to more speciality-oriented adult healthcare creates a "*care gap*" with serious consequences. This transition may be accompanied by instability in housing, unemployment, or reduced access to rehabilitation services [40]. Furthermore, limited resources—including restricted budgets, shortages of trained personnel, and the absence of multidisciplinary adult care teams—remain major obstacles to providing high-quality, holistic care [41].

18.2.3 End-of-Life Decision-Making

End-of-life decision-making, particularly for individuals with severe disabilities, requires nuanced discussions with the patient and family, respect for autonomy (where cognitive capacity is intact), and careful consideration of the patient's best interests [42]. When cognitive impairment is present, the process of obtaining IC becomes more complex and may necessitate the involvement of legal guardians or family members [43]. In such cases, surrogate decision-makers must act in alignment with the patient's best interests, guided by ethical and medical principles. Key considerations include preserving dignity, reducing suffering, and evaluating quality of life [44].

Early and open conversations regarding values, goals, and preferences for end-of-life care—often referred to as *advance care planning*—are essential, even in the absence of acute illness [45]. These discussions allow patients and families to articulate their wills and document their future medical decisions. In pediatric contexts, factors such as the availability and appropriateness of palliative services, parental capacity to provide care, and the well-being of siblings play important roles in shaping decisions about the type and setting of end-of-life care [46].

A major challenge in end-of-life decisions for individuals with CP is the persistence of biases within the medical community. Healthcare providers may underestimate the actual quality of life of individuals with disabilities, sometimes equating CP with terminal illness or undervaluing their capacities [37, 47]. Such perspectives can lead to recommendations for withdrawing life-sustaining treatment, despite the absence of clear evidence that such actions align with the patient's values or best interests. Erroneous assumptions about quality of life, such as viewing disability through a catastrophic or deficit-based lens, constitute one of the most pervasive biases [48–50]. Cognitive and emotional biases—including misplaced pity, fatalistic attitudes, or implicit prejudices—may further distort decision-making and override the individual's own values and desires [51].

Limiting patient and family involvement in these decisions, or disproportionately deferring to family members' judgments of quality of life, are also common challenges [52]. In addition, "futility policies" and reliance on subjective judgments of quality of life can inadvertently redirect care towards palliative measures, contrary to the preferences of patients themselves [47]. Insufficient training of healthcare professionals, avoidance of end-of-life discussions due to discomfort with mortality, and communication barriers exacerbate these difficulties [53, 54].

Addressing these challenges requires raising awareness, providing ongoing professional education, and adopting patient-centered approaches that prioritize individual values and preferences [55]. Such measures are critical to ensuring ethical and equitable care for individuals with CP throughout their lives and at the end of life.

Multidisciplinary teams—including physicians, nurses, social workers, psychologists, and palliative care specialists—play a pivotal role in supporting patients and families during this process [56]. By offering comprehensive information, facilitating difficult conversations, and coordinating care, they ensure that decision-making is both ethically sound and empathetically delivered. Effective and compassionate communication with families about prognosis, treatment options, and support is particularly vital when the patient lacks decision-making capacity [45, 56].

18.3 Ethical Considerations in Research Involving Patients with Cerebral Palsy

Ethical concerns in research involving individuals with disabilities and cognitive impairments, including CP, represent a complex and multifaceted domain. These issues arise from the inherent vulnerability of these populations, the unique dynamics within their families, and widespread misconceptions regarding potential treatments [57]. Consequently, such research requires careful attention to participants' rights, dignity, and overall well-being [58]. A central challenge lies in balancing the advancement of scientific knowledge with the obligation to safeguard vulnerable populations. Ultimately, the primary objective must be to ensure ethical participation—facilitating valuable knowledge generation while simultaneously protecting participants' autonomy and minimizing their exposure to harm [59].

People with disabilities, particularly those with cognitive impairments, are usually classified as a vulnerable population due to factors such as reduced decision-making capacity in some cases, power imbalances with researchers, and heightened susceptibility to manipulation, coercion or undue influence. Research Ethics Committees and investigators share the responsibility of protecting these participants' rights and welfare. Respect for persons dictates that all individuals must be regarded as autonomous agents -unless clear evidence proves othrewise-, while those with limited autonomy are entitled to additional safeguards. Such safeguards encompass preventing exploitation, protecting privacy and confidentiality, ensuring fair participant selection, minimizing risks, and maximizing benefits [59]. In practice, however, the absence of consensus on ethical approaches and the lack of clear guidelines for conducting research with these populations often generate considerable challenges [60].

Families of individuals with CP are frequently placed in vulnerable positions due to psychological, social, and financial pressures. These conditions may compromise their ability to critically evaluate treatment and research options, potentially driving them toward decisions based on inadequate information or unrealistic expectations. Consequently, families may be more susceptible to manipulation and exploitation, particularly in the context of treatment decisions and research participation. For example, some actors may exploit parents' desperation by offering overly optimistic portrayals of interventions or by perpetuating "therapeutic misconception," steering families toward unproven treatments or inappropriate studies. Parents themselves may also request unvalidated interventions out of hope for improvement. To prevent therapeutic misconception, it is essential that both the individual and their family clearly understand that the defining purpose of clinical research is to generate generalizable knowledge, not to guarantee direct therapeutic benefit. Researchers must explicitly communicate that studies may involve placebo controls or non-therapeutic interventions, and that participation is designed to advance future treatment options for others rather than assure benefit to the participant [57, 61]. These realities highlight the critical need for comprehensive support to empower families in making informed and independent decisions.

Misinterpretation of information can lead to poor parental decisions that not only waste financial resources but also delay access to effective therapies and may even harm the child. Physicians and therapists play a central role in providing accurate information and supporting families throughout this process. Clinicians must communicate the truth regarding diagnosis, prognosis, and potential treatment outcomes with sensitivity, patience, and an awareness of families' emotional states. Delivering a prognosis that is realistic yet not entirely discouraging—while simultaneously motivating families to work toward improving the child's condition—can be a valuable strategy. The goal is to help families remain realistic without losing hope. Furthermore, clinicians and researchers must warn families about misleading claims made by profit-driven actors and support them in critically interpreting available information. Examples include hyperbaric oxygen therapy and stem cell interventions, both of which remain under investigation and must be approached with caution. Although studies have examined community perceptions of stem cell therapy for CP, substantial ethical concerns and methodological risks remain unresolved [57, 61].

Clinical trials involving patients with CP—especially those with cognitive impairments—often compromise the individual's capacity to provide valid IC. Patients with cognitive impairments may be unable to fully comprehend research procedures, associated risks and benefits, or the implications of participation. However, it is vital that even such participants be involved in the decision-making process as much as their capacity permits. Information such asthe study's purpose, the intended use of collected data, and their right to withdraw at any stage should be tailored to their level of capacity for understanding such information. For example such information should be presented in simple, accessible language [62]. The 'Subjective' standard for nature, details and amount of of information disclosed to participants is the acceptable disclosure standard compared with other disclosure standards such as 'reasonable patient' standards. The concept of "consent-as-process" underscores the importance of ongoing assessment of capacity and comprehension over time [63]. In cases where participants cannot provide full consent, obtaining consent from an authorized legal representative (such as a parent or guardian) becomes necessary. Given that parents themselves may be vulnerable to false hopes, researchers must ensure that their consent is genuinely informed and that they fully understand the differences between clinical care and research participation [57, 61]. Research Ethics Committees - known as Institutional Review Boards (IRBs) in some countries- play a critical role in reviewing study protocols to guarantee adequate protections for these participants [64].

Qualitative research with individuals with CP—particularly interviews—raises additional ethical considerations requiring sensitive and adaptive approaches. The goal of such methods is to amplify participants' voices and capture their lived experiences, perspectives that have historically been overlooked or articulated on their behalf by others [65]. Individuals with disabilities, particularly those with cognitive or speech impairments, often encounter substantial barriers to verbal communication. These barriers can complicate interviews and may even exclude participants from research altogether, as some investigators perceive them as "impossible" to interview. To overcome this, researchers must employ flexible and creative strategies to enable meaningful participation. This may include responsive communication techniques tailored to the individual's needs, involvement of family members or caregivers as intermediaries, and the use of visual tools such as pictures or diagrams to simplify concepts and facilitate expression. Additionally, conducting "walk-along" interviews in familiar environments [65], or using email-based interviews, when possible, as alternatives to face-to-face conversations can expand accessibility [66]. Open-ended, indirect questioning may also help participants express their views more freely. Attention to power dynamics is essential; adopting a non-directive, participatory approach allows individuals to act not merely as respondents but as experts in their own lives. At the same time, dual roles (e.g., clinician-researcher) should be avoided as they may blur ethical boundaries [67].

Maintaining confidentiality and data security in qualitative research with individuals with CP is of paramount importance, given their heightened vulnerability to breaches of privacy. Researchers must establish rigorous data management protocols to protect participants' identities [62].

Ultimately, research involving individuals with disabilities and cognitive impairments demands a deep commitment to ethical principles and innovative methodologies. Despite the challenges, such studies are essential for advancing knowledge and improving the lives of these populations. By ensuring robust IC, safeguarding vulnerable participants, employing adaptive strategies, and conducting continuous ethical evaluation, we can guarantee that their voices are heard and that their participation in research is both meaningful and morally sound.

18.4 Other Ethical Considerations

18.4.1 Social and Economic Challenges

Individuals with CP and their families face significant challenges within the public health landscape, necessitating attention to principles of justice, equitable access, and social support [68]. These challenges include unequal access to healthcare services, the impact of social and economic disparities, and the need for active community and family involvement in policy development. Health equity refers to the absence of avoidable health disparities, which can be addressed through reasonable means [69]. Social and economic inequalities profoundly influence the prevalence, severity, and health outcomes of Individuals with CP and their families. People with disabilities often encounter more barriers to healthcare access compared to non-disabled peers, frequently resulting in unmet needs [70].

Barriers include limited provider knowledge, physical inaccessibility, fragmented continuity of care, and difficulties transitioning from pediatric to adult services. For instance, adults with CP may struggle to find specialists experienced in managing adult CP, face a lack of continuous care, and lose long-standing relationships with pediatric providers [71, 72].

Addressing these challenges requires meaningful community and family participation in the development, implementation, and evaluation of health services, particularly for individuals with disabilities. Such engagement can improve health outcomes, promote equity, enhance service access, communication, acceptability, quality, and accountability. Community involvement is recognized as a core principle in primary healthcare and is strongly associated with improved health outcomes [73].

Caring for Individuals with severe CP raises fundamental questions about the purpose of medical interventions, extending beyond physiological mechanisms to encompass social and humanistic considerations [74]. Perhaps the most pressing challenge is the considerable financial and emotional burden on families [75], which can negatively affect overall family quality of life and psychosocial well-being, making it a public health concern. The economic impact extends beyond direct medical costs (medications, rehabilitation, assistive devices, specialized care) to indirect costs such as lost income and diminished quality of life for parents and unaffected siblings. For example, in China, the estimated annual economic burden per CP case is approximately 4,188,500 yuan, with the majority (around 3,982,700 yuan) being indirect costs [76]. In Denmark, lifetime costs of CP are estimated at roughly 860,000 euros for men and 800,000 euros for women, largely attributable to social care, especially during childhood [77]. Higher costs are associated with increased motor impairment (as classified by the Gross Motor Function Classification System, GMFCS) and comorbidities [78]. In the United States, lifetime costs for individuals born with CP in 2000 were estimated at $11.5 billion in 2003 [79], including both direct medical expenses and indirect costs, primarily for rehabilitation and home care. In resource-limited settings, healthcare costs may be prohibitively high, disrupting caregivers' social and economic participation [80]. Strong social support and coping strategies among caregivers positively impact life satisfaction and resilience to caregiving stress [81]. Families with children with CP also face additional daily expenses related to housing adaptations, accessible transportation, and higher utility usage [82].

18.4.2 Impact on Healthy Siblings

Living with a sibling affected by CP can have significant psychological, social, and emotional consequences for siblings without disabilities. Studies indicate that the presence of a child with CP influences parent–sibling relationships among typically developing children [83]. In other words, sometimes parental attention may prioritize the child with CP, leaving siblings with less guidance and support. Typically developing siblings often must assume greater independence early in life, as they navigate daily responsibilities with limited parental oversight. Given the intensive caregiving demands for the child with CP, these siblings frequently have minimal time to express their needs or share experiences with parents [84].

Research shows that parents' primary focus is often on the child with a disability, sometimes resulting in some levels of neglect of other children and contributing to behavioral problems, including aggression, delinquent behavior [85], anxiety and depression [86], social stigma, fear about the future, anger, and excessive responsibility among siblings without CP [87]. Most studies are from high-income countries with social support structures for children with CP; low- and middle-income countries, despite relatively high prevalence, often provide limited data in this regard [88].

Family dynamics shift in the presence of a child with CP. Limitations on family social and recreational activities may contribute to social isolation, affecting siblings without CP. Older siblings often reach psychological maturity earlier and assume heavier responsibilities. Parental interventions—particularly by mothers—are typically more intensive in sibling interactions, especially when children are younger and social skills are still developing. This may restrict autonomy and freedom for unaffected siblings. Over the long term, siblings may assume lifelong caregiving roles, particularly as parents age or lose capacity. These responsibilities, while rooted in familial commitment and emotional bonds, impose significant personal burdens [89].

Given these outcomes, support for siblings of children with CP is crucial. Early interventions to identify challenges and provide psychosocial assistance can improve overall family quality of life. Education and awareness from neurologists, peadiatricians, physiotherapists and other professionals play a key role. Understanding CP, stress management techniques, and coping strategies help siblings adapt. Encouraging active participation in care planning and shared family activities not only strengthens sibling bonds but also supports the independence and development of the child with CP [90].

18.4.3 Abuse and Neglect of Individuals with Cerebral Palsy

Children with CP are at a higher risk of various forms of abuse, particularly neglect [81]. Children with CP often have severe physical limitations that make routine tasks like feeding, bathing, and mobility dependent on caregivers [91]. Factors such as parental stress, caregiver vulnerabilities, and poor adult-child interactions can exacerbate this risk [92]. In some cases, low family socioeconomic status further increases the likelihood of neglect and abuse [93].

Neglect can have wide-ranging negative consequences. Physically, lack of proper care can worsen functional limitations [94]—for instance, inadequate access to physiotherapy, occupational therapy, or speech therapy may accelerate muscle contractures, weaken muscles, impair mobility, and delay cognitive and communication skill development. Nutritional neglect can result in malnutrition, underweight, or obesity, all of which compromise health and increase vulnerability to secondary illnesses [95, 96]. Poor hygiene may lead to recurrent skin infections, pressure sores, and dental problems, requiring complex and costly medical interventions.

Cognitively and emotionally, neglect can significantly impair development. Insufficient attention to educational and supportive needs may delay cognitive growth, hinder learning, and reduce academic achievement. Social interactions and exposure to educational opportunities, critical for full development, may be limited. Emotional neglect, including inadequate affection, attention, or support, can lead to depression, anxiety, low self-esteem, and behavioral issues. These problems may hinder social communication, participation in community activities, and independence [97].

Socially, neglected children may struggle to form healthy, stable relationships with peers and adults, feeling isolated or rejected, which negatively affects overall quality of life [98]. Such neglect perpetuates cycles of health and social inequities, placing additional burdens on healthcare and social support systems. Another important consideration is that in some contexts children with motor impairments, especially in inclusive school settings, are often placed alongside peers with cognitive disabilities. This close interaction can create complex challenges for their motor, social, and emotional development. For these reasons, early identification and well-designed interventions are essential to support the overall health and well-being of children and adolescents with CP.

In high-income countries, concerns about child abuse or neglect usually involve social services [99]. However, in resource-limited settings, low-quality social services pose serious challenges [99, 100], including shortages of trained personnel, cultural barriers, and limited service availability.

Beyond environmental factors, individuals with CP may experience social marginalization even within their families, despite having cognitive capacity. Causes include lack of public awareness about the diversity of CP, poor understanding of how to communicate with people with disabilities, inaccessible environments, and societal prejudice toward visible physical impairments [25]. Experiencing discrimination and rejection from family and community members can adversely affect health and well-being. Negative attitudes often stem from myths and misinformation. Psychosocial support through family counseling and education can challenge misconceptions and improve social inclusion [101].

18.4.4 Pregnancy and Childbirth Challenges in Individuals with Cerebral Palsy

Pregnancy and childbirth in women with CP present a broad range of challenges, beginning with issues related to menstrual health. Managing menstruation in adolescent and young women with CP can be particularly difficult. Beyond the physical aspects, assistance from caregivers in personal hygiene can intensify privacy concerns [102]. Many parents report lacking sufficient knowledge about available menstrual management options, and even pediatricians may not adequately address this topic [103].

Although some studies indicate that women with CP may experience less severe menstrual symptoms [104], discomfort can be amplified and may interfere with functional abilities [105]. Early puberty is also observed in some patients with CP [106], which not only increases the physical burden but also adds psychological and social stress on families, especially in cases of severe disability [107]. Other relevant issues include poor genital hygiene [104], increased seizure frequency in women with coexisting epilepsy during menstruation [108], and limited sexual health education [103]. Timely intervention and education at this stage are therefore crucial.

Pregnancy itself introduces additional complexities. Functional abilities may decline during pregnancy, including decreased muscle strength, increased spasticity, bladder dysfunction, and severe fatigue. Many women require new assistive devices to manage pain, prevent falls, and maintain daily independence—even those who were previously mobile without assistance [109]. These changes directly impact quality of life and autonomy.

Women with CP are also at a higher risk for adverse pregnancy outcomes. Preterm birth is among the most common complications, along with increased likelihood of cesarean delivery, labor induction, low Apgar scores in newborns, abnormal fetal growth, and, in some cases, stillbirth [107]. Addressing these challenges necessitates specialized, multidisciplinary care. Key aspects include educating women and their families, boosting maternal confidence in newborn care, and empowering women to manage personal needs independently. Research shows that careful preconception planning and active involvement of specialists familiar with disability care significantly improve outcomes and reduce risks [110].

18.4.5 Hysterectomy in Individuals with Cerebral Palsy

Hysterectomy is performed to treat a variety of conditions, including uterine fibroids, refractory bleeding, uterine prolapse, endometriosis, and malignancies. However, non-therapeutic hysterectomy in women with intellectual or developmental disabilities happens, despite global efforts to align their rights with the principles of the Universal Declaration of Human Rights [111]. Demographic data indicate that certain groups of women with disabilities undergo hysterectomy at higher rates than women without disabilities, often at younger ages [112, 113]. Precise statistics specifically for women with CP are limited, with most evidence coming from case reports, small patient cohorts [112], or ethical and legal discussions.

Clinical guidelines emphasize that hysterectomy should only be considered when less invasive options—such as pharmacologic interventions for menstrual suppression or regulation (e.g., combined oral contraceptives, progestins, intrauterine devices, or endometrial ablation)—are ineffective or unsuitable. Hysterectomy is recognized as a "final intervention," with significant long-term consequences, and should never be the first-line option unless medically necessary [114].

Nevertheless, some care systems and countries report non-therapeutic hysterectomies in women with developmental or intellectual disabilities [111], which raises serious ethical and legal concerns. Clinically, the reasons for hysterectomy in women with CP are generally similar to the general population. However, unique considerations in this group include difficulties managing menstrual hygiene or cooperating with contraception due to physical or cognitive limitations. Families or care teams in some cases may consider surgery if the individual cannot independently manage menstruation or if her physical condition complicates menstrual care.

The ethical dimension of this issue is critical. Historical cases of sterilization or non-consensual surgeries in women with intellectual or physical disabilities have created heightened sensitivity. From a medical ethics and human rights perspective, any request for hysterectomy in a person with a disability must undergo rigorous review and extensive ethics evaluation and consultation. This includes examining whether the patient can provide IC, whether there are tangible benefits for the individual herself (not solely for caregivers or family), and whether all alternatives have been fully considered [115].

Whenever possible, the individual should actively participate in decision-making, with the use of assistive communication tools if needed. If the patient cannot assess or decide for herself, final decisions should involve a multidisciplinary team, a clear legal representative, and, if necessary, review by an ethics committee or judicial body [116]. Transparency in documenting the reasons, considered options, and rationale for excluding alternatives, along with recording actual benefits and burdens for the patient, is fundamental to ethical practice [117].

18.4.6 Challenges of Pseudoscience and Complementary Medicine in Cerebral Palsy

Alongside the various physical, psychological, social, emotional, and financial challenges faced by individuals with CP, family acceptance plays a critical role in navigating these issues. While in some societies, family acceptance is influenced by the child's condition, parental optimism, and access to healthcare and educational services, in other societies, cultural beliefs, stigma, prejudice, and discrimination strongly affect family acceptance [118].

Families often have strong beliefs in the benefits of complementary therapies and show a high commitment to exploring any intervention that could help their child. However, parental knowledge about the range and potential applications of complementary and alternative medicine (CAM) is often limited. Concerns exist regarding safety, efficacy, practical challenges such as cost and time, and unknown side effects [119].

The use of CAM presents multiple ethical dilemmas for healthcare providers, particularly when patients integrate these treatments into their care. The lack of robust research on most of CAM methods, combined with its increasing popularity and the provider's ethical obligation to consider patient preferences, creates a complex ethical situation. Providers must be aware of existing CAM interventions, the quality of supporting evidence (efficacy), potential risks or adverse effects (non-maleficence), and ensure equitable access to care that may benefit each individual with CP [120].

Additionally, healthcare providers should cultivate a close, trusting relationship with patients, remaining open to the potential insights CAM may offer into clinical practice, while actively emphasis the significance of scientific evidence in accepting any therapeutic claims. They should transparently discuss such treatment options with families, highlighting the current state of knowledge regarding efficacy [121]. Parents want to help their child by any possible means and therefore could be vulnerable to unrealistic therapeutic claims that provide false hopes. To overcome such situations they require clear information, guidance, and practical support to make informed decisions about complementary therapies.

18.5 Conclusion

CP is more than just a motor or neurological disorder; it sits at the intersection of medicine, human rights, social justice, and ethics. The ethical challenges surrounding CP touch every aspect of life, affecting patients, families, and the professionals who care for them.

In the Clinical Care domain, it is crucial to recognize that CP exists on a spectrum rather than fitting a single stereotype. Respecting autonomy remains essential, even when cognitive impairments are present, and supported decision-making should guide choices instead of making decisions on behalf of the individual. Palliative care should be introduced at diagnosis, not only in the final stages of life, and conversations about end-of-life decisions must be handled sensitively, free of bias, and mindful of assumptions about quality of life.

In Research, the inherent vulnerability of individuals with CP and their families calls for careful planning when obtaining informed consent. Clear communication, transparency about the difference between research and therapy, and avoiding the promise of unproven treatments (for example, some experimental stem cell interventions) are ethical necessities. Research should prioritize the voices of individuals with CP, ensuring they can actively participate in shaping the studies that affect them.

In Public Health, the impact of CP extends beyond medical care, encompassing significant economic and psychosocial burdens on families. Inequities in access to services, especially during the transition from childhood to adulthood and in low- and middle-income countries, raise serious ethical concerns. Policies should be developed with the direct involvement of individuals with disabilities and their families, addressing issues like reproductive health, protection against abuse or neglect, and the well-being of siblings. Careful consideration of complementary and alternative therapies through education and transparent communication is also essential.

Ultimately, an ethical approach to CP requires moving beyond a purely medical perspective. Individuals with CP should be recognized first as human beings with dignity and rights, not just as patients. This chapter offers guidance for clinicians, researchers, and policymakers to improve care and advance knowledge while keeping the well-being, autonomy, and rights of individuals with CP and their families at the center. Achieving this vision depends on ongoing education to challenge biases, strengthening support systems, developing tailored ethical guidelines, and promoting research that genuinely includes the voices of those living with CP.

References

1. Surman G, Hemming K, Platt MJ, Parkes J, Green A, Hutton J, et al. Children with cerebral palsy: severity and trends over time. Paediatr Perinat Epidemiol. 2009;23:513–21.
2. Cerebral palsy. Nat Rev Dis Primers. 2016;2:15083. https://doi.org/10.1038/nrdp.2015.83.
3. Olusanya BO, Nair M, Boo NY, Davis AC, Hadders-Algra M, Wright SM. Cerebral palsy in young children: bridging the global data gap. Lancet Glob Health. 2025;13:e1663.
4. Olusanya BO, Gladstone M, Wright SM, Hadders-Algra M, Boo N-Y, Nair M, et al. Cerebral palsy and developmental intellectual disability in children younger than 5 years: findings from the GBD-WHO Rehabilitation Database 2019. Front Public Health. 2022;10:894546.
5. Oskoui M, Coutinho F, Dykeman J, Jetté N, Pringsheim T. An update on the prevalence of cerebral palsy: a systematic review and meta-analysis. Dev Med Child Neurol. 2013;55:509–19.
6. Patel DR, Neelakantan M, Pandher K, Merrick J. Cerebral palsy in children: a clinical overview. Transl Pediatr. 2020;9:S125–35. https://doi.org/10.21037/tp.2020.01.01.

7. Whitney DG, Kamdar NS, Ng S, Hurvitz EA, Peterson MD. Prevalence of high-burden medical conditions and health care resource utilization and costs among adults with cerebral palsy. Clin Epidemiol. 2019;11:469–81.
8. Shih ST, Tonmukayakul U, Imms C, Reddihough D, Graham HK, Cox L, et al. Economic evaluation and cost of interventions for cerebral palsy: a systematic review. Dev Med Child Neurol. 2018;60:543–58.
9. Nova Diaz DM, Arana Rivera P, Sánchez Iriso E, Aguilera-Albesa S. The economic and social burden of pediatric cerebral palsy in Spain: a cost-of-illness study. Front Public Health. 2025;13:1589114.
10. Dan B. New ethical issues in cerebral palsy. Front Neurol. 2021;12:650653.
11. Gooshki ES. Defensive medicine: a serious threat to Iran's healthcare system. Iran J Med Ethics Hist Med. 2025;17:7.
12. WMA – The World Medical Association. WMA declaration of Lisbon on the rights of the patient. n.d. https://www.wma.net/policies-post/wma-declaration-of-lisbon-on-the-rights-of-the-patient/. Accessed 28 Sept 2025.
13. Convention on the Rights of Persons with Disabilities (CRPD). 2006. https://chr-observatories.uwazi.io/en/entity. Accessed 28 Sept 2025.
14. OHCHR. Convention on the rights of persons with disabilities. Article 12 – equal recognition before the law. OHCHR. n.d. https://www.ohchr.org/en/instruments-mechanisms/instruments/convention-rights-persons-disabilities. Accessed 23 Sept 2025.
15. Weller P. Legal capacity and access to justice: the right to participation in the CRPD. Laws. 2016;5:13.
16. Appelbaum PS, Grisso T. MacArthur competence assessment tool for clinical research (MacCAT-CR). Professional Resource Press/Professional Resource Exchange; 2001.
17. Webb P, Davidson G, Edge R, Falls D, Keenan F, Kelly B, et al. Key components of supporting and assessing decision making ability. Int J Law Psychiatry. 2020;72:101613.
18. Peter M, Maddocks S, Tang C, Camp PG. Simplicity: using the power of plain language to encourage patient-centered communication. Phys Ther. 2024;104:pzad103.
19. Richlin BC, Chow K, Cosetti MK. Augmentative and alternative communication (AAC) in pediatric cochlear implant recipients with complex needs: a scoping review. Int J Pediatr Otorhinolaryngol. 2023;171:111610.
20. Van Goidsenhoven L, De Schauwer E. Relational ethics, informed consent, and informed assent in participatory research with children with complex communication needs. Dev Med Child Neurol. 2022;64:1323–9.
21. Selwyn CN, Lathan EC, Richie F, Gigler ME, Langhinrichsen-Rohling J. Bitten by the system that cared for them: towards a trauma-informed understanding of patients' healthcare engagement. J Trauma Dissociation. 2021;22:636–52.
22. Massetti T, Crocetta TB, Guarnieri R, da Silva TD, Leal AF, Voos MC, et al. A didactic approach to presenting verbal and visual information to children participating in research protocols: the comic book informed assent. Clinics (Sao Paulo). 2018;73:e207. https://doi.org/10.6061/clinics/2018/e207.
23. Thompson S, Cannon M, Wickenden M. Exploring critical issues in the ethical involvement of children with disabilities in evidence generation and use. UNICEF; 2020.
24. Yin Foo R, Guppy M, Johnston LM. Intelligence assessments for children with cerebral palsy: a systematic review. Dev Med Child Neurol. 2013;55:911–8.
25. Smith KJ, Burke J, Lawrence R, Oputa E, Bailey R. The experience of cerebral palsy stigma amongst adults living in the UK and Ireland: a qualitative co-designed project. PLoS One. 2025;20:e0331562.
26. Nario-Redmond MR, Kemerling AA, Silverman A. Hostile, benevolent, and ambivalent ableism: contemporary manifestations. J Soc Issues. 2019;75:726–56.
27. Coceski M, Hocking DR, Abu-Rayya HM, Sherwell S, Reid SM, Reddihough DS, et al. WISC-V motor-free cognitive profile and predictive factors in adolescents with cerebral palsy. Res Dev Disabil. 2021;113:103934.

28. OHCHR. Convention on the rights of persons with disabilities. Article 3 – general principles. OHCHR. 2006. https://www.ohchr.org/en/instruments-mechanisms/instruments/convention-rights-persons-disabilities. Accessed 23 Sept 2025.
29. Gillam L. The zone of parental discretion: an ethical tool for dealing with disagreement between parents and doctors about medical treatment for a child. Clin Ethics. 2016;11:1–8.
30. Sharma R, Sharma G, Sharma D, Kumar P, Sharma J. To assess the need of palliative care in children with life limiting diseases using paediatric palliative screening scale (PaPaS scale). JMSCR. 2018;6:191–7.
31. Aishammari YFH, Alharbi MN, Alanazi HF, Aldhahawi BK, Alshammari FM, Alsuwaydan RH, et al. Palliative care and end-of-life health practice. Int J Health Med Sci. 2018;1:39–46.
32. Jones KB, Wilson B, Weedon D, Bilder D. Care of adults with Intellectual and developmental disabilities: cerebral palsy. FP Essent. 2015;439:26–30.
33. Ezhumalai S, Kuppusamy CV. Palliative care for chronic neurological disorders: a case series and literature review. Indian J Psychiatr Soc Work. 2024:88–97.
34. Swarnakar R, Yadav SL. A combined comprehensive palliative and rehabilitative care plan for a child with cerebral palsy. Cureus. 2024;16:e75010.
35. Bindels de Heus G, Ball L, Michiels E, Moll H, Niks E, van Walraven S. Paediatric palliative care: multidisciplinary and pro-active. Ned Tijdschr Geneeskd. 2017;161:D857.
36. Smith KJ, Peterson MD, O'Connell NE, Victor C, Liverani S, Anokye N, et al. Risk of depression and anxiety in adults with cerebral palsy. JAMA Neurol. 2019;76:294–300.
37. Murphy KP. Cerebral palsy, non-communicable diseases, and lifespan care. Dev Med Child Neurol. 2018;60:733.
38. Poojari DP, Umakanth S, Maiya GA, Rao BK, Khurana S, Attal R, et al. Effect of family-centered care interventions on well-being of caregivers of children with cerebral palsy: a systematic review. F1000Res. 2024;12:790.
39. Hurvitz EA, Whitney DG, Waldron-Perrine B, Ryan D, Haapala HJ, Schmidt M, et al. Navigating the pathway to care in adults with cerebral palsy. Front Neurol. 2021;12:734139.
40. Mitchell DL, Shlobin NA, Winterhalter E, Lam SK, Raskin JS. Gaps in transitional care to adulthood for patients with cerebral palsy: a systematic review. Childs Nerv Syst. 2023;39:3083–101.
41. Field B, Scheinberg A, Cruickshank A. Health care services for adults with cerebral palsy. Aust Fam Physician. 2010;39:165–7.
42. Dygert L, Lewis A. Who should make medical decisions when a patient lacks an advance directive? Neurohospitalist. 2022;12:5–7.
43. Wagemans AM, Van Schrojenstein Lantman-de Valk HM, Proot IM, Metsemakers J, Tuffrey-Wijne I, Curfs LM. End-of-life decisions for people with intellectual disabilities, an interview study with patient representatives. Palliat Med. 2013;27:765–71.
44. Zaal-Schuller IH, Willems DL, Ewals FV, Van Goudoever J, De Vos M. Considering quality of life in end-of-life decisions for severely disabled children. Res Dev Disabil. 2018;73:67–75.
45. Khalid F, Ng Voon SI, Ong LC, Lim WK, Li L, Adnan A, et al. Advance care plan discussion among parents of children with cerebral palsy. Dev Med Child Neurol. 2022;64:1025–33.
46. Crowe A, Hurley F, Kiernan G, Kerr H, Corcoran Y, Price J, et al. Decision-making regarding place of end-of-life care for children with life-limiting and life-threatening conditions: a systematic integrative review. BMC Palliat Care. 2025;24:24.
47. Coleman D. Disability perspectives on public policy in advance care planning. BMJ Support Palliat Care. 2012;2:171.
48. Hurst DJ, Potter J, Naumann P, Baig JA, Evatt M, Lockhart JS, et al. Barriers to patient involvement in decision-making in advanced cancer care: culture as an amplifier. Narrat Inq Bioeth. 2022;12:77–92.
49. Kripke CC. Patients with disabilities: avoiding unconscious bias when discussing goals of care. Am Fam Physician. 2017;96:192–5.
50. Saposnik G, Redelmeier D, Ruff CC, Tobler PN. Cognitive biases associated with medical decisions: a systematic review. BMC Med Inform Decis Mak. 2016;16:138.

51. Budd MA, Haque OS, Stein MA. Biases in the evaluation of self-harm in patients with disability due to spinal cord injury. Spinal Cord Ser Cases. 2020;6:43.
52. Voss H, Loxton A, Anderson J, Watson J. "It was one of those complicated cases": health practitioners' perspectives and practices of providing end-of-life care for people with profound intellectual and multiple disability. BMC Palliat Care. 2021;20:177.
53. FitzGerald C, Hurst S. Implicit bias in healthcare professionals: a systematic review. BMC Med Ethics. 2017;18:19.
54. Hemsley B, Meredith J, Bryant L, Wilson NJ, Higgins I, Georgiou A, et al. An integrative review of stakeholder views on Advance Care Directives (ACD): barriers and facilitators to initiation, documentation, storage, and implementation. Patient Educ Couns. 2019;102:1067–79.
55. Atkins CG, Das S. What should clinicians and patients know about the clinical gaze, disability, and iatrogenic harm when making decisions? AMA J Ethics. 2022;24:762–7.
56. Li F, Santhanam G. G473 (P) End of life care in children with neurodisability and concurrent palliative care needs: an audit of local paediatric palliative services. Arch Dis Child. 2019;104:A190.3–A191.
57. Mietola R, Miettinen S, Vehmas S. Voiceless subjects? Research ethics and persons with profound intellectual disabilities. Int J Soc Res Methodol. 2017;20:263–74.
58. Cobigo V, Potvin LA, Fulford C, Chalghoumi H, Hanna M, Plourde N, et al. A conversation with research ethics boards about inclusive research with persons with intellectual and developmental disabilities. Res Involv Particip Cogn Disabil Differ Ethics Auton Incl Innov. 2019:185.
59. Freedman RI. Ethical challenges in the conduct of research involving persons with mental retardation. Ment Retard. 2001;39:130–41.
60. McDonald KE, Kidney CA. What is right? Ethics in intellectual disabilities research. J Policy Pract Intellect Disabil. 2012;9:27–39.
61. Goldsmith L, Skirton H. Research involving people with a learning disability–methodological challenges and ethical considerations. J Res Nurs. 2015;20:435–46.
62. Saleem A, Saleem I, Younus D, Khalid N, Naeem S, Fatima S, et al. Addressing research ethical dilemmas on cognitively impaired mentally ill patients (CIMI): insights from a prisma-guided review: ethics on conducting research on CIMI patients. Found Univ Med J. 2024;6:45–53.
63. Quinn H, Long R-E. Consent-as-method: capacity to consent of cognitively disabled people and research ethics review. Can J Disabil Stud. 2024;13:87–119.
64. Shore D. Ethical issues in schizophrenia research: a commentary on some current concerns. Schizophr Bull. 2006;32:26.
65. McFarland B, Bryant L, Wark S, Morales-Boyce T. Adaptive interviewing for the inclusion of people with intellectual disability in qualitative research. J Appl Res Intellect Disabil. 2024;37:e13182.
66. Ison NL. Having their say: email interviews for research data collection with people who have verbal communication impairment. Int J Soc Res Methodol. 2009;12:161–72.
67. Moyle W. Unstructured interviews: challenges when participants have a major depressive illness. J Adv Nurs. 2002;39:266–73.
68. Lariviere-Bastien D, Racine E. Ethics in health care services for young persons with neurodevelopmental disabilities: a focus on cerebral palsy. J Child Neurol. 2011;26:1221–9.
69. Ostojic K, Karem I, Paget SP, Berg A, Dee-Price B, Lingam R, et al. Social determinants of health for children with cerebral palsy and their families. Dev Med Child Neurol. 2024;66:32–40.
70. Shah P, Thornton I, Turrin D, Hipskind JE. Informed consent. In: StatPearls. Treasure Island: StatPearls Publishing; 2024.
71. Brandon E, Ballantyne M, Penner M, Lauzon A, McCarvill E. Accessing primary health care services for transition-aged young adults with cerebral palsy; perspectives of young adults, parents, and physicians. J Transit Med. 2019;1:20190004.

72. Lilly H, Bitzel M, Pejnovic T, Schnell J, Doty A. Barriers and characteristics for successful transition to adult healthcare for individuals with cerebral palsy: a systematic review. Phys Ther Rev. 2019;24:195–207.
73. Anaby D, Pozniak K. Participation-based intervention in childhood disability: a family-centred approach. Dev Med Child Neurol. 2019;61:502.
74. Diniz D. The ethical dilemmas of human life: the hospital history of children with serious cerebral palsy. Cad Saude Publica. 1996;12:345–55.
75. Henry G, Webb A, Galea C, Pearce A, Balde I, Garrity F, et al. Out-of-pocket costs for families and people living with cerebral palsy in Australia. PLoS One. 2023;18:e0288865.
76. Bian C, Peng F, Guo H, Chen K. [Retracted] investigation on quality of life and economic burden of children with cerebral palsy in Changzhou. J Healthcare Eng. 2022;2022:1519689.
77. Kruse M, Michelsen SI, Flachs EM, Brønnum-Hansen H, Madsen M, Uldall P. Lifetime costs of cerebral palsy. Dev Med Child Neurol. 2009;51:622–8.
78. Easton T, Boyd RN, Scuffham PA, Downes MJ. Health care resource use in preschool children with cerebral palsy. Dev Med Child Neurol. 2024;66:1476–84.
79. Honeycutt A, Dunlap L, Chen H, Homsi G, Grosse S, Schendel D. Economic costs associated with mental retardation, cerebral palsy, hearing loss, and vision impairment–United States, 2003. MMWR Morb Mortal Wkly Rep. 2004;53:57–9.
80. Umar UI, Adamu H, Abdulkareem A. Economic evaluation of cerebral palsy in a resource-challenged setting. Niger J Basic Clin Sci. 2020;17:50–6.
81. Dertli S, Aydin AS, Gunay U. Care burden, perceived social support, coping attitudes and life satisfaction of mothers with children with cerebral palsy. Child Care Health Dev. 2024;50:e13297.
82. Roos G, Alecu A, Austgulen M. Everyday household costs of raising a child with cerebral palsy. Eur J Pub Health. 2024;34:ckae144–2175.
83. Louis PT, Kumar N. Perceived parental differential treatment, cognition, behaviour and family cohesiveness among siblings of children with cerebral palsy? A family-mediated intervention to understand "displaced" children. Int J Disabil Hum Dev. 2016;15:243–50.
84. Huang Y, Kellett U, St JW. Being concerned: caregiving for Taiwanese mothers of a child with cerebral palsy. J Clin Nurs. 2012;21:189–97.
85. Ross P, Cuskelly M. Adjustment, sibling problems and coping strategies of brothers and sisters of children with autistic spectrum disorder. J Intellect Dev Disabil. 2006;31:77–86.
86. Elsakka E, Abdelhady M, Anwar S. Depression and anxiety among siblings of children with cerebral palsy. J High Inst Public Health. 2022;52:24–32.
87. Mukhwana T. Psychological experiences of non-cerebral palsy siblings. LAP LAMBERT Academic Publishing; 2016.
88. Dogbe JA, Kyeremateng JDA, Opoku MP, Nketsia W, Hammond C. 'There is family tension, but they understand…': familial and sibling relationships following the diagnosis of cerebral palsy in children in Ghana. Int J Dev Disabil. 2022;68:35–46. https://doi.org/10.1080/20473869.2019.1573572.
89. Dew A, Llewellyn G, Balandin S. Exploring the later life relationship between adults with cerebral palsy and their non-disabled siblings. Disabil Rehabil. 2014;36:756–64.
90. Lostelius PV, Ståhle-Öberg L, Fjellman-Wiklund A. Pain in children with cerebral palsy–adolescent siblings' awareness of pain and perceived influence on their family. Eur J Phys. 2019;21:164–70.
91. Dantas MSDA, Pontes JF, de Assis WD, Collet N. Family's abilities and difficulties in caring for children with cerebral palsy. Rev Gaucha Enferm. 2012;33:73–80.
92. Grayson A, J. Family resource centers: A way to grow. Virginia Child Protection Newsletter. 1990;30,1:3–8.
93. Martins PC, Matos CD, Sani AI. Parental stress and risk of child abuse: the role of socioeconomic status. Child Youth Serv Rev. 2023;148:106879.
94. Mayston MJ. People with cerebral palsy: effects of and perspectives for therapy. Neural Plast. 2001;8:51–69.
95. Foster BA, Lane JE, Massey E, Noelck M, Green S, Austin JP. The impact of malnutrition on hospitalized children with cerebral palsy. Hosp Pediatr. 2020;10:1087–95.

96. Reyes FI, Salemi JL, Dongarwar D, Magazine CB, Salihu HM. Prevalence, trends, and correlates of malnutrition among hospitalized children with cerebral palsy. Dev Med Child Neurol. 2019;61:1432–8.
97. Elkholi SM, Awad SS, Alotaibi MH. Neglect of psychological care for children with cerebral palsy and their families and its impact on their occupational engagement in Saudi Arabia. Medicina. 2024;60:1216.
98. Kendrick-Allwood SR, Murphy MM, Shin KS, Minaz A, Walker LK, Maitre NL. Social determinants of health in cerebral palsy. J Clin Med. 2024;13:7081.
99. Alyamy SMA, Aldawsari FSM, Al Joarah ASA, Alyami HMH, Al Enzi MAH, Aldosari SFM, et al. Crisis of care: how social workers can mitigate the impact of limited community resources on patient well. J Int Crisis Risk Commun Res. 2024;7:565.
100. FardAzar FE, Choopani A, Ahmad S, Teymourlouy A, Arkian S. Challenges of health care reforms (HCRS) in low and middle-income countries (LMICS): a qualitative systematic review. Preprint (Version 1). Available at Research Square. https://doi.org/10.21203/rs.3.rs-510547/v1.
101. Dako-Gyeke M, Boateng DA, Mills AA, Kodom RB, Appiah-Kubi J. Known by the children's condition: associative stigma among family carers of children with cerebral palsy. Glob Soc Welf. 2021;8:379–92.
102. Burke LM, Kalpakjian CZ, Smith YR, Quint EH. Gynecologic issues of adolescents with Down syndrome, autism, and cerebral palsy. J Pediatr Adolesc Gynecol. 2010;23:11–5.
103. Gray SH, Byrne R, Christensen S, Williams D, Wylie M, Fowler E, et al. Women with cerebral palsy: a qualitative study about their experiences with sexual and reproductive health education and services. J Pediatr Rehabil Med. 2021;14:285–93.
104. Türker D, Doğan H, Coban O, Goksuluk MB, Özengin N, Ün Yıldırım N. Menstrual health and genital hygiene status in adolescent girls and young women with cerebral palsy. Women Health. 2023;63:243–50.
105. Flavin M, Shore BJ, Miller P, Gray S. Hormonal contraceptive prescription in young women with cerebral palsy. J Adolesc Health. 2019;65:405–9.
106. Dural Ö, Taş İS, Akhan SE. Management of menstrual and gynecologic concerns in girls with special needs. J Clin Res Pediatr Endocrinol. 2020;12:41.
107. Zacharin M, Savasi I, Grover S. The impact of menstruation in adolescents with disabilities related to cerebral palsy. Arch Dis Child. 2010;95:526–30.
108. Alouf B. Care of the the adolescent female with cerebral palsy. Int J Disabil Hum Dev. 2007;6:3–10.
109. Deeksha H, Pajai S, Acharya N, Mohammad S. Pregnancy in women with cerebral palsy. Cureus. 2023;15:e36502.
110. Dave FG, Ansar H, Singhal T. PMM. 77 Care of pregnant women with physical disabilities. Arch Dis Child Fetal Neonatal Ed. 2014;99:A147.
111. Márquez-González H, Valdez-Martínez E, Bedolla M. Clinical, epidemiologic and ethical aspects of hysterectomy in young females with intellectual disability: a multi-centre study of public hospitals in Mexico City. Front Public Health. 2021;9:746399.
112. Amir N, Mitra M, Leung K, Simas TAM. Complications following hysterectomy in women with intellectual and developmental disabilities. Disabil Health J. 2022;15:101213.
113. Products – Data Briefs – Number 494. 2024. https://doi.org/10.15620/cdc:145592.
114. Rana A. Hysterectomy of mentally disabled female: an ethical dilemma. J Clin Res Bioeth. 2020;11:357.
115. Schickler R, Whittum M, Fanarjian N, Rapkin R, Nguyen BT. The history of female surgical sterilization: a social and ethics perspective. J Gynecol Surg. 2021;37:465–9.
116. Kirkpatrick L, Collins A, Harrison E, Miller E, Patterson C, Sogawa Y, et al. Pediatric neurologists' perspectives on sexual and reproductive health care for adolescent and young adult women with epilepsy and intellectual disability. J Child Neurol. 2022;37:56–63.
117. Pradhan M, Dileep K, Nair A, Al Sawafi KM. Forced surgeries in the mentally challenged females: ethical consideration and a narrative review of literature. Cureus. 2022;14:e26935.

118. Andromeda A, Hartini N, Suryanto S. Challenges and acceptance of families caring for children with cerebral palsy: a scoping review. Int J Care Caring. 2024;1:1–17.
119. Wray J, Edwards V, Wyatt K, Maddick A, Logan S, Franck L. Parents' attitudes toward the use of complementary therapy by their children with moderate or severe cerebral palsy. J Altern Complement Med. 2014;20:130–5.
120. Oskoui M, Ng P, Zaman M, Buckley D, Kirton A, van Rensburg E, et al. Complementary and alternative therapy use in children with cerebral palsy. Can J Neurol Sci. 2021;48:408–14.
121. Majnemer A, Shikako-Thomas K, Shevell MI, Poulin C, Lach L, Schmitz N, et al. Pursuit of complementary and alternative medicine treatments in adolescents with cerebral palsy. J Child Neurol. 2013;28:1443–7.

Global and Cross-Cultural Perspectives 19

Kaveh Same and Saeed Pourhassan

19.1 Introduction

"This case study will focus on the *evolution* of finding [a] meaningful occupation for a young man." This sentence marks the opening words of a case report penned by the mother of a 27-year-old patient with cerebral palsy—herself a former occupational therapist—as the family navigates the challenges posed by society and culture—and opportunities offered by them—in order for their son to find a meaningful job suitable to his abilities and likings [1]. Born prematurely by 14 weeks, Patrick weighed 1 pound, 14 ounces at birth and was immediately admitted to the NICU. He was ultimately diagnosed with spastic diplegic cerebral palsy, seizure disorder, retinopathy of prematurity with no light perception, and profound intellectual delay, leading to him being non-verbal.

Surveying the available options proved finding an appropriate choice not to be easy, as most were either not compatible with his unique set of abilities and disabilities or were not to his liking. From job locations without barrier-free access to activities unsuitable for an individual without vision, nothing ideal was ultimately found. Eventually, instead of trying to rule out the possibilities deemed unfit, the caregivers started—in his mother's words—to "look at what an individual *could* do, not what they *couldn't* do."

K. Same
Michael Ogon Laboratory for Orthopaedic Research, Orthopaedic Hospital Speising, Vienna, Austria

Doctoral Programme MedUni Vienna, Medical University of Vienna, Vienna, Austria
e-mail: kaveh.same@oss.at

S. Pourhassan (✉)
Internal Medicine Department, School of Medicine, Shariati Hospital, Tehran University of Medical Sciences, Tehran, Iran

A. Presedo et al. (eds.), *Enhancing Quality of Life in Patients with Cerebral Palsy*, https://doi.org/10.1007/978-3-032-20967-2_19

Patrick was adept at a particular hand motion that enabled him to *squish* or mix stuff—a gesture he enjoyed doing repetitively—and he regularly used an assistive device for pouring liquids or powders in containers. He also had an environmental control unit that enabled him to control different devices around him. Drawing on such abilities, an idea slowly emerged for a business model that centered around him creating packaged mixtures of different dry or powdered ingredients that could then be used to create different food items, delicacies, or pet treats. Initially selling the jars at the family business or at school, his business slowly expanded to other venues such as town fairs or seasonal outdoor markets, and more recently, an online shop.

Twenty-seven at the time of article publication, Patrick continues to take care of his business with the help of his family and a dedicated job coach. An overall success story, the case showcases not only the difficulties of navigating a society that is not always compatible with, or even accepting of, an individual with special needs or disabilities but also signifies the importance and impact of proper attention and empowerment in ensuring social inclusion and prosperity for such individuals.

19.1.1 Cerebral Palsy

First characterized by Dr. Little in the eighteenth century, cerebral palsy (CP) is a common physical and developmental condition with a wide variety of symptoms and differing severities. An international panel held in 2006 provided the following definition for the condition: "Cerebral palsy (CP) describes a group of permanent disorders of the development of movement and posture, causing activity limitation, that are attributed to non-progressive disturbances that occurred in the developing fetal or infant brain" [2]. Encompassing a wide range of clinical symptoms and phenotypes, the disease is often classified based on the type of involvement—spastic versus non-spastic—or the limbs affected—hemiplegia, paraplegia, or quadriplegia [3]. More sophisticated classifications also exist, but their usefulness is debated, especially due to low inter-rater reliability and the tendency of the disease to evolve over time.

Diagnosis has traditionally relied on thorough neurological examinations and was typically feasible no earlier than the first or second year of life. Since the disease is believed to be present from birth or very early in the neonatal period—at least in the majority of cases—the ability to establish a definitive diagnosis as early as possible would be immensely beneficial. Early diagnosis would enable the implementation of treatment approaches and necessary lifestyle adjustments sooner, thereby taking advantage of the high plasticity of the nervous system during early life [3]. In recent years, modern clinical or paraclinical tools have made it possible to achieve a reliable diagnosis before 5 months of age. Neonatal magnetic resonance imaging (MRI), the Prechtl Qualitative Assessment of General Movements (GMA), and Hammersmith Infant Neurologic Examination (HINE) all provide excellent sensitivity, with GMA having a sensitivity of 98% [4].

19.1.2 History of the Disease

Cerebral palsy is believed to have been known to some capacity since ancient times, as drawings have survived from the fifth century BC that depict individuals affected with what seems to be spastic CP [5]. As mentioned earlier, however, the modern description of the disease is often credited to Dr. William John Little—himself a polio survivor suffering from an equinus deformity—who made tremendous efforts in establishing surgical correction of physical deformities as a viable treatment approach in such cases [6]. The term *Cerebral Palsy* is believed to have been coined by the English physician Sir William Osler in 1889 in his description of 151 patients affected by the condition [7].

From such early attempts to define CP, it took almost an entire century for a unified definition to be offered by the Little Club in the twentieth century. Alternative disease definitions and classifications were also offered by other scientific bodies over time, including the Spastic Society, and by the Surveillance of Cerebral Palsy in Europe (SCPE). A more recent definition of the condition, as adopted by the International Workshop on Definition and Classification of CP, revised some of the details and emphasized recognizing the fact that CP is more than merely a motor disability, acknowledging that often other impairments may accompany CP [2, 6].

19.1.3 Epidemiology and Burden

Prevalence of CP is significant as it not only indicates the number of individuals with the condition, but also acts as a measure of overall maternal, prenatal, and perinatal care. The overall prevalence of the disease seems to have remained stable through the years, a finding somewhat surprising, especially considering the significant advances in the fields of maternal and perinatal care, and the observed decrease in early child mortality rates [8]. In Europe, the overall prevalence rates per 1000 live births vary from 1.04 to 2.52 [9]. The Center for Disease Control and Prevention in Atlanta reports a relatively higher prevalence of 3.6 in one of the few population-based studies in the United States [10]. Based on global reports, overall and etiology-specific rates appear to vary significantly, particularly in developing countries [8].

A systematic review by McIntyre and colleagues included the data from 41 different studies from 27 countries (6 of which were countries with low or middle income and the rest among the high-income countries). The results reported a birth prevalence of 2 per 1000 in high-income countries and 3 per 1000 for low- or middle-income countries [11]. This was considerably lower than the estimates based on the Global Burden of Disease data, which reported a global average prevalence of 9 per 1000, with high-income countries having a reported prevalence of 6 individuals per 1000 [12].

19.1.4 Cultural Differences and Socioeconomic Status

As a condition significantly affected by the conditions experienced by the mother and the embryo during the prenatal period, as well as perinatal and early-life health conditions of the child, CP is believed to be significantly influenced by the socioeconomic status of the family and that of the community. Indeed, a recently published report estimated about 96% of all children born with CP to be from low- to middle-income countries [13]. Furthermore, as the condition affects the individual's ability to communicate and function effectively in society, cultural beliefs and norms are also believed to play an important role in the individual's quality of life and even in their disease prognosis. The rest of the chapter will focus on the differences that exist in these regards between different populations and will try to create an overview of the global conditions. Also, we will try to answer how such differences impact the lives of patients with cerebral palsy.

19.2 Cultural Differences

There is little doubt that cultural beliefs and norms have a profound effect on the degree of acceptance, and hence inclusion, that a society will offer to people with different disabilities. Such differences not only determine the person's chance of growth and prosperity in that society but can even impact their access to the required treatments and health services. As a disease defined by the existence of physical—and sometimes mental—disabilities, and in many cases significantly affecting the patients' ability to communicate effectively with other people, CP is greatly influenced by the differences in social culture.

19.2.1 Differing Views on Disability

In today's world, talks of *inclusion* are everywhere, from media to politics, people are trying—or at least pretending to try—to appeal to the noble ideas of equal participation and inclusion for all members of society, regardless of their individual differences from what a more conservative society might consider *normal* or *average*. This is especially important for people with different kinds of disabilities, as historically, social stigma and negative attitudes towards their condition have been an important factor in hindering their independence and meaningful integration into society. Indeed, our struggles seem to be fruitful, as studies have demonstrated that social perception and acceptance have improved for people with disability in the past decades—at least in developed countries [14].

An interesting work by Westerbrook et al. investigated the differences in attitudes towards different disabilities in a multicultural setting. Based on the results, although general cultural views had a significant impact on the social stigma placed on certain disabilities, and populations were found to demonstrate differing amounts of *overall* negative attitudes towards disability, the hierarchy by which different conditions were ranked in each society was found to be surprisingly similar—conditions such as asthma and diabetes were the most, and AIDS, mental retardation, cerebral palsy, and psychiatric disorders the least accepted conditions in all cases [15]. Such results indicate that different populations may not have different views towards specific conditions but rather differ in their overall acceptance of disability.

Indeed, a study in non-Western societies found that cultures that have higher levels of productivity in proportion to their population, demonstrate more equality in resource distribution, and put less cultural emphasis on competitiveness and merits of personal achievement, are those with more accepting attitudes towards disabilities [16]. A society similar to the democratic social structure found in many developed European countries.

Focusing on mental disabilities and looking from a somewhat different point of view, McKearney et al. argue that the degree of acceptance observed in a society for each particular disability might not in fact originate from the ability of the individual to *function* from an objective point of view, but rather from the extend by which their behaviors and actions follow what is *anticipated* or *expected* by other members of the society, especially their close relatives and caregivers [17]. This is significant as it opens new ways by which the cultural views can be influenced to become more favorable towards people with differing degrees of disability.

19.2.2 Cultural Differences and Cerebral Palsy

The impact of cultural and societal beliefs and traditions on a person with CP can—and probably should—be viewed from different points of view. Such social *norms* not only cast judgments on the individual's perceived *worth* in their society and the extent to which they may be accepted among them, but also impose the weight of their views on the parents and those close to the patient. At its best, in a culture accepting of people with disabilities and far from damaging beliefs, such an effect might lead to social inclusion of the person by focusing on their strengths instead of their shortcomings, provide support to their caregivers through official and unofficial means, and—by holding the said caregivers to high standards—demand adequate attention and support from them regarding their child. On the other hand, in a society with a value system hostile towards such people, the effects of cultural judgment can severely compromise the individual's prospects and limit the extent of their growth and social integration.

A study focusing on the emotional response of Taiwanese mothers upon learning a diagnosis of CP in their children, highlights the social setting and cultural background in which they occur, as believing a significant portion of the emotional burden and distress experienced by them to originate not from the objective difficulties of raising a physically—and mentally—disabled child, but in reality from the social stigma attached to the situation [18]. Of the 15 mothers interviewed in the study, many expressed that they had experienced distress and fear out of concern for being blamed for their child's condition, or for the child to be shunned from the family. The authors state that such emotions might stem from the emphasis of the Chinese traditional culture on the importance of having a strong and healthy family that the elders can be proud of and depend on upon their old age, and as a result how having children with CP can be viewed not only as a fault of the mother, but also the children themselves to be considered undependable and therefore worthless.

Another study focusing on health beliefs surrounding CP in pediatric patients among their caregivers in the African nation of Botswana, found that not only traditional *folk* beliefs regarding the origin and cause of CP affect the families'—most importantly the mothers'—perception through the eye of their society, but also in some occasions posed real challenges in their pursuit of receiving proper care for their child [19]. Women in the study expressed concern that society thought of their child's illness as a result of them "having been unfaithful to their man," "having worn trousers," or "having worked too much." Furthermore, several stated that they found it difficult to seek the needed medical care for their children due to the people's negative reactions or stares when they saw their child.

The significance of cultural influences in the prognosis of CP is not a newly understood concept. In a comprehensive study by Victor Sanua in 1970, the attitude of 205 CP patients towards their disease was examined in eight European countries [20]. Their main hypothesis was that psychological and sociocultural forces have a significant impact on the individual's response to their disability. Using the Attitude Towards Disabled Persons (ATDP) scale [21] as their main measurement, an expansive battery of physical and psychological tests was also administered as part of the study. ATDP is a twenty-item scale developed to assess the view of the individual towards disabilities and disabled people. A higher score on the scale would mean a more favorable attitude towards disability and less prejudice towards the disabled. Aiming to assess the extent to which the views of patients echoed those of their caregivers, the ATDP scale was also administered to the professional and non-professional staff present at each visited center. The results were also compared with those of a similar study performed on a population of individuals with different disabilities and their non-disabled peers in the United States.

The results obtained from CP patients indicated a discrepancy between the male and female respondents in the less developed countries surveyed, with girls having lower scores—and hence a less favorable attitude towards their disability—compared with boys. Such a difference was not observed in the more technologically advanced countries in the study, and was also absent from the results of the US population. The authors concluded that a culture imposing a socially subservient role on the female sex also seems to result in them having a less favorable attitude towards their disability. Indeed, as an exception to the pattern, Yugoslavian girls, who had significantly higher levels of education than boys, were also found to have markedly higher scores.

As for the non-CP participants, females were found to show overall less prejudice towards people with disability—a stark distinction from their attitudes towards their own disability in the CP group, which again might stem from the cultural norms of compassion and care geared towards them. Interestingly, such a discrepancy between the sexes was not observed in the results from the most advanced countries in the study, or those from the US population.

Overall, the results clearly indicate the importance—and extent—of the influence of cultural norms and beliefs on society's attitude towards individuals with CP, and the patients themselves towards their disability. Such a profound effect warrants the need for careful consideration of such influences both in individual treatment planning and in social policy making.

19.3 Socioeconomic Status

In the seemingly never-ending struggle of health as a right versus a commodity, and despite our efforts otherwise, one cannot overlook the effect of socioeconomic status on virtually all aspects of health and disease. As with countless other conditions, physical and mental disabilities such as cerebral palsy seem to be no exception, as economic and social status can profoundly impact their burden and prognosis.

19.3.1 Effects on Disability

Assessing the impact of socioeconomic status (SES) on different aspects of disability, a population-based study on more than 100,000 people in Bangladesh indicated that not only were those with a higher SES significantly more likely to have access to and use healthcare services, but they were also meaningfully less likely to develop disabilities in the first place [22].

Focusing on socioeconomic (SE) determinants of disability, another study on a large population in Chile concluded that while the exact relation between the presence of each specific disability and different aspects of SES varied with every disability, the three *classic* SE factors of *Income*, *education*, and *occupation* were consistently among the most important associated factors regardless of disability type [23]. Using the same rationale, a study including over 19,000 people from 19 European countries assessed the underlying determinants of the observed discrepancy between different levels of SES and the existence of self-reported disabilities while considering the individual's highest education level to be an overall representative of their SES. The results suggested that three main groups of determinants—namely, *occupational factors*, *behavioral factors*, and *living conditions*—explained much of the observed inequality [24].

The observation that SES can be a source of inequality and disparity not just in the prognosis and management of disabilities, but also in their reported presence, proves the need for careful consideration of its effect on all aspects of disease management when dealing with a patient with disability. Indeed, it has been shown that while having a disabled child can lead to significantly worse health in the mother in families with a lower SES, as the SES improves, so does the maternal health indices, eventually approximating those of a mother with a healthy child [25]. Such findings indicate that the long-held belief of disabilities being a source of burden may not be true, as it seems that rather than the disability itself, the *burden* originates from dysfunctional social constructs leading to a limited availability of resources and an unfavorable SE standing.

19.3.2 Socioeconomic Status and Cerebral Palsy

"I am what I am because of who we all are." The concept of *ubuntu* has been an integral part of social interactions in many African nations for centuries. The fact that for every change regarding a particular issue to be effective and persistent, all the aspects and contributing parties should be included. Recognizing its importance, therapists in South Africa who care for individuals with CP aim not only to involve the entire family—rather than just the patient—in their efforts, but also to organize community-based supports to compensate for the limited number of trained professionals.

The true effectiveness of such an approach can only be understood by examining the effects of SES and living conditions on different aspects of CP. In a large-scale study on the Australian population, the results indicated that while advances in healthcare interventions—particularly maternal and perinatal care—in the last 20 years, have significantly impacted the prevalence of CP in the country as evident by a nearly 40% decline in CP prevalence, the proportion of individuals with CP that lived in remote or very remote areas of the country was significantly larger than the population proportion that resided in these areas [26].

A study based on data from the Quebec Cerebral Palsy Registry (REPACQ) and including 483 children with CP born between 1999 and 2010, aimed to assess several outcomes such as gross motor function, manual ability, CP subtype, and comorbidities. Furthermore, both maternal education level—as an indicator of individual-level SES—and neighborhood deprivation were also measured. The results demonstrated a clear socioeconomic gradient in mobility outcomes. Children from socioeconomically disadvantaged families, particularly those whose mothers had not completed high school, were more likely to be non-ambulant and to have poor manual ability. Area-level deprivation further compounded risk, but only among children of mothers with higher education levels—suggesting that in families already disadvantaged at the individual level, neighborhood effects added little additional risk. The strongest associations were observed among preterm children, where living in deprived neighborhoods was linked to a higher likelihood of spastic quadriparesis and severe motor impairment [27].

Aiming to further assess the effects of SES on CP, other teams have also compared patterns of the disease between high- and low-resource countries. In a study including 300 preschool-aged children from Australia and Bangladesh, children were assessed regarding motor function and disease subtype classification, as well as the presence of perinatal risk factors. Results revealed striking differences between the two populations. Australian children were more likely to have mild motor impairment, whereas Bangladeshi children showed greater representation in the most severe categories. Motor subtype distribution also differed significantly: spastic CP predominated in Australia, while dystonic and athetoid types were more common in Bangladesh. Risk factors associated with poor gross motor outcomes included low Apgar scores, seizures, lethargy, and term birth in the Bangladesh cohort. Cognitive impairments were reported more frequently in Bangladeshi children, while visual impairments were more common in the Australian group [28]. The authors concluded that the patterns of motor severity, comorbidities, and associated risk factors differ markedly between high- and low-resource settings. These findings underscore the influence of differing aspects of SE status—*environmental*, *perinatal*, and *healthcare* factors—in shaping CP outcomes.

Coming back to the situation in South Africa, in a community where a significant portion of the population suffers from economical and educational poverty, and with documented and tangible effects of SES in the occurrence and outcome of CP, such approaches try to leverage the cultural strengths to minimize the negative impacts of a low SES on the condition, thereby fostering resilience and promoting more sustainable outcomes for both the individuals and their families [29]. Indeed, while socioeconomic conditions play a significant role in the presence and determination of type, severity, and outcome of cerebral palsy, and while the disease is shown to affect all aspects of the patient's quality of life, present evidence suggests that appropriate and scientifically designed interventions can have a substantial effect in improving the conditions for those affected [30].

19.4 Recommendations

19.4.1 For Parents and Caregivers

- Seek early diagnosis and intervention: Whenever possible, access diagnostic tools early, as early therapy maximizes developmental potential.
- Advocate for inclusion: Engaging actively with schools, community organizations, and local disability advocacy groups can improve opportunities for integration and reduce stigma.
- Leverage community networks: Families should use cultural, religious, and neighborhood support systems to share caregiving responsibilities and reduce caregiver burnout.
- Prioritize education: For children with CP, even modest educational attainment is strongly associated with greater independence, higher self-esteem, and better long-term outcomes.

19.4.2 For Healthcare Professionals and Policy Makers

- Adopt a family-centered approach: Involve not only the patient but also caregivers and siblings in therapy planning, recognizing their central role in long-term outcomes.

- Respect cultural contexts: Understanding patients' cultural backgrounds allows clinicians to address stigma, counteract harmful beliefs, and adapt interventions to local realities.
- Promote interdisciplinary collaboration: Work closely with physiotherapists, speech therapists, occupational therapists, and psychologists to provide comprehensive care.
- Support community-based rehabilitation: In resource-limited settings, help design scalable, low-cost interventions that empower caregivers to continue therapy at home.
- Invest in early detection programs: Training healthcare workers to identify early signs of CP can significantly improve outcomes and reduce long-term costs.
- Reduce socioeconomic disparities: Policies addressing maternal health, nutrition, and education will reduce CP prevalence and improve quality of life for affected families.
- Combat stigma through public campaigns: Shifting societal attitudes toward disability is essential for inclusion, employment opportunities, and social participation.
- Expand rehabilitation infrastructure: Funding community-based programs, especially in rural or impoverished areas, ensures equitable access to care.
- Integrate CP into broader disability frameworks: Policymaking should avoid siloing CP as a rare condition and instead address it within national strategies on disability rights, social protection, and inclusive education.

19.5 Conclusions

Cerebral palsy (CP) is one of the most extensively studied yet persistently complex conditions in medicine. From its early descriptions by Dr. William John Little to its modern definitions refined through international consensus, CP has remained emblematic of how biological, social, cultural, and economic determinants intertwine in shaping health outcomes. Despite significant progress in perinatal and neonatal care worldwide, prevalence rates remain remarkably stable, reminding us that CP is not solely a biomedical phenomenon, but rather a condition profoundly influenced by societal structures.

Cultural beliefs have a direct and often underestimated impact on how CP is perceived and managed. Stigma, fatalistic attitudes, or cultural misattributions of blame not only add psychological burden to families but can also hinder timely access to healthcare services. Furthermore, socioeconomic status (SES) also appears to be one of the most consistent predictors of outcome. Families with greater access to financial, educational, and social resources experience better health outcomes, whereas poverty compounds the challenges of caregiving, access to rehabilitation, and long-term integration into society.

Ultimately, cerebral palsy is not just a neurological disorder—it is a societal challenge. Its prevalence, prognosis, and lived experience are shaped as much by MRI scans and physical therapy sessions as they are by education, income distribution, cultural acceptance, and political will. In this light, addressing CP requires coordinated action across multiple levels of society. A future where children with CP thrive is one in which medicine, culture, and policy intersect harmoniously—a future built on the recognition that resilience does not arise solely from the individual but from the collective strength of families, communities, and nations.

References

1. Lewis MA. Purely Patrick: a case study report. Work. 2019;62(3):427–34.
2. Rosenbaum P, et al. A report: the definition and classification of cerebral palsy April 2006. Dev Med Child Neurol Suppl. 2007;109:8–14.
3. Michael-Asalu A, et al. Cerebral palsy: diagnosis, epidemiology, genetics, and clinical update. Adv Pediatr. 2019;66:189–208.
4. Novak I, et al. Early, accurate diagnosis and early intervention in cerebral palsy: advances in diagnosis and treatment. JAMA Pediatr. 2017;171(9):897–907.
5. Richer P, Charcot J-M. Les Difformes et les malades dans l'art, par J.-M. Charcot... et Paul Richer. Lecrosnier et Babé; 1889.
6. Pakula AT, Braun KVN, Yeargin-Allsopp M. Cerebral palsy: classification and epidemiology. Phys Med Rehabil Clin. 2009;20(3):425–52.
7. Osler, W., Cerebral palsies of children. 1889: Mac Keith Press.
8. Himmelmann K, et al. Epidemiology of cerebral palsy. In: Cerebral palsy. Springer; 2020. p. 131–46.
9. EURO-PERISTAT Project, W.S.E. and EURONEOSTAT. European Perinatal Health Report. 2008. Available from. http://www.europeristat.com.
10. Yeargin-Allsopp M, et al. Prevalence of cerebral palsy in 8-year-old children in three areas of the United States in 2002: a multisite collaboration. Pediatrics. 2008;121(3):547–54.
11. McIntyre S, et al. Global prevalence of cerebral palsy: a systematic analysis. Dev Med Child Neurol. 2022;64(12):1494–506.
12. Olusanya BO, et al. Global prevalence of developmental disabilities in children and adolescents: a systematic umbrella review. Front Public Health. 2023;11:1122009.
13. Olusanya BO, et al. Cerebral palsy in young children: bridging the global data gap. Lancet Glob Health. 2025;13:e1663.
14. Leichenko S. The ICD survey of disabled Americans: bringing disabled Americans into the mainstream. A nationwide survey of 1,000 disabled people. Study No. 854009. Louis Harris and Associates; 1986.
15. Westbrook MT, Legge V, Pennay M. Attitudes towards disabilities in a multicultural society. Soc Sci Med. 1993;36(5):615–23.
16. Scheer J, Groce N. Impairment as a human constant: cross-cultural and historical perspectives on variation. J Soc Issues. 1988;44(1):23–37.
17. McKearney P, Zogas A. Mentally fit: negotiating the boundaries of cognitive disability. Taylor & Francis; 2021. p. 111–5.
18. Huang YP, Kellett UM, St John W. Cerebral palsy: experiences of mothers after learning their child's diagnosis. J Adv Nurs. 2010;66(6):1213–21.
19. Patel P, et al. Health beliefs regarding pediatric cerebral palsy among caregivers in Botswana: a qualitative study. Child Care Health Dev. 2017;43(6):861–8.
20. Sanua VD. A cross cultural study of cerebral palsy. Soc Sci Med (1967). 1970;4(5):461–512.
21. Yuker HE. The measurement of attitudes toward disabled persons. Human Resources Center. 1970. 100–102.
22. Rahman M, et al. Socioeconomic inequalities in disability prevalence and health service use in Bangladesh. Sci Rep. 2025;15(1):23363.
23. Zitko Melo P, Cabieses Valdes B. Socioeconomic determinants of disability in Chile. Disabil Health J. 2011;4(4):271–82.

24. Pérez-Hernández B, et al. Socioeconomic inequalities in disability in Europe: contribution of behavioral, work-related and living conditions. Eur J Pub Health. 2019;29(4):640–7.
25. Bixby LE. Disability is not a burden: the relationship between early childhood disability and maternal health depends on family socioeconomic status. J Health Soc Behav. 2023;64(3):354–69.
26. Smithers-Sheedy H, et al. Cerebral palsy in Australia: birth prevalence, 1995–2016, and differences by residential remoteness: a population-based register study. Med J Aust. 2024;221(10):533–9.
27. Oskoui M, et al. Variation in cerebral palsy profile by socio-economic status. Dev Med Child Neurol. 2016;58(2):160–6.
28. Benfer KA, et al. Motor severity in children with cerebral palsy studied in a high-resource and low-resource country. Pediatrics. 2014;134(6):e1594–602.
29. Levin K. 'I am what I am because of who we all are': international perspectives on rehabilitation: South Africa. Pediatr Rehabil. 2006;9(3):285–92.
30. Marwa G, et al. Quality of life and its predicting factors for Tunisian children with cerebral palsy. Afr J Disabil. 2022;11:1046.

Research and Future Directions 20

Fatemeh Moghadas

Abbreviations

Cerebral palsy	CP
Magnetic Resonance Imaging	MRI
Magnetic Resonance Spectroscopy	MRS
Intelligence Quotient	IQ
Diffuse Excessive High Signal Intensity	DEHSI
Proton MRS	H-MRS
N-acetylaspartate	NAA
Creatine	Cr
Choline	Cho
Excitatory Amino Acid Transporter 2	EAAT2
Deoxyribonucleic acid	DNA
Ribonucleic acid	RNA
micro Ribonucleic Acid	miRNA
Tumor Necrosis Factor-α	TNF-α
beta subunit of human Chorionic Gonadotropin	βhCG
Pregnancy-Associated Plasma Protein-A	PAPP-A
Alpha-Fetoprotein	AFP
General Movement Assessment	GMA
Artificial Intelligence	AI
Magnetoencephalography	MEG
Electroencephalography	EEG
Near-Infrared Spectroscopy	NIRS

F. Moghadas (✉)
Neurology Research Center, Kerman University of Medical Sciences, Kerman, Iran
e-mail: f.moghadas@kmu.ac.ir

A. Presedo et al. (eds.), *Enhancing Quality of Life in Patients with Cerebral Palsy*, https://doi.org/10.1007/978-3-032-20967-2_20

Repetitive Transcranial Magnetic Stimulation	rTMS
Transcranial Direct Current Stimulation	tDCS

20.1 Introduction

Cerebral palsy (CP) is a spectrum of neurologic disorders characterized by prominent motor impairments, caused by nonprogressive injury to the developing brain. These injuries can occur at different time frames early in life, including prenatal, intrapartum, and postpartum periods. The cause of CP can be multifactorial, and in the majority of cases, unknown [1].

As the most common cause of childhood disability, CP is frequently associated with other comorbidities such as epilepsy, hearing loss, intellectual disability, feeding difficulties, and sensory impairments [2]. This disease, with an estimated birth prevalence of 1.6 in 1000 live births in high-income countries and a twofold greater birth prevalence in middle- and low-income countries, places a noteworthy burden on both families and societies [3].

Recently, many studies have been conducted to explore new diagnostic and therapeutic methods for early diagnosis and treatment of CP. This chapter aims to explore recent advances and the next promising topics in CP research, focusing on early diagnosis, early interventions, and patient care, with the hope that these current and future developments will benefit individuals, families, and societies.

This chapter is organized into two main sections. The first section reviews newly adopted biomarkers that may aid the early diagnosis of CP, highlighting imaging, genetic, and other biomarkers with promising potential. The second section surveys recent treatment approaches and therapeutic interventions currently under investigation, aimed at managing CP and enhancing patients' quality of life.

20.2 Novel Diagnostic Modalities

CP is a clinical diagnosis. Nevertheless, for all children diagnosed with CP, a diagnostic evaluation should be performed to identify the underlying cause or to rule out other conditions. Typically, CP is diagnosed in children between 12 and 24 months [4, 5].

Neuroscience studies have shown that brain development continues postnatally. The infant's interaction with the environment can drive neuromotor system development, as well as the development of muscles, ligaments, and bones [6–8]. Accordingly, early diagnosis of CP can offer significant advantages, particularly during the critical window of brain development. Furthermore, the sooner the diagnosis is made, the sooner the intervention can begin. The earlier intervention has the advantage of maximizing neuroplasticity and minimizing secondary musculoskeletal and developmental modifications [9–11]. Early intervention should be done with the following goals [12]:

1. Better outcome in motor function, cognition, and communication;
2. Minimizing secondary impairments and complications;
3. Better caregiver mental health and reducing anxiety and depression.

Given the impact of early intervention on outcomes for patients with CP, recent research has focused on new modalities to facilitate earlier diagnosis, some of which suggest that a diagnosis may be possible as early as the corrected age of 6 months.

In this section, the modalities employed for early diagnosis of CP are examined. The discussion begins with emerging imaging biomarkers, followed by an exploration of genetic biomarkers. Then, other indicators, such as biochemical, prenatal, movement-based, and neurophysiological biomarkers, are briefly discussed.

20.2.1 Imaging Biomarkers

Imaging modalities are among the most researched methods, which have shown promising results in early diagnosis of CP. Advanced modes of Magnetic Resonance Imaging (MRI), such as diffusion MRI, brain morphometry, and Magnetic Resonance Spectroscopy (MRS), are examples of these biomarkers [1, 13, 14]. Compared to structural MRI, these new modes, besides having greater sensitivity, objectivity, and being more quantitative in detecting injuries, can also evaluate the brain microstructure and some metabolites that can indicate neural damage [15]. Here, these new modalities and their role in the early detection of CP are briefly reviewed.

20.2.1.1 Diffusion MRI

Diffusion MRI measures the water molecules' diffusion in the brain's microstructure. In a normal brain, water molecules move more freely longitudinally along the axons than perpendicular to them. Diffusion properties of the brain can reflect axonal and myelin integrity and are altered in cases of brain injuries that break down the organelles and membranes [16]. Overall, increased radial (perpendicular) diffusivity can be a sign of demyelination or delayed myelination, while improper axial (longitudinal) diffusivity can be an indicator of axonal immaturity, injury, or necrosis [17]. Diffusion tensor tractography, a 3-dimensional interpretation of diffusion MRI, can be used to visualize different white matter pathways involved in the pathophysiology of CP [18]. Therefore, this modality can be useful in the early diagnosis of CP.

Using diffusion MRI, different sensory and motor pathway abnormalities have been identified in patients with CP. Impairments in the corticospinal tract, posterior and superior thalamic radiations (encompassing both motor and sensory components), as well as the posterior midbody and isthmus of the corpus callosum, are commonly observed in individuals with cerebral palsy [19–23]. Various combinations of abnormal diffusivity in these pathways are reported as an early indicator of CP. Nevertheless, the roles of these parameters in the early and accurate diagnosis of CP should be further studied.

20.2.1.2 Brain Morphometry

Deformation-based morphometry is an MRI-based technique to measure different anatomical parts of the brain volumes to detect subtle macroscopic differences in brain shape and volume [24, 25]. Brain morphometry of preterm infants at term-equivalent age can be used as a prognostic biomarker of developmental outcome in these children [13].

Previous research has shown that brain volume can be reduced in the context of preterm brain injury [26, 27]. This brain volume reduction is associated with both developmental impairment and reduced Intelligence Quotient (IQ) [28–30]. Volume reduction is observed in both white matter and gray matter of the brain, particularly in the sensorimotor cortex. Nevertheless, subcortical gray matter in the basal ganglia, cortical gray matter of the amygdala and hippocampus, dorsomedial nucleus of the thalamus, and posterior corpus callosum white matter are among regions with volume reduction in preterm children [30, 31]. Other measures, including the third ventricle's width and ventricles' enlargement, were also associated with speech and motor development, respectively [32].

Brain MRI at term-equivalent age in preterm infants can also show different degrees of diffuse excessive high signal intensity (DEHSI) on T2-weighted imaging. DEHSI is characterized by hyperintense white matter signal abnormalities in periventricular and subcortical regions, exceeding the typical distribution of normal periventricular crossroads–transient fetal brain structures containing intersecting developing fiber systems [33, 34]. DEHSI volumes, especially in the centrum semiovale, measured by quantitative MRI methods, can be an early predictor of future cognitive and language impairments in preterm neonates, and thus may be a potential biomarker for the early diagnosis of CP [34, 35].

20.2.1.3 Proton Magnetic Resonance Spectroscopy

MRS, a non-invasive imaging technique that uses similar principles as MRI, is a useful tool for determining the brain's biochemistry. Considering the high gyromagnetic ratio of protons and their abundance in most of the body's molecules, proton MRS (H-MRS) is the most popular method for studying the biochemical content of the tissues [36]. N-acetylaspartate (NAA), creatine (Cr), and choline (Cho) are the most considered metabolites in evaluating brain chemical content. NAA is an indicator of neuronal integrity, while Cr is an energy marker, used to monitor energy metabolism in brain tissue [37, 38]. Cho, on the other hand, is maximum during the prenatal period, decreases with early neurodevelopment, and stands at a stable level after birth [37]. Some studies showed Cho's neuroprotective effect in brain injuries and claimed that it can improve brain recovery [39].

The biochemical content of the brain in high-risk infants for CP, including low birth weight infants, is a prominent area of research. Several biomarkers in different brain regions have been proposed to be predictive of neurodevelopmental impairment in high-risk neonates. However, the most frequently observed finding was a reduced NAA concentration, which was associated with neurodevelopmental impairment in subsequent years [14, 40–47]. It is noteworthy that the NAA/Cho ratio in the central white matter and deep gray matter of neonates was the strongest predictor of neurodevelopmental impairment [13, 48, 49].

20.2.2 Genetic, Epigenetic, and Transcriptomic Biomarkers

20.2.2.1 Genetic Testing

In addition to advances in imaging techniques for early diagnosis of CP, growing evidence highlights the significant role of genetics in CP. Higher risk of CP in monozygotic twins in comparison to dizygotic ones, and the fact that CP is more prevalent in consanguineous than nonconsanguineous families [50] highlight the role of genetics in the pathophysiology of CP and open new paths to its earlier diagnosis. Genetic testing in CP patients also offers other advantages, such as the opportunity for early diagnosis and treatment of progressive and treatable disorders, and planning for future pregnancies [51].

Exome sequencing is the current method for studying the genes contributing to CP. With genetic evaluation of patients with CP, the following three situations are possible [51, 52]:

1. Detection of genes known for specific monogenic diseases such as leukoencephalopathies, neurometabolic, neurodegenerative, and neuromuscular diseases. These disorders can mimic CP's clinical features.
2. Detection of monogenic disorders whose clinical features are well-matched with CP.
3. Detection of genetic variants that increase the patient's brain susceptibility to environmental factors.

Studies have identified monogenic pathological variants in 11% to 40% of CP patients [53–56]. This proportion is higher in patients with cryptogenic CP – those without identifiable environmental risk factors–compared to CP patients with known risk factors (35% versus 7%) [54].

Surprisingly, recent studies revealed that genetic susceptibility can also be seen in CP patients with identifiable environmental risk factors [57]. There are genetic variants that make patients more vulnerable to environmental factors such as preterm birth, intrauterine growth restriction, multiple gestations, and perinatal asphyxia. For example, an underlying genetic predisposition is proposed to have a role in the outcome of neonates with hypoxic-ischemic encephalopathy as a result of perinatal asphyxia, as well as the patient's response to this condition's standard treatment (therapeutic hypothermia) [58–62]. The association of gene variants in Excitatory Amino Acid Transporter 2 (EAAT2) and Cyclo-oxygenase-1/2 with CP in patients with a history of preterm birth could be another example [63, 64].

Considering the cost of genetic testing and the fact that this test is not widely available, selecting the CP patient for genetic evaluation is an active field of research [51]. In previous studies, it has been shown that some features, such as dyskinesia without spasticity, are strongly associated with genetic CP [65]. Additional characteristics have also been reported to be associated with genetic variants in CP patients. These include a normal brain MRI, no history of preterm birth, intellectual disability, communication difficulties, parental consanguinity, and bilateral motor symptoms [65, 66].

While recent studies have focused on CP as a polygenic disorder [67], more research is needed to understand the genetic characteristics of CP.

20.2.2.2 Epigenetics

Epigenetics is defined as the process of regulating gene expression without modifying the structure of Deoxyribonucleic Acid (DNA) [68] and includes alterations such as DNA methylation, histone modifications, and non-coding Ribonucleic Acid (RNA) regulation [69]. It has a major role in regulating gene expression in cases of cellular stress or disease [70, 71]. Recent studies have suggested epigenetics as a biomarker for earlier diagnosis of CP [72–74]. For example, DNA methylation, the process of adding a methyl group to the cytosine base in DNA [75], is altered in particular genes in CP patients, exhibiting either hypomethylation or hypermethylation. Some of these genes are involved in immune signaling pathways [72, 76–78]. Plasma level of micro Ribonucleic Acid (miRNA) has also been introduced as a potential biomarker for predicting CP [72, 79]. However, studies in this field, particularly on histone modifications, are limited and should be expanded to confirm their clinical relevance.

20.2.2.3 Transcriptomes

Transcriptomes, the complete set of RNA transcripts, have been proposed as potential biomarkers for the early detection of CP. Investigating transcriptomic profiles in patients at risk for CP is another promising and rapidly advancing area of research [73, 80].

20.2.3 Biochemical and Metabolomic Biomarkers

Many studies have shown that the elevated level of inflammatory biomarkers such as interleukin-6, interleukin-8, interleukin-1β, Tumor Necrosis Factor-α (TNF-α), TNF-α-receptor-1, and intercellular adhesion molecule-1 are associated with increased risk of developing CP [73, 81–86]. Besides, limited studies have introduced neuregulin-1 as a neuroprotector during fetal development, which was associated with a lower risk of CP in preterm children [87]. However, most studies in this field have evaluated inflammatory biomarkers in preschool and school-aged children or adults. To establish their applicability in the early diagnosis of CP, further investigations are needed.

Studying the metabolome, including metabolic pathways and associated metabolites within biological systems, is another promising biomarker for early detection of CP. There are studies evaluating metabolomic biomarkers of neurologic outcomes in patients with perinatal asphyxia and hypoxic ischemic encephalopathy, such as particular amino acids, acylcarnitines, glycerophospholipid classes, and energy-related metabolites, including succinate, glycerol, ketones, acetone, and 3-hydroxybutyrate [88, 89]. Additionally, the metabolomic profiles of low-birth-weight newborns differ from those of normal-weight newborns [90, 91].

To date, studies investigating the metabolomic profiles of individuals with CP remain limited. However, existing research has identified distinct metabolomic profiles in CP patients compared to normal individuals, both at rest and following physical activity [92, 93]. These findings underscore the potential of metabolomics as a compelling area of investigation for the early diagnosis of CP.

20.2.4 Prenatal Biomarkers

Limited studies have evaluated the association between pregnancy screening biomarkers and the risk of CP. Lower levels of the beta subunit of human Chorionic Gonadotropin (βhCG) and Pregnancy-Associated Plasma Protein-A (PAPP-A) in first-trimester screening tests [94–96], and higher levels of Alpha-Fetoprotein (AFP) and inhibin in second-trimester tests were detected in mothers of CP patients [97]. A combination of low βhCG and PAPP-A concentration has improved this association in the first trimester [95, 98]. Also, CP pregnancies were more likely when both AFP and inhibin levels were elevated [97]. These data emphasize the importance of early pregnancy and placentation in certain causal pathways to CP, making this a promising area for future research.

20.2.5 Movement-Based Biomarkers

Fidgety movements are spontaneous movements in newborns and young infants. Evaluating these actions using the General Movement Assessment (GMA), a method involving systematic observation of movements in infants as young as 3–5 months, has been shown to effectively predict future CP risk [99, 100]. Nevertheless, these observations are subjective and need trained experts to evaluate the risk of CP [101]. This task can be easily performed by Artificial Intelligence (AI) today.

New advancements in the field of AI, specifically in deep learning and computer vision, provide new avenues to early detection of CP. In certain studies, patients' skeletal data were extracted from video recordings using pose estimation algorithms [102, 103]. In these studies, deep learning algorithms were used to process this data to obtain spatio-temporal information of the infant's movements required for CP prediction [104, 105]. Furthermore, this information can serve as a disease-specific movement biomarker for AI-assisted early detection of CP. Despite its outstanding capabilities, AI is not yet clinically validated and requires further study in clinical settings [106].

20.2.6 Neurophysiological Biomarkers

Magnetoencephalography (MEG), high-density electroencephalography (EEG), and near-infrared spectroscopy (NIRS) are neurophysiological techniques currently under investigation for both the early diagnosis and rehabilitation planning of CP. A brief overview of each method and its potential applications is presented below.

MEG is a noninvasive, high-resolution neurophysiological imaging technique that detects magnetic fields generated by ionic currents within brain tissue [107]. Recent studies using MEG in CP patients may yield new findings about the pathophysiology of CP, and the results can be used as a biomarker, as well as helping to design new interventions [13, 107–110].

High-density EEG is another investigated tool that can lead to the development of new biomarkers for the early detection of CP [111, 112]. EEG can also help to evaluate the effectiveness of rehabilitation and other interventions in CP patients [113, 114].

NIRS, a noninvasive technique for continuously measuring oxygenation and perfusion of tissues, including the brain, can be used in various ways for patients with or at high risk of CP: as a monitoring tool for high-risk infants [115], a potential biomarker for early detection of CP [13], and for planning rehabilitation and predicting outcomes in CP patients [116–118].

Although recent studies have yielded promising results in the field of neurophysiological biomarkers, further research is needed to establish their clinical relevance.

20.3 Novel and Promising Management Strategies

Alongside traditional treatments such as physiotherapy, occupational therapy, oral muscle relaxants, and botulinum toxin, some new therapeutic interventions have been developed recently, including intrathecal baclofen injections, selective dorsal rhizotomy, and sensory integration therapies [119, 120]. Ongoing studies have reported encouraging findings, opening the path for innovative therapies.

This section reviews selected studies and examines the therapeutic potential of the new methods to enhance the quality of life for individuals with CP. It begins with an overview of emerging pharmacologic therapies currently under investigation, followed by a review of the novel and promising method of stem cell therapy. Subsequently, recent findings on the role of neuromodulation in patients with CP are discussed. Finally, the section explores new advances in neurorehabilitation and assistive communication technologies, highlighting their potential to enhance functional outcomes in CP patients.

20.3.1 Pharmacologic Therapies

New pharmacologic agents are under investigation for the prevention and treatment of CP. Darbepoetin alfa and erythropoietin (both erythropoiesis-stimulating agents) have been studied in neonates with hypoxic-ischemic encephalopathy or prematurity. While some studies reported improvements in neurodevelopmental outcomes and even a decreased risk of CP following administration of these agents in the first week of life [121–125], others questioned the long-term effects of these agents on cognition, especially regarding erythropoietin [126–128]. Accordingly, more detailed studies are needed to confirm the neuroprotective effects of these agents and their optimal dose.

Other agents, such as citicoline (oral and injectable), intramuscular piracetam, cerebrolysin, and nandrolone decanoate, have been reported to improve motor development in CP patients [129]. However, the studies are limited to case reports, and clinical trials are necessary to determine their effectiveness.

20.3.2 Stem Cell Therapy

Stem Cell therapy is a promising field for the future treatment of CP [130]. Most clinical trials used the umbilical cord blood/umbilical cord stem cells for this purpose, while bone marrow was the second common source for stem cells [131]. These types of stem cells, especially umbilical cord blood, are safe, efficient, and pose no ethical concern. These stem cells are also accessible, easy to preserve, and their proliferation is non-neoplastic [132]. Intrathecal and intravenous injection were the most prevalent routes of administration [131]. Studies have shown an improvement in gross motor functions following this treatment [131, 133, 134]. Although limited in number, there are studies, particularly those utilizing stem cells derived from sources other than umbilical cord blood, that have reported enhancements in fine motor skills, cognitive abilities, language development, and muscle tone [130, 131]. Furthermore, additional clinical trials are necessary to establish the efficacy and safety of this method before it can be routinely implemented in clinical practice.

20.3.3 Non-invasive Neuromodulation

Neuromodulation is a technique to alter neuronal activity by delivering electrical, electromagnetic, or chemical stimulation to different parts of the nervous system [135]. While extensively explored in some psychiatric disorders, these methods are currently under investigation in neurologic diseases. The most studied non-invasive neuromodulation devices in CP patients are Repetitive Transcranial Magnetic Stimulation (rTMS), Transcranial Direct Current Stimulation (tDCS), and transcutaneous spinal neuromodulation.

Studies using rTMS in children with CP have shown improvement in the patients' motor function and language ability. However, the duration and persistence of this effect are uncertain. In addition, the studies' small sample size and inconsistent results make the results non-generalizable [136]. Furthermore, more qualified studies, especially those comparing the effect of rTMS to sham stimulation, are required before its routine application in clinical settings.

Studies evaluating the effect of tDCS in CP patients on improving upper limb function have revealed promising results. However, limited studies have evaluated its effectiveness on lower limb function, gait, balance, cognition, and language ability. Despite the potential effect of tDCS in these domains based on case reports and small studies, its clinical relevance needs to be studied further [136].

The other non-invasive neuromodulation method, transcutaneous spinal neuromodulation, is usually used in patients with spinal cord injury. But recent studies have examined its effect in combination with activity-based neurorehabilitation therapy on enhancing voluntary sensorimotor function in CP patients and produced promising results [137]. Considering that the studies are limited to case series and small trials, more extensive studies are needed to confirm this method's clinical application.

20.3.4 Advanced Neurorehabilitation and Communication Devices

Advances in robotics have a role in the rehabilitation of CP patients. Robot-assisted gait training has the advantage of longer duration, repetition, and constant speed and pattern over traditional gait rehabilitation. Lower limb robotic exoskeletons can improve the quality of life in patients with CP [138]. Despite the extensive literature on these techniques, further review studies are needed to investigate their efficacy. The other research focus in this field is upper limb robotic assistance and also social robots, which can improve communication in CP patients [139, 140].

Virtual reality, a technology for making imagination as real as reality, is a development in the field of rehabilitation. It provides an environment that facilitates patients' engagement in functional activities. This technology has been used in CP patients to help them as a strategy for managing pain [139, 141]. Although recent studies have shown its promising effect in improving upper extremity function, motor performance, and balance, more studies are needed to confirm its effectiveness in CP patients [142–144].

Augmentative and alternative communication devices are new technological devices helping speech-impaired CP patients to communicate and express their thoughts [139]. Although most studies have shown these devices' efficacy in improving the communication of CP patients, more thorough methodological studies are required to investigate their detailed efficacy on different aspects of communication [145].

Different mobile applications have been developed to help CP patients either in caregiver training, executing occupational and physiotherapy methods, identifying pain in non-communicating patients, or enhancing affected arm utilization in daily tasks [146, 147]. While these applications are already beneficial, they can evolve further by adopting user-centered designs, making therapy more engaging, data-driven, and widely accessible.

20.4 Parent and Caregiver Support

Recent progress in CP research is driving meaningful improvements in patient care, while easing the physical, emotional, and financial challenges experienced by patients and their families. A major focus has been on earlier diagnosis, which not only enables timely intervention but also supports parents in planning future pregnancies with greater confidence. Meanwhile, progress in therapeutic strategies, particularly the integration of AI into CP management, has shown encouraging potential for enhancing patient outcomes. Nonetheless, it is important to note that many of these diagnostic and treatment approaches remain under investigation and require further validation before they can be widely adopted in clinical practice.

20.5 Conclusion

New advances in early diagnosis and treatment of CP will reshape its future management. Developments such as AI-assisted video analysis, genetic, and epigenetic testing have been the most promising early diagnostic techniques.

Stem cell therapy and robotic rehabilitation have the potential to improve CP patients' motor function, cognition, and quality of life. Nevertheless, besides the issues such as cost and accessibility, the performance of these methods requires further clinical validation.

Finally, all of these advancements can be more effective in the case of adopting a multidisciplinary approach. Researchers, clinicians, policy-makers, caregivers, and CP patients should collaborate to translate these innovations into worldwide benefits. Together, we can create a brighter future for people with CP, featuring better treatments, greater independence, and new hope.

References

1. Smigelski GD. Cerebral palsy: current concepts and a glimpse into the future. Jaapa. 2025;38(3):30–5.
2. Baxter P, Morris C, Rosenbaum P, Paneth N, Leviton A, Goldstein M, et al. The definition and classification of cerebral palsy. Dev Med Child Neurol. 2007;109:8–14.
3. Tonmukayakul U, Shih ST, Bourke-Taylor H, Imms C, Reddihough D, Cox L, et al. Systematic review of the economic impact of cerebral palsy. Res Dev Disabil. 2018;80:93–101.
4. Granild-Jensen JB, Rackauskaite G, Flachs EM, Uldall P. Predictors for early diagnosis of cerebral palsy from national registry data. Dev Med Child Neurol. 2015;57(10):931–5.
5. Hubermann L, Boychuck Z, Shevell M, Majnemer A. Age at referral of children for initial diagnosis of cerebral palsy and rehabilitation: current practices. J Child Neurol. 2016;31(3):364–9.
6. Shepherd RB. Cerebral palsy in infancy: targeted activity to optimize early growth and development. Elsevier Health Sciences; 2013.
7. Eliasson AC, Holmefur M. The influence of early modified constraint-induced movement therapy training on the longitudinal development of hand function in children with unilateral cerebral palsy. Dev Med Child Neurol. 2015;57(1):89–94.

8. Herskind A, Greisen G, Nielsen JB. Early identification and intervention in cerebral palsy. Dev Med Child Neurol. 2015;57(1):29–36.
9. Eyre J. Corticospinal tract development and activity-dependent plasticity. In: Cerebral Palsy in Infancy: targeted activity to optimize early growth and development, vol. 53; 2013.
10. Martin JH, Chakrabarty S, Friel KM. Harnessing activity-dependent plasticity to repair the damaged corticospinal tract in an animal model of cerebral palsy. Dev Med Child Neurol. 2011;53:9–13.
11. Spittle A, Orton J, Doyle LW, Boyd R. Early developmental intervention programs post hospital discharge to prevent motor and cognitive impairments in preterm infants. In: Cochrane Database Syst Rev, vol. 12; 2007. p. CD005495.
12. Novak I, Morgan C, Adde L, Blackman J, Boyd RN, Brunstrom-Hernandez J, et al. Early, accurate diagnosis and early intervention in cerebral palsy: advances in diagnosis and treatment. JAMA Pediatr. 2017;171(9):897–907.
13. Parikh NA. Advanced neuroimaging and its role in predicting neurodevelopmental outcomes in very preterm infants. Semin Perinatol. 2016;40(8):530–41.
14. Anderson PJ, Cheong JL, Thompson DK. The predictive validity of neonatal MRI for neurodevelopmental outcome in very preterm children. Semin Perinatol. 2015;39(2):147–58.
15. Parikh NA, Hershey A, Altaye M. Early detection of cerebral palsy using sensorimotor tract biomarkers in very preterm infants. Pediatr Neurol. 2019;98:53–60.
16. Le Bihan D. Apparent diffusion coefficient and beyond: what diffusion MR imaging can tell us about tissue structure. Radiology. 2013;268:318–22.
17. Winklewski PJ, Sabisz A, Naumczyk P, Jodzio K, Szurowska E, Szarmach A. Understanding the physiopathology behind axial and radial diffusivity changes—what do we know? Front Neurol. 2018;9:92.
18. Jeurissen B, Descoteaux M, Mori S, Leemans A. Diffusion MRI fiber tractography of the brain. NMR Biomed. 2019;32(4):e3785.
19. Hoon JA, Lawrie JW, Melhem E, Reinhardt E, Van Zijl P, Solaiyappan M, et al. Diffusion tensor imaging of periventricular leukomalacia shows affected sensory cortex white matter pathways. Neurology. 2002;59(5):752–6.
20. Hoon AH Jr, Stashinko EE, Nagae LM, Lin DD, Keller J, Bastian A, et al. Sensory and motor deficits in children with cerebral palsy born preterm correlate with diffusion tensor imaging abnormalities in thalamocortical pathways. Dev Med Child Neurol. 2009;51(9):697–704.
21. Scheck SM, Boyd RN, Rose SE. New insights into the pathology of white matter tracts in cerebral palsy from diffusion magnetic resonance imaging: a systematic review. Dev Med Child Neurol. 2012;54(8):684–96.
22. Kaur S, Powell S, He L, Pierson CR, Parikh NA. Reliability and repeatability of quantitative tractography methods for mapping structural white matter connectivity in preterm and term infants at term-equivalent age. PLoS One. 2014;9(1):e85807.
23. Teli R, Hay M, Hershey A, Kumar M, Yin H, Parikh NA. Postnatal microstructural developmental trajectory of corpus callosum subregions and relationship to clinical factors in very preterm infants. Sci Rep. 2018;8(1):7550.
24. Boardman JP, Bhatia K, Counsell S, Allsop J, Kapellou O, Rutherford MA, et al., editors. An evaluation of deformation-based morphometry applied to the developing human brain and detection of volumetric changes associated with preterm birth. Medical Image Computing and Computer-Assisted Intervention-MICCAI 2003: 6th International Conference, Montréal, November 15–18, 2003 Proceedings 6; 2003: Springer.
25. Boardman JP, Counsell SJ, Rueckert D, Kapellou O, Bhatia KK, Aljabar P, et al. Abnormal deep grey matter development following preterm birth detected using deformation-based morphometry. NeuroImage. 2006;32(1):70–8.
26. Inder TE, Huppi PS, Warfield S, Kikinis R, Zientara GP, Barnes PD, et al. Periventricular white matter injury in the premature infant is followed by reduced cerebral cortical gray matter volume at term. Ann Neurol. 1999;46(5):755–60.
27. Woodward LJ, Anderson PJ, Austin NC, Howard K, Inder TE. Neonatal MRI to predict neurodevelopmental outcomes in preterm infants. N Engl J Med. 2006;355(7):685–94.

28. Cheong JL, Hunt RW, Anderson PJ, Howard K, Thompson DK, Wang HX, et al. Head growth in preterm infants: correlation with magnetic resonance imaging and neurodevelopmental outcome. Pediatrics. 2008;121(6):e1534–e40.
29. Northam GB, Liégeois F, Chong WK, S. Wyatt J, Baldeweg T. Total brain white matter is a major determinant of IQ in adolescents born preterm. Ann Neurol. 2011;69(4):702–11.
30. Peterson BS, Vohr B, Staib LH, Cannistraci CJ, Dolberg A, Schneider KC, et al. Regional brain volume abnormalities and long-term cognitive outcome in preterm infants. JAMA. 2000;284(15):1939–47.
31. Boardman JP, Craven C, Valappil S, Counsell SJ, Dyet LE, Rueckert D, et al. A common neonatal image phenotype predicts adverse neurodevelopmental outcome in children born preterm. NeuroImage. 2010;52(2):409–14.
32. Kułak P, Maciorkowska E, Gościk E. Volumetric magnetic resonance imaging study of brain and cerebellum in children with cerebral palsy. Biomed Res Int. 2016;2016:5961928.
33. Milos RI, Jovanov-Milošević N, Mitter C, Bobić-Rasonja M, Pogledic I, Gruber GM, et al. Developmental dynamics of the periventricular parietal crossroads of growing cortical pathways in the fetal brain – in vivo fetal MRI with histological correlation. NeuroImage. 2020;210:116553.
34. He L, Parikh NA. Atlas-guided quantification of white matter signal abnormalities on term-equivalent age MRI in very preterm infants: findings predict language and cognitive development at two years of age. PLoS One. 2013;8(12):e85475.
35. Parikh NA, He L, Bonfante-Mejia E, Hochhauser L, Wilder PE, Burson K, et al. Automatically quantified diffuse excessive high signal intensity on MRI predicts cognitive development in preterm infants. Pediatr Neurol. 2013;49(6):424–30.
36. Hui SC, Andescavage N, Limperopoulos C. The role of proton magnetic resonance spectroscopy in neonatal and fetal brain research. J Magn Reson Imaging. 2025;61:2404.
37. Perdue MV, DeMayo MM, Bell TK, Boudes E, Bagshawe M, Harris AD, et al. Changes in brain metabolite levels across childhood. NeuroImage. 2023;274:120087.
38. Zhu H, Barker PB. MR spectroscopy and spectroscopic imaging of the brain. In: Magnetic resonance neuroimaging: methods and protocols; 2010. p. 203–26.
39. Blusztajn JK, Slack BE, Mellott TJ. Neuroprotective actions of dietary choline. Nutrients. 2017;9(8):815.
40. Bapat R, Narayana PA, Zhou Y, Parikh NA. Magnetic resonance spectroscopy at term-equivalent age in extremely preterm infants: association with cognitive and language development. Pediatr Neurol. 2014;51(1):53–9.
41. Hyodo R, Sato Y, Ito M, Sugiyama Y, Ogawa C, Kawai H, et al. Magnetic resonance spectroscopy in preterm infants: association with neurodevelopmental outcomes. Arch Dis Child Fetal Neonatal Ed. 2018;103(3):F238–F44.
42. Hart A, Smith M, Whitby E, Alladi S, Wilkinson S, Paley M, et al. Diffusion-weighted imaging and magnetic resonance proton spectroscopy following preterm birth. Clin Radiol. 2014;69(8):870–9.
43. Van Kooij BJ, Benders MJ, Anbeek P, Van Haastert IC, De Vries LS, Groenendaal F. Cerebellar volume and proton magnetic resonance spectroscopy at term, and neurodevelopment at 2 years of age in preterm infants. Dev Med Child Neurol. 2012;54(3):260–6.
44. Kendall GS, Melbourne A, Johnson S, Price D, Bainbridge A, Gunny R, et al. White matter NAA/Cho and Cho/Cr ratios at MR spectroscopy are predictive of motor outcome in preterm infants. Radiology. 2014;271(1):230–8.
45. Gire C, Berbis J, Dequin M, Marret S, Muller J-B, Saliba E, et al. A correlation between magnetic resonance spectroscopy (1-H MRS) and the neurodevelopment of two-year-olds born preterm in an EPIRMEX cohort study. Front Pediatr. 2022;10:936130.
46. Chau V, Synnes A, Grunau RE, Poskitt KJ, Brant R, Miller SP. Abnormal brain maturation in preterm neonates associated with adverse developmental outcomes. Neurology. 2013;81(24):2082–9.

47. Tomiyasu M, Shibasaki J, Kawaguchi H, Enokizono M, Toyoshima K, Obata T, et al. Altered brain metabolite concentration and delayed neurodevelopment in preterm neonates. Pediatr Res. 2022;91(1):197–203.
48. Cebeci B, Alderliesten T, Wijnen JP, van der Aa NE, Benders MJ, de Vries LS, et al. Brain proton magnetic resonance spectroscopy and neurodevelopment after preterm birth: a systematic review. Pediatr Res. 2022;91(6):1322–33.
49. Laccetta G, De Nardo MC, Cellitti R, Angeloni U, Terrin G. 1H-magnetic resonance spectroscopy and its role in predicting neurodevelopmental impairment in preterm neonates: a systematic review. Neuroradiol J. 2022;35(6):667–77.
50. Michael-Asalu A, Taylor G, Campbell H, Lelea L-L, Kirby RS. Cerebral palsy: diagnosis, epidemiology, genetics, and clinical update. Adv Pediatr. 2019;66:189–208.
51. Basu AP, Low K, Ratnaike T, Rowitch D. Genetic investigations in cerebral palsy. Dev Med Child Neurol. 2025;67(2):177–85.
52. Fahey MC, Maclennan AH, Kretzschmar D, Gecz J, Kruer MC. The genetic basis of cerebral palsy. Dev Med Child Neurol. 2017;59(5):462–9.
53. Chopra M, Gable DL, Love-Nichols J, Tsao A, Rockowitz S, Sliz P, et al. Mendelian etiologies identified with whole exome sequencing in cerebral palsy. Ann Clin Transl Neurol. 2022;9(2):193–205.
54. Srivastava S, Lewis SA, Cohen JS, Zhang B, Aravamuthan BR, Chopra M, et al. Molecular diagnostic yield of exome sequencing and chromosomal microarray in cerebral palsy: a systematic review and meta-analysis. JAMA Neurol. 2022;79(12):1287–95.
55. Gonzalez-Mantilla PJ, Hu Y, Myers SM, Finucane BM, Ledbetter DH, Martin CL, et al. Diagnostic yield of exome sequencing in cerebral palsy and implications for genetic testing guidelines: a systematic review and meta-analysis. JAMA Pediatr. 2023;177(5):472–8.
56. Takezawa Y, Kikuchi A, Haginoya K, Niihori T, Numata-Uematsu Y, Inui T, et al. Genomic analysis identifies masqueraders of full-term cerebral palsy. Ann Clin Transl Neurol. 2018;5(5):538–51.
57. May HJ, Fasheun JA, Bain JM, Baugh EH, Bier LE, Revah-Politi A, et al. Genetic testing in individuals with cerebral palsy. Dev Med Child Neurol. 2021;63(12):1448–55.
58. Wang Y, Xu Y, Zhou C, Cheng Y, Qiao N, Shang Q, et al. Exome sequencing reveals genetic heterogeneity and clinically actionable findings in children with cerebral palsy. Nat Med. 2024;30(5):1395–405.
59. Morell AS, Monsell SE, Cornet MC, Wisnowski JL, McKinstry RC, Mathur AM, et al. Genetic and congenital anomalies in infants with hypoxic-ischemic encephalopathy. Pediatr Neurol. 2024;154:44–50.
60. Woodward KE, Murthy P, Mineyko A, Mohammad K, Esser MJ. Identifying genetic susceptibility in neonates with hypoxic-ischemic encephalopathy: a retrospective case series. J Child Neurol. 2023;38(1–2):16–24.
61. Merchant N, Azzopardi D. Early predictors of outcome in infants treated with hypothermia for hypoxic-ischaemic encephalopathy. Dev Med Child Neurol. 2015;57(Suppl 3):8–16.
62. Packer CH, Hersh AR, Sargent JA, Caughey AB. Therapeutic hypothermia in severe hypoxic-ischemic encephalopathy: a cost-effectiveness analysis. J Matern Fetal Neonatal Med. 2022;35(5):890–7.
63. Kapitanović Vidak H, Catela Ivković T, Vidak Z, Kapitanović S. COX-1 and COX-2 polymorphisms in susceptibility to cerebral palsy in very preterm infants. Mol Neurobiol. 2017;54(2):930–8.
64. Rajatileka S, Odd D, Robinson MT, Spittle AC, Dwomoh L, Williams M, et al. Variants of the EAAT2 glutamate transporter gene promoter are associated with cerebral palsy in preterm infants. Mol Neurobiol. 2018;55(3):2013–24.
65. Janzing AM, Eklund E, De Koning TJ, Eggink H. Clinical characteristics suggestive of a genetic cause in cerebral palsy: a systematic review. Pediatr Neurol. 2024;153:144–51.
66. Fehlings DL, Zarrei M, Engchuan W, Sondheimer N, Thiruvahindrapuram B, MacDonald JR, et al. Comprehensive whole-genome sequence analyses provide insights into the genomic architecture of cerebral palsy. Nat Genet. 2024;56(4):585–94.

67. Hale AT, Akinnusotu O, He J, Wang J, Hibshman N, Shannon CN, et al. Genome-wide association study identifies genetic risk factors for spastic cerebral palsy. Neurosurgery. 2021;89(3):435–42.
68. Bird A. Perceptions of epigenetics. London: Nature Publishing Group; 2007.
69. Chuang JC, Jones PA. Epigenetics and microRNAs. Pediatr Res. 2007;61(7):24–9.
70. Barker DJ. The origins of the developmental origins theory. J Intern Med. 2007;261(5):412–7.
71. Dolinoy DC, Weidman JR, Jirtle RL. Epigenetic gene regulation: linking early developmental environment to adult disease. Reprod Toxicol. 2007;23(3):297–307.
72. Romero B, Robinson KG, Batish M, Akins RE. An emerging role for epigenetics in cerebral palsy. J Pers Med. 2021;11(11):1187.
73. Savasan ZA, Kim SK, Oh KJ, Graham SF. Advances in cerebral palsy biomarkers. Adv Clin Chem. 2021;100:139–69.
74. Akins R. Epigenetic biomarkers for spastic cerebral palsy. 2023.
75. Holliday R, Grigg G. DNA methylation and mutation. Mutat Res/Fundam Mol Mech Mutagen. 1993;285(1):61–7.
76. Jiao Z, Jiang Z, Wang J, Xu H, Zhang Q, Liu S, et al. Whole-genome scale identification of methylation markers specific for cerebral palsy in monozygotic discordant twins. Mol Med Rep. 2017;16(6):9423–30.
77. Mohandas N, Bass-Stringer S, Maksimovic J, Crompton K, Loke YJ, Walstab J, et al. Epigenome-wide analysis in newborn blood spots from monozygotic twins discordant for cerebral palsy reveals consistent regional differences in DNA methylation. Clin Epigenetics. 2018;10(1):25.
78. Bahado-Singh RO, Vishweswaraiah S, Aydas B, Mishra NK, Guda C, Radhakrishna U. Deep learning/artificial intelligence and blood-based DNA epigenomic prediction of cerebral palsy. Int J Mol Sci. 2019;20(9):2075.
79. Chapman S, Farina L, Kronforst K, Dizon M. MicroRNA profile differences in neonates at risk for cerebral palsy. Phys Med Rehabil Int. 2018;5(3):1148.
80. Ho NT, Furge K, Fu W, Busik J, Khoo SK, Lu Q, et al. Gene expression in archived newborn blood spots distinguishes infants who will later develop cerebral palsy from matched controls. Pediatr Res. 2013;73(1):450–6.
81. Magalhães RC, Moreira JM, Vieira ÉLM, Rocha NP, Miranda DM, Simoes e Silva AC. Urinary levels of IL-1β and GDNF in preterm neonates as potential biomarkers of motor development: a prospective study. Mediat Inflamm. 2017;2017(1):8201423.
82. Yoon BH, Romero R, Park JS, Kim CJ, Kim SH, Choi J-H, et al. Fetal exposure to an intra-amniotic inflammation and the development of cerebral palsy at the age of three years. Am J Obstet Gynecol. 2000;182(3):675–81.
83. Kuban KC, O'Shea TM, Allred EN, Paneth N, Hirtz D, Fichorova RN, et al. Systemic inflammation and cerebral palsy risk in extremely preterm infants. J Child Neurol. 2014;29(12):1692–8.
84. Yanni D, Korzeniewski SJ, Allred EN, Fichorova RN, O'Shea TM, Kuban K, et al. Both antenatal and postnatal inflammation contribute information about the risk of brain damage in extremely preterm newborns. Pediatr Res. 2017;82(4):691–6.
85. Carlo WA, McDonald SA, Tyson JE, Stoll BJ, Ehrenkranz RA, Shankaran S, et al. Cytokines and neurodevelopmental outcomes in extremely low birth weight infants. J Pediatr. 2011;159(6):919–25.e3.
86. Magalhaes RC, Moreira JM, Lauar AO, da Silva AAS, Teixeira AL, e Silva ACS. Inflammatory biomarkers in children with cerebral palsy: a systematic review. Res Dev Disabil. 2019;95:103508.
87. Hoffmann I, Bueter W, Zscheppang K, Brinkhaus M-J, Liese A, Riemke S, et al. Neuregulin-1, the fetal endothelium, and brain damage in preterm newborns. Brain Behav Immun. 2010;24(5):784–91.
88. Walsh BH, Broadhurst DI, Mandal R, Wishart DS, Boylan GB, Kenny LC, et al. The metabolomic profile of umbilical cord blood in neonatal hypoxic ischaemic encephalopathy. PLoS One. 2012;7(12):e50520.

89. Reinke SN, Walsh BH, Boylan GB, Sykes BD, Kenny LC, Murray DM, et al. 1H NMR derived metabolomic profile of neonatal asphyxia in umbilical cord serum: implications for hypoxic ischemic encephalopathy. J Proteome Res. 2013;12(9):4230–9.
90. Favretto D, Cosmi E, Ragazzi E, Visentin S, Tucci M, Fais P, et al. Cord blood metabolomic profiling in intrauterine growth restriction. Anal Bioanal Chem. 2012;402(3):1109–21.
91. Ivorra C, García-Vicent C, Chaves FJ, Monleón D, Morales JM, Lurbe E. Metabolomic profiling in blood from umbilical cords of low birth weight newborns. J Transl Med. 2012;10(1):142.
92. Wang D, Song J, Cheng Y, Xu Y, Song L, Qiao Y, et al. Targeting the metabolic profile of amino acids to identify the key metabolic characteristics in cerebral palsy. Front Mol Neurosci. 2023;16:1237745.
93. Hanaoka C, Pichika R, Dayanidhi S, Jayabalan P. Serum metabolomics after exercise in ambulatory individuals with cerebral palsy. Dev Med Child Neurol. 2025;67(5):639–47.
94. Eskild A, Monkerud L, Jukic AM, Åsvold BO, Lie KK. Maternal concentrations of human chorionic gonadotropin (hCG) and risk for cerebral palsy (CP) in the child. A case control study. Eur J Obstet Gynecol Reprod Biol. 2018;228:203–8.
95. Peris M, Reid SM, Dobie S, Bonacquisto L, Shepherd DA, Amor DJ. First-trimester maternal serum biomarkers and the risk of cerebral palsy. Dev Med Child Neurol. 2021;63(2):183–9.
96. Larsen ML, Rackauskaite G, Pihl K, Uldall P, Greisen G, Krebs L, et al. First-trimester biomarkers and the risk of cerebral palsy. Early Hum Dev. 2022;167:105564.
97. Peris M, Reid SM, Dobie S, Bonacquisto L, Shepherd DA, Amor DJ. Second trimester maternal serum biomarkers and the risk of cerebral palsy. Prenat Diagn. 2021;41(9):1101–10.
98. Lentejas JPR, Velayo CL. Association of first-trimester screening biomarkers and the prevalence of cerebral palsy and other neurodevelopmental conditions: a systematic review. Sci Engg J. 2024;17(Supplement):155–62.
99. Prechtl HF, Einspieler C, Cioni G, Bos AF, Ferrari F, Sontheimer D. An early marker for neurological deficits after perinatal brain lesions. Lancet. 1997;349(9062):1361–3.
100. Ricci E, Einspieler C, Craig AK. Feasibility of using the general movements assessment of infants in the United States. Phys Occup Ther Pediatr. 2018;38(3):269–79.
101. Silva N, Zhang D, Kulvicius T, Gail A, Barreiros C, Lindstaedt S, et al. The future of general movement assessment: the role of computer vision and machine learning–a scoping review. Res Dev Disabil. 2021;110:103854.
102. Dubey S, Dixit M. A comprehensive survey on human pose estimation approaches. Multimedia Systems. 2023;29(1):167–95.
103. Knap P. Human modelling and pose estimation overview. arXiv preprint arXiv:240619290. 2024.
104. Zhang H, Ho ES, Shum HP. Cp-agcn: Pytorch-based attention informed graph convolutional network for identifying infants at risk of cerebral palsy. Software Impacts. 2022;14:100419.
105. Groos D, Adde L, Aubert S, Boswell L, De Regnier R-A, Fjørtoft T, et al. Development and validation of a deep learning method to predict cerebral palsy from spontaneous movements in infants at high risk. JAMA Netw Open. 2022;5(7):e2221325-e.
106. Pellano KN, Strümke I, Groos D, Adde L, Haugen P, Ihlen EAF. Towards biomarker discovery for early cerebral palsy detection: evaluating explanations through kinematic perturbations. arXiv preprint arXiv:250316452. 2025.
107. Wilson TW, Heinrichs-Graham E, Proskovec AL, McDermott TJ. Neuroimaging with magnetoencephalography: a dynamic view of brain pathophysiology. Transl Res. 2016;175:17–36.
108. Pihko E, Nevalainen P, Vaalto S, Laaksonen K, Mäenpää H, Valanne L, et al. Reactivity of sensorimotor oscillations is altered in children with hemiplegic cerebral palsy: a magnetoencephalographic study. Hum Brain Mapp. 2014;35(8):4105–17.
109. Démas J, Bourguignon M, Périvier M, De Tiège X, Dinomais M, Van Bogaert P. Mu rhythm: state of the art with special focus on cerebral palsy. Ann Phys Rehabil Med. 2020;63(5):439–46.

110. Kurz MJ, Becker KM, Heinrichs-Graham E, Wilson TW. Neurophysiological abnormalities in the sensorimotor cortices during the motor planning and movement execution stages of children with cerebral palsy. Dev Med Child Neurol. 2014;56(11):1072–7.
111. Bakheet D, Alotaibi N, Konn D, Vollmer B, Maharatna K. Prediction of cerebral palsy in newborns with hypoxic-ischemic encephalopathy using multivariate EEG analysis and machine learning. IEEE Access. 2021;9:137833–46.
112. Rajak BL, Gupta M, Bhatia D, Mukherjee A, Paul S, Sinha TK. Power spectral analysis of EEG as a potential marker in the diagnosis of spastic cerebral palsy cases. Int J Biomed Eng Sci. 2016;3(3):23–9.
113. Rajak BL, Gupta M, Bhatia D, Mukherjee A, Paul S, Sinha TK. Power spectrum density analysis of EEG signals in spastic cerebral palsy patients by inducing r-TMS therapy. J Biomed Eng Technol. 2016;4(1):7–11.
114. Kułak W, Sobaniec W, Boćkowski L, Sołowiej E, Śmigielska-Kuzia J, Artemowicz B, et al. Neurophysiologic studies of brain plasticity in children with cerebral palsy. Depression. 2005;27:28.
115. Jeon GW. Clinical application of near-infrared spectroscopy in neonates. Neonatal Med. 2019;26(3):121–7.
116. Cao J, Khan B, Hervey N, Tian F, Delgado MR, Clegg NJ, et al. Evaluation of cortical plasticity in children with cerebral palsy undergoing constraint-induced movement therapy based on functional near-infrared spectroscopy. J Biomed Opt. 2015;20(4):046009.
117. Sukal-Moulton T, de Campos AC, Alter KE, Huppert TJ, Damiano DL. Relationship between sensorimotor cortical activation as assessed by functional near infrared spectroscopy and lower extremity motor coordination in bilateral cerebral palsy. NeuroImage Clin. 2018;20:275–85.
118. Chaudhary U, Hall M, Gonzalez J, Elbaum L, Bloyer M, Godavarty A. Motor response investigation in individuals with cerebral palsy using near infrared spectroscopy: pilot study. Appl Opt. 2014;53(3):503–10.
119. Rana M, Upadhyay J, Rana A, Durgapal S, Jantwal A. A systematic review on etiology, epidemiology, and treatment of cerebral palsy. Int J Nutr Pharmacol Neurol Dis. 2017;7(4):76–83.
120. Mittal R, Dhiman S, Ahmed S, Sharma R, Khan MH, Ajmera P, et al. Impact of sensory-based therapy on problems with balance and posture in children with cerebral palsy: a systematic review and meta-analysis. Discover Public Health. 2024;21(1):197.
121. Ohls RK, Cannon DC, Phillips J, Caprihan A, Patel S, Winter S, et al. Preschool assessment of preterm infants treated with darbepoetin and erythropoietin. Pediatrics. 2016;137(3):e20153859.
122. Ohls RK, Kamath-Rayne BD, Christensen RD, Wiedmeier SE, Rosenberg A, Fuller J, et al. Cognitive outcomes of preterm infants randomized to darbepoetin, erythropoietin, or placebo. Pediatrics. 2014;133(6):1023–30.
123. Razak A, Hussain A. Erythropoietin in perinatal hypoxic-ischemic encephalopathy: a systematic review and meta-analysis. J Perinat Med. 2019;47(4):478–89.
124. Patel S, Ohls RK. Darbepoetin administration in term and preterm neonates. Clin Perinatol. 2015;42(3):557–66.
125. DuPont TL, Baserga M, Lowe J, Zamora T, Beauman S, Ohls RK. Darbepoetin as a neuroprotective agent in mild neonatal encephalopathy: a randomized, placebo-controlled, feasibility trial. J Perinatol. 2021;41(6):1339–46.
126. Wu YW, Comstock BA, Gonzalez FF, Mayock DE, Goodman AM, Maitre NL, et al. Trial of erythropoietin for hypoxic–ischemic encephalopathy in newborns. N Engl J Med. 2022;387(2):148–59.
127. Ohls RK, Das A, Tan S, Lowe JR, Schibler K, Beauman SS, et al. Darbepoetin, red cell mass, and neuroprotection in preterm infants: a randomized clinical trial. JAMA Pediatr. 2025;179:836.
128. Perrone S, Lembo C, Gironi F, Petrolini C, Catalucci T, Corbo G, et al. Erythropoietin as a neuroprotective drug for newborn infants: ten years after the first use. Antioxidants. 2022;11(4):652.

129. Al-Mosawi A. Cerebral palsy: A unique illustrated experience. Med Res Chronicles. 2020;7(4):217–39.
130. Akat A, Karaöz E. A systematic review of cell therapy modalities and outcomes in cerebral palsy. Mol Cell Biochem. 2025;480(2):891–922.
131. Lv Z-Y, Li Y, Liu J. Progress in clinical trials of stem cell therapy for cerebral palsy. Neural Regen Res. 2021;16(7):1377–82.
132. Jiao Y, Li X-y, Liu J. A new approach to cerebral palsy treatment: discussion of the effective components of umbilical cord blood and its mechanisms of action. Cell Transplant. 2019;28(5):497–509.
133. Eggenberger S, Boucard C, Schoeberlein A, Guzman R, Limacher A, Surbek D, et al. Stem cell treatment and cerebral palsy: systemic review and meta-analysis. World J Stem Cells. 2019;11(10):891.
134. Qu J, Zhou L, Zhang H, Han D, Luo Y, Chen J, et al. Efficacy and safety of stem cell therapy in cerebral palsy: a systematic review and meta-analysis. Front Bioeng Biotechnol. 2022;10:1006845.
135. Johnson MD, Lim HH, Netoff TI, Connolly AT, Johnson N, Roy A, et al. Neuromodulation for brain disorders: challenges and opportunities. IEEE Trans Biomed Eng. 2013;60(3):610–24.
136. Singh S, Bhattacharjee S, Udupa K. Neuromodulation interventions in paediatric neurological disorders: a contemporary review of scientific advancements. J Pediatr Neonat Med. 2024;6(1)
137. Sachdeva R, Girshin K, Shirkhani Y, Gad P, Edgerton VR. Combining spinal neuromodulation and activity based neurorehabilitation therapy improves sensorimotor function in cerebral palsy. Front Rehabil Sci. 2023;4:1216281.
138. Cherni Y, Ballaz L, Lemaire J, Dal Maso F, Begon M. Effect of low dose robotic-gait training on walking capacity in children and adolescents with cerebral palsy. Neurophysiol Clin. 2020;50(6):507–19.
139. Paul S, Nahar A, Bhagawati M, Kunwar AJ. A review on recent advances of cerebral palsy. Oxidative Med Cell Longev. 2022;2022(1):2622310.
140. Papakostas GA, Sidiropoulos GK, Papadopoulou CI, Vrochidou E, Kaburlasos VG, Papadopoulou MT, et al. Social robots in special education: a systematic review. Electronics. 2021;10(12):1398.
141. Chen Y, Fanchiang HD, Howard A. Effectiveness of virtual reality in children with cerebral palsy: a systematic review and meta-analysis of randomized controlled trials. Phys Ther. 2018;98(1):63–77.
142. Bell J, Decker B, Eichmann A, Palkovich C, Reji C. Effectiveness of virtual reality for upper extremity function and motor performance of children with cerebral palsy: a systematic review. Am J Occup Ther. 2024;78(2):7802180180.
143. Komariah M, Amirah S, Abdurrahman MF, Handimulya MFS, Platini H, Maulana S, et al. Effectivity of virtual reality to improve balance, motor function, activities of daily living, and upper limb function in children with cerebral palsy: a systematic review and meta-analysis. Ther Clin Risk Manag. 2024;Volume 20:95–109.
144. Ravi D, Kumar N, Singhi P. Effectiveness of virtual reality rehabilitation for children and adolescents with cerebral palsy: an updated evidence-based systematic review. Physiotherapy. 2017;103(3):245–58.
145. Avagyan A, Mkrtchyan H, Shafa FA, Mathew JA, Petrosyan T. Effectiveness and determinant variables of augmentative and alternative communication interventions in cerebral palsy patients with communication deficit: a systematic review. Codas. 2021;33(5):e20200244.
146. Gozali E, Asr RT, Kashani K, Rahimi B. Effect of smart mobile applications in the care of children with cerebral palsy. Iran Biomed J. 2024;28:3.
147. Sabater-Gárriz Á, Gaya-Morey FX, Buades-Rubio JM, Manresa-Yee C, Riquelme I, Montoya P, et al. Design of a mobile application based on artificial intelligence to identify pain in non-communicating individuals with cerebral palsy. Res Dev Disabil. 2025;164:105058.

MIX
Papier aus verantwortungsvollen Quellen
Paper from responsible sources
FSC® C105338

FSC
www.fsc.org

If you have any concerns about our products,
you can contact us on
ProductSafety@springernature.com

In case Publisher is established outside the EU,
the EU authorized representative is:
Springer Nature Customer Service Center GmbH
Europaplatz 3, 69115 Heidelberg, Germany

Printed by Libri Plureos GmbH
in Hamburg, Germany